ELK GROVE VILLAGE PUBLIC LIBRARY
1001 WELLINGTON AVE
ELK GROVE VILLAGE, IL 60007
(847) 439-0447

THE ENCYCLOPEDIA OF

ALCOHOLISM AND ALCOHOL ABUSE

THE ENCYCLOPEDIA OF

ALCOHOLISM AND ALCOHOL ABUSE

Mark S. Gold, M.D.
and
Christine Adamec

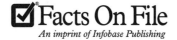

An imprint of Infobase Publishing

The Encyclopedia of Alcoholism and Alcohol Abuse

Facts On File
An imprint of Infobase Publishing, Inc.
132 West 31st Street
New York NY 10001

Library of Congress Cataloging-in-Publication Data
Gold, Mark S.
The encyclopedia of alcoholism and alcohol abuse / by Mark S. Gold and Christine Adamec.
p. ; cm.
Includes bibliographical references and index.
ISBN-13: 978-0-8160-7709-0 (hardcover : alk. paper)
ISBN-10: 0-8160-7709-6 (hardcover : alk. paper) 1. Alcoholism—Encyclopedias.
I. Adamec, Christine A., 1949– II. Title.
[DNLM: 1. Alcoholism—Encyclopedias—English. WM 13 G6176e 2010]
HV5017.G65 2010
362.29203—dc22   2009037200

Facts On File books are available at special discounts when purchased in bulk quantities for businesses, associations, institutions, or sales promotions. Please call our Special Sales Department in New York at (212) 967-8800 or (800) 322-8755.

You can find Facts On File on the World Wide Web at http://www.factsonfile.com

Text design by Annie O'Donnell
Composition by Hermitage Publishing Services
Cover printed by Sheridan Books, Inc., Ann Arbor, Mich.
Book printed by Sheridan Books, Inc., Ann Arbor, Mich.
Date printed: July 2010
Printed in the United States of America

10 9 8 7 6 5 4 3 2 1

This book is printed on acid-free paper.

CONTENTS

FOREWORD

Alcohol is the most popular psychoactive substance in the world, and this has been true for millennia. It is also one of the most damaging and dangerous substances known to humans, second only to the harmful effects inflicted on the human body by tobacco smoking. At the same time, the judicious and moderate use of alcohol has been widely reported as clearly effective at preventing or delaying aging, heart disease, and stroke and other cardiovascular manifestations of disease. Drinking red wine has been correlated with all sorts of health benefits, such that the likely "French-effect" chemicals, resveratrol and resveratrol-related pharmaceuticals, are likely to be evaluated in clinical trials soon. It is now clear that in males, alcohol has significant positive effects, and in women the beneficial effects of alcohol are tempered by the increased risk for breast cancer. Alcohol also reduces social inhibitions and anxiety and produces an overall feeling of well-being. It is an important element in social, political, and religious rituals, at which, without it, most participants would find the ceremony essentially meaningless. For example, what is a Catholic mass without wine? Yet the use of alcohol is proscribed by many prominent faiths, most notably Islam, arguably the fastest-growing religion in the world.

Alcohol is a legal substance, and one that is easily obtained, often even by those who are lawfully forbidden from its use, such as individuals in the United States who are younger than the age of 21. It is this group, the underage population, which concerns many experts, particularly high school or college students who drink. Developmentally, the teenage brain is not ready for alcohol, and binge-drinking episodes appear to sow the seeds for later alcohol abuse and early alcoholism. Teen and college drinking is a major problem. Young adults who drink risk accidents, injury, and death and also many dire consequences, including contracting sexually transmitted diseases, initiating unplanned pregnancies, and suffering from violence engendered by inhibitions that are markedly decreased by alcohol. In the worst case, young people who binge drink die of alcohol poisoning or they drive drunk and kill or harm others.

There are some who support the lowering of the drinking age to 18 years, arguing that an 18-year-old can vote and go to war, and, thus, it is only fair that an 18-year-old should be able to consume alcohol too. However, the minimum drinking age restriction has saved thousands of lives since its inception, and rescinding it would not be consistent with Hippocrates' admonition to "First, do no harm."

Of course, the limitation of 21 years does not prevent all young people from drinking, but deaths due to drinking and driving have decreased so much over the past decade that in many states, drugged driving exceeds or contributes to the majority of arrests for driving under the influence. The law helps by serving as a mental barrier for many people, just as many (but not all) adults refrained from drinking during Prohibition in the 1920s because alcohol was illegal. This reduced drinking from the very high level that preceded that period.

A major problem with alcohol arises when people become addicted to (or "dependent on") this substance; at that point, the problem of alcoholism is extremely difficult to treat. Prior to the onset of alcoholism, however, when the individual has begun abusing alcohol but has not yet become addicted, an early drinking problem is often treatable with what is referred to as a brief intervention with a trusted physician. Many studies have confirmed this fact, yet some physicians are uncomfortable talking freely about alcohol and drugs with their patients. In general, physicians are used to the doctor-patient relationship being very truthful. So it is not a surprise that they are uncomfortable asking questions that provoke defensive responses and to which many patients routinely lie or deny or minimize. Yet, asking their patients about their use of alcohol, providing an office-based brief intervention, or even challenging unhealthy use when it is identified can help patients reduce their abuse or dependence.

Many people have confused and contradictory attitudes toward alcohol. On the one hand, among many families and friends, alcohol is a substance that is often approved for celebrations, such as graduations, birthdays, and holidays. On the other hand, the extreme use of alcohol and the concomitant embarrassing drunken behaviors of family members, coworkers, and others are subject to gossip and criticism, and the alcoholic person is often "convicted" by a jury of his or her peers as guilty when unable to refrain from drinking to excess. Most experts know that alcohol dependence is a disease. Some laypeople regard alcoholism as a disease, while others view it as a moral failing or a weakness.

Females who drink are often particularly stigmatized, and this has been true for centuries. The alcoholic man who stops drinking is lionized as a hero; in contrast, the societal attitude toward the female alcoholic in remission is that she should have known better than ever to drink to excess in the first place.

Yet there are reasons for excessive drinking. For example, some individuals apparently have a genetic predisposition toward alcoholism, and if they drink, they are likely to drink to excess. Some experts believe that it is the feeling of euphoria that they seek to duplicate, while others believe that alcohol-

ics are often individuals with untreated depression or anxiety who turn to alcohol for some emotional relief and escape, however transient. Others drink one or two drinks on occasion and have no particular affinity toward alcohol; clearly there is no family history of alcoholism in this group.

In this book, my coauthor and I cover the key issues of alcoholism and alcohol abuse today, including the latest research on who are the major users and abusers (in terms of gender, age, and other factors), what are the effects of their use on themselves and others, and how alcoholism is treated. Medications are available for treatment, but the most effective means to resolve alcoholism is with the assistance of Alcoholics Anonymous.

We also describe in detail the common psychiatric "comorbidities" (disorders that occur concurrently) that occur with alcohol dependence. For example, anxiety disorders and depression frequently occur with alcoholism, and it is often difficult to tease out which disorder came first, the alcoholism or the comorbid psychiatric disorder. Adults with attention-deficit/hyperactivity disorder (ADHD) and antisocial personality disorder (ASPD) have an increased risk for an alcohol use disorder. In addition, often there are multiple psychiatric comorbidities, making diagnosis and treatment challenging for the physician.

We also cover the physical effects of alcohol abuse and alcoholism on the body, including an increased risk for cancer and many other diseases. The alcoholic is unlikely to take needed medication and is at risk for harm from existing untreated diseases, including such common and chronic diseases as diabetes and hypertension. An estimated 80 percent of all alcoholics also smoke, further escalating the risk for disability and death. Alcohol dependence is also harmful to the brain and can lead to an alcoholic dementia.

The actions of the person who abuses alcohol are not performed in a vacuum and affect many people around them, including strangers. For example, the individual who drives drunk may kill or permanently maim others that he or she crashes into with a motor vehicle. For years, drunk drivers repeatedly drove drunk with few legal repercussions, until bereaved mothers started Mothers Against Drunk Driving (MADD). Our book discusses drunk driving, its consequences and its punishments, in detail.

Individuals who abuse or depend on alcohol are more likely to behave aggressively toward others, exhibiting violence toward their spouses, partners, their own children, and the children of others. Our book discusses violence and child abuse that stem from abuse of and dependence on alcohol.

I am a medical school professor and chair of the psychiatry department at a prestigious medical school. I am also a researcher and addiction expert who has studied substance use, abuse, and dependence for many years, as well as mentored young scientists in this area of research. I am well versed in the pros and cons of the use of alcohol as well as the devastation that alcohol dependence inflicts upon the individual sufferer and those around him or her. It is my hope that readers will find the answers that they need from the information provided in my book.

As of this writing, progress on the full effects of alcohol on the brain and behavior is rapidly ongoing, and these findings will ultimately result in the development of newer and more powerful medications to help block the effects of alcohol and prevent relapse. In the meantime, I have been guided by the exceptionally good five-year outcomes that have been reported with physician alcoholics as well as by the experiences over more than the past two decades at the Betty Ford Center in understanding effective interventions and gold standard treatment and follow-up.

—Mark S. Gold, M.D.
Donald R. Dizney Eminent Scholar
and Distinguished Professor,
University of Florida College of Medicine &
McKnight Brain Institute Departments of
Psychiatry, Neuroscience, Anesthesiology,
Community Health & Family Medicine
Chairman of the Department of Psychiatry

ACKNOWLEDGMENTS

Special thanks from the authors to Paula J. Edge, Addictions Editorial Program Assistant at the Department of Psychiatry, University of Florida, for her extensive assistance in locating crucial journal articles, suggesting numerous extremely helpful articles, and dedicating many hours to reading and proofing the text.

INTRODUCTION
A History of Alcohol Abuse and Dependence

Whether alcohol is consumed as beer, brandy, hard cider, wine, distilled spirits, or any other form, it is an intoxicating substance that has been used and often abused by many millions of people over millennia. In addition, countless numbers of individuals throughout time have also developed an addiction to alcohol. The modern terms for an addiction to alcohol are *alcohol dependence* or *alcoholism.* The ancient Egyptians enjoyed their beer, sometimes to considerable excess, in the same manner as some ancient Romans copiously over imbibed their wine. In the 11th century C.E., physician Simeon Seth of the Byzantine court wrote that drinking wine caused liver inflammation, a condition that he treated with pomegranate syrup.

It may greatly surprise many people to learn that the early Pilgrims who colonized America were regular alcohol consumers, and when the Pilgrims landed at Plymouth Rock in 1620, they had a major crisis involving alcohol: They had just run out of beer, which was their primary source of liquid replenishment. Freshwater was unavailable, and there was no such thing as purified bottled water at that time. William Bradford, the leader of the Pilgrims, purportedly fervently begged the ship's captain and the crew to give the colonists at least some portion of their own beer supply. At first, their pleas were to no avail. Finally, the captain chose to give up his own portion of beer to the Pilgrims, agreeing to drink only water on his trip back home. This was no small sacrifice, because stored water frequently became contaminated on long journeys, while beer would remain potable (drinkable and safe) during the long trek homeward.

Since the time of the Pilgrims, alcohol has played a considerable role in U.S. history, and at some points in the past, excessive drinking was very common by 21st-century standards. As a result, throughout the nation's history, many attempts have been made to ban all sales of alcohol by various states (starting with the Maine Liquor Law in 1851). The most notable success of the "drys" (those who strongly favored banning all alcohol, in contrast to the "wets" who supported the continued sale and use of alcohol) occurred with the passage of the Eighteenth Amendment (commonly referred to as Prohibition) in 1920. This statute banned alcohol through the entire United States. However, the Eighteenth Amendment was repealed 13 years later in 1933 with the passage of the Twenty-first Amendment. The loss of tax revenues to the states, the flagrant abuse of alcohol that had occurred despite the ban, the rise of violent organized crime groups dealing in bootleg (illegal) liquor, and other reasons ultimately led to the repeal of Prohibition.

Alcohol itself is a substance that once was viewed as "God's good creature" by none other than Puritan preacher Cotton Mather, who perceived alcohol as a benign and healthful substance that everyone, including children and pregnant women, should drink on a regular basis. Of course, at other times the public has held a radically different perception of alcohol. For example, in the late 19th century, alcohol in general, as well as rum in particular, was perceived as an inherently wicked substance. "Demon rum" was believed by some to be a severely and instantly addictive substance to any person who foolishly chose to imbibe it, and thus it was also believed to be a substance that should be actively avoided by all right-thinking individuals. In later years, Alcoholics Anonymous originators and devotees adopted the idea of alcohol as an irresistible substance for some individuals, for whom their only salvation or relief was abstinence. (This belief in abstinence and sobriety for alcoholics is now supported by considerable research.)

It is instructive and often helpful to learn from the beliefs and practices of people in the past. This historical overview will discuss the varying views of alcohol, alcohol abuse and alcoholism, and alcoholics throughout history, starting with Europe in the Middle Ages and with an emphasis on alcohol use and abuse from the colonial period to the present in the United States. Attitudes toward the alcohol abuser and alcoholic have also changed through time in an almost cyclical fashion, and this introduction covers varying societal views of the alcoholic as well as attitudes toward his or her family members and associates. For example, at different points in time, the alcoholic person has been viewed as a moral degenerate, an ill person, a weak person, an evil person, a person with an uncontrolled disease, and so on. In today's society, many individuals regard alcohol dependence as a disease, but there are still those who perceive alcoholism as a moral weakness.

Similarly, views of society toward the alcoholic's family members (particularly the spouse) have varied as well. For example, at different points in history, the spouses of drunken men have been viewed as tragic victims, as people who are part of the problem, or even as individuals who somehow "drove" the alcoholic person to drink. Attitudes have generally been even more unfavorable toward women alcoholics, who have been viewed as weak, sluttish, evil, bad mothers, or, much less frequently, as simply individuals who need help from their addiction. This introduction provides a discussion of varying attitudes toward female alcohol abusers and alcoholics through time.

In looking at times past, it is important to consider societal views toward alcohol at the time in question rather than to overlay modern views on the Pilgrims who landed at Plymouth Rock, Victorian men and women, and other historical cultures or groups. When the views of the people at the time and the reasons behind them are known, their behavior is often much more understandable.

Finally, the introduction has a separate section on treatment of alcoholic abusers through the ages, which has ranged from bleeding the alcoholic (a treatment for many ailments in the 18th century) to spiking his drink with ipecac syrup or other noxious substances that induced extreme vomiting to counseling and social support and other measures.

Societal Views toward the Alcoholic

Throughout history, some individuals have abused alcohol while others have become dependent on alcohol. Similar to attitudes toward those with problems with drug abuse and drug addiction, attitudes toward those who abuse or are dependent on alcohol have changed throughout history in a seemingly cyclical fashion. Sometimes the alcohol abuser has been viewed benevolently, particularly if he or she is a young person, while the alcoholic may be perceived as a victim of his or her culture or sometimes of alcohol itself. From this perspective, individuals were believed to need to be led to treatment by others who were more enlightened.

Alternatively, at various points in history, the alcoholic has been seen as one who is so severely flawed in character or personality that he or she will never agree to treatment, and consequently there is no point in trying to help him or her, since failure is inevitable. In the most extreme case, the alcoholic has been viewed as someone who actually chooses to be evil and sometimes as one who should be shunned by society or incarcerated away from nice people. One common denominator among these various viewpoints is that the alcoholic person either cannot or will not choose to receive treatment in order to recover.

Of course, alcoholism is not a positive trait in anyone, but it is important to realize that there are factors that move some individuals toward a risk for alcohol dependence, such as genetics and environmental factors (parents and/or peers who are heavy drinkers). There are also protective factors leading people away from alcohol abuse and dependence (such as non drinking parents and peers). At the same time, there are treatments available that can help those with alcohol dependence.

Another view of heavy drinkers or alcohol-dependent individuals is that the person is a free thinker who is exhibiting individual spirit. People who hold this view may see excessive drinking among some people, such as the stereotypical hard-drinking writer or artist or the macho man who really knows how to hold his liquor, as benevolent. In reality the ability of hard-drinking people to drink more than others results from building up a tolerance to alcohol, not from any secret knowledge the individual has acquired.

At different times in American history, the substance of alcohol itself was considered either good or evil. When it was good, it was perceived as a substance that was safe and healthful to drink and as a pain reliever. When it was evil, it was believed to be as addicting as heroin is known to be in modern times. With this underlying view, no one was exempt from becoming addicted. The belief that alcohol itself is very dangerous to all people helps explain why the substance was banned outright during the Prohibition years.

Others believed that not everyone was prone to becoming addicted to alcohol, but that some individuals inexplicably were drawn to alcohol and then they subsequently, and inevitably, became addicted. According to this belief, the first sip of alcohol triggered the addiction. For such individuals this led to a ruinous life unless they were able, with help, to overcome their addiction.

The Nonalcoholic Spouse of the Alcoholic: Victim or Enabler?
Societal views toward the nonalcoholic spouse or partner of the alcohol-dependent person have changed through time. In the early part of the 20th century, wives were often viewed as the innocent victims of men who were entrapped into the evils of drinking. This attitude shifted in the 1950s and beyond, when professional articles began to appear that questioned whether the male alcoholic's problems were at least partially caused by marital dysfunction. Women with alcoholic spouses were advised to look within themselves for the root cause of the problem.

In her book *Love on the Rocks,* Lori Rotskoff said, "This view was common among mental health experts by the late 1940s and the early 1950s, especially those schooled in psychoanalytic theory, which became increasingly popular during this period." Rotskoff also added that "psychiatric social workers perceived the wife's behavior as a sign of neurosis that existed *prior to* the onset of the partner's alcohol abuse."

Terms such as *enabling* were created to refer to particular behaviors that allow alcoholic behavior to continue. The prevailing belief (and one that is still held by many individuals today) was that if the enabling ended, then the alcohol-dependent person would have to face up to his problem (it is usually regarded as a male problem), thereby gaining the insight and the desire to seek treatment. Yet even with spouses and family members out of the picture, the alcoholic must acknowledge that a problem exists and seek treatment for it.

Women partners of alcoholic males were advised not to regard themselves as victims but instead to learn how to deal with their spouse's problem by joining self-help groups such as Al-Anon and sending their adolescent children to Alateen (sister groups to Alcoholics Anonymous). In many ways, however, nonalcoholic spouses were regarded more as part of the problem than as part of the solution. Despite working hard to avoid enabling their spouse or partner and faithfully attending Al-Anon meetings and receiving therapy, many women often found their spouse's alcoholic behavior continued anyway. Some women concluded that they must not be trying hard enough, thinking that they were somehow still "driving" their male partners to drink.

Females with Drinking Problems
The issue of gender must also be considered in any historical overview of alcoholism. In the late 19th and early 20th centuries, alcoholic behavior, or even

drinking any alcohol, was regarded as a male pastime. As a result, women who drank a little were viewed as aberrant and women who drank to excess were extremely aberrant. Some saw a woman who consumed alcohol as evil and/or a temptress whose underlying goal was to lure men (especially married men or healthy, unmarried men) away from their families and into a life of dissolute drunkenness.

This was also the time frame when the "cult of domesticity," as it has been phrased by some authors, became an important part of accepted family life. The father was perceived as the sole breadwinner, while the mother was assumed to be the stay-at-home caregiver of children and manager of the home. A drunken husband and father threatened this ideal scenario, but a drunken mother was considered unspeakably evil. Some writers of the time said that such a person was so bad that she was not worthy of a tombstone when she died.

In the 1800s, women who became intoxicated in public could be punished severely. Carolyn S. Carter, in her article on historical attitudes toward alcoholic women, published in 1997 in *Affilia,* noted that "chronically drunk or alcoholic women could be committed to insane asylums, lose their children, or be subject to involuntary hysterectomies."

Some historians believe that the very underpinnings of the relatively new middle class in the United States at that time depended heavily on the idealized image of the woman as a gentle and kind homemaker. Such an image clashed mightily with the view of a thuggish drunk woman who neglected or abused her own children. One way that the ideal image could still be held and yet somehow reconciled with those women who drank, says Scott Martin in *Devil of the Domestic Sphere,* was for alcohol itself to be demonized. Alcohol was then viewed as a substance so incredibly and inherently powerful and with such a malevolent impact that it could bring down saintly women who, for whatever reason (sometimes through trickery), had imbibed alcohol and then subsequently become addicted to it.

Martin described this view: "Women were different from men; the monster alcohol exploited those very differences to compromise woman's moral nature and transmogrify her into a horrible creature that resembled but outstripped the most degraded male drunkard."

Women who were heavy drinkers or alcoholics were seen as sexually depraved creatures who usually became prostitutes. Mark Edwards Lender, in his chapter in *Alcohol Interventions,* wrote: "Everything the country believed about women on one hand, and about alcoholics on the other, left it unprepared to envision women with drinking problems as real women. Women were virtuous and pure, alcoholics were degraded; women defended the home; alcoholics imperiled it; and while mothers strove to raise their children in a moral environment, drunkards were constant impediments to the task. Thus, to be an alcoholic was to behave in a way that was so far removed from public expectations of women in the nineteenth century that society could account for it only as a form of the most extreme deviance."

Even a male recovered alcoholic was appalled at the treatment of female alcoholics in the 19th century. In his book *Eleven Years a Drunkard,* published in 1877, T. Doner wrote:

> Hopeless, indeed, seems the condition of fallen women. Men can reform; society welcomes them back to the path of virtue; a veil is cast over their conduct, and their vows of amendment are accepted and their promises to reform are hailed with great delight. But, alas! for poor women who have been tempted to sin by rum. For them there are no calls to come home; no sheltering arm; no acceptance of confessions and promises to amend. We may call them the hopeless class. For all others we have hope: The drunken man can throw down the filthy cup and reform; he can take his place again in society and be welcomed back. But for the poor woman, after she once becomes debased by this fiery liquid, there seems to be no space for acceptance; for her there is no hope and prayer. How seldom we attempt to reach and rescue her! For her there is no refuge.

Some propagandists who were opposed to the use of alcohol were worried about the sexual debauchery that they felt certain went hand-in-hand with the use of alcohol. For example, they believed drinking might lead to interracial sexual experiences (at that time, this was a highly horrific thought), and they described with fear the potential risk of intoxicated black men ravishing white women or of drunken white women who willingly succumbed to the physical embraces of black adult males.

Ironically, some women of that time *were* actually addicted to laudanum, a concoction that usually included a combination of both alcohol and an opiate. It was frequently prescribed by many physicians of the time for virtually any complaint that a woman could have (headaches, menstrual problems, and so on). But laudanum was a sedative, and as a result, it usually kept women at home and inactive, whereas alcohol was feared by some as a substance that would transform normal women into lustful and adulterous creatures who neglected their children. Since "home and hearth" were extremely important values at the time, alcohol in general and drinking women in particular were viewed with horror and repulsion.

A Look at Alcohol Use in the Past and to Modern Times

Ancient cultures sometimes used alcohol (as well as psychoactive drugs) as part of their religious ceremonies and rites, as with the Egyptians and the first known alcoholic beverage, barley beer. However, this introduction will start with the Middle Ages in Europe and concentrate on alcohol use, abuse, and alcoholism in colonial America to the present.

Alcohol Use and Abuse in Medieval and Early Modern Europe According to author A. Lynn Martin, from about 1300 to 1700 in England, France, and Italy, alcohol was ubiquitous, and it was used for almost every reason—as well as for no particular reason at all. Until it became a fashion to boil water for tea and coffee, water was often contaminated and very unsafe, and thus, men, women, and children consumed wine and ale to survive. After the introduction of hops, they also consumed beer. Of course, some people consumed more alcohol than others, and sometimes peasants found it difficult to obtain alcohol. As well, excessive drinking by women was generally frowned

upon, although the idea of abstention from alcohol was not considered feasible or reasonable.

In the 18th century, gin became extremely cheap in Europe and particularly in England, and alcohol abuse and alcoholism became so rampant that many people became alarmed. According to A. Lynn Martin, the annual per capita consumption of gin increased from 1.2 million gallons in 1700 to 8.2 million gallons by 1743. Consumption was so heavy that the period from about 1721 to 1751 was referred to as the "gin craze" years. Individuals in Holland as well as England heavily imbibed gin during this period. At one time, there were an estimated 7,000 gin shops in the city of London alone.

People engaged in binge-drinking contests, which were common, and some contestants died of apparent alcohol poisoning. According to James R. McIntosh in *Alcohol and Temperance in Modern History,* "Street vendors offered a ladle of gin at a half pence, from a kettle being pushed in a wheelbarrow-like vehicle. Shops of all sorts sold gin. Signs appeared advertising 'drunk for a penny, dead drunk for two pence and straw for nothing,' the last being a generous offer of bedding."

In 1751, politicians decided to raise the price of licenses to sell gin, and they also banned gin distillers from selling their product directly to the public or to unlicensed retailers. These laws brought the consumption of gin down to previous levels from before the "gin craze."

Alcohol Use and Abuse in Colonial America Contrary to modern popular belief, the original settlers of the colonies that ultimately became the United States were liberal in their use of alcohol, and experts estimate they consumed an average of at least twice (and possibly three times) as much alcohol as is the average consumption of individuals in the 21st century. Despite this, individuals of that time disapproved of public drunkenness.

According to author Peter Mancall, "During the colonial period, when average consumption of distilled beverages was approximately seven shots per day, abusive drinking was typically linked to moral failings: drunkenness, scorned in the Bible, was a sign of degeneration and savagery. Those who could not control their desires were denied entry into public houses, thereby not only losing the opportunity for tippling but also forfeiting the personal and political relationships that so often formed in such buildings."

However, the context of the time must be taken into consideration. The Pilgrims did not have bottled water, soft drinks, or other purified beverages to consume, and they depended heavily on beer for liquid. They did eventually discover, to their astonishment, that much of the water in the new world was potable, in contrast to the contaminated water in their homeland; however, habits die hard and they largely kept to drinking beer although learning to appreciate hard cider and rum as well.

At this time alcohol was also used as a means for individuals to tolerate pain before the development of narcotics and other pain remedies. Public drunkenness was frowned upon but what went on behind closed doors was often another matter altogether. Few people considered drinking bad, and almost no one supported the idea of not drinking alcoholic beverages; abstemious behavior was seen as weird and aberrant. However, some prominent individuals, such as Benjamin Franklin, advised to avoid drinking to excess—although he also remarked that the alcoholic beverages of the time (beer, applejack, sherry, brandy, and various liqueurs) were safer to consume than was drinking the water in Philadelphia or Boston. At that time, colonists drank beer and sherry with their breakfast and beer at lunch. Dinner was accompanied by wine or liqueurs.

Catherine Gilbert Murdock wrote: "Brought to the English colonies with the first settlers, beer, hard cider, and rum were integral to colonial life. Alcohol constituted most of the limited pharmacopoeia of the era. It numbed pain, eased headaches, lowered fever, cured infection, soothed troubled minds, and revised low spirits. In a culture still reliant on medieval community and ritual, drink bound men together in times of sorrow and joy."

Gilbert Murdock continues, "As in Europe, alcohol purified or replaced tainted water and milk—a function it would serve throughout the nineteenth century wherever wells were fouled and dairies questionable. Colonists considered alcohol essential to manual labor; indeed to day-to-day survival. They drank upon waking, with breakfast, lunch,

and dinner; during 'grog time' pauses in shop and field work; and at every social event. Employers often paid laborers in drink or drinking binges." It was not until the Industrial Revolution and the mechanization of many tasks that employers decided that it was not cost-effective or smart to pay their employees with alcohol while they were on the job.

In the early days of the colonies, the colonists brewed their own beer, eventually also creating distilled spirits (known then as "ardent spirits") from corn and other items that were available. Hard cider, which had up to a 7 percent alcohol content, was also popular in the northern colonies, while peach brandies were more favored in Virginia and Georgia.

Rum was another popular beverage, and some individuals became wealthy with importing distilled molasses to be made into rum. Rum was also traded with the Native Americans, to their ultimate sorrow, because some of them developed a dependence on alcohol. Victor Stolberg says, however, that many colonies forbade the colonists from giving or selling alcohol to Native Americans for any reason. This rule was sometimes violated: For example, Joseph Borne was removed as a missionary to the Wampanoag Indians in Massachusetts in 1740 for giving them a pint of rum for medicinal purposes.

According to Stolberg, rum was used medicinally as well for many different functions; for example, in 1639, rum with root bark was used to treat gout and fever and rum-soaked cherries were believed to treat colds. (Possibly the vitamin C-rich cherries helped improve the colds, while the rum helped the sick person to sleep.) However, when the colonists rebelled against England, their rum supply was cut off, so they began distilling whiskey from grain imported from the Midwest, and according to W. J. Rorabaugh, whiskey was depicted as a patriotic drink by 1790.

Alcohol was also commonly consumed at election time in the colonial years and through much of the 19th century, when individuals running for office "treated" potential voters to copious quantities of alcohol. (Later, alcohol became a different type of factor in elections when some individuals opted only for "dry" candidates who favored temperance, despite their party affiliation.) Even during voting, alcohol consumption was common.

According to Mark Lender and James Kirby Martin in their book *Drinking in America*, "Polling places [the places where people voted] themselves were rarely dry: There was only one poll per county and after making the long trek to do his citizen's duty, the voter expected some tangible reward. He usually got it. This meant that in order to qualify as a Founding Father, George Washington, John Marshall, Thomas Jefferson, and other Revolutionary leaders must have provided many a drink for the multitude."

Beer was another popular beverage, and according to Stolberg, there were two breweries in Virginia in 1629. By 1810, there were 132 breweries nationwide producing 185,000 barrels of beer each year. By 1850, 750,000 barrels of beer were produced by 431 breweries. Production increased to a million barrels per year by 1860.

Blacks were restricted from drinking, and most of the colonies passed laws prohibiting giving or selling liquor to any slaves. Despite this, sometimes slaves did acquire alcohol and drink to excess.

Alcohol Consumption 1790–1840 According to researcher W. J. Rorabaugh, alcohol consumption in America was at its all-time high between 1790 and 1830, when, as he put it, "Americans seem to have indulged in a veritable alcoholic binge." Perhaps copious drinking was a common practice because, as Rorabaugh explains, most people during this time believed that alcohol was healthy and both stimulating and relaxing, as did individuals in colonial America. Another factor in heavy drinking was that alcohol was inexpensive; cheap whiskey (grain alcohol) became readily available because of the very low prices of grain in the Midwest. This grain was transported to states where it was made into distilled spirits. At one point, the price of alcohol fell to less than the price for coffee, tea, milk, or other alcoholic beverages.

In their book *The Serpent in the Cup,* Debra J. Rosenthal and Davis S. Reynolds agreed that alcohol consumption in 1830 was at an astonishingly high level. These authors wrote, "By 1830 the average American consumed the equivalent of over four gallons of absolute alcohol a year—an astonishing amount, especially since many liquors were adulterated by brain-ravaging additives such as lead, logwood, and tartaric acid. Alcoholic beverages were served at virtually all social gatherings."

See Table 1 for Rorabaugh's estimate of per capita (per person) consumption among individuals

TABLE 1
CONSUMPTION OF ALCOHOLIC BEVERAGES AND ABSOLUTE ALCOHOL, PER CAPITA OF POPULATION AGED 15 YEARS AND OLDER, IN U.S. GALLONS, USA, BY YEAR

	Spirits*		Wine*		Cider*		Beer*		Total
	Bev.	Absolute Alcohol	Bev.	Absolute Alcohol	Bev.	Absolute Alcohol	Bev.	Absolute Alcohol	Absolute Alcohol
1790	5.1	2.3	0.6	0.1	34.0	3.4	Not available	Not available	5.8
1795	5.9	2.7	0.6	0.1	34.0	3.4	Not available	Not available	6.2
1800	7.2	3.3	0.6	0.1	32.0	3.2	Not available	Not available	6.6
1805	8.2	3.7	0.6	0.1	30.0	3.0	Not available	Not available	6.8
1810	8.7	3.9	0.4	0.1	30.0	3.0	1.3	0.1	7.1
1815	9.2	3.7	0.4	0.1	30.0	3.0	Not available	Not available	6.8
1820	8.7	3.9	0.4	0.1	28.0	2.8	Not available	Not available	6.8
1825	9.2	4.1	0.4	0.1	28.0	2.8	Not available	Not available	7.0

(continues)

(continued)

	Spirits*		Wine*		Cider*		Beer*		Total
	Bev.	Absolute Alcohol	Bev.	Absolute Alcohol	Bev.	Absolute Alcohol	Bev.	Absolute Alcohol	Absolute Alcohol
1830	9.5	4.3	0.5	0.1	27.0	2.7	Not available	Not available	7.1
1835	7.6	3.4	0.5	0.1	15.0	1.5	Not available	Not available	5.0
1840	5.5	2.5	0.5	0.1	4.0	0.4	2.3	0.1	3.1
1845	3.7	1.6	0.3	0.1	Not available from this point on		2.4	0.1	1.8
1850	3.6	1.6	0.3	0.1			2.7	0.1	1.8
1855	3.7	1.6	0.3	0.1			4.6	0.2	2.0
1860	3.9	1.7	0.5	0.1			6.4	0.3	2.1
1865	3.5	1.6	0.5	0.1			5.8	0.3	2.0
1870	3.1	1.4	0.5	0.1			8.6	0.4	1.9
1875	2.8	1.2	0.8	0.1			10.1	0.5	1.8
1880	2.4	1.1	1.0	0.2			11.1	0.6	1.9
1885	2.2	1.0	0.8	0.1			18.0	0.9	2.0
1890	2.2	1.0	0.6	0.1			20.6	1.0	2.1
1895	1.8	0.8	0.6	0.1			23.4	1.2	2.1
1900	1.8	0.9	0.6	0.1			23.6	1.2	2.1
1905	1.9	0.9	0.7	0.1			25.9	1.3	2.3
1910	2.1	0.9	0.9	0.2			29.2	1.5	2.6
1915	1.8	0.8	0.7	0.1			29.7	1.5	2.4
1920	2.1	0.9	Prohibition years						
1925	2.0	0.9	Prohibition years						
1930	2.0	0.9	Prohibition years						
1935	1.5	0.7	0.4	0.1			15.0	0.7	1.5
1940	1.3	0.6	0.9	0.2			17.2	0.8	1.6
1945	1.5	0.7	1.1	0.2			24.2	1.1	2.0
1950	1.5	0.7	1.1	0.2			24.1	1.1	2.0
1955	1.6	0.7	1.3	0.2			22.8	1.0	1.9
1960	1.9	0.8	1.3	0.2			22.1	1.0	2.0
1965	2.1	1.0	1.3	0.2			22.8	1.0	2.2
1970	2.5	1.1	1.8	0.3			25.7	1.2	2.5

*The absolute alcohol content of spirits was estimated as 45 percent; in wine, 18 percent, cider, 10 percent; and beer, 5 percent.

Source: Reprinted with permission from *Journal of Studies on Alcohol,* vol. 37, pp. 357–364, 1976 (presently *Journal of Studies on Alcohol and Drugs*). Copyright by Alcohol Research Documentation, Inc., Rutgers Center of Alcohol Studies, Piscataway, NJ 08854.

aged 15 years old and older in terms of the gallons of alcohol consumed every five years from 1790 to 1970, including the per person amount consumed of distilled spirits, wine, cider (up to 1840), and beer. The table also includes the amount of absolute alcohol for spirits, wine, cider, and beer, for a comparison basis. For example, in 1830, a very heavy year of drinking, the per capita rate for distilled spirits was 9.5 gallons.

The average per capita consumption of wine in 1830 was 0.5 gallons (with an absolute alcohol content of 0.1), and the average per capita consumption of hard cider was 27.0 gallons (with an average absolute alcohol of 2.7). (Beer consumption was not reported for that year.) The total absolute alcohol consumption in 1830 per capita

was 7.1 gallons. By comparison, in 2005, according to the National Institute on Alcohol Abuse and Alcoholism, the average per capita ethanol consumption of wine was 0.36 and the total for all absolute alcohol content for all alcoholic beverages was 2.24 gallons in 2005.

In considering the per capita consumption of alcohol of all people in the United States, the rate for spirits was 5.2 gallons in 1830. This is another important measure of alcohol consumption because many people drank at that time, including men, women, and children. The total per capita consumption of absolute alcohol at that time was 3.9 gallons per year, much higher than the years to come. (See Table 2 for the per capita alcohol consumption of the entire population.)

TABLE 2
CONSUMPTION OF ALCOHOLIC BEVERAGES AND ABSOLUTE ALCOHOL, PER CAPITA, OF TOTAL POPULATION, IN U.S. GALLONS, USA, BY YEAR

	Spirits*		Wine*		Cider*		Beer*		Total
	Bev.	Absolute Alcohol	Bev.	Absolute Alcohol	Bev.	Absolute Alcohol	Bev.	Absolute Alcohol	Absolute Alcohol
1790	2.7	1.2	0.3	0.1	18.0	1.8	Not available	Not available	3.1
1795	3.1	1.4	0.3	0.1	18.0	1.8	Not available	Not available	3.3
1800	3.8	1.7	0.3	0.1	17.0	1.7	Not available	Not available	3.5
1805	4.3	1.9	0.3	0.1	16.0	1.6	Not available	Not available	3.6
1810	4.6	2.1	0.2	<0.05	16.0	1.6	0.7	<0.05	3.7
1815	4.4	2.0	0.2	<0.05	16.0	1.6	Not available	Not available	3.6
1820	4.7	2.1	0.2	<0.05	15.0	1.5	Not available	Not available	3.6
1825	5.0	2.2	0.2	<0.05	15.0	1.5	Not available	Not available	3.7
1830	5.2	2.3	0.3	0.1	15.0	1.5	Not available	Not available	3.9
1835	4.2	1.9	0.3	0.1	8.5	0.8	Not available	Not available	2.8
1840	3.1	1.4	0.3	0.1	2.0	0.2	1.3	0.1	1.8
1845	2.1	0.9	0.2	<0.05	Not available from this point on		1.4	0.1	1.0
1850	2.1	0.9	0.2	<0.05			1.6	0.1	1.0
1855	2.2	1.0	0.2	<0.05			2.7	0.1	1.1
1860	2.3	1.0	0.3	0.1			3.8	0.2	1.3
1865	2.1	0.9	0.3	0.1			3.5	0.2	1.2
1870	1.9	0.9	0.3	0.1			5.2	0.3	1.3

(continues)

(continued)

	Spirits*		Wine*		Cider*		Beer*		Total
	Bev.	Absolute Alcohol	Bev.	Absolute Alcohol	Bev.	Absolute Alcohol	Bev.	Absolute Alcohol	Absolute Alcohol
1875	1.7	0.8	0.5	0.1			6.2	0.3	1.2
1880	1.5	0.7	0.6	0.1			6.9	0.3	1.1
1885	1.4	0.6	0.5	0.1			11.4	0.6	1.3
1890	1.4	0.6	0.4	0.1			13.3	0.7	1.4
1895	1.2	0.5	0.4	0.1			15.2	0.8	1.4
1900	1.2	0.5	0.4	0.1			15.5	0.8	1.4
1905	1.3	0.6	0.5	0.1			17.3	0.9	1.6
1910	1.4	0.6	0.6	0.1			19.8	1.0	1.7
1915	1.2	0.5	0.5	0.1			20.2	1.0	1.6
1920	1.4	0.6	Not available (Prohibition)	Not available			Not available (Prohibition)	Not available	0.6
1925	1.4	0.6	Not available	Not available			Not available	Not available	0.6
1930	1.4	0.6	Not available	Not available			Not available	Not available	0.6
1935	1.1	0.5	0.3	0.1			10.9	0.5	1.1
1940	1.0	0.4	0.7	0.1			12.9	0.6	1.1
1945	1.1	0.5	0.8	0.1			17.9	0.8	1.4
1950	1.1	0.5	0.8	0.1			17.6	0.8	1.4
1955	1.1	0.5	0.9	0.2			16.2	0.7	1.4
1960	1.3	0.6	0.9	0.2			15.2	0.7	1.5
1965	1.5	0.7	0.9	0.2			16.0	0.7	1.6
1970	1.8	0.8	1.3	0.2			18.4	0.8	1.8

*The absolute alcohol content of spirits was estimated as 45 percent; in wine, 18 percent, cider, 10 percent; and beer, 5 percent.
Source: Rorabaugh, W. J., "Estimated U.S. Alcoholic Beverage Consumption, 1790–1860." *Journal of Studies on Alcohol* 37, no. 1 (1976): 360.
Reprinted with permission from *Journal of Studies on Alcohol*, vol. 37, pp. 357–364, 1976 (presently *Journal of Studies on Alcohol and Drugs*).
Copyright by Alcohol Research Documentation, Inc., Rutgers Center of Alcohol Studies, Piscataway, NJ 08854.

Dr. Benjamin Rush and His Views on Alcoholism

In 1784, Benjamin Rush, M.D., a noted and influential physician from Philadelphia and one of the signers of the Declaration of Independence, published his book, *Medical Inquiries and Observations upon the Diseases of the Mind*. This book included Rush's views on alcoholism and his forward-thinking ideas on temperance. Rush, the former surgeon general of the Continental Army during the Revolution, was the first prominent physician of his time (and for many years beyond his time) to see alcoholism as a disease and also as a problem that required treatment. He urged the establishment of special hospitals specifically designed to treat alcoholics, which he called "sober houses."

Today Rush is viewed as the father of American psychiatry. However, Dr. Rush was primarily concerned with the health risks of distilled spirits, and he saw no problem with drinking beer, wine, or hard cider. Today it is known that individuals can become dependent on these substances as well.

Rush said of alcoholism, "The use of strong drink is at first the effect of free agency. From habit it takes place and from necessity. That this is the case, I infer from persons who are inordinately devoted to the use of ardent spirits being irreclaimable, by all the considerations which domestic obligations, friendship, reputation, property, and sometimes even by those which religion and the love of life, can suggest to them. An instance of insensibility to the last, in an habitual drunkard, occurred some years ago in Philadelphia. When strongly urged, by one of his friends, to leave off drinking, he said, 'Were a keg of rum in one corner of a room, and were a cannon constantly discharging balls between me and it, I could not refrain from passing before that cannon, in order to get at the rum.'"

Rush continued, "Who can calculate the extensive influence of a drunken husband or wife upon the property and morals of their families, and of the waste of the former, and corruption of the latter, upon the order and happiness of society?" Who indeed?

"Patent" Medications Were Often Laced with Alcohol In the late 19th and early 20th centuries, and before the passage of the Pure Food and Drug Act in the United States in 1906, many drugs were sold directly to consumers with no controls or information about their content. They were so-called patent medicines (which often were *not* patented, confusingly) and often they were heavily laced with alcohol. For example, Lydia Pinkham's Vegetable Compound was 20 percent alcohol (40 proof), as was Hall's Tonic. In addition, syrups administered to sick or even teething children often contained alcohol or morphine (unbeknownst to the parents), and they were extremely dangerous and sometimes fatal for sick children. Manufacturers had no requirement to reveal any of the ingredients of their products, so if the product contained anything that might be objectionable to anyone (such as alcohol or narcotics), that information was not provided on the label or anywhere in advertisements.

Many women, including some members of the strident, anti-alcohol Woman's Christian Temperance Union, consumed Lydia Pinkham's remedy for just about any ailment they had. According to author John Parascandola, in 1904 the editor of the *Ladies' Home Journal* wrote to 50 Woman's Christian Temperance Union members to find out if any of them used any patent medicines. He discovered that 75 percent of them used patent medicines with an alcohol content ranging from 1/8 to 1/2. They were not hypocrites; they really did not know what was in their "medicine."

Parascandola says that alcohol was a common key ingredient in patent medicines that were called "bitters." For example, Hostetter's bitters included about 40 percent alcohol (80 proof) as well as some herbs. Ironically, Mr. Hostetter was allegedly a temperance supporter, but he rationalized that he needed to include alcohol as both a solvent and preservative.

Another popular potion, the Balm of Gilead, was 70 percent alcohol, and it was a remedy endorsed by some members of the clergy. (Again, it is highly unlikely that they were aware of the high alcohol content of the drug.)

It should also be mentioned that most physicians opposed the use of patent medications, but they did not have the power to ban their use. It is probably also true that their patients did not tell their doctors about their use of these drugs, particularly if their doctor expressed any negative views toward them.

After the passage of the Pure Food and Drug Act and the legal requirement to reveal the ingredients of drugs to consumers, the sales of patent medications eventually fell off. It is interesting to note as a point of comparison, however, that in the 21st century, many consumers spend large sums purchasing unregulated, "alternative" herbal remedies, often not discussing these purchases with their physicians. Apparently the hope for quick-fix miracle cures for many disorders is still present in modern-day society.

Temperance in the Early Nineteenth Century
Contrary to what is popularly believed in the 21st century, the temperance movement (primarily those who completely opposed the sale of any

alcohol) did not spring to life in the latter part of the 19th century. Women and men were actively involved in the temperance movement well before the Civil War. The movement centered in the northeast, but temperance was an issue that individuals throughout the United States could agree on. However, and confusingly, some temperance supporters advocated total abstinence while others urged moderation. Still others were opposed to distilled spirits, but felt that wine and beer were acceptable in moderation. However, eventually the movement coalesced into an abstinence-only core belief.

The Good Creature of God, Transformed into Demon Rum   In the late 18th and early 19th centuries, alcohol was fondly referred to by some as "God's good creature" because it provided a sanitary beverage that also helped warm the blood on cold winter's nights and eased some of the pain from often back-breaking labor. Excessive drinking was frowned upon, but moderate drinking was the norm. This situation began to change with the mechanization of labor and when prominent and wealthy businessmen realized they were losing money because of intoxicated workers. This group, combined with genuinely sincere advocates of temperance, were a formidable force, and finally in the early 20th century, they were unstoppable. But prior to that time, the temperance advocates made major inroads. For example, alcohol was banned altogether in Maine in 1851. The ban was first lifted and then reinstated. About 12 states followed Maine's lead, passing "Maine laws" by themselves, and becoming "dry" states.

The Role of Taverns and Saloons in the Past   One of the first establishments that the Pilgrims created was the tavern (which often included an inn where travelers stayed). The tavern was an establishment that served as a central place for people (mostly men) to get together and learn the latest gossip and talk about politics and local problems and issues. It was a central and integral part of the community. About the 18th century tavern, Lender and Martin wrote: "Taverns filled a variety of practical social needs. In many areas, they were the most convenient retail outlets for

liquor—and often the only place where travelers could find food and lodging. They provided all localities with a forum for social intercourse, which often included political, religious, or other gatherings. Before and during the Revolution, for example, inns were favorite places for political discussions, and they served as rallying points for the militia and as recruiting stations for the Continental army. Innkeepers ideally reflected the high public status accorded their establishments, and in reality they often did. Publicans were commonly among a town's most prominent citizens and not infrequently were deacons."

Later in the 19th century, however, many taverns devolved into places that were frequented by prostitutes, and some individuals began to perceive the tavern (or "saloon") as the primary problem causing alcoholism and alcohol abuse. Those who worried about taverns and their influence used flyers and other means to depict taverns (often accurately) as dens of iniquity. Some temperance-minded individuals urged lawmakers to refuse to license new taverns and to revoke the licenses of existing taverns. Yet many men found taverns to be their primary social outlet, and they perceived collegial drinking as a particularly male activity. (Women who drank were generally frowned upon.)

According to Lender and Martin, successful brewers often also owned taverns in the late 19th century, then called saloons, and these businessmen sold as much alcohol as they possibly could. Said Lender and Martin, "Many saloons lured customers with offers of a 'free lunch'—usually well-salted to inspire drinking (the saloon 'bouncer' was generally on hand to discourage hearty appetites). New patrons were also given free drinks. As one Brewer's Association spokesman explained, this tactic extended even to children: A few cents spent on free drinks for boys was a good investment; the money would be amply recovered as these youths became habitual drinkers!"

Beer also became very inexpensive, and as a result, it replaced whiskey and other distilled spirits as the favorite drink of those who imbibed, as well as those who abused or were dependent on alcohol. Brewers opened saloons, as did some immigrants from Ireland and other locations. The

Irish and other Europeans were heavily "wet," compared to the "dry" temperance supporters.

Saloons in large cities were also places where politics were discussed as well as where the local ballot boxes could be stuffed. As a result, saloons became the target of temperance authorities such as the Woman's Christian Temperance Union (WCTU).

Temperance in the Mid- to Late Nineteenth Century

The movement to ban alcohol and ostensibly, to save the family, was spearheaded by such temperance leaders as Woman's Christian Temperance Union leader Frances Willard, who led the organization from 1879 until she died in 1898. Her motto was "Do Everything," and the WCTU led very active campaigns advocating for a wide variety of civic changes: public water fountains, girl's precision drill teams, and mandatory temperance education in public schools. However, they were strongly preceded in this movement by patriarchal organizations such as the Washingtonians and the Sons of Temperance. The Good Templars, in contrast, allowed female members. Of course, the Woman's Christian Temperance Union was dominated by female members.

One of the earliest temperance movements, according to Stolberg, was the Massachusetts Society for the Suppression of Intemperance, formed in 1813 by Lyman Beecher, a Protestant minister. This was a group of clergy and leading community members who hoped to prevent the "lower social class" from drinking. This group disbanded in 1823, not succeeding in their mission.

The Washingtonians Launched by six formerly hard-drinking men, the Washingtonians became a movement that attracted an astonishing 600,000 people who signed sobriety pledges. The organization also had sister organizations: Martha Washington groups for women. According to author William White, the Washingtonian movement all started with an argument at a tavern when the proprietor stated that temperance lecturers were all a bunch of hypocrites. Several of the men wondered if this was true, so they decided to attend a tem-

perance lecture to discover for themselves if there was anything to it. Apparently they were considerably moved by the lecture because subsequently they and two of their fellow drinkers decided to form their own organization. They created their own pledge, which read: "We, whose names are annexed, desirous of forming a society for mutual benefit, and to guard against a pernicious practice which is injurious to our health, standing and families, do pledge ourselves as gentlemen that we will not drink any spirituous or malt liquor, wine, or cider." The members as well as the leaders of the Washingtonians were drawn from working class individuals, meeting weekly.

Author William White describes the weekly meetings of the Washingtonians in his book *Slaying the Dragon,* and his description of these meetings sounds remarkably like the format of today's Alcoholics Anonymous meetings: "Instead of the debates, formal speeches, and abstract principles that had been on the standard temperance meeting agenda, the main bill of fare at a Washingtonian meeting was *experience sharing*—confessions of alcoholic debauchery followed by glorious accounts of personal reformation. Following these opening presentations by established members, newly arrived alcoholics with bloated faces and trembling hands were offered the opportunity to join. As each newcomer came forward, he was asked to tell a little of his own story, then sign the abstinence pledge amid the cheers of onlookers. This ritual of public confession and public signing of the pledge carried great emotional power for those participating. It evoked, at least temporarily, what would be described one hundred years later as ego deflation or surrender."

The Washingtonians organization ultimately spurred more than 600,000 people to sign pledges of sobriety, and thousands of their members marched in temperance parades. However, by 1845, the movement had lost most of its momentum. Some experts have theorized that conflicts with religious groups were responsible for the decline of the movement, while others said the organization had a weak internal structure or that other reasons were responsible for its demise. Many former members of the Washingtonians joined the Sons of Temperance, another fraternal order that was founded in 1842 and grew to about 250,000 members.

The Independent Order of the Good Templars

The Independent Order of the Good Templars, otherwise known simply as the Good Templars, was an extremely large and powerful organization that operated in the mid- to late 19th century. It was also an early impetus to the eventual passage of Prohibition. The Independent Order of Good Templars (IOGT) was created in Oneida County in upstate New York in 1851, when several members of a discontented faction of another fraternal society, the Order of Good Templars, decided to break off and begin another organization.

Two lodges were launched in Utica, and eleven lodges were started within Oneida county, according to Peirce and Thompson, authors of the *History of the Independent Order of Good Templars*. These authors attributed much of the credit of the initial growth of the organization to Nathaniel Curtis, a reformed alcoholic from Ithaca, New York, who had taken the pledge of sobriety with the Washingtonians. It was also Curtis who decided that it was important for women to become members of the Good Templars.

In 1868, the Templars had more than a half million male and female members in the United States and Canada. By 1876, the IOGT boasted of having initiated more than 3 million members worldwide, with members in the United States, Canada, Australia, New Zealand, Sweden, Britain, and elsewhere. The name of the organization was changed to the International Order of the Good Templars, to acknowledge the many members in other countries.

A fraternal society in the 19th century, with many of the same accoutrements of other fraternal organizations, such as secret handshakes, rituals, and ranks, the Good Templars was uniquely different in several ways. First, it required its members to take a vow of sobriety, and it also supported the prohibition of the sale of alcohol. Second, it allowed females full membership, unheard of at that time, calling their male members "brothers" and their female members "sisters." During the Civil War, female members were credited with holding the organization together. However, some females complained that they did not have full equal status with men.

Despite this complaint, their role exceeded that of any other fraternal organization in the United States at that time. Other fraternal organizations let women join auxiliaries of the main membership, at best. Some female members who cut their teeth in leadership roles within the Good Templars later became members and leaders of the Woman's Christian Temperance Union.

The Anti-Saloon League

The Ohio Anti-Saloon League was created in 1893, according to K. Austin Kerr, followed by the American Anti-Saloon League in 1895. A nonpartisan approach to achieving prohibition, the Anti-Saloon League was the brainchild of Reverend Howard Hyde Russell, a former attorney who decided to become a minister. Russell believed that by supporting all candidates who were "dry," despite their political party, the organization could attain political power. At this time in history, the temperance movement was in disarray, and the Prohibition political party had little chance of gaining political power. Prohibitionists in the North and South continued to argue about civil rights for freed slaves in the South, and they could not unite on a single party platform. Russell decided to attack the places that sold alcohol—the saloons—in a concerted attack to achieve his ultimate goal of the prohibition of alcohol.

Saloon owners greatly underestimated the power of the Anti-Saloon League (ASL), and they failed to unite against it. In addition, powerful organizations such as the United Brewers' Association thought they had nothing to worry about because they made only beer, apparently not realizing that the Anti-Saloon League and other temperance groups wanted to ban *all* alcoholic beverages. When they finally realized that they had a serious political problem, saloon owners tried to be more vigilant about what occurred on their premises, no longer allowing gambling or prostitution and generally cleaning up their moral acts. But it was too late. The prohibition movement was steamrollering ahead by that point.

Said authors Lender and Martin, "The league proved that it could marshal votes for anyone—

Republican or Democrat—who was willing to vote dry. Both the major parties rapidly awoke to the electoral power of the league, and it soon became apparent that the political fortunes of the anti-liquor crusade would not have to depend on any single party—and certainly not on the small and ineffectual Prohibition party."

Wayne Wheeler led this effort for the Anti-Saloon League, and "Wheelerism" became synonymous at that time with heavy and effective politicking. Wheeler actually drafted the implementing legislation which was known as the National Prohibition Act, but it was named after Andrew Volstead, a congressman from Minnesota. The Volstead Act banned not only the use of distilled spirits, but also the use of wine and beer, and it also provided federal regulations overseeing the use of sacramental wine in the churches.

The Anti-Saloon League, the primary temperance organization in 1910, was more powerful and effective than the Woman's Christian Temperance Union. It obtained its funding from churches, and according to Iain Gately, author of *Drink,* the ASL received financial support from 60,000 congregations, which provided 2 million dollars per year, a significant amount of money at that time.

Gately said, "The donations it gathered from its supporters were spent on propaganda, and its publishing arm spewed out over 250 million pages of temperance writing each month. This blizzard of print was directed at white Protestant men and women in the old western and northeastern states. These people were beginning to resent the changes that were occurring in America and to be ready to accept that drunkenness might be behind such phenomena as industrialization, the rise of mega-cities, and their population with hordes of Roman Catholic immigrants."

The group relied heavily on propaganda. They used a combination of anti-immigrant rhetoric, racism, and whatever else might work to win voters. For example, they attempted to link alcohol use in people's mind with the spread of venereal diseases such as gonorrhea and syphilis, which at that time were diseases that were incurable and prevalent.

The mood of the population at the time was ripe for change, and the ASL whipped the voters into a frenzy. Even the famous author Jack London, himself a notorious heavy drinker, wrote an anti-alcohol book that was based on his alcoholic memories. In his book, *John Barleycorn,* he stated that the first time that he was intoxicated he was only five years old. He said that his father frequently took him to saloons as a child, and it impressed him deeply and negatively. London said that by the age of 15 he was a heavy drinker. He eventually came to believe that only Prohibition would save others from the life of alcoholism that he had experienced.

The greatest success of the league was the passage of the Eighteenth Amendment, which it was instrumental in passing. However, it was unable to prevent the repeal of Prohibition and subsequently lost its power, since it was essentially a one-issue organization and that one issue could not be re-won.

The Woman's Christian Temperance Union (WCTU)
No account of temperance would be complete without a description of the Woman's Christian Temperance Union. Formed in 1874 in Cleveland, Ohio, this organization dominated the information received by the public about alcohol, alcohol abuse, and alcoholism in the latter part of the 19th century and the early 20th century. (The organization still exists today, although it is a mere shadow of its former self.)

The WCTU sought to punish public drunkenness with incarceration and did not buy into the idea that alcoholism was a disease. Instead, WCTU members saw it as a moral failing and believed the only true course against it was abstinence. To the WCTU, intemperance was a serious and direct assault on the home and the family. They believed in the view of the man as the breadwinner and were distressed at the thought that drinking males deprived their family of income as well as of their company. They actively attempted to redefine the male role from an image of swaggering and drinking males to the truly "masculine" males who supported and paid attention to their families. They wore white ribbons to identify themselves as WCTU members.

WCTU members were extremely diligent at bringing their message of sobriety to young people, working with Sunday schools at first, and then public schools; for example, the organization created their Department for the Promotion of Purity in Literature and Art in 1883, whose mission was to promote their temperance views and censor the views of all those who opposed them. The WCTU, under Frances Willard and others, eventually expanded their views to women's suffrage, realizing that there was much more power available to those who could vote.

Carry Nation was a dramatic individual and a pivotal figure in the late 19th century temperance movement. She founded a county division of the WCTU in Kansas, and she closed down many illegal saloons. Then in 1899, she decided to go even further, because she said that God had ordered her to do so. The "hachetations" of Carry Nation (her own invented word) struck terror in the heart of many saloon keepers across the country. Nation entered saloons and used her hatchet to smash and destroy as much of a saloon as she possibly could before getting arrested and hauled off to jail. She was relentless.

Nation believed that alcohol itself was evil, and she was convinced that the banning of alcohol and the destruction of saloons that sold this substance were the only ways to save wives and children from suffering from unhappy lives. According to Gilbert Murdock, Nation died in 1911, apparently of congenital syphilis.

Immigrants and Their Impact on Temperance

During the early 20th century, the large influx of immigrants from Europe also influenced temperance movements. Some immigrants, particularly Germans, Italians, and Irish, were loath to give up alcohol, and they actively resented movements toward restrictions against or the prohibition of alcohol.

Prohibition

Prohibition was not necessarily a "failure," as many have written since that time, if failure is measured solely in terms of the drinking population. Contrary to popular belief, Prohibition was not a period of drunken abandonment for most Americans, and in fact, alcohol consumption dropped to about half

its previous level. Many people stopped drinking, some because they wanted to obey the law and some because they did not want to be poisoned by illegal alcohol (a valid fear at the time) such as "bathtub gin" or moonshine. Many of those who continued to drink drank illegally imported Canadian whiskey. On the other hand, Prohibition could be regarded as a "failure" because many people *did* continue to drink, and illegal elements (such as organized crime) became involved in alcohol smuggling and developed criminal organizations that exist to this day. For these reasons, Prohibition deserves its own section.

Prohibition was hard-fought, both by the "drys" and the "wets." After years of pushing for a ban on alcohol, the drys finally won with the passage of the Eighteenth Amendment. Prohibition officially began on January 16, 1920 and lasted until its repeal on December 5, 1933, nearly 13 years later, with the passage of the Twenty-first Amendment. According to authors Lender and Martin, "In 1916, after a tremendous push from all dry organizations, the general elections sent so many league [Anti-Saloon League] endorsed candidates to the House and Senate that action on a prohibitory amendment to the Constitution was virtually assured."

Alcohol had been previously banned temporarily in 1917 with the entry of the United States into World War I, in part to deal with grain shortages and also in part to ensure sober soldiers. However, despite the pre-Prohibition ban, millions of people had continued to drink anyway.

It should also be noted that during Prohibition, physicians were allowed to write prescriptions for alcohol and many did. According to some sources, before Prohibition ended, doctors were writing 10 million prescriptions (for medicinal purposes) a year.

World War I was another factor in the passage of the Eighteenth Amendment, and its advocates actively equated support for "wets" as anti-patriotic. Many brewers in the United States had German names, and this fact was noted disparagingly by dry leaders.

Prior to the repeal of Prohibition, many politicians bemoaned the loss of tax revenue from all the alcohol consumed during Prohibition. Because the Great Depression continued to affect the United

States severely in 1933, advocates of repeal discussed not only the increased revenues that legalization of alcohol would provide, but also jobs that would be created at a time when unemployment was at a shocking 25 percent of all Americans. In addition (and very ironically), because Prohibition banned the sale of alcohol, many people had begun drinking at home. Whereas in the pre-Prohibition years, heavy drinking was primarily limited to men (or at least, that is what temperance supporters believed), now both men and women began drinking. Some experts say it was the invention of the cocktail, or the mixed drink, that enticed women into drinking. The cocktail was largely created to disguise the bad taste of illegal alcohol, but it made drinking seem glamorous and fun. The general appeal of the cocktail has persisted to the present day, although the formulations and the type of alcohol used varies.

Was Prohibition a Mistake? After Prohibition laws were discarded, many people believed (and still believe today) that Prohibition was a major mistake. Yet some historians argue with this view. Says Catherine Gilbert Murdock, "According to popular opinion, the attempt by small-minded moralists to eliminate a drug so easily manufactured, so readily transported, and so essential to the national psyche was doomed from the beginning. Yet alcohol abuse in the nineteenth and early twentieth centuries existed on a scale Americans today have trouble conceptualizing. Public drunkards were a pathetic, everyday spectacle in villages and cities throughout America. Drink really did kill men and ruin families, and millions of citizens felt that the best way to meet the crisis would be to eliminate alcoholic beverages. Moreover, the nation's abusive drinking patterns were strictly gendered. At the very most, 20 percent of the alcoholic population was female. Historically, it is not America that has had a drinking problem, it is American men."

Other experts have stated that death rates from acute and chronic alcoholism dropped subsequent to the passage of Prohibition. For example, according to Haven Emerson, M.D., in his article in 1932 for the *Annals of the American Academy of Political and Social Science*, death rates for white males per 100,000 individuals fell from 7.9 in 1911 to 5.2

in 1924. In addition, death rates from cirrhosis of the liver fell from 16.8 per 100,000 in 1911 among white males to 7.7 in 1924. Haven also noted that admissions to state hospitals for alcoholic psychosis in New York dropped from 11.5 percent in 1910 to 3.0 percent in 1920, rising to 6.5 percent in 1931. In Massachusetts, the rate dropped by more than half, from 14.6 percent in 1910 to 6.4 percent in 1922, then increasing to 7.7 percent in 1929.

Emerson concluded, "While we do not know the per capita consumption of alcohol in this country since prohibition, the lowering of death rates and sick rates from causes related to alcoholism offers strong presumptive evidence that prohibition has accomplished a reduction in the beverage use of alcohol in the United States."

According to author Jack S. Blocker, in his 2006 article for the *American Journal of Public Health*, Prohibition had a major positive effect on many people. Said Blocker, "Death rates from cirrhosis and alcoholism, alcoholic psychosis hospital admissions, and drunkenness arrests all declined steeply during the later years of the 1910s, when both the cultural and the legal climate were increasingly inhospitable to drink, and in the early years after National Prohibition went into effect. They rose after that, but generally did not reach the peaks recorded during the period 1900 to 1915." According to Blocker, even after the repeal of Prohibition, per capita annual consumption levels were less than half that of the pre-Prohibition period. Consumption did not reach the pre-Prohibition peak of alcohol use again until the 1970s.

Blocker concluded, "Perhaps the most powerful legacy of National Prohibition is the widely held belief that it did not work. I agree with other historians who have argued that this belief is false. Prohibition did work in lowering per capita consumption. The lowered level of consumption during the quarter century following Repeal, together with the large minority of abstainers, suggests that Prohibition did socialize or maintain a significant portion of the population in temperate or abstemious habits."

The Idealized View Did Not Work as Reformers Had Hoped Prohibition may or may not have been a mistake, but it did not work out as its supporters envisioned. The proponents of Prohibition fervently believed prior to its passage that banning alcohol would mean that alcohol abuse and alcoholism would become a remnant of the past; however, they were quickly proven very wrong. People who wanted to drink either drank at home with alcohol that they or their friends had produced themselves ("bathtub gin"), or they frequented clubs known as "speakeasies" or "blind pigs," which offered bootlegged alcohol and where one had to know the password to gain entrance.

Another problem was that since alcohol production was illegal, the federal and state governments had no control over its manufacture, and some individuals added dangerous and life-threatening adulterants to the alcohol, such as kerosene.

The "Wets" Prevail: The End of Prohibition

Prohibition ended when the "wets" overcame the "drys" in terms of their political power. The death of Prohibition was partly a desire to allow self-determination and let adults engage in what was considered adult behavior. But the reason Prohibition was overturned was more of an economic reason: to obtain the tax revenues from the lawful sale of alcoholic beverages in the face of the Great Depression. There were also some individuals whose primary support for repeal was their belief that excise taxes on alcohol could replace other taxes, such as income taxes. (History proved them wrong. Rarely does a new tax mean that an old tax is repealed.)

The Creation of Alcoholics Anonymous

Surgeon Robert Smith and stock analyst William Wilson (known for many years as "Dr. Bob" and "Bill W.") were two alcoholics who initially launched Alcoholics Anonymous in 1935. The beginning of this organization was somewhat similar to that of the Washingtonians, who were also alcoholics who decided to reform. The two men met in Atlantic City in 1935 when Dr. Smith was attending a medical convention, introduced by mutual contacts. The two realized that to carry their message of sobriety, they needed to tell their stories to others. They also realized that to stay sober themselves, they needed to help other people stay sober.

Smith and Wilson agreed that by themselves they were helpless against their addiction to alcohol, and they hoped that by sharing their story with others with the same problem, they could remain sober. The name of the organization was created in 1939. Alcoholics Anonymous (AA) was a self-help organization with only two requirements: the sincere desire to stop drinking and also the willingness to help others who were dependent on alcohol. AA also revived the notion that alcoholism was a disease, rather than an immoral choice made by weak or degenerate individuals. Wilson drafted what was to be referred to as the AA "Big Book," inculcating their major principles and beliefs. Supposedly the printer was ordered to use the thickest paper possible so that the book would seem big and important to the reforming alcoholics who would read it. Physicians were disinterested in the book, but a groundswell of support grew through meetings of alcoholics in cities on the East Coast.

Alcoholics Anonymous was and continues to be a great success. By the late 1970s, more than 500,000 people had joined the organization. There were also two other organizations that were created as spinoffs of Alcoholics Anonymous, including Al-Anon, founded to help the families of alcoholics, and Alateen, for the adolescent family members of alcoholics. Some groups and individuals have criticized AA for its emphasis on the importance of abstinence, and others have stated that the group is oriented more towards white, middle-class alcoholics. Yet the group has many black, Hispanic, and other minority members, so the criticism seems unfounded.

Many alcoholism treatment groups require membership in AA, as do many courts; for example, if a person has been found guilty of driving while intoxicated, the court may require the person to attend AA meetings as part of his or her sentence.

AA does not work with everyone, but it has had many successes, and it is one very important means for alcoholics to regain control of their lives.

Drunk-driving Laws

The first drunk-driving law was passed in New York in 1910, followed by laws against drunk driving enacted in California in 1911 and many other states thereafter. Today all states have laws against driving while intoxicated. According to Robert H. Voas and John H. Lacey in their paper on impaired-driving laws in the United States, the issue of drunk driving was first recognized in 1904, about five years after the first highway fatality. Voas and Lacey say that by 1924, Connecticut was jailing about 254 drivers per year for driving while intoxicated (DWI).

In the early years of laws against drunk driving, there were no means provided to police officials on how to determine whether individuals were drunk, because there were no blood tests for alcohol abuse nor were there breath tests or any other means to verify intoxication. As a result, the police officer had to decide for himself whether the person was sufficiently intoxicated to be arrested. General judgment and field sobriety tests were used; for example, common symptoms of intoxication are slurred speech, flushed face, and a staggering gait. Field sobriety tests involve asking the driver to get out of the car and walk a straight line, touch his or her nose with the eyes closed, and so forth. These tasks, much easier to perform when a person is sober, are far more difficult to achieve when an individual is intoxicated.

Voas and Lacey say that just prior to World War II, chemical tests to measure intoxication, such as blood alcohol tests, were first introduced in the United States. Indiana was the first state to provide for chemical tests in 1939 and Maine, New York, and Oregon soon followed with state laws on blood alcohol levels. The first tests considered a blood alcohol level of 0.15 to be proof of intoxication, which is nearly twice the level of legal intoxication used in the 21st century, or a blood alcohol concentration (BAC) level of 0.08. Lower levels of a BAC were also considered intoxication but only if accompanied by supporting verbal testimony.

By the mid-1970s, roadside breath tests were available to police departments, making the verification of intoxication much faster and easier. The Alco-Sensor was the first breath test to be used in the United States. More advanced breath tests were subsequently developed. In later years, the alcohol interlock safety device was developed, and some states required its use by drivers convicted of driving under the influence. The interlock safety device requires the driver to blow into a device in order to start their car. If alcohol is present, the car ignition will remain locked.

However, for many years, there were few penalties for drunk driving. This all changed with the development of the organization Mothers Against Drunk Driving (MADD), created by two mothers, including Candy Lightner in Sacramento, California, after a drunk driver killed her daughter Cari, age 13, and received a penalty of only two years in prison after pleading guilty. Lightner, along with another mother, Cindy Lamb of Maryland, whose five-and-a-half-month-old daughter, Laura, was left paraplegic after a drunk driver hit their car, began the organization to publicize their plight.

The drunk driver who killed Lightner's daughter had received five previous convictions for drunk driving. Lightner's story and her campaign created a nationwide sensation and furor and convinced most Americans in the 1980s that driving while intoxicated should be punished, particularly if someone died as a result of an accident with a drunk driver who was at fault or if the driver had repeat offenses.

According to Ralph Hingson and colleagues in the *American Journal of Public Health,* in 1981, Maine implemented what was considered to be the most stringent drunk-driving law in the nation. At that time, a blood alcohol level of 0.10 percent or greater was considered evidence of drunken driving. Individuals who refused to take a blood or breath test had their driver's licenses suspended for 180 days. In 1982, Massachusetts created a new category of law: vehicular homicide under the influence. Individuals convicted of this offense automatically had their licenses revoked for 10 years and received at least one year in prison and a fine of $500–$5,000, according to Hingson et al.

In 2000, President Bill Clinton signed a bill into law requiring states to enact laws making a blood alcohol concentration of 0.08 or greater as the level of intoxication for drivers. States had until 2003 to pass such a law or lose highway funding, and all states did pass such laws.

World War II through the End of the Twentieth Century

Prior to the United States entering World War II, those supporting Prohibition thought they had yet another chance to ban alcohol. They actively sought to promote the idea that the troops needed to be fully sober in order to preserve the freedom of Americans. This time, it did not work, and the "wets" prevailed.

According to author Lori Rotskoff, during World War II, the brewers were especially clever, linking alcohol to patriotism and what "our boys" were fighting for back home, such as steaks in the backyard and a cold beer. Another concept that was heavily promoted by all who favored retaining the sale of alcohol was the idea of moderation in drinking, which was strongly used in advertisements and any mention of alcohol. Drinking in moderation was perceived as a good thing. Excessive drinking and alcoholism was still considered bad, if it was considered at all.

The banning of alcohol was clearly a thing of the past. Or was it? After the passage of the National Underage Drinking Act in 1984, underage soldiers were lawfully banned from drinking in most cases. However, research has shown that military members, particularly Marines, are a very hard-drinking group. Some studies have shown that the military has a major problem with alcohol, which may be embedded in military culture, according to some experts.

Betty Ford: A Change Maker Who Admitted to Problems with Alcoholism   In 1978, Betty Ford, wife of President Gerald Ford, openly admitted to having problems with alcohol as well as prescription drugs and receiving rehabilitative treatment, shocking many people. Part of the shock came from surprise that Mrs. Ford had such a problem, but probably the greater part of the shock was that she openly admitted it to the public. Prior to that time, the problems of female drinkers (as well as women who abused prescription drugs) generally

were hidden and not discussed. If they were discussed, the underlying assumption was that only weak or bad women had such problems. Robert DuPont, who also served as the first director of the National Institute on Drug Abuse, said, "She made it [addiction] a disease that a good person could have and get well from."

The Betty Ford Center was opened in 1982 in Rancho Mirage, California, and the organization celebrated its 25th anniversary in 2007. According to author Carl Sherman in his article on the Ford Center, "The respectability of a former first lady, a popular image of elegance, and the glamour of A-list clientele that have included prominent entertainers (Elizabeth Taylor, Robert Mitchum, Liza Minnelli, and Johnny Cash) and sports figures, such as Mickey Mantle, have helped neutralize the stigma of addiction treatment." The Betty Ford Center is not just a place for celebrities, however, and of the more than 26,000 clients, many average individuals have received treatment in the clinic.

According to Jerome L. Short, Colleen J. Shogan, and Nicole M. Owings in their article about Betty Ford, "The larger impact of her efforts was to help break down the stigma associated with psychological disorders by speaking out about her anxiety and substance abuse, obtaining professional help, and making treatment more widely available to others."

The Idea of Alcoholism as a Disease   After the initial views of the colonial physician Benjamin Rush on alcoholism as a disease, little was done to advance this idea, and the average person viewed the alcohol-dependent person as evil and depraved or weak. Then in 1870, according to author Sarah W. Tracy, a group of clergy, physicians, and businessmen in New York City, Philadelphia, Boston, and Chicago formed the American Association for the Cure of Inebriates. They declared that "intemperance" was a disease that was either inherited or acquired, and that it could be cured. They recommended the establishment of asylums for alcoholics and recommended that every large city have a local home for inebriates (chronic alcoholics) and that each state should have at least one asylum. They further recommended that law enforcement officials should view intemperance as a disease that should be managed by other than fines and jails.

According to Stolberg, in 1922, about 13 percent of all psychiatric hospital admissions were for alcoholism.

In the 1940s, Elvin Morton Jellinek, a professor at Yale, described his theories on the cause of alcoholism. Jellinek's views are no longer accepted and are offered as historical information only. Jellinek said there were five different types of alcoholics, including alpha alcoholics, beta alcoholics, gamma alcoholics, delta alcoholics, and epsilon alcoholics.

An alpha alcoholic was someone who used alcohol to loosen up or to cope with stress. He or she need not have a physical tolerance for alcohol, although one could develop. Jellinek said that beta drinkers were alcoholics who developed health problems because of their excessive drinking. As with alpha alcoholics, betas did not physically depend on alcohol and drank for social reasons and despite the health problems that drinking caused them. Jellinek said that the most common alcoholic was the gamma alcoholic, who had increasing health and social problems because of his or her heavy alcohol consumption. An alpha drinker could become a gamma alcoholic. The delta alcoholic, according to Jellinek, was a person who drank all day long, had a physical dependence on alcohol, and also had a tolerance such that he or she needed to consume increasing amounts of alcohol to achieve the same level of intoxication. The epsilon alcoholic was a person who went on binges of drinking but who abstained from alcohol between those binges.

Although Jellinek's typologies were not adopted by medical organizations, such organizations did begin to formally accept the idea that alcoholism was a disease; for example, in the mid-1950s, the American Medical Association with the American Hospital Association issued joint policy statements that alcoholism was a disease.

Methods of Treatment of Alcoholism throughout History

As views toward alcoholism have changed throughout history, so have the means attempted to treat alcohol dependence. Today, medications, psycho-therapy, and attendance at Alcoholics Anonymous meetings are the primary means to help alcoholics. But past treatment methods were very different. These have ranged from such aversive methods as putting a worm or insect in the alcoholic's drink to cause revulsion to alcohol to advertisements for various potions wives could secretly place in their husbands' drinks to cause them to stop drinking. These were usually substances that led to copious vomiting, such as syrup of ipecac, and were dangerous. But at that time, drugs were freely sold without the constraints of the Food and Drug Administration or other federal government rules and regulations.

The Keeley Method   One extremely popular past method of treatment for alcoholism was the "Keeley Cure," or Bi-Chloride of Gold Cure developed by Dr. Leslie E. Keeley. It did not work at all other than with those who responded to the placebo effect, or the strong belief that it would work because of extreme confidence in the drug. There have been many different sham treatments for alcoholism, but this treatment is described because so many people (as many as 500,000 alcoholics from 1880–1920) bought into it. Dr. Keeley became a wealthy man as a result of his so-called cure.

Keeley was an Irishman who had relocated to the United States. He became a doctor and was a surgeon in the Union Army of the Civil War. Keeley developed his chemical compound in Illinois, and he boasted in 1879, "Drunkenness is a disease and I can cure it." Keeley believed that alcoholism was caused by toxins from alcohol, cocaine, tobacco, and opiates, and he said that his compound would rid the body of these toxins and transform the alcoholic into a sober person. According to author Sarah W. Tracy, Keeley provided four injections daily to his inpatients.

He refused to divulge his specific formula to anyone, insisting that it worked. Patients came from all over the United States for the Keeley treatment, which lasted a month. Keeley claimed a 95 percent success rate, a very dubious claim. Some doctors of the time waggishly said that if it worked 95 percent of the time, that meant 95 percent of the patients died.

Some people believed they knew the ingredients of the Keeley cure. Tracy wrote of a Keeley facility located in Canada: "Three or four times a day, men lined up in the main building (called the 'shot tower') for their hypodermic injections of strychnine (supposedly mixed with incidental amounts of gold and sodium chloride). Every two hours, patients took a dram of tonic (called 'the dope'), which was said to contain atropine, strychnine, cinchona, glycerin, and gold and sodium chloride. One had to possess a strong constitution to withstand the treatment."

Patients who were reluctant or refused to take their "medicine" were allowed and even encouraged to consume alcohol to the full extent that they wished but they were secretly given drugs that caused extreme vomiting, to create in them an aversion to alcohol. In modern times disulfiram, also called Antabuse, is used in this manner, although patients are fully aware of the effects of consuming alcohol when they take it.

Many of Keeley's patients relapsed; the 118 treatment institutions dropped down to 50 facilities by 1900, and they were eventually shut down altogether.

Aversive Treatments   In the late 19th and early 20th centuries, some physicians used shock therapy to treat patients with alcoholism. The Swedish Treatment was one aversive method used in the 1890s. It comprised giving the patient massive quantities of alcohol to induce an aversion. Said author William White, "All meals and all snacks, regardless of fare, were saturated with whiskey. Patients wore whiskey-sprayed clothes and slept in whiskey-saturated sheets. The goal was to satiate and sicken the appetite for alcohol and leave one begging for pure water." There is no record of whether this treatment worked on anyone, although it likely did work on at least a few people.

Unusual and Bizarre Treatments   According to author Mark Keller, some physicians in the 1940s and 1950s viewed alcoholism as an endocrine disorder and used treatments of adrenal steroids and adrenocorticotropic hormone (ACTH). Other physicians used injections of alcohol to treat alcoholism as well as injections of antihistamines or oxygen as well as treatment with carbon dioxide inhalation and neurosurgery.

Sometimes the drugs that were used to "cure" the alcoholism were themselves very harmful substances, such as cocaine and marijuana. Others who treated alcoholism thought that all the alcoholic really needed was a healthy diet. Some of them concluded that red meat induced a craving for alcohol, and therefore it must be eliminated entirely from the diet to rid the person of the craving.

Inebriate Hospitals and Insane Asylums   One method of treating alcoholics was to put them in asylums for up to a year or longer, where they could not gain any access to alcohol. These facilities were called inebriate hospitals. In other cases, alcoholics were placed in insane asylums with psychotic individuals and other alcoholics. Said Mark Keller in his chapter in *Alcohol Interventions*, "Like all treatments, apparently the long institutional confinement also produced its fair share of remissions. Some alcoholics emerged as confirmed abstainers."

Some alcoholics were sent to "lunatic asylums" for the mentally ill, and they were also put on restricted diets as a form of punishment for their alcohol excesses. The cold shower punishment was a common treatment for alcoholism at hospitals of the time. Poverty-stricken alcoholics in the early 19th century were also often warehoused into almshouses, along with mentally ill people, the blind, those with syphilis, and others that society did not know what to do about (sometimes including orphaned children). Sometimes alcoholics were placed in overcrowded prisons.

Lobotomies and Enforced Sterilizations   In the early 20th century, some institutionalized alcoholic women were told that if they wished to leave the institution where they had been placed because of their alcohol dependence, then they would have to undergo sterilization. Doctors reasoned that these women would have children who were alcoholic if the women were not sterilized, and thus sterilizing them would save the world from more alcoholics. Interestingly, the same logic was not applied to male alcoholics, many of whom also bore children.

Another treatment for some alcoholics was the frontal lobotomy, which involves severing connections to the prefrontal cortex in the brain. It was first performed as a cure for alcoholism by physicians Walter Freeman and James Watts in 1936. The treatment failed, and according to William White in his book *Slaying the Dragon*, one patient who had just received a lobotomy reacted this way: "Following the procedure, the patient dressed and, pulling a hat down over his bandaged head, slipped out of the hospital in search of a drink. Freeman and Watts spent Christmas Eve, 1936, searching the bars for this patient, who they eventually found and returned to the hospital in a state of extreme intoxication."

The Twenty-first Century

Although the very hard-drinking days of some past centuries appear to be long gone, there are still problems with alcohol abuse and alcohol dependence in the United States and in many other countries today. For example, according to the Substance Abuse and Mental Health Services Administration (SAMHSA), in 2007, about 7.3 million minor children (10.3 percent of all children) in the United States lived with a parent who either abused or was dependent on alcohol.

Although print and signage advertising of alcohol has been sharply curtailed by pressure groups concerned about the effect of advertisements promoting alcohol as something "cool" to adolescents and underage youths, underage drinking remains a problem. The influence of alcohol is nowhere more prevalent than on the college campus, where fraternities and sororities, as well as students who are unaffiliated with "Greek" organizations, hold keg parties and engage in almost ritualistic binge drinking. But the problem may not start in college. Many students begin their drinking in high school or even earlier.

Adolescents and Drinking   Studies have shown that many adolescents begin drinking in high school and some start drinking before they reach their 13th birthday. Early initiators of drinking (before age 14) have an increased risk for alcohol dependence in young adulthood and adulthood.

They also have a seven-fold increase in risk for unintentional injuries and are more likely to become involved in alcohol-related violence up to age 21 and beyond.

Underage-drinking laws have had a positive impact on adolescents, based on research by James C. Fell and colleagues published in 2009 in *Alcoholism: Clinical and Experimental Research*. According to the researchers' analysis of state drinking laws over the period 1982 to 2004, the laws against those under age 21 purchasing and possessing alcohol as well as the zero-tolerance law prohibiting drivers from having a very low (or any, depending on the state) level of blood alcohol have saved an estimated 732 lives per year nationwide. The researchers also recommended that all states should adopt the "use and lose" law on the books in 37 states as of 2004. Under this law, if underage drivers violate alcohol laws, their driver's license will be suspended. The researchers estimated that adopting such a law in every state would save an additional 165 lives per year.

College Students   Heavy drinking and binge drinking are major problems on many college campuses in the 21st century, and these problems continue unresolved despite efforts to stem the tide of alcohol abuse. (Note that most binge drinkers are not alcoholics, although binge drinking can have many serious health consequences.) In one study by J. R. Knight and colleagues, the researchers found that of 14,000 students who were surveyed, 31 percent met the criteria for alcohol abuse, and also 6 percent met the criteria for alcohol dependence.

A study by Carlos Blanco et al., published in 2008 in the *Archives of General Psychiatry*, demonstrated that college students had a greater risk for developing a problem with alcohol abuse and alcohol dependence than did their noncollege peers. For example, of the 2,188 college students surveyed, about 8 percent had a problem with alcohol abuse, and even more disturbingly, about 13 percent of the students were alcoholics. In contrast, about 7 percent of 2,904 noncollege students of the same age had a problem with alcohol abuse and 10 percent were alcoholics.

Clearly, alcohol is a problem for both groups, although apparently a greater problem among college students. Other studies have confirmed that many college students have a serious problem with heavy drinking, including binge drinking. Drinking has become an ingrained part of the culture of many college campuses. Some college students also engage in the practice of binge drinking and even excessive drinking to the point of suffering from alcohol poisoning, a condition in which the liver cannot process alcohol as fast as it is consumed. Alcohol poisoning can cause death.

Some college students engage in extreme binge drinking, or drinking 10 or more drinks in a row on one occasion in the past two weeks. According to the Monitoring the Future results for 2007, 26 percent of college males and 6 percent of college females engaged in this behavior in 2005–07. In addition, 12 percent of college males and less than 1 percent (0.8 percent) of college females downed 15 or more drinks in a row on one occasion. College men are also more likely to engage in daily drinking than women in college; the Monitoring the Future survey found that 6.2 percent of college men drank every day in 2007, compared to 3.1 percent of college women.

The Monitoring the Future study researchers also noted that throughout the 28 years that college students have been surveyed, they have consistently reported episodes of binge drinking. Say the researchers, "It is interesting to conjecture why college students did not show much decline in heavy drinking for a decade (1981–1991) while their noncollege peers and 12th graders did. One possibility is that campuses provided some insulation from the effects of changes in the drinking age laws that took place during that interval."

Similarly, entrenched on many college campuses is a culture of binge drinking which has proven impervious to many social trends (and intervention attempts) regarding excessive alcohol use. It is also true that some college students are of the legal drinking age while others are not, while in high school, it is illegal for *all* students to consume alcohol. This can make enforcement of the laws confusing and difficult, especially since many underage drinkers carry false IDs that purportedly "prove" that they are 21 or older.

The idea that these individuals were heavy drinkers before they got to college and just con-

tinued their prior drinking patterns is open to challenge. Instead, for some individuals, it is apparently the excessive drinking behavior of their peers that affects them.

According to the survey authors, "We have shown that this differential change after high school is largely attributable to college students' greater likelihood of leaving the parental home and smaller likelihood of getting married in the four years after graduating from high school." The authors also noted that membership in a fraternity or sorority also increases the risk for binge drinking as well as for the use of marijuana.

Some individuals believe that a dialogue should be opened about lowering the drinking age because of the problem college students have with heavy drinking. The Amethyst Initiative, an organization of college presidents based in Washington, D.C., says that "a culture of dangerous, clandestine 'binge drinking'—often conducted off-campus—has developed. Alcohol education that mandates abstinence as the only legal option has not resulted in significant constructive behavioral change among our students. Adults under 21 are deemed capable of voting, signing contracts, serving on juries, and enlisting in the military, but are told they are not mature enough to have a beer. By choosing to use fake IDs, students make ethical compromises that erode respect for the law." There are about 100 college presidents who are members of this organization, including presidents of Dartmouth, Duke, Ohio State, and many others.

The idea of lowering the drinking age infuriates members of MADD, who regard it as irresponsible to even consider lowering the drinking age. They are concerned that drinking will become an even worse problem if the drinking age were lowered.

One possible benefit to lowering the drinking age is that the "forbidden fruit" aura surrounding drinking would be eliminated on college campuses, because most people in college are age 18 and older. There would also no longer be a two-tiered system of those who are 21 and older and thus legally allowed to drink and those who are younger than 21 and who could be criminally prosecuted for their drinking behavior. However, at the same time, it can be argued that if the drinking age were lowered to age 18, then people who were 16 and 17 would be obtaining fake IDs and drinking to even greater excess than as of this writing. It is likely this debate, as with debates about decriminalizing marijuana use, will continue for the foreseeable future.

Alcohol and Young Adults   Statistics provided by the Substance Abuse and Mental Health Administration make it very clear that young adults up to about the age of 25 are the heaviest drinkers of any age group in the United States. They also have the greatest rate of binge drinking. Among young adults, many college students have a particular problem with alcohol abuse. Underage drinking is also a major problem, and in some cases children as young as 13 years old (or younger) are taking their first drink and starting what often becomes a disastrous drinking "career."

Binge Drinking   Binge drinking, which is generally defined as consuming five drinks on at least one occasion for men and four drinks on one occasion for women in the past 30 days, is primarily a problem among young adults and college students, although some adolescents also engage in binge drinking. Most binge drinkers consume beer; according to a study by Naimi et al. that was published in the *American Journal of Preventive Medicine* in 2007, 74.4 percent of binge drinkers drank only beer or mostly beer. Some people believe (clearly, an erroneous belief) that since beer has a significantly lower alcohol content than distilled spirits, that it is somehow safer. However, when beer is drunk to excess, it can often be a very dangerous substance.

Binge drinking is a serious problem in the 21st century, responsible for many problems in society, such as individuals who drive while intoxicated, injuring themselves and others. Aggressive behavior is much more common among those who binge drink, in the form of harm to sexual partners, children, and even casual acquaintances. Excessive drinking may cause some men to believe that they have an "excuse" to sexually assault women, because they have misread the cues women have sent and also because they may believe that intoxication is itself an excuse for aggressive and even criminal behavior.

In 2006, an estimated 12.7 percent of individuals ages 18–44 engaged in binge drinking. The risk for binge drinking was highest among American Indians or Alaska Natives (12.2 percent) and lowest among Asians (3.7 percent). The risk for males was much higher (14.4 percent) than for females (4.1 percent). See Table 3 for further details.

As Table 3 shows, binge drinking has slightly decreased among many groups since 1997; for example, the rate of binge drinking among all persons 18–44 years of age in 1997 was 13.2 percent, and it dropped slightly to 12.7 percent by 2006; however, this newer rate is still problematic for many reasons. It is also interesting to note that binge drinking is less common among the poor; for example, 8.4 percent of men and women below 100 percent of the poverty level were binge drinkers in 2006, compared to 9.5 percent of those who earned 200 percent or more of the poverty level.

Parents and Children Who Drink at Home   Studies have shown that the attitude of their parents toward alcohol affects children. In addition, their parents' attitude toward underage drinking also affects children; if parents observe their own underage children drinking in the home and do nothing to stop them (and worse, sometimes even encourage this behavior), then adolescents and children receive the clear message that it is acceptable to drink, and they often will drink. Yet underage drinking is illegal and children who drink can be arrested, as sometimes can their parents for providing them with alcohol or sometimes for acquiescing to the use of alcohol in the home. Parents who state or think that there is nothing they can do could be asked, if their child were carrying around a gun, would they say that there was nothing they could do or would they demand that the gun be removed from the home as soon as possible? It is unlikely that they would tolerate this behavior.

Alcohol and Other Drugs: A Troublesome Combination   Another major problem among many people who are dependent on alcohol is that they are also dependent on another drug. The drug may be a stimulant, such as cocaine, or it

TABLE 3
BINGE DRINKING AMONG ADULTS 18 YEARS OF AGE AND OLDER, BY SELECTED CHARACTERISTICS:
UNITED STATES, 1997–2006, BY PERCENT OF ADULTS

Characteristic	1997	2000	2005	2006
18 years and older	9.8	8.7	8.8	9.1
Both sexes				
Age				
All persons:				
18–44 years	13.2	12.2	12.7	12.7
18–24 years	15.2	15.5	15.7	15.9
25–44 years	12.6	11.1	11.6	11.6
45–64 years	7.6	6.4	6.3	7.2
55–64 years	5.8	5.4	4.4	5.2
65 years and older	2.2	1.8	1.7	2.1
65–74 years	3.0	2.5	2.7	3.2
75 years and older	1.1	0.9	0.7	0.9
Race				
White only	10.3	9.2	9.6	10.0
Black or African American only	6.5	6.5	5.6	6.2
American Indian or Alaska Native only	17.4	12.1	11.9	12.2
Asian only	4.8	3.6	3.8	3.7
2 or more races	Unknown	15.9	9.0	9.4
Hispanic origin and race				
Hispanic or Latino	11.2	9.0	8.4	8.4
Mexican	12.6	10.8	9.9	9.6
Not Hispanic or Latino	9.5	8.8	9.0	9.4
White only	10.3	9.3	9.9	10.4
Black or African American only	6.5	6.5	5.6	6.2
Percent of poverty level				
Below 100 percent	9.7	8.6	8.1	8.4
100 percent-less than 200 percent	9.8	8.0	8.4	8.8
200 percent or more	9.7	8.9	9.1	9.5
Males				
Age				
All males, 18 and older	15.8	14.4	14.2	14.4
18–44 years	21.1	19.6	19.8	19.2
18–24 years	22.9	22.9	22.8	21.7
25–44 years	20.6	18.5	18.8	18.3
45–64 years	12.7	11.3	10.6	12.1
55–64 years	14.5	12.3	12.7	13.9
65 years and older	10.0	9.8	7.5	9.7
65–74 years	4.7	3.7	3.5	3.8
75 years and older	2.5	2.0	1.4	1.9
Race (males)				
White only	16.7	14.9	15.2	15.5
Black or African American only	11.0	12.4	10.5	11.6

Characteristic	1997	2000	2005	2006
American Indian or Alaska Native only	30.4	14.0	19.0	Unknown
Asian only	7.5	5.9	5.7	5.7
2 or more races	Unknown	23.7	13.2	12.1
Hispanic origin and race				
Hispanic or Latino	18.8	15.9	14.4	13.5
Mexican	21.9	19.1	17.3	15.8
Not Hispanic or Latino	15.5	14.3	14.3	14.7
Percent of poverty level				
Below 100 percent	16.5	15.7	14.4	14.7
100-less than 200 percent	16.4	13.3	14.0	14.1
200 percent or more	15.6	14.5	14.2	14.4
Females				
Age				
All females, 18 and older	3.9	3.3	3.7	4.1
18–44 years	5.5	5.2	5.7	6.4
18–24 years	7.6	8.3	8.8	10.3
25–44 years	4.9	4.2	4.7	5.1
45–64 years	2.9	1.9	2.4	2.6
45–54 years	3.3	2.1	3.0	3.6
55–64 years and older	2.1	1.5	1.6	1.3
65 years and older	0.4	0.4	Unknown	0.8
65–74 years	Unknown	Unknown	Unknown	1.4
75 years and older	Unknown	Unknown	Unknown	Unknown
Race				
White only	4.2	3.7	4.2	4.8
Black or African American only	2.9	1.9	1.7	2.0
American Indian or Alaska Native only	Unknown	Unknown	Unknown	Unknown
Asian only	Unknown	Unknown	Unknown	Unknown
2 or more races	Unknown	8.2	Unknown	Unknown
Hispanic origin and race				
Hispanic or Latino	3.5	2.1	2.2	3.1
Mexican	3.2	2.2	2.3	2.5
Not Hispanic or Latino	4.0	3.6	4.1	4.5
Percent of poverty level				
Below 100 percent	5.1	3.6	3.7	3.8
100-less than 200 percent	4.0	3.5	3.7	3.8
200 percent or more	3.7	3.4	3.9	4.6

Adapted from: National Center for Health Statistics. *Health, United States, 2008 with Chartbook.* Hyattsville, Md.: National Center for Health Statistics. Pages 308–309.

could be a sedating drug such as benzodiazepine. (When used legally, benzodiazepines are anti-anxiety drugs.) The combination of illegal drugs or misused prescription drugs and alcohol is very dangerous and can be lethal.

Studies in Canada have shown that up to 30 percent of fatally injured drivers were using a combination of alcohol and drugs. A 2008 survey in Canada by Douglas J. Beirnes, published in 2009 by the Canadian Centre on Substance Abuse, found that 15.5 percent of drivers tested positive for alcohol, drugs, or both alcohol and drugs. The researchers found that alcohol use was most commonly found during weekends and late at night, while drug use was evenly distributed. Research in the United States and Canada has found that most drivers who abuse alcohol and drugs are males.

Moderate Drinking: A Health Boon to Some

Many studies have shown that moderate drinking, or the consumption of no more than one to two drinks per day, may confer a health benefit, particularly in terms of preserving healthy cardiac function. Other research shows that moderate drinking may be protective against the development of type 2 diabetes. Among people already diagnosed with diabetes, moderate drinking may provide a protective factor against heart disease as well; however, some studies show that moderate drinking may lead to hypoglycemia.

When health benefits are found with moderate drinking, these benefits are generally the most pronounced in middle-aged and older individuals, among whom moderate drinking may provide a protective benefit greater than abstinence offers. However, if the moderate drinker escalates drinking to a higher level, the health benefits are lost.

Twenty-first Century Treatment

Fortunately, enforced lobotomies and sterilizations and the other horrors of treatment for alcoholism are no longer lawful in the United States, and most people view them with horror. Today, hospitals, specialty clinics, and outpatient facilities treat individuals with alcohol dependence with medications such as naltrexone, acamprosate, and disulfiram, as well as with psychotherapy.

Disulfiram, a drug used to induce aversion to alcohol, is still used today. This drug has an interesting history. It was first developed in 1947, when Danish researchers Erik Jacobsen and Jens Hald were testing it as a treatment to kill parasitic worms. They each tried the drug to see if it was toxic to them and did not notice any effects at all. However, later that day, the two researchers decided to go out and have a few drinks, and both quickly became extremely ill, with copious nausea and vomiting. After they recovered, Jacobsen and

Hald realized that the drug might work far better as a treatment for alcoholism. (It is unknown if disulfiram works against parasites.)

However, compliance with a disulfiram regimen is notably poor, because the drug makes the user extremely ill even from a tiny amount of alcohol. Medication compliance among alcoholics is also poor among medications such as naltrexone and acamprosate, which do not cause severe nausea.

Psychotherapy is another important form of treatment. Inpatient and outpatient facilities offer group and individual psychotherapy, as well as encourage individuals to attend frequent meetings of Alcoholics Anonymous. However, the broad majority of alcoholics refuse to seek any treatment whatsoever, failing to recognize that they have a problem and continuing to consume alcohol until it eventually takes its toll on their bodies with liver disease, cancer, pancreatitis, brain damage, and many other severe medical problems. Some people with alcohol dependence also suffer from degenerative mental diseases, such as Wernicke-Korsakoff syndrome, which leads to incurable dementia.

Words That Have Been Used to Denote the Person Dependent on Alcohol

Through the past few centuries in the United States, many words and phrases have been used, often pejoratively, to denote the person with alcohol dependence. Some key words and phrases are listed below. Some have fallen out of use (such as *dipsomaniac* or *inebriate*), while many are still used today, usually in a negative manner to convey contempt, such as *drunk*, *drunkard*, and *sot*. In general, the most judgment-free term as of this writing is "person with alcohol dependence."

alcohol addict
alcoholic
"alkie"
dipsomaniac
drunk
drunkard
drunken bum
drunken degenerate
drunken fool
habitual drinker
inebriate

person with alcohol dependence
problem drinker
Skid Row bum
sot
wino

References

Amethyst Initiative. Statement. Available online. URL: http://www.amethystinitiative.org/statement. Accessed March 1, 2009.

Beirness, Douglas J., and Erin E. Beasley. *Alcohol and Drug Use Among Drivers: British Columbia Roadside Survey, 2008.* Ottawa, Ontario: Canadian Centre on Substance Abuse, 2009.

Berridge, Virginia, and Sarah Mars. "History of Addictions." *Journal of Epidemiology and Public Health* 58 (2003): 747–750.

Blanco, Carlos, M.D., et al. "Mental Health of College Students and Their Non-College-Attending Peers: Results from the National Epidemiologic Study on Alcohol and Related Conditions." *Archives of General Psychiatry* 65, no. 12 (2008): 1,429–1,437.

Blocker, Jack S., Jr. "Did Prohibition Really Work: Alcohol Prohibition as a Public Health Innovation." *American Journal of Public Health* 96, no. 2 (2006): 233–243.

Blocker, Jack S., Jr., David M. Fahey, and Ian R. Tyrrell, eds. *Alcohol and Temperance in Modern History: An International Encyclopedia.* Santa Barbara, Calif.: ABC Clio, 2003.

Carter, Carolyn S. "Ladies Don't: A Historical Perspective on Attitudes Toward Alcoholic Women." *Affilia* 12, no. 4 (1997): 471–485.

Cook, Sharon Anne. "Educating for Temperance: The Woman's Christian Temperance Union and Ontario Children, 1880–1916." *Historical Studies in Education* 5, no. 2 (1993): 251–277.

Corley, T. A. B. "Interactions between the British and American Patent Medicine Industries 1708–1914." *Business and Economic History* 16 (1987): 111–129.

Doner, T. *Eleven Years a Drunkard: The Life of Thomas Doner.* Sycamore, Ill.: Doner, 1877.

Edison, A. J. *An Overview of Alcohol Use, Abuse, and Alcoholism.* Washington, D.C.: National Defense University, Fort McNair, 1993.

Emerson, Haven. "Prohibition and Mortality and Morbidity." *The Annals of the American Academy of Political and Social Science* 163, no. 53 (1932): 53–60.

Fahey, David M. "Temperance Internationalism: Guy Hayler and the World Prohibition Federation." *The Social History of Alcohol and Drugs* 20 (2006): 247–275.

———. *Temperance & Racism: John Bull, Johnny Reb and the Good Templars.* Lexington: University Press of Kentucky, 1996.

Fell, James C., et al. "The Impact of Underage Drinking Laws on Alcohol-Related Fatal Crashes of Young Drivers." *Alcoholism: Clinical and Experimental Research* 33, no. 7 (2009): 1–12.

Felton, Eric. "Celebrating Cinco de Drinko." *Wall Street Journal* (28 November 2008). Available online. URL: http://online.wsj.com/article/SB/22790942540265309.html. Accessed November 29, 2008.

Ferry, Darren. "'To the Interests and Conscience of the Great Mass of the Community': The Evolution of Temperance Societies in Nineteenth-Century Central Canada." *Journal of the Canadian Historical Association* 14, no. 1 (2003): 137–163.

Gately, Iain. *Drink: A Cultural History of Alcohol.* New York: Gotham Books, 2008.

Gwinnell, Esther, M.D., and Christine Adamec. *The Encyclopedia of Drug Abuse.* New York: Facts On File, Inc., 2008

Hingson, Ralph, et al. "Effects of Maine's 1981 and Massachusetts' 1982 Law Driving-Under-The-Influence Legislation." *American Journal of Public Health* 77, no. 5 (1987): 593–597.

Johnston, Lloyd D., Patrick M. O'Malley, Jerald G. Bachman, and John E. Schulenberg. *Monitoring the Future: National Results on Adolescent Drug Use. Overview of Key Findings, 2007.* Bethesda, Md.: National Institute on Drug Abuse. 2008.

Johnston, Lloyd D., et al. *Monitoring the Future: National Survey Results on Drug Use, 1975–2007. Volume II. College Students and Adults Age 19–45.* Bethesda, Md.: National Institute on Drug Abuse, 2008.

Katcher, Brian S. "Benjamin Rush's Educational Campaign Against Hard Drinking." *American Journal of Public Health* 83, no. 2 (1993): 273–281.

Keller, Mark. "A Historical Overview of Alcohol and Alcoholism." *Cancer Research* 39 (1979): 2,822–2,829.

———. "The Old and the New in the Treatment of Alcoholism." In *Alcohol Interventions: Historical and Sociocultural Approaches,* edited by David L. Strug, S. Pryadarsini, and Merton M. Hyman, 23–40. New York: Haworth Press, 1986.

Keniston, James M., M.D. "Alcoholic Psychoses in Hospitals for the Insane." *American Journal of Insanity* 65 (1909): 525–532.

Kent, Holly M. "'Our Good Angel': Women, Moral Influence, and the Nation in Antebellum American Pirate Novels." *Lumina: A Journal of Historical and Cultural Studies* 14 (2008): 50–58.

Kerr, K. Austin. "Organizing for Reform: The Anti-Saloon League and Innovation in Politics." *American Quarterly* 32, no. 1 (1980): 37–53.

Khantzian, Edward J., M.D. "How AA and Psychotherapy Can Work Together." *Psychiatric Times* 16, no. 7 (July 1, 1999). Available online. URL: http://www.psychiatrictimes.com/psychotherapy/article/10168/50026. Accessed April 15, 2009.

Knight, J. R., et al. "Alcohol Abuse and Dependence Among U.S. College Students." *Journal of Studies on Alcohol* 63, no. 3 (2002): 263–270.

Krasnick Warsh, Cheryl, ed. *Drink in Canada: Historical Essays.* Montreal, Canada: McGill-Queens University Press, 1993.

Lakins, Nekisha E., Robin A. LaVallee, Gerald D. Williams, and Hsiao-ye Yi. *Surveillance Report #82: Apparent Per Capita Alcohol Consumption: National, State, and Regional Trends, 1977–2005.* National Institute on Alcohol Abuse and Alcoholism. Rockville, Md.: National Institutes of Health, August 2007.

Lender, Mark Edwards. "A Special Stigma: Women and Alcoholism in the Late 19th and Early 20th Centuries." In *Alcohol Interventions: Historical and Sociocultural Approaches,* edited by David L. Strug, S. Pryadarsini, and Merton M. Hyman, 41–58. New York: Haworth Press, 1986.

Lender, Mark Edwards, and James Kirby Martin. *Drinking in America: A History. The Revised and Expanded Edition.* New York: Free Press 1987.

Levine, Harry Gene. "The Alcohol Problem in America: From Temperance to Alcoholism." *British Journal of Addictions* 79 (1984): 108–119.

———. "The Discovery of Addiction: Changing Conceptions of Habitual Drunkenness in America." *Journal of Studies on Alcohol* 39, no. 1 (1978): 143–174.

———. "Temperance Cultures: Concern about Alcohol Problems in Nordic and English-speaking Cultures." In *The Nature of Alcohol and Drug-Related Problems,* edited by Malcom Lader, Griffith Edwards, and D. Colin Drummon, 16–36. New York: Oxford University Press, 1993.

Levinthal, Charles F. *Drugs, Society, and Criminal Justice.* New York: Pearson Education, 2006.

Mancall, Peter C. "'I Was Addicted to Drinking Rum.'" In *Altering American Consciousness: The History of Alcohol and Drug Use in the United States 1800–2000,* edited by Sarah W. Tracy and Caroline Jean Acker, 91–107. Amherst: University of Massachusetts Press, 2004.

Martin, A. Lynn. *Alcohol, Sex, and Gender in Late Medieval and Early Modern Europe.* London: Palgrave, 2001.

Martin, Scott C. *Devil of the Domestic Sphere: Temperance, Gender, and Middle-Class Ideology, 1800–1860.* DeKalb: Northern Illinois University Press, 2008.

McIntosh, James R. "Elvin Morton Jellinek." In *Alcohol and Temperance in Modern History: An International Encyclopedia,* Vol. 1, edited by Jack S. Blocker, David M. Fahey, and Ian R. Tyrrell, 32–35. Santa Barbara, Calif.: ABC Clio, 2003.

———. "Gin Craze." In *Alcohol and Temperance in Modern History: An International Encyclopedia.* Vol. 1, edited by Jack S. Blocker, David M. Fahey and Ian R. Tyrrell, 265–267. Santa Barbara, Calif.: ABC Clio, 2003.

Miller, Norman S., M.D., and Mark S. Gold, M.D. *Alcohol.* New York: Plenum Medical Book Company, 1991.

Murdock, Catherine Gilbert. *Domesticating Drink: Women, Men, and Alcohol in America, 1870–1940.* Baltimore, Md.: Johns Hopkins University Press, 1998.

Naimi, T. S., et al. "What Do Binge Drinkers Drink? Implications for Alcohol Control Policy." *American Journal of Preventive Medicine* 33, no. 3 (2007): 188–193.

National Center for Health Statistics. *Health, United States, 2008 with Chartbook.* Hyattsville, Md.: National Center for Health Statistics, 2009.

Parascandola, John. "Patent Medicines in Nineteenth-Century America." *Caduceus: A Museum Quarterly for the Health Sciences* 1, no. 1 (Spring 1985): 1–41.

Peirce, Isaac Newton, and Silvanus Phillips Thompson. *History of the Independent Order of Good Templars.* Birmingham: Grand Lodge of England. 1873.

Pennock, Pamela. "The Evolution of U.S. Temperance Movements Since Repeal: A Comparison of Two Campaigns to Control Alcoholic Beverage Marketing, 1950s and 1980s. In *The Social History of Alcohol and Drugs* 20 (2005) 14–65.

Porter, Eugene O. "An Outline of the Temperance Movement." *The Historian* 7, no. 1 (1944): 54–67.

Reynolds, David S., and Debra J. Rosenthal, eds. *The Serpent in the Cup: Temperance in American Literature.* Amherst: University of Massachusetts Press, 1997.

Rorabaugh, W. J. "Estimated U.S. Alcoholic Beverage Consumption, 1790–1860." *Journal of Studies on Alcohol* 37, no. 3 (1976): 357–364.

Rosenthal, Debra J., and Davis S. Reynolds. Introduction to *The Serpent in the Cup: Temperance in American Literature,* edited by David S. Reynolds, and Debra J. Rosenthal, 1–9. Amherst: University of Massachusetts Press. 1997.

Rotskoff, Lori. *Love on the Rocks: Men, Women, and Alcohol in Post–World War II America.* Chapel Hill: University of North Carolina Press, 2002.

Rush, Benjamin. *Medical Inquiries and Observations upon the Diseases of the Mind.* Philadelphia: Kimber & Richardson, 1812.

Sherman, Carl. "Ford Center Hailed for Impact on Addiction Tx." *Clinical Psychiatry News* 35, no. 3 (2007): 26.

Short, Jerome L., Colleen J. Shogan, and Nicole M. Owings. "The Influence of First Ladies on Mental Health Policy." *White House Studies* 5, no. 1 (2005): 65–76.

Stolberg, Victor B. "A Review of Perspectives on Alcohol and Alcoholism in the History of American Health and Medicine." *Journal of Ethnicity in Substance Abuse* 5, no. 4 (2006): 39–106.

Straussner, Shulamith Lala, Ashenberg and Patricia Rose Attia. "Women's Addiction and Treatment through a Historical Lens." In Shulasmith Lala Ashenberg Straussner and Stephanie Brown, *The Handbook of Addiction Treatment for Women,* edited by New York: Jossey-Bass, 2002.

Strug, David L., S. Priyadarsini, and Merton M. Hyman, eds. *Alcohol Interventions: Historical and Sociocultural Approaches.* New York: The Haworth Press, 1986.

Substance Abuse and Mental Health Services Administration. "Children Living with Substance-Dependent or Substance-Abusing Parents: 2002 to 2007." *The NSDUH Report* (April 16, 2009): 1–4.

Tracy, Sarah W. *Alcoholism in America: From Reconstruction to Prohibition.* Baltimore, Md.: Johns Hopkins University Press, 2005.

Tracy, Sarah W., and Caroline Jean Acer, eds. *Altering American Consciousness: The History of Alcohol and Drug Use in the United States, 1800–2000.* Amherst: University of Massachusetts Press, 2004.

Tyrrell, Ian. *Woman's World, Woman's Empire: The Woman's Christian Temperance Union in International Perspective 1880–1930.* Chapel Hill: University of North Carolina Press, 1991.

Voas, Robert B., and John L. Lacey. "Issues in the Enforcement of Impaired Driving Laws in the United States." In *Surgeon General's Workshop on Drunk Driving: Background Papers,* 136–156, 1989. Available online. URL: http://profiles.nlm.nih.gov/NN/B/C/Y/D/_/nnbcyd.pdf. Accessed April 19, 2009.

White, William L. "Pre-A.A. Alcoholic Mutual Aid Societies." *Alcoholism Treatment Quarterly* 19, no. 2 (2001): 1–21.

———. *Slaying the Dragon: The History of Addiction Treatment and Recovery in America.* Bloomington, Ill.: Chestnut Hills Publication, 1998.

ENTRIES A–Z

abstinence Completely refraining from the consumption of all alcoholic beverages, including beer, wine, distilled spirits, or any other items that contain alcohol. Most rehabilitation plans for individuals who are alcoholics, as well as twelve-step groups, such as Alcoholics Anonymous, stress that it is very important for an alcohol-dependent person to avoid consuming *any* alcohol and on a permanent basis. That is, they can never drink again in their lives. These experts believe that if the formerly active alcoholic has even one drink (or even one sip of one alcoholic drink), it will cause a cascade of unconscious events that inevitably leads to the person's consuming one drink after another until he or she has become intoxicated and has relapsed into alcohol dependence. They believe that the person will drink repeatedly unless or until he or she returns to abstinence.

In the 19th and early 20th centuries, organizations such as the Good Templars, the Woman's Christian Temperance Union, and many other groups strongly supported abstinence from all alcohol as well as making the sale of alcohol illegal.

Individuals who are dependent on alcohol find abstinence particularly difficult, and many of them gain emotional support through their attendance at support group meetings offered by groups such as Alcoholics Anonymous. There are twelve steps in the Alcoholics Anonymous process towards rehabilitation, although no one is ever considered "cured"; instead, participants still call themselves "alcoholics" even if they have abstained from consuming alcohol for many years. They continue to fear that taking even one drink could lead them into addiction again.

The person who is alcohol-dependent has centered his or her life around drinking. It is not only an addiction, but it is also a habit that is associated with the places that he or she has frequented (bars, parties, clubs) where the individual drinks, as well as the people with whom he or she has associated, often including others who are heavy drinkers or alcoholics. The individual must learn to dissociate himself or herself from such places and people. This is especially difficult if members of his or her family consider drinking to be a normal and acceptable activity.

Medications are sometimes used to promote abstinence. An aversive medication given to treat alcoholics, DISULFIRAM (Antabuse), has severe side effects, such that if the individual consumes any alcohol, it causes severe vomiting. This includes the consumption of any alcohol in food (such as added wine) or even the minute amount of alcohol that may be included in mouthwash and other common products. Disulfiram is still used at some treatment centers nationwide and is also prescribed by some physicians for their patients on an outpatient basis.

Other medications are also used to promote abstinence, but they do not cause extreme side effects. Instead, these drugs are primarily designed to decrease the individual's psychological craving for alcohol. Acamprosate (Campral) and NALTREXONE (ReVia, Vivitriol) are the primary examples of such drugs.

See also ALCOHOL ABUSE; ALCOHOLISM/ALCOHOL DEPENDENCE AND ALCOHOL ABUSE; ALCOHOLISM MUTUAL AID SOCIETIES; BINGE DRINKING; CODEPENDENCY; DENIAL; EXCESSIVE DRINKING AND HEALTH CONSEQUENCES; EXCESSIVE DRINKING AND NEGATIVE SOCIAL CONSEQUENCES; IMPAIRED PHYSICIANS; MODERATE DRINKING AND HEALTH BENEFITS; TREATMENT.

acetaldehyde The initial metabolic byproduct of alcohol consumption. According to researchers, ethanol (the substance in alcohol that causes intoxication) is oxidized to acetaldehyde in the human brain, and this action may be responsible for the effects of ethanol on the central nervous system. However, this is a theory that is yet to be proven and research continues.

It is known that alcohol is metabolized in the body by four key enzymes, including aldehyde dehydrogenase (ALDH), alcohol dehydrogenase (ADH), cytochrome P450 (CYP2E1), and catalase. It is believed that genetic variations of these enzymes affect not only the consumption of alcohol but also may lead to tissue damage that is caused by alcohol and alcoholism. The liver is the primary organ involved in metabolizing alcohol, but the stomach is also involved, as well as the brain.

When acetaldehyde has been directly administered into the brain by researchers, effects that mimic the use of alcohol occurred, according to Quertemont and Didone. High doses were sedating and caused impairment of movement and memory. Lower doses caused behavioral effects, such as stimulation and reinforcement that were similar to the effect of addicting drugs.

Acetaldehyde is greatly increased when individuals with alcohol dependence are treated with aversive drugs such as DISULFIRAM (Antabuse). This drug prevents the oxidization of acetaldehyde from alcohol, and it causes the blood concentrations to increase to five to 10 times the normal rate. This toxicity leads to the extreme nausea and vomiting that is exhibited by the individual taking disulfiram when he or she consumes even a small quantity of alcohol. This is also why disulfiram is effective, assuming it is taken. As might be expected in light of disulfiram's unpleasant effect, medication compliance is an issue.

Some experts believe that acetaldehyde has a carcinogenic (cancer-causing) effect in some individuals, based on animal studies. According to Dirk W. Lachenmeier and his colleagues in an article on the carcinogenicity of acetaldehyde, published in *Addiction* in 2009, acetaldehyde is also present in alcohol and is not solely a product of the metabolizing of alcohol. The researchers found acetaldehyde within various forms of alcohol, such as beer, wine, whiskey, vodka, brandy, rum, and other forms. They also pointed out that acetaldehyde may be found in nonalcoholic items as well, such as fruit yogurt, fruit juices, candy, soft drinks, and margarine.

According to the authors, "The life-time cancer risks for acetaldehyde from alcoholic beverages greatly exceed the usual limits for cancer risks from the environment set between 1 : 10,000 and 1 : 1,000,000. Alcohol consumption has thus been identified as a direct source of acetaldehyde exposure, which in conjunction with other sources (food flavourings, tobacco) results in a magnitude of risk requiring intervention. An initial public health measure could be to reduce the acetaldehyde content in alcoholic beverages as low as technologically possible, and to restrict its use as a food flavour additive."

See also ALCOHOL ABUSE; ALCOHOL FLUSHING RESPONSE; ALCOHOLISM/ALCOHOL DEPENDENCE; CANCER; DISULFIRAM; TREATMENT.

Lachenmeier, Dirk W., Fotis Kanteres, and Jürgen Rehm. "Carcinogenicity of Acetaldehyde in Alcoholic Beverages: Risk Assessment Outside Ethanol Metabolism." *Addiction* 104, no. 4 (2009): 533–550.

Quertemont, Etienne, and Vincent Didone. "Role of Acetaldehyde in Mediating the Pharmacological and Behavioral Effects of Alcohol." *Alcohol Research & Health* 29, no. 4 (2006): 258–265.

Zakhari, Samir. "Overview: How Is Alcohol Metabolized by the Body?" *Alcohol Research & Health* 29, no. 4 (2006): 245–254.

addictive personality A controversial term used to describe a type of person who is prone to developing addictions. Experts do not agree on what traits may comprise an addictive personality, and some experts believe that the concept is not valid. However, some studies have found a correlation between some psychiatric disorders and the risk for ALCOHOL ABUSE and alcohol dependence. It is also true that some studies have found a correlation between alcohol abuse and individuals in some specific careers or OCCUPATIONS.

According to the 2002 report from the Task Force of the National Advisory Council on Alcohol Abuse and Alcoholism on drinking in college, "Decades of research have failed to identify an 'addictive personality.' However, certain personality traits have been related to drinking habit. For example, sensation-seeking has been related to higher rates of consumption, while religiosity has been related to lower rates. Personality traits are typically seen as mediating or moderating the relationship between biological, psychological, social, and environmental factors and subsequent alcohol use and misuse."

Individuals with some psychiatric disorders seem more prone to developing a problem with substance abuse, particularly individuals with untreated ATTENTION-DEFICIT/HYPERACTIVITY DISORDER or IMPULSE CONTROL DISORDERS (particularly PATHOLOGICAL GAMBLING and INTERMITTENT EXPLOSIVE DISORDER,) as well as those with other serious psychiatric disorders, such as DEPRESSION or some ANXIETY DISORDERS, and in some PERSONALITY DISORDERS, such as ANTISOCIAL PERSONALITY DISORDER or borderline personality disorder.

Researchers are focused heavily on early onset (teenage) drinking as the largest environmental risk factor in addictions. Genes matter a great deal, but teenage BINGE DRINKING creates a risk when none would have otherwise existed.

Another population that often has a problem with alcohol abuse and alcoholism is those who are incarcerated in prison. According to a study of 320 newly incarcerated men and women in the Iowa Prison system, reported in 2008 in the *Journal of the American Academy of Psychiatry Law,* 90 percent of the inmates had substance use disorders. Among the men, 77.7 percent had alcohol use disorders, while 55.3 percent of the women were diagnosed with an alcohol use disorder.

According to the authors, "This study confirms the high frequency of mental and addictive disorders in incarcerated offenders, findings generally consistent with reports from other prison-based findings."

The researchers also found a high rate of mood disorders and anxiety disorders among the inmates; for example, 46.4 percent of the women and 36.4 percent of the men had an anxiety disorder, and 37.5 percent of the women and 33.3 percent of the men had a mood disorder. The researchers also reported a high rate of antisocial personality disorder occurring among 37 percent of the incarcerated men and 27 percent of the incarcerated women.

See also ALCOHOLISM/ALCOHOL DEPENDENCE AND ALCOHOL ABUSE; GENETICS AND ALCOHOL; IMPAIRED PHYSICIANS; PSYCHIATRIC COMORBIDITIES.

Gunter, Tracy D., et al. "Frequency of Mental and Addictive Disorders among 320 Men and Women Entering the Iowa Prison System: Use of the MINI-Plus." *Jour-*

nal of the American Academy of Psychiatry Law 36, no. 1 (2008): 27–34.

Task Force of the National Advisory Council on Alcohol Abuse and Alcoholism. *High Risk Drinking in College: What We Know and What We Need to Learn: Final Report on Contexts and Consequences.* Washington, D.C.: National Institute on Alcohol Abuse and Alcoholism, April 2002.

adolescents and drinking   See AGE AND ALCOHOL; UNDERAGE DRINKING.

adoption and twin studies and alcohol   Research studies that compare the outcomes either for adopted individuals (such as adoption studies) or for twins (preferably identical twins who were raised apart since birth or shortly thereafter) as study subjects, in an attempt to avoid the bias that the environment may create. Many possible outcomes are considered for adopted individuals or twins, one of which is alcohol dependence.

A combination of adoption, twin, and family studies indicate a heritability of up to 50 percent for alcoholism. This means that when a person becomes an alcoholic, as much as 50 percent of the cause may be a genetic predisposition to alcoholism. Of course it also means that individuals born to alcoholic parents are *not* foredoomed to alcoholism in adulthood. Many complex factors may increase the risk for alcoholism in an individual in addition to their genetic risks, such as CHILD ABUSE AND NEGLECT, their peer associations, and other influences in their lives.

Adoption Studies

Sir Francis Galton was the first researcher to use adoption studies, in about 1876. (Galton also used twin studies.) With adoption studies, the researchers may compare the prevalence of a social problem such as alcoholism in adopted adults to the prevalence of alcoholism found in the birth parents of the adopted individuals. They often also compare the prevalence to that within the general public. It is assumed that alcoholic birth parents may provide the adopted-out child with a genetic predisposition toward drinking, if a significant proportion of both the birth parents and the adopted adults in the study are alcoholics. Research has generally borne out this finding, particularly for males.

Some adoption studies also consider the rate of alcoholism in the adoptive parents as well. In general, however, the alcoholism of the birth parents apparently plays a much greater role than the alcohol dependence of the adoptive parent in the ultimate appearance of alcohol use disorders in the adopted adult.

Most large-scale adoption studies are performed in Finland, Sweden, and Denmark, where adoption records are openly available to researchers. In contrast, most adoptions in the United States are confidential adoptions, and in most cases, even the adopted adult does not know the identity of his or her biological mother or father, nor do the birth parents know the legal name of the adopted adult.

The majority of adoption studies consider data at one point in time only, while researchers performing longitudinal studies revisit the same population and make comparisons to their past findings every several years. One such study is the Colorado Adoption Project. Many researchers have used the data from the Colorado Adoption Project.

One potential problem with adoption studies, as pointed out by the authors of *The Encyclopedia of Adoption,* is that some adoption studies include some major inherent (although unplanned) biases; for example, these studies may include a population of children adopted as infants along with children who were adopted as older children and who may have been abused and/or neglected or living in poor orphanage conditions. Thus, the abuse or neglect that the children adopted at older ages experienced may have been more significant to the development of later problems such as alcoholism than was the adoptive or genetic status of the individual. It is also true that pathology (diseases or unhealthy conditions) is generally studied in adoption studies (and twin studies), and some individuals make the grand leap that because of this fact, adopted children are more prone to pathology.

Said David Howe in his book *Patterns of Adoption:* "The choice of behaviours by scientists is often that which also concerns policy makers and practitioners: education, mental health and antisocial behavior. To this extent, the knowledge produced about adopted children's development appears a little unbalanced, concentrating mainly on the disturbed and the deviant. More 'normal' behaviours receive less attention. Thus, a digest of behavioural genetic research that might interest adoption workers needs to be read with this distortion in mind. By association, one can have the feeling that because these scientists write a lot about schizophrenia or crime using adoption as one of their 'natural experiments,' then adoptions themselves are beset with these behaviours. This, of course, is not the case."

Twin Studies

Twin studies are often used to compare the outcome of one identical twin (and sometimes one fraternal twin) to the other twin, since they share the same genes. It is often assumed that if one identical twin has a healthy life and the other twin has severe pathology, this then means that the problems of the non-healthy twin were caused by the environment, rather than by an inherited predisposition.

In one study of identical twins who were separated as infants, one being adopted and the other raised by the biological parent, reported in *Psychiatry* in 1998, the researchers found that the twin who was reared by the biological mother was more likely to abuse alcohol than the adopted twin. The researchers speculated that the better socioeconomic status of the adopted twin reduced the risk for alcohol abuse.

See also ADDICTIVE PERSONALITY; ALCOHOL AND ALCOHOL USE; FAMILIES AND ALCOHOL; GENETICS AND ALCOHOL; UNDERAGE DRINKING.

Adamec, Christine, and Laurie C. Miller, M.D. *The Encyclopedia of Adoption.* 3rd Ed. New York: Facts On File, Inc., 2006.

Howe, David. *Patterns of Adoption: Nature, Nurture and Psychosocial Development.* Oxford, U.K.: Blackwell Science, 1998.

Li, Ting-Kai, M.D. "The Genetics of Alcoholism." *Alcohol Alert* 60 (July 2003): 1–4.

Smyer, Michael A., et al. "Childhood Adoption: Long-Term Effects in Adulthood." *Psychiatry* 61, no. 3 (Fall 1998): 191–205.

adult children of alcoholics See AGE AND ALCOHOL; FAMILIES AND ALCOHOL.

advertising of alcohol Promotion of alcohol products to individuals that the manufacturer hopes will purchase their products. Some experts are concerned that such advertising may affect underage drinkers and young adults. Advertising includes print, television, radio, Internet, and any other available media, such as public signs. In general, advertisers of alcohol products depict drinking individuals as beautiful and glamorous or athletic people. Whatever image is used, the individual is shown clearly having a wonderful time. Such images are cultivated by advertisers in an effort to induce people to buy their products.

Individuals who are concerned about the impact of advertising on alcohol consumption, particularly the marketing of alcohol consumed in UNDERAGE DRINKING, seek to create stricter regulations to limit alcohol advertising that appears to target adolescents and young adults. For example, some groups are concerned about specific "energy drinks" that combine alcohol with caffeine and other substances and which seem to be aimed at young adults or other underage individuals.

In their study on alcohol marketing to youth, researchers for the Center on Alcohol Marketing and Youth at Georgetown University analyzed data from 2001 to 2007. They found that the impact of television alcohol advertisements had increased, and that from 2001 to 2007, youths ages 12 to 20 years old saw 38 percent more ads. Most of the growth was due to advertisements for distilled sprits. The researchers also found that most of the youth overexposure was on cable television. The researchers also found that more than 40 percent of alcohol advertisements that were exposed to youth were placed on youth-oriented programming, or programs directed to those ages 12–20 years old.

According to the researchers, alcohol spending on advertisements increased on cable television networks from $156.8 million spent for 51,109 ads in 2001 to $391.6 million for 168,318 ads by 2007. Spending for ads on beer and ale dominated. The number of ads for beer and ale on cable networks increased from 36,834 in 2001 to 90,630 ads in 2007. The number of ads for distilled spirits on cable TV increased hugely from 1,973 ads in 2001 to 62,776 ads in 2007. Wine ads were relatively flat on cable TV: there were 9,166 ads in 2001 and that number increased to 10,577 ads by 2007.

The researchers said, "The prevalence and the toll of underage drinking in the United States remain high. Evidence that alcohol advertising plays a role in the problems grows stronger each year."

In another study published in *Alcohol & Alcoholism* in 2009, researchers Rutger C.M.E. Engels and colleagues found that the portrayals of alcohol in advertising and in movies on television directly affected alcohol consumption. The subjects in the study were 80 male university students, and the subjects that viewed alcohol in movies and in advertisements drank an average 1.5 glasses more of alcohol than the subjects who watched movies and saw advertisements with no depictions of alcohol. Said the researchers, "This study—for the first time—shows a causal link between exposure to drinking models and alcohol commercials on acute alcohol consumption."

Research performed by Auden C. McClure, M.D., and colleagues and published in the *American Journal of Preventive Medicine* in 2006 reported their study of the effect of the ownership of alcohol-branded merchandise and the onset of adolescent drinking. The researchers found that of 2,406 adolescents who had never consumed alcohol, 15 percent later initiated alcohol use and 14 percent owned alcohol-branded items. Ownership of such items correlated with exposure to peers who were drinking, male gender, having tried SMOKING, having lower levels of academic achievement, having higher levels of rebelliousness and sensation-seeking, and having less restrictive parents. At follow-up of the formerly nondrinking adolescents, the teenage owners of the alcohol-branded items had higher rates of alcohol initiation (25.5 percent) compared to nonowners (13.1 percent). The researchers concluded that those who owned alcohol-branded items were significantly more likely to have started using alcohol.

The researchers noted that further research was needed to determine whether owning the items appeared causal and whether the use of the alcohol-branded items had influenced drinking behavior. (It may be possible that those adolescents who are more likely to begin to drink are also more likely to wish to own alcohol-branded merchandise, which is why more research is needed.) However, until further research is performed, it seems logical that parents and others should not give adolescents T-shirts or other items that are branded with the name of any form of alcohol.

See also AGE AND ALCOHOL; UNDERAGE DRINKING.

Center on Alcohol Marketing and Youth. *Youth Exposure to Alcohol Advertising on Television, 2001 to 2007.* Washington, D.C.: Georgetown University. June 24, 2008. Available online. URL: http://www.camy.org/research/tv0608/tv0608.pdf. Accessed August 1, 2009.

Engels, C. M. E. Rutger, et al. "Alcohol Portrayal on Television Affects Actual Drinking Behavior." *Alcohol & Alcoholism* 44, no. 3 (2009): 244–249.

McClure, Auden C., M.D., Sonya Dal Cin, Jennifer Gibson, and James D. Sargent, M.D. "Ownership of Alcohol-Branded Merchandise and Initiation of Teen Drinking." *American Journal of Preventive Medicine* 30, no. 4 (2006): 277–283.

Snyder, Leslie B., et al. "Effects of Alcohol Advertising Exposure on Drinking Among Youth." *Archives of Pediatric & Adolescent Medicine* 160 (January 2006): 18–24.

age and alcohol   One of the major factors affecting whether a person drinks to excess is an individual's age, and the risk for heavy drinking as well as BINGE DRINKING is generally the highest among young adults, particularly COLLEGE STUDENTS. In addition, it is important to note that drinking behavior in adolescence or during childhood as well as adverse childhood events, such as physical abuse, are predictive for future alcohol dependence.

In many ways, the old saying "The child is the father to the man" (or, to be more egalitarian, the child is also mother to the woman) is relevant when it comes to drinking. Early drinking in adolescence greatly increases the risk for ALCOHOLISM in the same person as an adult male or female; for example, if the initiation of alcohol consumption starts before age 14 or 15, the individual is at an increased risk for alcohol dependence in adulthood, as well as for an elevated risk for accidental injuries that are caused by excessive alcohol consumption and the risks for many health problems that are associated with excessive drinking.

Some longitudinal research has demonstrated that the greater the number of adverse childhood events that occur to an individual, the higher the probability for alcoholism in adulthood. In addition, adverse childhood events are predictive for many behaviors, such as the early initiation of alcohol use or a later marriage to an alcoholic. Other research has shown that an overall depressed mood state in a preadolescent child is predictive for later alcohol abuse or dependence.

Young adults from ages 18 to 24 are generally the heaviest drinkers of all ages, and sometimes this heavy alcohol consumption is viewed as a rite of passage to adulthood. Yet extreme drinking can lead to many serious consequences, such as sexual and physical assaults, car crashes, and other negative consequences. (See EXCESSIVE DRINKING AND NEGATIVE SOCIAL CONSEQUENCES.) In considering middle-aged people, most individuals have established drinking patterns. Some middle-aged people are alcohol abusers and others are alcoholics. During this phase of life, alcoholics are starting to see the problematic health consequences of their alcohol dependence in terms of CIRRHOSIS and many other health problems.

Although they are less likely to abuse or be dependent on alcohol than younger people, sometimes elderly individuals drink to excess, risking many health problems when they do so. In some cases, the onset of heavy drinking occurs late in life. This circumstance is more likely to occur among older women, possibly because of personal and emotional losses, such as the death of a spouse or friends, relatives, or others they loved, as well as because of serious health problems that are difficult to manage and which may cause severe physical pain.

The Adverse Childhood Experiences Study and Alcohol

Dr. Robert Anda, a physician on the board of scientific advisors for the National Association for Children of Alcoholics, discussed both the health and social impacts of growing up with family members who abused alcohol as well as the impact of growing up under related adverse childhood experiences, such as CHILD ABUSE. Dr. Anda said that the Adverse Childhood Experiences (ACE) study was an ongoing study. In the first part of the study, there were 9,508 subjects and in the second part, there were 8,667 subjects. The subjects had an average age of 56 years and 75 percent were white. Most had graduated from college or high school.

The specific childhood experiences that the researchers identified as ACEs included childhood abuse (physical, sexual, and emotional abuse); childhood neglect (emotional and physical); growing up in a very dysfunctional household as evidenced by the child witnessing domestic violence; the presence of alcohol abuse or other substance abuse by members in the home; the presence of mentally ill or suicidal household members; parental marital discord as evidenced by separation or divorce; and crime in the home, as evidenced by a household member who went to prison.

The researchers found that the number of alcohol abusers in the childhood home was significant for whether study subjects experienced childhood abuse. As might be expected, the risk for child abuse was lowest if no one in the family abused alcohol. It increased if one person was an alcohol abuser and increased further if there were two or more alcohol abusers present.

Anda and colleagues also found that the ACE scores were highly interrelated and that as the ACE score (the number of adverse childhood experiences) increased, so did the risk for health and social problems throughout life. For example, the researchers found that increased ACE scores had a strong influence on later behaviors and conditions such as alcohol abuse, teenage pregnancy, smoking, illicit drug abuse, mental health, the stability of relationships, workforce performance, and the risk of revictimization.

In addition, ACEs also affected the adult children's risk for heart disease, chronic lung disease, LIVER DISEASE, SUICIDE, injuries, and infection with the human immunodeficiency virus (HIV) and other sexually transmitted diseases (STDs).

The greater the number of ACEs, then the greater is the risk for problems in adulthood related to alcohol dependence. For example, when the ACE score was 0, indicating that none of the specified adverse events had occurred in childhood, then the percentage of alcoholics in the adult children was 2.9 percent. When there was one ACE, the percentage of adult alcoholics in adulthood increased to 5.4 percent. For two ACEs, the percentage increased to 7.5 percent. For three ACEs, the percentage increased to 8.7 percent. If there were 4 or more ACEs among the subjects, then 14.5 percent of this population were alcoholics. A greater number of ACEs was also predictive for the early initiation of alcohol use, for problems with alcohol use, and for the individual marrying an alcoholic, all illustrated in Figure 1.

In another report on the ACE study, published in the *American Journal of Preventive Medicine* in 2005, Shanta R. Dube and colleagues reported on the impact of childhood sexual abuse in adulthood. They found that childhood sexual abuse had occurred to 16 percent of the males and 25 percent of the females in the study. Men and women who were exposed to childhood sexual abuse had a 40 percent increased risk of marrying a person with alcohol dependence, compared to those who were not exposed to childhood abuse. Risks of marrying an alcoholic were higher if intercourse had occurred during the abuse.

Depressed Mood in Childhood and Adult Alcohol Dependence

In another study of more than a thousand mostly African-American children in elementary school, most (75 percent) were followed into adulthood. The researchers found that a high level of depressed mood in preadolescent children was predictive for alcohol-related problems in late childhood and also for the development of alcohol dependence in young adulthood. Rosa M. Crum, M.D., and colleagues reported their findings in the *Archives of General Psychiatry* in 2008. According to the researchers, "We found no association with alcohol abuse. Early depressed mood appears to predict the transition from high-risk drinking to alcohol dependence but not to the occurrence of alcohol abuse without dependence."

The researchers also noted that "The vulnerability to increased risk for alcohol involvement extended across both life stages studied and was independent of potential causal determinants of maladaptive drinking, such as family income in childhood, heavy drinking among caregivers, peer alcohol use, level of conduct problems, and neighborhood disadvantage."

Early Initiation of Drinking and Effects

Excessive drinking and alcoholism in adulthood is often linked backward to the early initiation of drinking among adolescents; for example, researcher Ralph Hingson and colleagues reported in *Pediatrics* in 2001 that of college students who drank, those who began their drinking before age 14 were three times more likely to experience alcohol dependence at some point in their lives.

Risks of Early Drinking In another study by Hingson and colleagues, reported in the *Journal of the American Medical Association* in 2000 and based on 42,862 individuals, the researchers revealed

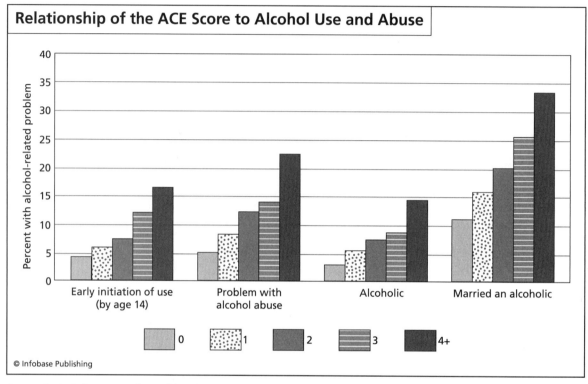

Relationship of the ACE Score to Alcohol Use and Abuse

© Infobase Publishing

Source: Anda, Robert, M.D. *The Health and Social Impact of Growing Up with Alcohol Abuse and Related Adverse Childhood Experiences.* Undated. Available online. URL: http://www.nacoa.net/pdfs/Anda%20NACoA%20Review_web.pdf. Accessed April 18, 2009.

that people who started drinking at an early age (younger than age 14) had an increased risk for suffering unintentional injuries while under the influence of alcohol. Said the researchers, "Compared with respondents who began drinking at age 21 years or older, those who began drinking prior to age 14 years were nearly 7 times more likely to report having been in situations that increased their chance of injury ever in their lifetime and in the past year. Persons drinking prior to age 14 years were also 12 times more likely to have ever been injured while under the influence of alcohol ever in their lifetime and in the past year."

Early drinkers are also more likely as adolescents to become involved in alcohol-related violence. For example, in a study by Ralph Hingson, Timothy Heeren, and Ronda Zakocs, reported in *Pediatrics* in 2001, the researchers found that individuals who started drinking before age 17 were significantly more likely to be involved in physical fights after

their drinking than those who started drinking when they were age 21 or older. The early drinkers were at least three times likelier to have been in a fight in the past year. The risk for physical violence was not only present among those under age 21 in the early drinkers group, but it continued until adulthood as well.

The researchers speculated on possible reasons for early drinking and physical fights. They said, "Studies show those who began drinking at an earlier age are more likely to drive after drinking and place themselves in situations that increase their risk of unintentional injury. Another explanation is that those who begin drinking earlier, because of their longer drinking experiences, may develop strong beliefs that alcohol will make them (and/or others who drink) more aggressive, which may foster violent behavior. Several studies have demonstrated these heightened alcohol beliefs are associated with increased episodes of alcohol-related aggression. Lastly, peer norms regarding alcohol use are known to be important predictors of adolescent alcohol misuse. It may be plausible, therefore, that persons who start drinking at an early age may also associate with others who engage in similar deviant behaviors and, thus, ascribe to social norms encouraging interpersonal violence that persist[s] through their adult ages."

Male Twins, Early Initiation of Alcohol Use, and Progression to Alcohol Dependence In a study of 1,269 male twins, with an average age of 20.1 years, researchers Carolyn E. Sartor and colleagues reported in *Addiction* in 2006 on the factors related to an early initiation of drinking as well as the progression to alcohol dependence. The twins were "genetically loaded," in that nearly half (46.2 percent) were the children of alcoholic fathers.

The researchers found that among the study subjects, the first drink occurred at an average 15.7 years and alcohol dependence had its onset at 19.1 years. They also found that CONDUCT DISORDER in the subjects was the only factor that predicted both the early initiation of drinking and the progression to alcohol dependence. Other risk factors identified with early initiation included a rapid development to alcoholism, SMOKING (nicotine dependence), the use of marijuana, and the diagnosis of generalized anxiety disorder (GAD). Factors associated with the early use of alcohol included the diagnosis of ATTENTION-DEFICIT/HYPERACTIVITY DISORDER (ADHD), maternal alcohol dependence, paternal alcohol dependence, parental divorce, and male gender.

Adolescent Drinking

Adolescence is generally defined as the period between ages 12 and 17 years, although some researchers define adolescence as a year or two later or earlier. Adolescents are much less sensitive to the negative after effects of excessive alcohol consumption than adults, such as a headache, hangover, extreme fatigue, nausea, and vomiting. This may make them less averse to drinking again after their first experience with alcohol. However, it is also true that adolescents who drink often have more difficulty with performing tasks than adults, such as driving a car or performing complex tasks, and they are also more likely to experience impairment with such tasks when they attempt them

while they are intoxicated. According to the Monitoring the Future study, 1.4 percent of students in the 10th grade drank alcohol every day in 2007, as did 3.1 percent of those in the 12th grade.

An estimated 9.7 percent of youths ages 12–17 engaged in binge drinking in 2007 according to the National Survey on Drug Use and Health. Research indicates that adolescent binge drinking can significantly affect an individual's earning power throughout life, especially among males. Researcher Francesco Renna found that binging on alcohol in adolescence reduced the probability of graduating from high school on time by 5.2 percent for females and 14.5 percent for males. Renna also found that the 1994 earnings of males who graduated from high school by May 1 of the year that they turned age 19 was about $10,000 a year greater than those who graduated later in life. (Over the course of a lifetime, this translates to about $400,000 less for those who graduated late compared to those who graduated on time.) Renna also found a direct correlation between adolescent binge drinking and late graduation (or no graduation) from high school.

Renna found that white adolescent males were the most likely to binge drink, and they were also more likely to have a father with an alcohol problem. (See UNDERAGE DRINKING.)

It is important to note that adolescents are strongly influenced by ADVERTISING, including branded material that they wear with logos and other promotional material for alcoholic beverages, such as T-shirts and other items. In a study by A. C. McClure and colleagues published in *Archives of Pediatrics & Adolescent Medicine* in 2009, the researchers found among never-drinking adolescents ages 10 to 14 years who subsequently obtained alcohol-branded merchandise, their susceptibility to start drinking was significantly increased, as was their binge drinking. In about a quarter of the cases, the adolescents purchased the branded items themselves. Clearly, adults should actively discourage adolescents from buying alcohol-branded merchandise.

Drinking in Young Adulthood

Young adulthood is generally defined as the period from age 18 to 29 years. The younger members of this group, or those who are ages 18–24 years, are generally much more likely to exhibit problematic alcohol consumption than younger or older cohorts, whether they are males or females or in college or not in college. According to the Monitoring the Future study, 5.6 percent of those ages 19–28 were daily drinkers in 2007. Among young adults ages 18–25 years, 41.8 percent engaged in binge drinking in 2007.

It is illegal for individuals under age 21 to possess alcohol in the United States, but despite this, many young people report that it is very easy for them to find someone to buy them alcohol or even to buy alcohol themselves. Sometimes they use a false identification or someone else's identification, whether or not the person resembles the young underage adult in any way.

Among young adults, studies have found that up to 13 percent of young adult males and 6 percent of females meet the diagnostic criteria for alcohol dependence; however, many may end their excessive drinking when they are older. Yet this early heavy drinking can continue to have consequences, as pointed out by Peter M. Monti and colleagues in their article on drinking among young adults for *Alcohol Research & Health* in 2004–05.

According to the researchers, "Even one episode of excessive drinking can have serious consequences that persist well beyond adolescence and young adulthood, such as alcohol-related car crashes, unintended pregnancies, and physical fights leading to arrest or jail. Young adults who engage in heavy episodic drinking (another term for binge drinking) are significantly more likely than those who do not drink heavily to get in trouble with police, damage property, sustain injuries, drive after drinking, and engage in unplanned and unprotected sexual activity."

College Students College students represent another category of adults who are at high risk for drinking. According to the National Survey on Drug Use and Health, young adults ages 18 to 22 years who were full-time college students in 2007 were more likely to abuse alcohol than their noncollege peers. For example, the percentage of past-month alcohol use was 63.7 percent for college students, compared to 53.5 percent for their same-age noncollege peers. Close to half of college students were binge drinkers in 2007 (43.7 percent), compared with 38.4 percent of their noncollege peers. With regard to heavy drinking, 17.2 percent of college students were heavy drinkers, compared to 12.9 percent of their noncollege peers. Studies have

shown that college students have a higher risk for alcohol abuse and alcohol dependence than their noncollege peers.

The Monitoring the Future survey results on college students and adults ages 19–45 years, published in 2008, and including some data on younger individuals, found a large and significant difference between 18-year-olds (who had a heavy drinking rate of 26 percent) and those ages 21–22, who had a heavy drinking rate of 46 percent. Then drinking fell off at each subsequent age, dropping to 19 percent by age 45.

Said the researchers, "We have interpreted this curvilinear relationship as reflecting an age effect—and not a cohort effect—because it seems to replicate across different graduating class cohorts, and also because it has been linked directly to age-related events such as leaving the parental home (which increases heavy drinking) and marriage (which decreases it), both of which are, in turn, related to attending college."

There may be some good news. In her 2005 article in the *Archives of General Psychiatry,* Wendy S. Slutske points out that although college students are more likely to receive a diagnosis of an alcohol use disorder (18.0 percent for alcohol abuse in 2001 from the National Household Survey on Drug Abuse) than their noncollege peers (15.1 percent), these subjects were not at a greater risk for alcohol dependence.

Slutske said, "The results of this study provide a more encouraging message about the consequences of college drinking than many of the recent reports—although college students suffer from some clinically significant consequences of their heavy/binge drinking, they do not appear to be at greater risk than their non-college attending peers for the more pervasive syndrome of problems that is characteristic of alcohol dependence. "

She also noted, however, that alcohol-related problems among college students often lead to severe consequences, and said that about 75 percent of the alcohol-related deaths among college students each year were due to the alcohol abuse symptom of being under the influence of alcohol when conditions were physically hazardous, such as when driving a car or operating machinery.

Military Veterans and Active Duty Military Young people who are MILITARY VETERANS and military personnel on active duty have a high risk for alcohol abuse as well as an increased risk for alcohol dependence, largely because of a military culture that encourages drinking. (However, individuals in the military are much less likely to abuse illicit drugs than their nonmilitary peers.)

Being sent to a war zone such as Iraq or Afghanistan can be extremely traumatic for young military individuals. Some military veterans may escalate their drinking behavior when they return home, possibly because of POSTTRAUMATIC STRESS DISORDER or an ineffective means of coping with the hardships and harms that they have seen in a combat zone, as well as other reasons.

Data from NESARC Research from the 2001–02 National Epidemiologic Survey on Alcohol and Related Conditions (NESARC) shows that among young adults ages 18–24, men (74.7 percent) were more likely to have engaged in drinking in the past year than women (66.8 percent), and whites were the heaviest drinkers (77.1 percent). However, when considering risky drinking either daily or weekly, the category of American Indian/Alaska Native had slightly higher rates for daily drinking than whites and significantly higher rates for exceeding weekly drinking limits. It should also be noted that rates were even higher among individuals ages 21–24 than among those ages 18–20 years. See Table 1 for further data.

Heavy Drinking in Young Adulthood May Have Long-term Effects through Life Many young individuals engage in heavy drinking or even binge drinking, giving up such drinking in their later years. According to a study of alcohol drinking trajectories, both an early initiation of drinking and heavy drinking in adolescence and young adulthood may increase the risk for the cardiovascular factors that are used to define metabolic syndrome.

In this study by Amy Z. Fan and colleagues on 2,818 ever-regular drinkers, published in the *Journal of Clinical Endocrinology & Metabolism* in 2008, the researchers identified different drinking patterns. One group included early-peak drinkers who had an early onset of drinking, and who drank heavily during adolescence and young adulthood, then tapered off their drinking in middle age. The other group was comprised of "stable trajectory drinkers" who maintained about the same levels of drinking from youth to middle age, and who drank less than the early-peak drinkers.

The researchers found that the early-peak drinkers had a greater risk for the symptoms of metabolic syndrome, including obesity, low levels of high-density lipoprotein cholesterol ("good" cholesterol), high levels of triglycerides, elevated blood pressure, and high fasting glucose levels.

Said the researchers, "The possibility that early binge drinking has long-term negative consequences for cardiovascular health is especially significant in view of current trends in alcohol use and episodic heavy drinking (or binge drinking). A report from a U.S. multistate survey indicates that binge drinking in late adolescence and early adulthood, such as that associated with the early-peak lifetime drinking trajectories observed here, may be increasing, especially among 18-to-20 year olds. Binge drinking has been associated with an increased risk of cardiovascular and other negative health outcomes."

Alcohol Consumption That Occurs in Middle Age

Alcohol abuse and alcohol dependence may continue in middle life, which is generally defined as ages 30–59 years. Some experts have recommended that initiating moderate drinking may be beneficial to middle-aged individuals because of its health benefits. (See MODERATE DRINKING AND HEALTH BENEFITS.)

According to Lisa Merlo, Ph.D., and Mark S. Gold, M.D., in their 2008 letter to the *American Journal of Medicine*, childhood exposure to alcohol, especially when it is marked by feelings of intoxication, is associated with a greater risk of problem drinking in adulthood by about age 30. This early exposure causes changes to the brain and has effects that may not have occurred except for the early exposure. The authors state that this risk is probably much less likely if the initiation of drinking occurs at a later age, because the neurobiology is more stable than among children. Say the authors, "The connections among pathways are well rehearsed and less amenable to change. Therefore, initial onset of alcohol consumption during middle age would be less likely to cause alcohol abuse or dependence." The authors recommended, however, that middle-aged patients should be educated about alcohol abuse and dependence and screened for problem drinking.

According to the National Institute on Alcohol Abuse and Alcoholism (NIAAA), individuals in their

TABLE 1
**PREVALENCE OF DRINKING, EXCEEDING THE DAILY DRINKING LEVELS IN THE PAST YEAR AMONG
THE TOTAL POPULATION OF YOUNG ADULTS AGES 18–20 AND 21–24, ACCORDING TO SEX,
RACE/ETHNICITY, AND COLLEGE ENROLLMENT STATUS, NESARC, 2001–2002**

Ages	Sex, Race/Ethnicity, College Enrollment Status	Past-Year Drinking, Percent	Exceeding Daily Drinking Limit, Percent	Exceeding Weekly Drinking Limit, Percent
18–24	Total	70.8	45.9	14.5
	Men	74.7	52.3	17.4
	Women	66.8	39.4	11.5
	White	77.1	52.5	17.3
	Black	60.1	29.0	8.9
	American Indian/Alaska Native	70.7	53.0	27.4
	Asian/NHOPI (Native Hawaiian/ Other Pacific Islander)	59.1	36.5	10.5
	Hispanic	60.4	37.3	8.5
	College, full-time	74.9	51.7	17.9
	College, part-time	76.3	45.9	14.6
	Noncollege	68.3	43.3	12.9
18–20	Total	64.2	40.8	12.6
	Men	68.4	46.8	15.6
	Women	59.7	34.5	9.4
	White	70.1	47.4	14.7
	Black	49.1	21.9	8.1
	American Indian/Alaska Native	64.9	44.3	29.4
	Asian/NHOPI (Native Hawaiian/ Other Pacific Islander)	55.2	30.6	8.9
	Hispanic	57.4	34.8	7.6
	College, full-time	68.4	44.5	14.7
	College, part-time	65.4	39.7	12.6
	Noncollege	62.4	39.4	11.8
21–24	Total	76.2	50.0	16.0
	Men	80.3	57.2	18.9
	Women	72.4	43.2	13.1
	White	82.9	56.8	19.5
	Black	69.9	35.3	9.7
	American Indian/Alaska Native	78.1	64.3	24.8
	Asian/NHOPI (Native Hawaiian/ Other Pacific Islander)	61.6	40.4	11.5
	Hispanic	62.7	39.2	9.1
	College, full-time	79.9	57.2	20.4
	College, part-time	81.6	48.8	15.6
	Noncollege	73.6	46.8	13.9

Source: Adapted from Chen, Chiung M., Mary C. Dufour, M.D., and Hsiao-ye Yi. "Alcohol Consumption among Young Adults Ages 18–24 in the United States: Results from the 2001–2002 NESARC Survey." *Alcohol Research & Health* 28, no. 4 (2004/2005): page 272.

middle years who are alcoholics are more likely to seek treatment for their alcohol dependence than younger individuals, and they are generally treated with psychotherapy and medications. (See TREAT-MENT.) Middle age is also the time when the physical effects of excessive chronic drinking often start to escalate and become troublesome to the individual in terms of alcoholic liver disease, PANCREATITIS, and some forms of CANCER, as well as damage to the individual's immune system and the brain. In addition, individuals may no longer be able to spring back from the effects of hangovers as in their youths, and as a result, they may miss work or perform poorly on the job, causing their jobs to be at risk.

Some middle-aged alcoholics are forced by circumstances to realize that alcohol dependence is an issue in their lives and they seek help from organizations such as Alcoholics Anonymous (AA); most AA members are middle-aged or older individuals.

According to the Monitoring the Future study, 64 percent of those who were 45 years old and high school graduates had at least one drink in the past 30 days and 8.8 percent reported daily drinking. Nineteen percent exhibited occasional heavy drinking (five or more drinks on at least one occasion in the past two weeks). Said the researchers, "The rate of occasional heavy drinking is much lower than was exhibited by members of this cohort when they were of high school and college ages."

Suicide and Middle-aged and Older Men According to L. Sher in his article for the *Quarterly Journal of Medicine* in 2006, middle-aged and older men (ages 50 and older) with both alcohol dependence and mood disorders have an especially high rate of suicide compared to individuals of other ages. This risk may be related to a decreased rate of serotonin activity in the brain.

Said Sher, "There are several different possible relationships between alcohol dependence and suicide: alcohol use may affect suicidal ideation and behavior; suicidal ideation may affect alcohol use; alcohol use and suicidal phenomena may affect each other; alcohol use may not itself affect suicide but may aggravate other factors that affect suicide; or alcohol use and suicidal behavior may each be affected by some third factor without themselves being directly affected, e.g. alcohol dependence and suicide may be manifestations of the same underlying disorder."

Sher recommends that all individuals with alcohol use disorders be evaluated for their possible suicide risk, especially in the early stages of withdrawal from alcohol or at the end of a drinking binge.

Consumption of Beer and Wine In a study of alcohol consumption that used data over a period of 50 years, the Framingham Study, researchers Yqing Zhang and colleagues provided data on middle-aged and elderly drinkers in the *American Journal of Medicine* in 2008. This study included 8,600 subjects. The researchers found a decrease in drinking among individuals ages 30–59 years with successive decreases for those born in the three time frames of 1900–19, 1920–39 and 1940–59. That is, the heaviest drinkers were those born in the years 1900–19. Lower levels of drinking occurred among those born 1920–39, and the least level of drinking was reported in those born in the years 1940–59.

The researchers also found that the proportion of beer consumed decreased as individuals aged, while the incidence of wine consumption increased among all age groups. In addition, the researchers found that there was a steady increase in abstinence as individuals aged, and by age 80 years, 60 percent of women and 40 percent of men were abstinent. (It should be noted that many of those who were not abstinent probably died before age 80.) However, the researchers found no decrease in alcohol use disorders as individuals in each birth group aged.

In another study that compared the alcohol dependence of beer drinkers and spirits drinkers, with an average age of 45 years, the researchers found that alcoholics with a preference for beer had a significantly greater adherence to treatment for alcohol dependence than did the drinkers who preferred spirits. According to Danilo Antonio Baltieri and colleagues in their article for *Alcohol* in 2009, the subjects who preferred spirits also had a greater severity of alcohol dependence, a higher craving for alcohol and a history of more frequent treatments for alcohol dependence than the beer drinkers.

Said the researchers, "Our study suggests that spirits preference drinkers should receive higher efforts during their [treatment] management, due to the fact that the compliance with treatment tends to be lower and that the severity of alcohol dependence is higher at the beginning of the treatment among these types of drinkers, as our study demonstrated."

Homeless Middle-Aged Alcoholics In the *Journal of the American Medical Association*, Mary E. Larimer and colleagues reported that 30–70 percent of homeless deaths in the United States were attributed to alcohol, and they also estimated that death rates among homeless adults were three to four times that of the rate among the general population. In their study of 95 housed participants and 39 on a housing waiting list, most of the subjects (94 percent) were male and the average age was 48 years. The subjects were ethnically diverse.

The researchers found that the cost of providing housing was significantly less than the cost of providing services to those who remained homeless and that the housed people exhibited significantly decreased rates of alcohol consumption and intoxication.

Said the researchers, "As with other studies of supportive housing for mentally ill homeless people, this study showed decrease in the use of expensive crisis-oriented systems like hospitals and jails." They also noted that providing housing increased the abstinence from alcohol, although the participants were not required to be abstinent from alcohol, nor were they required to obtain treatment for their alcoholism as a condition for receiving housing.

Drinking among Those Aged Sixty Years and Older

In general, older adults drink much less than their younger cohorts; however, some older adults drink to excess, and some people, particularly older women, have a late onset of problematic drinking, which may be triggered by the loss of their loved ones and the onset of DEPRESSION. Older adults metabolize alcohol significantly more slowly than younger individuals, and thus it takes much less alcohol to lead to intoxication. Binge-drinking rates are low among elderly individuals, with an estimated rate of 2 percent or less.

Older adults are more prone to the ill effects of excessive chronic drinking than younger individuals, and they may develop problems that are exacerbated by excessive alcohol use. These include such problems as hypertension, stroke, memory loss, mood disorders, and emotional and cognitive problems. In addition, they are at greater risk for harm from falls and sleep disorders than younger individuals, with or without alcohol consumption— although drinking to excess makes things worse.

In addition, research has demonstrated that older people are often poor judges of how impaired they are by alcohol. For example, in a study by Rebecca Gilbertson and colleagues, published in the 2009 issue of the *Journal of Studies on Alcohol and Drugs,* the researchers compared the psychomotor performance under the influence of alcohol of individuals ages 50–74 to those ages 25–35 years. They found that the older adults performed significantly more poorly on tasks while also perceiving better performance than they exhibited. Said the researchers, "These results reinforce the common knowledge that self-reported measures may not provide an accurate reflection of performance outcomes, and importantly, that older adults may be impaired even under a moderate dose of alcohol, although they may not be aware (i.e. report) of this impairment."

When older individuals seek treatment for their dependence, as about 10–15 percent do, they respond well if they are treated with individuals of about the same age, according to the NIAAA. Group therapy and individual cognitive-behavioral therapy has been shown to be effective among members of this group; however, medications to treat alcohol dependence do not appear to be as effective as they are in younger individuals.

Alcohol Abuse/Dependence among Elderly Is Often Misdiagnosed Sometimes alcoholism among older people is misdiagnosed by physicians, because doctors may make assumptions, such as that older women do not drink (sometimes they do; see ALCOHOL AND WOMEN), or that the older person is intellectually impaired when the person may be impaired by alcohol abuse or dependence.

In their article on alcohol use disorders (alcohol abuse and dependence) present in elderly people, published in the *British Medical Journal* in 2003, Henry O'Connell and colleagues assert that problematic drinking that occurs in older people is often misdiagnosed and under-detected. The researchers did an analysis of studies on elderly people and alcohol, and they found that there was a high rate of alcohol abuse and dependence among elderly inpatients (18 percent for medical inpatients and 23–44 percent for psychiatric inpatients). These rates are in sharp contrast to an estimated rate of

2–4 percent of alcohol abuse and dependence for individuals living in the community.

The researchers found that key risk factors associated with alcohol use disorders among the elderly included male gender, single marital status, social isolation, and being separated or divorced.

The primary reasons for under-detection and misdiagnosis varied; for example, health-care workers were apparently less likely to refer older people with alcohol problems for treatment. Said the authors, "Healthcare workers may perceive alcohol use disorders in older people as being understandable in the context of poor health and changing life circumstances, which leads to therapeutic nihilism when they [the healthcare workers] are confronted with such problems."

The researchers also noted that the presentation of alcohol disorders in the elderly can be atypical, and the individual may present with depression, confusion, or falls, or the disorder may be masked by physical or psychiatric illnesses. They also noted that "healthcare workers in all settings should be vigilant for the role of alcohol in the presentation of older people with physical and psychiatric illness, cognitive impairment, and social problems. A history of current and lifetime alcohol consumption should be ascertained, with a collateral history from a relative or spouse if possible."

Instruments to Measure Alcohol Disorders in Older People In their 2002 article on identifying older, at-risk drinkers in a primary care environment, published in the *Journal of Studies on Alcohol,* Alison A. Moore, M.D., and colleagues described the greater validity of some instruments than others to identify elderly individuals who were alcoholics. For example, they created several instruments themselves, including the Alcohol-Related Problems Survey (ARPS) and a shorter version that is known as the Short ARPS (shARPS). The researchers also tested the validity of the LEAD standard. (LEAD stood for "longitudinal evaluation done by experts employing all available data"). They found that the ARPS was valid 93 percent of the time and the shARPS was valid 92 percent of the time. In contrast, the LEAD was valid 63 percent of the time.

Other tests, such as the Alcohol Use Disorders Identification Test (AUDIT) or the Short Michigan Alcoholism Screening Test—Geriatric Version (SMAST-G) were compared to the LEAD, and they found that the AUDIT was sensitive and specific 28 percent of the time, and the rate for the SMAST-G was 52 percent.

The researchers concluded, "The ARPS and shARPS are quite sensitive in identifying older drinkers with a spectrum of alcohol use disorders. They are more sensitive than the AUDIT and the SMAST-G in identifying older persons who may be at risk or experiencing harm as a result of their alcohol use and comorbidities. They also provide information on specific risks associated with alcohol use not obtained by other screening measures and may therefore facilitate interventions by busy clinicians to reduce such risks."

Elderly People and Abuse As pointed out by Joseph Kandel, M.D., and Christine Adamec in *The Encyclopedia of Elder Care,* sometimes elderly people are abused by their spouses or adult children when those individuals are under the influence of alcohol. Often the older person is afraid to report the abuse, fearing that he or she has nowhere else to go and also not wanting the abusing individual to be removed from the home; for example, the elderly person may rely upon the abusive individual for money, food, and shelter. An indication of sexual abuse in an older woman is the presence of unexplained venereal diseases or tears in the vaginal area, as well as unexplained bruises in the breast. Examples of possible physical abuse include a caregiver's refusal for the older person to see the doctor alone or unexplained bruises, lacerations, or rope marks.

See also ALCOHOL AND MEN; EXCESSIVE DRINKING AND HEALTH CONSEQUENCES; PSYCHIATRIC COMORBIDITIES.

Anda, Robert, M.D. *The Health and Social Impact of Growing Up with Alcohol Abuse and Related Adverse Childhood Experiences: The Human and Economic Costs of the Status Quo.* Undated. Available online. URL: http://www. nacoa.net/pdfs/Anda%20NACoA%20Review_web. pdf. Accessed April 1, 2009.

Baltieri, Danilo Antonio, et al. "The Role of Alcoholic Beverage Preference in the Severity of Alcohol Dependence and Adherence to the Treatment." *Alcohol* 43, no. 3 (2009): 185–195.

Chen, Chiung M., Mary C. Dufour, M.D., and Hsiao-ye Yi. "Alcohol Consumption among Young Adults Ages 18–24 in the United States: Results from the 2001–

2002 NESARC Survey." *Alcohol Research & Health* 28, no. 4 (2004/2005): 269–280.

Crum, Rosa M., M.D., et al. "Depressed Mood in Childhood and Subsequent Alcohol Use through Adolescence and Young Adulthood." *Archives of General Psychiatry* 65, no. 6 (2008): 702–712.

Dube, Shanta R., et al. "Long-Term Consequences of Childhood Sexual Abuse by Gender of Victim." *American Journal of Preventive Medicine* 28, no. 5 (2005): 430–438.

Fan, Amy Z., et al. "Association of Lifetime Alcohol Drinking Trajectories with Cardiometabolic Risk." *Journal of Clinical Endocrinology & Metabolism* 93, no. 1 (2008): 154–161.

Gilbertson, Rebecca, et al. "Effects of Acute Alcohol Consumption in Older and Young Adults: Perceived Impairment Versus Psychomotor Performance." *Journal of Studies on Alcohol and Drugs* 70, no. 2 (2009): 242–252.

Hingson, Ralph, Timothy Heeren, and Ronda Zakocs. "Age of Drinking Onset and Involvement in Physical Fights After Drinking." *Pediatrics* 108, no. 4 (2001): 872–877.

Hingson, Ralph W., et al. "Age of Drinking Onset and Unintentional Injury Involvement After Drinking." *Journal of the American Medical Association* 284, no. 12 (2000): 1,527–1,533.

Hingson, Ralph, Timothy Heeren, Michael R. Winter and Henry Wechsler. "Early Age of First Drunkenness as a Factor in College Students' Unplanned and Unprotected Sex Attributable to Drinking." *Pediatrics* 111, no. 1 (2003): 34–41.

Johnston, L. D., et al. *Monitoring the Future National Survey Results on Drug Use, 1975–2007: Volume II, College Students and Adults Ages 19–45.* Bethesda, Md.: National Institute on Drug Abuse, October 2008.

Kandel, Joseph, M.D., and Christine Adamec. *The Encyclopedia of Elder Care.* New York: Facts On File, Inc., 2009.

Larimer, Mary E., et al. "Health Care and Public Service Use and Costs before and after Provision of Housing for Chronically Homeless Persons with Severe Alcohol Problems." *Journal of the American Medical Association* 301, no. 13 (2009): 1,349–1,357.

Lloyd, Donald A., and R. Jay Turner. "Cumulative Lifetime Adversities and Alcohol Dependence in Adolescence and Young Adulthood." *Drug and Alcohol Dependence* 93, no. 3 (2008): 217–226.

McClure, A. A., et al. "Alcohol-branded Merchandise and Its Association with Drinking Attitudes and Outcomes in U.S. Adolescents." *Archives of Pediatrics & Adolescent Medicine* 163, no. 2 (2009): 211–217.

Merlo, Lisa J., and Mark S. Gold, M.D. "Middle-age Initiation of Alcohol Consumption Unlikely to Cause Addiction." Letter to the Editor. *American Journal of Medicine* 121, no. 3 (2008): 201–206.

Monti, Peter M., et al. "Drinking Among Young Adults: Screening, Brief Intervention, and Outcome." *Alcohol Research & Health* 28, no. 4 (2004/2005): 236–244.

Moore, Alison A., et al. "Beyond Alcoholism: Identifying Older, At-Risk Drinkers in Primary Care." *Journal of Studies on Alcohol* 63, no. 3 (2002): 316–324.

National Institute on Alcohol Abuse and Alcoholism. "Alcohol Research: A Lifespan Perspective." *Alcohol Alert* 74, no. 1 (2008): 1–5.

O'Connell, Henry, et al. "Alcohol Use Disorders in Elderly People—Redefining an Age Old Problem in Old Age." *British Medical Journal* 327 (2003): 664–667.

Renna, Francesco. "The Economic Cost of Teen Drinking: Late Graduation and Lowered Earnings." *Health Economics* 16, no. 4 (2007): 407–419.

Sartor, Carolyn E., et al. "The Role of Childhood Risk Factors in Initiation of Alcohol Use and Progression to Alcohol Dependence." *Addiction* 102, no. 2 (2006): 216–225.

Sher, L. "Alcohol Consumption and Suicide." *Q Journal Med* 99, no. 1 (2006): 57–61.

Slutske, Wendy S. "Alcohol Use Disorders Among College Students and their Non-College-Attending Peers." *Archives of General Psychiatry* 62, no. 3 (2005): 321–327.

Zhang, Yuqing, et al. "Secular Trends in Alcohol Consumption over 50 Years: The Framingham Study." *American Journal of Medicine* 121, no. 8 (2008): 695–701.

age when drinking first started   See ADOLESCENTS AND DRINKING; ADVERTISING OF ALCOHOL; AGE AND ALCOHOL; UNDERAGE DRINKING.

aggressive behavior and alcohol   Alcohol often increases the level of aggression that an individual feels as well as the number and severity of aggressive actions that the drunken person exhibits. These acts are far more disruptive and violent than how these same individuals might behave if they were not under the influence of alcohol. Some individuals may combine other substances with alcohol, such as illicit substances (such as methamphetamine, steroids, or other illegal drugs), which may further intensify their aggressive impulses. (See ALCOHOL AND OTHER DRUGS.)

Some individuals who behave aggressively while under the influence of alcohol may have an ANTISOCIAL PERSONALITY DISORDER, while others may have INTERMITTENT EXPLOSIVE DISORDER (IED), which is a form of an IMPULSE CONTROL DISORDER. However, the individual need not have any underlying psychiatric diagnosis to behave more aggressively while under the influence of alcohol, because alcohol weakens brain mechanisms that normally inhibit impulsive behaviors. For example, one common problem is that alcohol intoxication can cause individuals to misread social cues of others and to perceive either insults or sexual come-ons when none were intended.

It is also more likely for acts of domestic violence to occur when the aggressor is intoxicated. Domestic violence is violence perpetrated by one individual upon another individual living in the home, often a spouse or partner. Acts of child maltreatment are also more common when an individual is under the influence of alcohol.

Some research has demonstrated that some individuals behave more aggressively when they consume alcohol in part because they *assume* that alcohol increases aggressive impulses. Some studies have shown that when people were told that they were consuming alcohol (but the substance was actually nonalcoholic), individuals behaved more aggressively than they normally did.

It is also true that the rate of victimization goes up significantly with excessive alcohol consumption by the victim. Individuals who drink to excess are more likely to be assaulted and otherwise victimized than others. This may be because they are less capable of saying "no" to physical or sexual aggressors, or they are unable to leave the scene where the aggressive acts take place.

Research on Alcohol and Aggression

In a study of intimate partner aggression among 303 men diagnosed with alcohol use disorders and their partners performed by Panuzio and colleagues, the researchers found that the physical and psychological aggression exhibited by men with alcohol use disorders were higher than among men without alcohol use disorders. They also found that the diagnosis of antisocial personality disorder was the strongest predictor for both male and female aggression among those with alcohol abuse or dependence.

Other factors that were predictive of aggression in this population were a higher severity of an alcohol problem, a poorer relationship adjustment, and higher psychopathic personality features. In this study, women subjects reported having suffered from more physical aggression than the men, while they also reported perpetrating more psychological abuse than did their male partners.

In another study of substance use and the risk for sexual and physical aggression among 2,170 young adults ages 23–29, published in *Violence and Victims* in 2004, researchers Steven C. Martino, Rebecca L. Collins, and Phyllis L. Ellickson studied whether marijuana or alcohol increased the risk for physical violence. They found that heavy alcohol use was predictive for female physical assault victimization, while marijuana use was associated with the sexual victimization of both men and women. The researchers said that although the users' own aggressive behavior was linked to victimization in the case of marijuana use, the same link was not found among female victims who were physically assaulted. However, they did find that alcohol use by female subjects was predictive of a risk for being physically assaulted.

See also ALCOHOL ABUSE; AGE AND ALCOHOL; ALCOHOL AND MEN; ALCOHOL AND WOMEN; ALCOHOLIC PSYCHOSIS; ALCOHOLISM/ALCOHOL DEPENDENCE; BINGE DRINKING; BIPOLAR DISORDER; CHILD ABUSE AND NEGLECT; CODEPENDENCY; COLLEGE STUDENTS; CONDUCT DISORDER; EXCESSIVE DRINKING AND NEGATIVE SOCIAL CONSEQUENCES; PSYCHIATRIC COMORBIDITIES; UNDERAGE DRINKING; VIOLENCE.

Adamec, Christine, *Impulse Control Disorders*. New York: Chelsea House, 2008.

Gwinell, Esther, M.D., and Christine Adamec. *The Encyclopedia of Drug Abuse*. New York: Facts On File, Inc., 2008.

Martino, Steven C., Rebecca L. Collins, and Phyllis L. Ellickson. "Substance Use and Vulnerability to Sexual and Physical Aggression: A Longitudinal Study of Young Adults." *Violence and Victims* 19, no. 5 (2004): 521–540.

National Institute on Alcohol Abuse and Alcoholism. "Alcohol, Violence, and Aggression." Alcohol Alert 38. October 1997. Available online. URL: http://pubs.niaaa.nih.gov/publications/aa38.htm. Accessed August 5, 2008.

Panuzio, Jillian. "Intimate Partner Aggression Reporting Concordance and Correlates of Agreement among Men with Alcohol Use Disorders and Their Female Partners." *Assessment* 13, no. 3 (2006): 266–279.

alcohol abuse   See ALCOHOLISM/ALCOHOL DEPENDENCE AND ALCOHOL ABUSE.

alcohol and alcohol use Alcohol is a drug that contains a substance known as ethanol that will, if consumed to excess, lead to intoxication and which may also eventually lead to ALCOHOL ABUSE or ALCOHOLISM/ALCOHOL DEPENDENCE in some individuals. ACETALDEHYDE, which may contribute to the effects of alcohol, is a substance produced within the body when the alcohol is metabolized. Alcohol is a depressant and a sedative. Beer, wine, and distilled spirits are different forms of alcohol, and they can all cause intoxication if sufficient quantities are consumed.

Basic Information about Alcohol

Alcohol (ethanol) is a colorless liquid that is produced through the fermentation of grains, fruits, or other organic materials. There are three primary forms of alcohol: beer, wine, or distilled spirits. (There are also some hybrid forms of alcohol that are available, such as liqueurs.) In terms of its intoxicating qualities, approximately five ounces (0.15 liter) of wine is equal to 12 ounces (0.35 liter) of beer and also equal to 1.5 ounces (0.04 liter) of distilled spirits. It is important to note that, contrary to popular belief, not all alcoholics are dependent on either distilled spirits or wine. For some alcoholics, beer is their beverage of choice. It is a relatively inexpensive and easy to obtain substance.

The alcohol content of distilled spirits is measured in "proof," and if a form of alcohol is, for example, 80 proof (as many distilled beverages are), then it is 40 percent alcohol. (The proof is twice the amount of alcohol in the distilled spirit.) In contrast, the alcohol content of beer and wine is specified by the percentage of alcohol that is present in the substance, and most wines contain 12–14 percent alcohol, while most beers have 3–6 percent alcohol. There are exceptions, and some beers have no alcohol content while others are very high in alcohol; for example, sake is a strong still beer that is made from rice, produced in Japan. It may have a 14–16 percent alcohol content.

In addition, some forms of wines, such as fortified wines such as sherry or Madeira, may have an alcoholic content that is up to 24 percent, while often aromatized wines such as vermouth may have an alcohol content ranging from 15–20 percent.

Some individuals ferment their own alcohol for personal consumption. However, once the process is mastered, it is relatively easy to increase production, which leads some people into trouble, especially with distilled spirits. It is against the law to sell privately made alcoholic beverages.

People consume alcohol primarily as a liquid, but it may also be found in some food. Alcoholics who are being treated with DISULFIRAM need to know if even minute quantities of alcohol are present in the foods and beverages that they ingest, especially when eating at a restaurant or someone's home, because the disulfiram prevents their bodies from metabolizing alcohol, and it will cause severe nausea and vomiting if they consume any alcohol.

Alcohol may also be present in household cooking items, such as vanilla or peppermint extract or other extracts, which may be up to 40 percent alcohol. Sometimes if severe alcoholics are unable to obtain their usual form of alcohol, they may resort to drinking such substances as vanilla extract or cough syrup containing alcohol.

The color of some forms of alcohol is derived from added ingredients and/or the aging process of the substance. Beer is fermented from a variety of grain malts and is usually flavored with hops. It is generally pale yellow in color, although the use of other malted grains may result in beers of a darker color. Most wine is derived from the naturally fermented juice of grapes. Red wines result from including the grape skin during some or all of the fermentation process, while white wines are fermented without the skins. White wines range in color from pale straw to deep brown and vary greatly in their sweetness.

In the case of distilled spirits, such as rum, tequila, whiskey, vodka, and other types of "hard liquor," the fermented product is either a wine or beer that is then distilled. The process of distillation involves heating the liquid so that the alcohol and other desired aromatics are separated into a vapor. The gaseous vapors of the distillate are then collected and condensed, and they are stored in liquid form. Then they are generally aged to improve or modify the flavor.

In a study in Denmark of the food-buying habits of individuals who purchase beer or wine by Ditte Johansen and colleagues and published in the *British Medical Journal* in 2006, the researchers analyzed the results of 3.5 million supermarket transactions over a six-month period. The researchers found that wine buyers were significantly more likely to purchase fruits and vegetables and poultry than beer buyers. Beer buyers were more likely to buy soft drinks, cold cuts, ready-made foods, and sugar than wine buyers. Said the researchers, "Our results support findings from the United States, Denmark, and France showing that wine drinkers tend to eat fruit, vegetables, and fish and use cooking oil more often and saturated fat less often than those who prefer other alcoholic drinks."

Says Michael Dietler of alcohol in his anthropological analysis of alcohol, "In the first place, it should be clear that the term does not describe a single, self-evident object. Rather, alcohol is a culturally specific, and quite recent, analytical category that lumps together an astonishing variety of disparate substances on the sole basis of the common presence of a chemical named ethanol (C_2H_3OH) that produces psychoactive effects. However, the chemical composition and properties of ethanol were identified only in the twentieth century, and, as noted above, the concept of alcohol as a collective term linking such things as beer, wine, and whiskey is a discursive product of the nineteenth-century temperance movement."

He also adds, "In brief, alcoholic drinks are not simply reducible to a uniform chemical substance with physiological effects. They constitute a form of material culture subject to almost unlimited possibilities for variation in terms of ingredients, techniques of preparation, patterns of association and exclusion, modes of serving and consumption, aesthetic and moral evaluations, expected behavior when drinking, styles of inebriation, and so forth."

Beer   Historians know that beer was produced by the ancient Egyptians, and anthropologists have deduced that some cultures created their own beer thousands of years prior to that time. The Egyptians used emmer (a form of wheat) without hops, a flavoring agent, reportedly avoiding the more bitter taste of hops. The colonists of early America were dependent on beer to drink because water was often not potable and there were no purification procedures or chemicals. For them, beer was safer to drink than water.

Breweries in the United States have used the same basic process of manufacturing for about 200 years. Raymond G. Anderson explains the modern process of brewing in this manner. "Brewing involves the warm aqueous extraction (mashing) of ground barley, [and] malt (often supplemented by other sources of carbohydrate) followed by separation of the soluble extract (wort), boiling with hops and fermentation by yeast to give a complex alcoholic solution which is clarified and sold as a sparkling beverage (beer) with an ethanol content of ca. [approximately] 3–10 percent by volume."

Other authors, Giuseppe Comi and Marisa Manzano, explain brewing this way: "The manufacture of beer is a biological process whereby barley and hops, both agricultural products, are converted by a complex biochemical process into beer by controlling biochemical reactions in the malting, mashing and fermentation stages."

In the 21st century, beer is made with barley, wheat, rice, hops, and corn. Differences in the ratio of the grains and hops as well as variations in the brewing process allow for many different types of beers to be created, including ale, stout, lager, porter, malt beer, pilsner beer and bock beer. Many beers include more than one form of cereal, and each is soaked separately and then mixed with the barley. The water that is used for the beer is also important, because it constitutes up to 90 percent of the beer.

The leading breweries in the United States are Anheuser Busch and MillerCoors. There are also many smaller breweries scattered throughout the country, offering their own specialty beers to consumers.

Some studies have shown that most binge drinkers are also beer drinkers. (See BINGE DRINKING.) Of course this does *not* mean that most people who drink beer are binge drinkers; many beer drinkers are moderate consumers.

Wine   Wine is an alcoholic liquid that is produced through the fermentation of grapes, fruits, or other plant parts. The ancient Greeks credited the god Dionysus with its creation, while the ancient Egyptians attributed wine to the god Osiris. In addition to grapes, wine may also be created from elderberries, blackberries, dandelions, and peaches, as well as any other fruit that ferments. Many people drink wine in moderation, and red wine in particular has proven health qualities for those who drink moderately because of an inherent substance known as resveratrol, which apparently has protective factors against cardiovascular disease. (It is likely that clinical studies will further advance the knowledge about this substance.) The protective factors that are associated with moderate wine drinking are more beneficial to men than women; women who drink even modestly have an increased risk for the development of breast cancer.

According to the *Sotheby's Wine Encyclopedia* by Tom Stevenson, the United States is the fourth largest wine-producing country worldwide, and California's wine production alone is more than twice as much as the fifth largest wine-producing country in the world: Australia.

Champagne is a sparkling wine that is naturally (or sometimes artificially) carbonated. Technically, champagne may be produced only in an area of France known as Champagne; however, most people view champagne as any type of sparkling wine. There are other forms of sparkling wines such as sparkling burgundy, Asti Spumante, and so forth.

Rosé is a pink wine (derived from red grapes and a form of red wine) but with minimal tannin content. (Tannin is a natural substance found in wine skins.) Pink champagne is a carbonated rosé.

Some people are wine connoisseurs, centering their lives around studying and consuming wine in moderation, while others drink only an occasional glass of wine. Still others are physically dependent on wine, and for those individuals, it is often not the quality of wine that is so important to them as much as the quantity.

Vineyards that grow wine-producing grapes are located worldwide, but are largely concentrated in Europe, primarily in France, Italy, and Germany. In the United States, the majority of wine (90 percent) is produced in California; however, there are also wineries located in every state, although wineries in many states must import grapes in order to produce their wine.

Some people mix wine with fruit juice, or they may purchase such mixtures as wine coolers, which include wine and carbonated water and are often served as iced drinks.

Distilled Spirits   A definition of distilled spirits is offered by Harriet Lembeck in *Grossman's Guide to Wines, Beers, and Spirits:* "A spirit is a potable alcoholic beverage obtained from the distillation of a liquid containing alcohol. It makes little difference whether the original liquid contains a small or a large amount of alcohol. Once the principles of distillation are applied, nearly all of the alcohol may be separated from the liquid. In addition, certain other flavor compounds may also be separated from the original liquid, and carried along with the alcohol. These are called 'congeners,' and they give spirits their distinct characteristics. If spirits are aged in wood, the wood also imparts congeners of its own."

Distilled spirits refer to alcohol that is distilled from either wines or beers, and which then is often aged in wood or metal casks; for example, rum is distilled from molasses or sugar cane and then may be aged for three or more years. Other forms of distilled spirits are tequila, vodka, whiskey, and gin. Brandy is distilled wine.

The process of distillation was first attributed to Albukassen, an Arabian alchemist; however, the substance was used only for medicinal purposes. Scotsman Robert Stein invented the continuous still in 1826. Rum was a popular commodity in the 18th and 19th centuries in the United States, primarily produced in New England, and often traded with slave traders for African slaves. Rum comes in a variety of dark and light flavors. Today rum is primarily used in mixed drinks.

In the 18th century, gin was very inexpensive, and it became so popular in England that it was given the nickname "mother's gin," because many women were passed out in the streets from drunkenness. William of Orange and subsequently Queen Anne raised taxes and duties on this product as well as creating regulatory laws, and the popularity of gin vastly subsided. Today, gin is primarily made in the United States, England, and the Netherlands. Sloe gin is not technically a gin at all, but rather it is a liqueur that is made with sloe berries that were steeped in gin.

Whiskey is distilled from fermented grain mash and then generally aged in wood. Bourbon is a popular form of whiskey that is aged in new charred-oak barrels which impart a distinct colorful flavor. Scotch whiskey is another form of whiskey.

Other Forms of Alcohol   Although most forms of alcohol fit readily into one of the three categories of beer, wine or distilled spirits, there are some that fit two categories; for example, liqueurs are brandies that have added flavorings, such as orange, peppermint, or other choices. Some people serve a liqueur over ice cream as a dessert, but most people use a liqueur as an after-dinner drink.

Mixed Drinks Mixed drinks, sometimes known as cocktails, are created by combining a distilled liquor with other ingredients, such as ice, tonic water or seltzer water, and/or fruit juice. Some mixed drink concoctions taste sweet and nonalcoholic (such as the Long Island Tea) and do not seem to have any alcohol in them; however, their potency can be deceivingly strong.

Some cocktails include more than one type of alcohol; for example, brandy is sometimes added to alcoholic beverages. Some mixed drinks are served primarily during winter holidays, such as Christmas and New Year's Eve; for example, the alcoholic eggnog includes the basics of alcohol, egg, milk, sugar, and nutmeg. (Many people purchase a nonalcoholic eggnog mixture in the supermarket during the holiday season and simply add alcohol to it.)

Mixed drinks may be served with or without ice, depending on the type of drink as well as the preference of the drinker; for example, the Martini is a gin or vodka drink that is iced while being prepared; it is then strained and served without ice. Some drinks are shaken or stirred, and there is a complex system that generally only bartenders (and sometimes few of them) fully understand.

Alcohol Abuse

Heavy drinking over a short period is called binge drinking. Very excessive alcohol consumption over a short period of time may lead to a very serious and even fatal condition known as ALCOHOL POISONING, in which the body is unable to metabolize the alcohol quickly enough. Among those who are binge drinkers, one study found that the beverage of choice is usually beer.

In their 2007 article in the *American Journal of Preventive Medicine,* researchers Timothy S. Naimi, M.D., and colleagues found that both males and females who binged chose beer most frequently, or 72.8 percent of males and 49.7 percent of females. In addition, binge drinkers of all ages most often

chose beer, whether Hispanic (74.9 percent), white (66.6 percent), or black (53.9 percent). People of all educational levels who binged on alcohol usually chose beer, or 75.3 percent of those with some high school, 72.2 percent of those who were high school graduates, 65.2 percent of those who had some college, and 60.9 percent of those who were college graduates. (More highly educated binge drinkers were also more likely to binge on distilled spirits or wine.)

The researchers found that whether family income was less than $25,000 per year, in a range of $42,500–$49,000, or $50,000 or more, the majority of people who binged on alcohol chose beer. Clearly, beer as a beverage plays a major role in binge drinking.

According to the National Institute of Alcohol Abuse and Alcoholism (NIAAA), in 2007 (latest data available as of this writing), an estimated 564,410 gallons of ethanol (the intoxicant in alcohol) were consumed in the United States. The per capita rate for individuals ages 14 and older was 2.31 gallons.

The highest per capita rate was seen in New Hampshire, or 4.22. (Note that in New Hampshire, the state has a monopoly on alcohol sales, and individuals from other states may purchase alcohol in the state because of lower prices.) The second highest rate was in the District of Columbia, or 3.95 gallons per capita. The lowest rate was seen in Utah, or a per capita rate of 1.33 gallons. The second lowest rate was in West Virginia, or 1.76 gallons per capita. See Table 1 for a state-by-state breakdown of the volume of beer, wine, and spirits, and the corresponding ethanol content consumed per capita in gallons.

Many people are able to consume alcohol occasionally, such as a glass or two of wine or beer, with little risk of developing an abuse or dependence on alcohol; however, others drink frequently and solely to achieve a state of intoxication, and thus they are at a greater risk for developing alcohol abuse or a dependence on alcohol. Individuals who spend a lot of time around others who drink heavily as well as individuals whose parents and/or siblings were or currently are heavy drinkers or alcoholics are more likely than others to develop a problem with drinking.

Users of Alcohol

Many people in the United States consume alcohol, and according to the National Survey on Drug Use and Health, in 2007, 51.1 percent of Americans ages 12 and older reported being current drinkers. This means that about 125.3 million people in the United States consume alcohol. More than a fifth of individuals ages 12 and older (23.3 percent) were binge drinkers in 2008. A binge drinker is a male who has five or more drinks on the same occasion on at least one day in the past 30 days or a female who has four or more drinks on the same occasion on at least one day in the past 30 days. By this definition, an estimated 57.8 million people in the United States are binge drinkers.

Heavy drinking is less common but still problematic. Heavy drinking refers to binge drinking that occurred on at least five days of the past 30 days. The National Survey on Drug Use and Health found that 6.9 percent of the population ages 12 and older were heavy drinkers, or 17 million people.

The rates of binge drinking and heavy drinking were much higher among young adults ages 18 to 25 years old in 2007; for example, the rate of binge drinking was 41.8 percent, while the rate of heavy drinking was 14.7 percent.

Most underage people ages 12 to 20 did not buy their own alcohol in 2007, according to the national survey. About a third (30.2 percent) purchased the alcohol, either buying it directly themselves (8.2 percent) or giving money to someone else to buy alcohol for them (21.8 percent). Of those who did not purchase their alcohol, 37.2 percent obtained the alcohol from an unrelated person aged 21 or older, while 20.7 percent purchased or received alcohol from another person under age 21. In 19.5 percent of the cases, the minor obtained alcohol from a parent, guardian, or other adult family member.

For ages 12 or older, there was a greater percentage of male drinkers (56.6 percent of males) than female drinkers (46.0 percent) in the United States in 2007. Among adolescents ages 12 to 17 years, the number of male drinkers (15.9 percent) was nearly identical to the rate for females (16.0 percent). Among young adults ages 18 to 25 years, 57.1 percent of females and 65.3 percent of males consumed alcohol in 2007.

Some pregnant women consume alcohol, despite the high risk to the fetus for FETAL ALCOHOL SYNDROME/FETAL ALCOHOL SPECTRUM DISORDERS and birth defects. Considering all pregnant women ages 15 to 44 years old, about 11.6 percent reported using alcohol. In addition, 3.7 percent reported binge drinking, and less than 1 percent (0.7 percent) reported being heavy drinkers.

In considering racial breakdowns of drinking, Caucasians are more likely to consume alcohol than individuals of other races; among individuals ages 12 and older, 56.1 percent of whites reported current use of alcohol in 2007. The next highest rate was found among persons reporting two or more races: 47.5 percent. In considering American Indians or Alaska Natives, 44.7 percent reported current alcohol use in 2007. The rate was 42.1 percent for Hispanics, 39.3 percent for blacks, and 35.2 percent for Asians.

Racial breakdowns for binge drinkers were not the same as among those who consumed alcohol; for example, the highest rate of binge drinking was among American Indians or Alaska Natives (28.2 percent), followed by whites (24.6 percent). This may sound counterintuitive, since American Indians or Alaska Natives did not have the highest percentage of current drinkers, but it means that, of those in this racial category who drink, a significant portion are binge drinkers.

Laws on Drinking Alcohol

In the United States, it is illegal for individuals younger than age 21 to purchase and/or to consume any amount of alcohol. It is also illegal for others to purchase or provide alcohol to those under 21 years, including their parents, friends, and other relatives, regardless of the occasion at which it is provided. There are no exceptions to state laws against drinking alcohol for individuals younger than 21 years, such as weddings, funerals, graduation parties, and so forth. It is also illegal to provide alcohol at no cost in a private home to those who are under age 21.

It is also true that some states have ZERO TOLERANCE LAWS, in which if individuals younger than age 21 are found to have a low amount of alcohol (or sometimes any alcohol) in their systems when driving, they are violating state law. This amount is usually much lower than the .08 percent blood alcohol concentration level that is the legal limit for those ages 21 and older.

Alcohol and Other Drugs (AOD)

If alcohol is mixed with other legal or illegal or prescribed or over-the-counter (OTC) substances, the individual may become very ill and in some cases, ALCOHOL AND OTHER DRUGS can cause an accidental overdose and may lead to death. Even a recommended minimum dosage of acetaminophen (Tylenol) can become harmful in conjunction with alcohol when both alcohol and acetaminophen are used frequently and concurrently. (See MEDICATION INTERACTIONS.) It should also be noted that many people who consume alcohol to excess also smoke tobacco, and the two substances (alcohol and nicotine) interact to decrease the likelihood of the person quitting either substance. Even among individuals undergoing inpatient rehabilitation, often there is little or no attempt by rehabilitative staff to help individuals stop smoking. (See SMOKING AND ALCOHOL.)

Underage Drinking

Drinking is perceived as a rite of passage by many young people. Most individuals in the United States do not forego drinking until the legal age of 21 years, instead, starting their drinking in early adolescence or even before then. (See UNDERAGE DRINKING.) According to the Substance Abuse and Mental Health Services Administration (SAMHSA) in their national survey on drug use and health for 2006, about 51 percent of Americans ages 12 years and older reported being current drinkers of alcohol.

Alcohol Dependence

In the late 19th and early 20th centuries, many people believed that alcohol was an addictive substance, much as heroin is known to be addictive today. Thus, it was believed that anyone who consumed alcohol would become addicted to it. However, this belief is not valid. Some people become dependent on alcohol while others who consume alcohol never develop dependence.

It is known from ADOPTION STUDIES that there is a genetic risk to alcoholism, and that if a biological parent is an alcoholic, the risk is increased for the adopted-out child to become an alcoholic as well, even when his or her adoptive parents are not alcoholics. It has also been shown through adoption studies that if the adoptive parents *are* alcoholics or alcohol abusers, if the biological parents were not alcoholics, then the risk for the child becoming an alcoholic as an adult is extremely low.

It is also known that individuals with psychiatric problems have a greater risk for developing alcoholism than those without such problems, particularly people with ANXIETY DISORDERS, DEPRESSION, ANTISOCIAL PERSONALITY DISORDER/ANTISOCIAL BEHAVIOR, BIPOLAR DISORDER, and SCHIZOPHRENIA.

The environment and the association with drinking peers play a role as well. Individuals who engage in early drinking as a result of peer pressure or for other reasons are more likely than others to develop a dependence on alcohol.

Study of Imaging Shows Effects of Alcohol on the Brain

A small study of 12 subjects using functional magnetic resonance imaging subsequent to administering alcohol intravenously to social drinkers imaged brain changes as the alcohol took effect. This study, reported in the *Journal of Neuroscience* in 2008 by researchers Jodi M. Gilman and colleagues, found that alcohol activated the striatal reward circuits of the brain while decreasing the response to fearful stimuli in the visual and limbic areas of the brain. The study showed both the pharmacologic rewards that alcohol generated in the brain and the antianxiety effects. The subjects had an average blood alcohol level of 0.072, and they achieved peak intoxication 25–45 minutes from the start of the infusion of alcohol.

Treatment of Alcohol Dependence

In 2007, an estimated 1.3 million people received treatment for the use of alcohol, and another 1.4 million received treatment for using both alcohol and illegal drugs, according to the National Survey on Drug Use and Health. Treatment options for these individuals included treatment at a self-help group as well as at a rehabilitation facility as an outpatient. Some individuals received inpatient rehabilitative services. In addition, some patients

TABLE 1
APPARENT ALCOHOL CONSUMPTION FOR STATES, CENSUS REGIONS, AND THE UNITED STATES, 2007.
(VOLUME AND ETHANOL IN THOUSANDS OF GALLONS, PER CAPITA ETHANOL
CONSUMPTION IN GALLONS, BASED ON POPULATION AGES 14 AND OLDER)

State or other geographic area	Beer			Wine			Spirits			All beverages	
	Volume	Ethanol	Per capita	Volume	Ethanol	Per capita	Volume	Ethanol	Per capita	Ethanol	Per capita
Alabama	103,905	4,676	1.24	6,381	823	0.22	5,117	2,103	0.56	7,602	2.02
Alaska	15,930	717	1.32	1,874	242	0.45	1,415	582	1.07	1,540	2.84
Arizona	152,116	6,845	1.36	13,032	1,681	0.33	9,341	3,839	0.76	12,366	2.45
Arkansas	54,473	2,451	1.07	3,008	388	0.17	3,320	1,365	0.60	4,204	1.84
California	694,575	31,256	1.07	125,250	16,157	0.55	51,001	20,961	0.72	68,375	2.34
Colorado	112,196	5,049	1.29	14,120	1,822	0.47	9,535	3,919	1.00	10,789	2.75
Connecticut	59,186	2,663	0.93	12,827	1,655	0.58	5,909	2,429	0.85	6,747	2.35
Delaware	21,735	978	1.39	3,250	16,157	0.59	2,135	877	1.25	2,275	3.23
District of Columbia	15,053	677	1.35	3,836	495	0.99	1,967	808	1.61	1,981	3.95
Florida	436,764	19,654	1.30	57,313	7,393	0.49	34,186	14,050	0.93	41,098	2.72
Georgia	195,525	8,799	1.16	14,995	1,934	0.26	11,784	4,843	0.64	15,576	2.06
Hawaii	31,358	1,411	1.34	4,008	517	0.49	2,046	841	0.80	2,769	2.62
Idaho	30,810	1,386	1.18	6,735	869	0.74	1,935	795	0.67	3,051	2.59
Illinois	282,149	12,697	1.22	32,742	4,224	0.41	18,455	7,585	0.73	24,506	2.36
Indiana	129,115	5,810	1.14	9,699	1,251	0.24	8,975	3,689	0.72	10,750	2.10
Iowa	75,735	3,408	1.40	3,220	415	0.17	3,992	1,641	0.67	5,464	2.24
Kansas	58,017	2,611	1.17	2,560	330	0.15	3,500	1,438	0.64	4,379	1.96
Kentucky	80,559	3,625	1.05	4,679	604	0.17	5,318	2,186	0.63	6,414	1.85
Louisiana	122,963	5,533	1.57	7,531	971	0.28	6,959	2,860	0.81	9,365	2.65
Maine	31,275	1,407	1.27	3,668	473	0.43	2,149	883	0.80	2,764	2.49
Maryland	103,401	4,653	1.01	12,738	1,643	0.36	9,418	3,871	0.84	10,167	2.21
Massachusetts	121,219	5,455	1.01	25,546	3,295	0.61	11,210	4,607	0.86	13,357	2.48
Michigan	202,770	9,125	1.11	19,018	2,453	0.30	15,532	6,384	0.78	17,962	2.19
Minnesota	108,608	4,887	1.16	10,520	1,357	0.32	9,999	4,110	0.97	10,354	2.45
Mississippi	75,600	3,402	1.46	2,171	280	0.12	3,876	1,593	0.68	5,275	2.26
Missouri	141,305	6,359	1.33	11,017	1,421	0.30	9,118	3,748	0.78	11,528	2.41
Montana	27,900	1,256	1.59	2,165	279	0.35	1,652	679	0.86	2,214	2.80
Nebraska	46,013	2,071	1.45	2,272	293	0.21	2,339	961	0.67	3,325	2.33
Nevada	77,411	3,483	1.71	10,061	1,298	0.64	6,280	2,581	1.27	7,362	3.61
New Hampshire	42,075	1,893	1.74	6,252	807	0.74	4,631	1,903	1.75	4,603	4.22
New Jersey	145,932	6,567	0.93	30,240	3,901	0.55	14,754	6,064	0.86	16,532	2.34
New Mexico	49,608	2,232	1.41	3,784	488	0.31	2,714	1,115	0.71	3,836	2.43
New York	328,061	14,763	0.92	57,880	7,467	0.46	26,594	10,930	0.68	33,159	2.06
North Carolina	189,055	8,507	1.16	15,636	2,017	0.28	10,052	4,131	0.56	14,656	2.00
North Dakota	18,427	829	1.57	959	124	0.23	1,394	573	1.08	1,526	2.88
Ohio	277,088	12,469	1.33	18,121	2,338	0.25	10,249	4,212	0.45	19,019	2.03
Oklahoma	76,208	3,429	1.18	3,936	508	0.17	4,080	1,677	0.58	5,614	1.93
Oregon	88,380	3,977	1.29	11,794	1,521	0.49	6,045	2,484	0.81	7,983	2.59

State or other geographic area	Beer			Wine			Spirits			All beverages	
	Volume	Ethanol	Per capita	Volume	Ethanol	Per capita	Volume	Ethanol	Per capita	Ethanol	Per capita
Pennsylvania	306,675	13,800	1.34	19,176	2,474	0.24	14,784	6,076	0.59	22,350	2.16
Rhode Island	22,005	990	1.13	3,669	473	0.54	1,916	787	0.90	2,251	2.56
South Carolina	114,300	5,144	1.43	6,825	880	0.24	6,711	2,758	0.77	8,782	2.44
South Dakota	21,668	975	1.51	1,092	141	0.22	1,346	553	0.86	1,669	2.59
Tennessee	126,428	5,689	1.13	7,784	1,004	0.20	6,814	2,801	0.56	9,494	1.89
Texas	585,365	26,341	1.41	39,223	5,060	0.27	25,595	10,519	0.56	41,921	2.25
Utah	33,615	1,513	0.75	2,490	321	0.16	2,097	862	0.43	2,665	1.33
Vermont	15,975	719	1.37	2,462	318	0.61	891	366	0.70	1,403	2.68
Virginia	158,732	7,143	1.13	20,053	2,587	0.41	8,897	3,657	0.58	13,386	2.13
Washington	130,388	5,867	1.11	20,435	2,636	0.50	9,488	3,900	0.74	12,403	2.35
West Virginia	41,648	1,874	1.24	1,215	157	0.10	1,566	644	0.42	2,675	1.76
Wisconsin	157,185	7,073	1.54	11,758	1,517	0.33	12,405	5,098	1.11	13,689	2.98
Wyoming	14,147	637	1.49	766	99	0.23	1,142	469	1.10	1,205	2.82
Regions											
Northeast	1,072,403	48,258	1.06	161,720	20,862	0.46	82,838	34,046	0.75	103,166	2.28
Midwest	1,518,080	68,314	1.27	122,978	15,864	0.29	97,305	39,992	0.74	124,170	2.30
South	2,501,715	112,577	1.26	210,575	27,164	0.30	147,795	60,744	0.68	200,485	2.25
West	1,458,435	65,630	1.17	216,556	27,936	0.50	104,555	41,972	0.77	136,560	2.43
United States, total	6,550,633	294,778	1.21	711,788	91,621	0.36	432,629	177,810	0.73	564,410	2.31

Source: Adapted from LaVallee, Robin A., Gerald D. Williams and Hsiao-ye Yi. *Surveillance Report #87: Apparent Per Capita Alcohol Consumption: National, State, and Regional Trends, 1977–2007.* National Institute on Alcohol Abuse and Alcoholism. Rockville, Md.: National Institutes of Health, September 2009. Pages 13–14.

received treatment as hospital inpatients, from private physician's offices, at hospital emergency rooms, or during the time when they were incarcerated in prison or jail.

According to the survey, an estimated 19.3 million people ages 12 and older needed treatment for an alcohol use problem in 2007, but they did not all receive it. Of this number, 1.6 million (about 8 percent of the people who needed treatment) actually obtained treatment at a specialty facility. The remaining 17.7 million people did not receive treatment.

Of those who did not receive any treatment, most subjects did not think that they needed treatment; only 4.8 percent of those who did not receive treatment felt that they needed to be treated. In addition, there were 1.4 million adolescents ages 12–17 years who needed treatment for an alcohol use problem in 2007; however, for reasons unknown,

only an estimated 82,000 did receive treatment at a specialty facility, and in contrast, 1.3 million youths needing treatment did not receive it.

Why Many People Are Alcoholics, Despite Modern Knowledge

Many people are alcoholics, and this has been true for centuries. Alcohol is legal and widely available, and the number of alcoholics per drinkers is strikingly similar between rich and poor, employed and unemployed, and other differences. Alcohol dependence is a pervasive disease, which often starts with early drinking and afflicts mostly those with alcoholism in their families. Alcoholics drink the majority of alcohol, and individuals arrested for drunk driving are likely to have driven drunk in the past.

Alcoholism is chronic, lifelong, and relapsing. While treatment has improved and success in treatment is common, many people with alcohol dependence still do not seek or receive treatment for their alcoholism, and it is abundantly clear that the problem of alcoholism is still a major one in society today—despite knowledge and understanding of alcohol far greater than at any time in the past. For example, scientists know exactly how alcohol affects the brain, down to the neurochemicals and the brain pathways. They also know the effects of alcohol on the brain and the body, and they are well aware of the process of addiction and how it works. Yet this knowledge, so far, does not translate into an alleviation of the problem of alcohol dependence. There are several reasons for this, including these key reasons:

- the failure of alcoholics to obtain treatment
- the failure of some treatments
- the high relapse rate among many alcoholics

The Failure to Obtain Treatment One reason for this failure to receive treatment is that the alcoholic must believe that he or she has a problem before seeking treatment. Most people drink and few people become alcoholic. Not being able to moderate the use of alcohol and the loss of control over alcohol, so common among alcoholics, is incomprehensible to many people. Another reason is that individuals who realize that they are alcohol-dependent may fear seeking treatment, afraid (sometimes rightfully so) that acknowledging the need for treatment and taking the time required to receive it could cost them their job and/or their income.

A much less common reason for a failure to seek treatment among those who accept that they need treatment is that some alcohol-dependent people say they are unable to find an expert or a facility that is willing or able to treat them. This may be true for some categories of individuals, such as pregnant women, elderly people, or people with a dual diagnosis, such as both alcohol and drug dependence or a diagnosis of alcoholism and a serious psychiatric problem, such as bipolar disorder or schizophrenia.

The Failure of Some Treatments Treatments for alcoholism are not always effective. First, treatment may fail and then the patient has a slip that

becomes a full blown relapse. Experts attribute some of the successes in treating physicians who are alcoholics to the early identification of slips and prompt responses.

Medications such as naltrexone and acamprosate can help some individuals, but they do not work for all alcoholics, and they are also costly and may be beyond the individual's financial resources unless insurance coverage is available. Psychotherapy may be ineffective for some individuals because they lack the intelligence, insight, and/or desire to assess and change their behavior. Even the best resources and the most dedicated professionals cannot overcome such problems.

The High Relapse Rate among Many Alcoholics Relapses are so common among alcoholics that they are often considered part of the diagnosis of alcoholism. Slips of using alcohol are common and often proceed to a relapse. Relapse may seem like it is part of the process toward recovery. However, some individuals continually relapse and never truly attain a sustained state of recovery. There are many possible explanations for this, such as the same reasons why some treatments for alcoholism fail: the individual lacks the intelligence, insight, or desire to change. Another reason for relapses is that many alcoholics who receive treatment return to their former environment, which may be heavily populated with family members and friends who view drinking as normal and acceptable and who thwart a policy of abstinence. Alcoholics also often have other psychiatric problems which may not have been identified or treated, such as depression or anxiety disorders. The psychological pain such disorders cause may lead the person to seek the emotional oblivion of alcohol.

See also ADVERTISING OF ALCOHOL; AGE AND ALCOHOL; AGGRESSIVE BEHAVIOR AND ALCOHOL; ALCOHOL AND MEN; ALCOHOL AND WOMEN; ATTENTION-DEFICIT/HYPERACTIVITY DISORDER; CANCER; COLLEGE STUDENTS; DRIVING UNDER THE INFLUENCE/DRIVING WHILE INTOXICATED; GENETICS AND ALCOHOL; PERSONALITY DISORDERS; STAGES OF CHANGE; TREATMENT; VIOLENCE.

Anderson, Raymond G. "Current Practice in Malting, Brewing and Distilling." In *Cereal Biotechnology,* edited by Peter C. Morris and James H. Bryce, 183–215. Cambridge: United Kingdom, 2000.

Comi, Giuseppe, and Marisa Manzano. "Beer Production." In *Molecular Techniques in the Microbial Ecology
of Fermented Foods*, edited by Luca Coclin and Danilo
Ercolini, 193–207. New York: Springer, 2008.

Dietler, Michael. "Alcohol: Anthropological/Archaeo-
logical Perspectives." *Annual Review Anthropology* 35
(2006): 229–249.

Gilman, Jodi M., et al. "Why We Like to Drink: A Functional Magnetic Resonance Imaging Study of the
Rewarding and Anxiolytic Effects of Alcohol." *Journal
of Neuroscience* 28, no. 18 (2008): 4,583–4,591.

Johansen, Ditte, et al. "Food Buying Habits of People
Who Buy Wine or Beer: Cross Sectional Study." *British
Medical Journal* x (2006). Available online. URL: http://
www.bmj.com/cgi/reprint/332/7540/519.   Accessed
August 9, 2009.

Lakins, Nekisha E., Robin A. LaVallee, Gerald D. Williams,
and Hsiao-ye Yi. *Surveillance Report #82: Apparent Per
Capita Alcohol Consumption: National, State, and Regional
Trends, 1977–2005.* National Institute on Alcohol Abuse
and Alcoholism. Rockville, Md.: National Institutes of
Health, August 2007.

Lembeck, Harriet. *Grossman's Guide to Wines, Beers, and Spirits.* 7th rev. ed. New York: Wiley Publishing, Inc., 1983.

Naimi, T. S. et al. "What Do Binge Drinkers Drink? Implications for Alcohol Control Policy." *American Journal of
Preventive Medicine* 33, no. 3 (2007): 188–193.

Stevenson, Tom. *The Sotheby's Wine Encyclopedia.* New
York: DK Publishing, 2007.

Substance Abuse and Mental Health Services Administration. *Results from the 2007 National Survey on Drug Use
and Health: National Findings.* Rockville, Md.: Office of
Applied Studies, 2008.

alcohol and men Alcohol is the most popular
drug in the United States, and men drink 74 percent of all the alcohol consumed in the country,
according to the National Institute on Alcohol
Abuse and Alcoholism (NIAAA). This may be true
at least partly because many men in the United
States (and in other countries) are socialized to
think that drinking is a manly activity, that a man is
admired if he can "hold" his liquor, and that drinking alcohol makes social events much more fun.

As a result, many men of all ages in the United
States accept these concepts as valid. However,
with regard to the assumed manliness of drinking,
there are increasing numbers of females engaging
in drinking alcohol, and some experts believe that
females are starting to catch up to men in terms of

drinking; consequently, such a change may challenge gender stereotypes regarding alcohol. (See
ALCOHOL AND WOMEN.) In addition, an increasing
ability to consume alcohol could indicate a tolerance
to alcohol, one of the signs of ALCOHOLISM, and not
a trait to admire. It is also true that some men have
an inherited ability to become intoxicated later than
other men, and this trait may lead to an increased
risk for dependence. (See GENETICS AND ALCOHOL.)

As for whether alcohol makes social events
more fun, alcohol *does* often loosen inhibitions, and
thus it can allow some men to enhance their pleasure. But the reality is that alcohol is a depressant
drug rather than a euphoria-inducing substance,
so eventually, the initially elevated mood stemming from decreased inhibitions will come back
down again. In some men, excessive quantities of
alcohol lead to excessively decreased inhibitions
and may also lead to increased aggressive behavior.
Some men abuse or neglect their partners or their
children (or their partner's children) while they
are under the influence of alcohol. Alcohol dependence leads to health problems, as well as job loss,
divorce, and many other problems for many men.

Men are nearly four times more likely to die of
events directly linked to alcohol abuse than women
and about four times more likely to die of alcohol
dependence. According to the Centers for Disease
Control and Prevention (CDC), about 75 percent
of male alcohol-related deaths occur to those who
are age 35 and older. However, an estimated 4,675
people under age 21, including 3,636 males, died
of alcohol-related causes in 2005, according to the
CDC. The greatest cause of death for young men
under age 21 is motor vehicle crashes, and 1,522
boys and young men died from alcohol-related car
crashes in 2005, along with 554 girls and young
women. In addition, 1,055 young men died of
alcohol-related homicides, compared to 172 girls
and young women. Finally, about 398 male youths
died from alcohol-related suicides, compared to 82
female youths.

In general, men are more likely to consume
alcohol than women, and they are also more likely
to abuse alcohol, to engage in BINGE DRINKING, and
to become dependent on alcohol than women. The
one exception, based on data from the Substance
Abuse and Mental Health Services Administration

(SAMHSA) is among females ages 12 to 17 years old, who have a slightly higher rate of alcohol abuse or dependence (6.0 percent) than males of the same age (5.5 percent). See Table 1 for further information. As also can be seen from this chart, the highest rate of alcohol use disorders (alcohol abuse and dependence together) was found among males ages 18 to 25 years, or 22 percent.

Among convicted inmates, large percentages admit to having used alcohol and/or drugs when they committed their offense. Most are male, although female inmates are more likely to be violent than women not in jail. There are several cases in which gender differences are somewhat blurred; for example, female COLLEGE STUDENTS frequently drink to excess or engage in binge drinking (although males usually drink more often and in greater quantities) and female prisoners have almost as high a rate of alcohol dependence as do male prisoners.

Some studies have shown that a greater percentage of men than women respond to increased stress with heavy drinking; for example, in a study by Deborah A. Dawson, Bridget F. Grant, and W. June Ruan, reported in *Alcohol & Alcoholism* in 2005, the researchers found that drinking five or more drinks for men increased by 24 percent with each added stressor. In contrast, heavy drinking among women (four or more drinks) increased by 13 percent with each additional stressor.

The excessive drinking of some men is harmful to themselves and others; for example, men have a higher rate of alcohol-related deaths and hospitalizations than women, and when they are drivers in fatal motor vehicle crashes, men are nearly twice as likely as women to have been intoxicated at the time of the crash. Alcohol consumption also increases the risk for CANCER of the esophagus, mouth, throat, liver, and colon in men. Excessive drinking increases the risk for other health problems; for example, greater numbers of men die of alcohol-induced stroke than women, as well as from chronic PANCREATITIS, and liver CIRRHOSIS.

TABLE 1
PERCENTAGES OF PAST YEAR ALCOHOL DEPENDENCE OR ABUSE AMONG PERSONS AGES 12 OR OLDER, BY GENDER AND DEMOGRAPHIC CHARACTERISTICS: 2004–2005

Demographic Characteristic	Male	Female
Age group		
12 to 17	5.5	6.0
18 to 25	22.0	12.9
26 to 49	12.4	5.4
50 and older	5.0	1.6
Race/Ethnicity		
White	10.6	5.6
Black or African American	9.7	3.5
American Indian or Alaska Native	19.5	13.7
Native Hawaiian or Other Pacific Islander	12.8	5.7
Asian	5.4	2.3
Two or more races	9.9	7.7
Hispanic or Latino	12.1	3.8
Family income		
Less than $20,000	14.0	6.0
$20,000–$49,999	10.3	4.6
$50,000–$74,999	9.3	4.6
$75,000 or more	9.7	5.2

Adapted from Office of Applied Studies, "Gender Differences in Alcohol Use and Alcohol Dependence or Abuse: 2004 and 2005. NSDUH Report. August 2, 2007. Page 2.

Among acute conditions that are alcohol-related, greater numbers of men than women die from alcohol abuse linked to ALCOHOL POISONING, drowning, homicide, motor vehicle accidents, and SUI- CIDE. See Table 2 for causes of alcohol-attributable deaths. Also see Table 3 for the numbers of years of life lost because of these causes; for example, an estimated total of 1,729,877 years were lost to

TABLE 2
ALCOHOL-ATTRIBUTABLE DEATHS, ALL AGES, MEDIUM AND HIGH AVERAGE DAILY CONSUMPTION, UNITED STATES, 2001–2005, BY CAUSE AND GENDER. AVERAGE DEATHS PER YEAR

	Male	Female	Total
Total for All Causes	**57,429**	**22,217**	**79,646**
Acute pancreatitis	366	320	695
Alcohol abuse	1,868	514	2,382
Alcohol cardiomyopathy	389	59	448
Alcohol dependence syndrome	3,037	820	3,857
Alcohol polyneuropathy	1	0	1
Alcohol-induced chronic pancreatitis	248	63	311
Alcoholic gastritis	17	4	21
Alcoholic liver disease	8,938	3,281	12,219
Alcoholic myopathy	1	0	1
Alcoholic psychosis	568	183	751
Breast cancer (females only)	0	355	355
Chronic hepatitis	2	2	4
Chronic pancreatitis	118	112	229
Degeneration of nervous system due to alcohol	77	14	91
Epilepsy	102	88	191
Esophageal cancer	426	52	478
Esophageal varices	53	20	74
Fetal alcohol syndrome	2	1	3
Fetus and newborn affected by maternal use of alcohol	0	1	1
Gastroesophageal hemorrhage	16	13	29
Hypertension	753	610	1,363
Ischemic heart disease	609	277	886
Laryngeal cancer	207	30	237
Liver cancer	598	187	786
Liver cirrhosis, unspecified	4,134	2,921	7,055
Low birth weight, premature, IUGR, death	108	52	160
Oropharyngeal cancer	320	56	376
Portal hypertension	26	14	40
Prostate cancer (males only)	232	0	232
Psoriasis	Less than 1	Less than 1	Less than 1
Spontaneous abortion (females only)	0	Less than 1	Less than 1
Stroke, hemorrhagic	1,472	303	1,775
Stroke, ischemic	495	181	676
Superventricular cardiac dysrhythmia	85	102	187
Subtotal	**25,269**	**10,646**	**35,915**

(continues)

(continued)

	Male	Female	Total
Acute Causes			
Air-space transport	104	21	125
Alcohol poisoning	292	78	370
Aspiration	109	95	204
Child maltreatment	96	72	168
Drowning	716	152	868
Fall injuries	2,888	2,644	5,532
Fire injuries	692	466	1,158
Homicide	108	15	123
Hypothermia	182	87	269
Motor-vehicle nontraffic crashes	147	36	183
Motor-vehicle traffic crashes	10,802	3,016	13,819
Occupational and machine injuries	130	7	137
Other road vehicle crashes	165	45	210
Poisoning (not alcohol)	3,669	1,747	5,416
Suicide	5,778	1,457	7,235
Suicide by and exposure to alcohol	22	9	31
Water transport	87	11	98
Subtotal	**32,159**	**11,572**	**43,731**

Note that totals may be slightly off because of rounding up or down.
Adapted from computer-generated report from the Alcohol-Related Disease Impact (ARDI) software, available online. URL: https://apps.need.cdcgov/ardi. Accessed May 12, 2009. Go to https://apps.nccd.cedc.gov/ardi/HomePage.aspx for the latest information.

TABLE 3
ALCOHOL-ATTRIBUTABLE YEARS OF POTENTIAL LIVES LOST, ALL AGES, ANNUAL AVERAGE, 2001–2005, BASED ON MEDIUM AND HIGH CONSUMPTION OF ALCOHOL

	Male	Female	Total
Total for All Causes	**1,729,877**	**627,667**	**2,357,544**
Acute pancreatitis	6,900	5,241	12,141
Alcohol abuse	8,952	1,539	10,491
Alcohol cardiomyopathy	8,952	1,539	10,491
Alcohol dependence syndrome	77,851	24,167	102,018
Alcohol polyneuropathy	22	0	22
Alcohol-induced chronic pancreatitis	6,851	1,895	8,746
Alcoholic gastritis	386	118	505
Alcoholic liver disease	215,817	93,438	309,255
Alcoholic myopathy	22	0	22
Alcoholic psychosis	12,354	4,219	16,573
Breast cancer (females only)	0	6,802	6,802
Chronic hepatitis	40	33	73
Chronic pancreatitis	2,502	2,146	4,648
Degeneration of nervous system due to alcohol	1,389	307	1,696

	Male	Female	Total
Epilepsy	3,033	2,468	5,501
Esophageal cancer	6,695	791	7,485
Esophageal varices	1,130	392	1,523
Fetal alcohol syndrome	143	73	216
Fetus and newborn affected by maternal use of alcohol	0	80	80
Gastroesophageal hemorrhage	253	164	416
Hypertension	11,405	7,169	18,574
Ischemic heart disease	7,708	2,957	10,665
Laryngeal cancer	3,209	522	3,731
Liver cancer	10,077	2,900	12,977
Liver cirrhosis, unspecified	84,254	56,753	141,007
Low birth weight, premature, IUGR, death	8,069	4,165	12,234
Oropharyngeal cancer	5,589	884	6,473
Portal hypertension	489	310	799
Prostate cancer (males only)	2,211	0	2,211
Psoriasis	2	1	3
Spontaneous abortion (females only)	0	8	8
Stroke, hemorrhagic	23,191	4,750	27,940
Stroke, ischemic	5,160	1,773	6,933
Superventricular cardiac dysrhythmia	736	874	1,610
Subtotal	**557,464**	**243,001**	**800,465**
Acute Causes			
Air-space transport	3,159	791	3,949
Alcohol poisoning	10,194	2,882	13,076
Aspiration	2,074	1,712	3,786
Child maltreatment	6,774	5,459	12,232
Drowning	26,497	4,870	31,367
Fall injuries	43,690	28,998	72,688
Fire injuries	17,923	11,794	29,716
Homicide	268,760	68,002	336,763
Hypothermia	4,264	1,485	5,749
Motor-vehicle nontraffic crashes	4,769	1,114	5,883
Motor-vehicle traffic crashes	442,719	135,010	577,729
Occupational and machine injuries	3,614	214	3,828
Other road vehicle crashes	5,664	1,572	7,237
Poisoning (not alcohol)	135,420	66,375	201,795
Suicide	188,937	53,022	241,959
Suicide by and exposure to alcohol	730	329	1,059
Water transport	3,021	472	3,493
Subtotal	**1,172,413**	**384,666**	**1,557,079**

Note that totals may be slightly off because of rounding up or down.
Adapted from computer-generated report from the Alcohol-Related Disease Impact (ARDI) software, available online. URL: https://apps.need.cdcgov/ardi. Accessed May 12, 2009. Go to https://apps.nccd.cedc.gov/ardi/HomePage.aspx for the latest information.

males as a result of alcohol-related causes due to medium and high alcohol consumption in 2005, compared to an estimated 627,667 years of life lost to females, based on a normal life expectancy of men and women.

According to Susan Nolen-Hoeksema in her article on gender differences in risk factors and consequences for alcohol use in *Clinical Psychology Review* in 2004, men are more likely than women to score high on ratings of sensation-seeking, impulsivity, and behavioral undercontrol. These behaviors may be linked to an increased risk for alcohol-related problems such as heavy drinking.

Some researchers have looked at alcohol use among members of the military, and R. Gregory Lande and colleagues compared the drinking behavior of men and women in the Army in their article for the *Journal of the American Osteopathic Association.* They found that military men were more likely to engage in binge drinking than military women and were also more likely to drive while intoxicated.

Some researchers have found that PSYCHIATRIC COMORBIDITIES, particularly the diagnosis of ANTI-SOCIAL PERSONALITY DISORDER (which is much more common among men than women), are predictive for the presence of alcohol dependence.

The research news about men and alcohol is not solely negative; for example, research published in 2009 by Marinette Streppel and colleagues in the *Journal of Epidemiology and Community Health* that followed Dutch men for more than 40 years found that men drinking 20 grams of alcohol per day (about a half glass of wine or beer) increased their life expectancy by 2 ½ years at age 50 compared to nondrinking men. In addition, the men who consumed *only* wine (and 70 percent of the wine that was consumed was red wine) added five years to their life expectancy. Researchers speculated that the cardioprotective effect of wine may be related to polyphenol compounds in the wine, or natural chemicals such as flavonoids or tannin.

Binge Drinking and Heavy Alcohol Use among Men

According to the Centers for Disease Control and Prevention (CDC), men average about 12.5 binge drinking episodes per year compared to the annual 2.7 binge drinking episodes of women. However, although binge drinkers are at risk for alcoholism, not all binge drinkers are alcoholics. According to the SAMHSA, only 18.5 percent of binge drinkers meet the criteria for alcohol dependence.

Another category of alcohol consumption is known as heavy alcohol use, which is defined as drinking five or more drinks on the same occasion on each of five or more days in the past 30 days, and according to SAMHSA, nearly half (44.7 percent) of heavy drinkers met the criteria for alcohol dependence. All heavy drinkers *are* also binge drinkers because binge drinkers consume five or more drinks on at least one occasion in the past 30 days, while heavy drinkers binge drink even more frequently: on at least five days out of the last 30 days. Thus, heavy drinkers binge even more than typical binge drinkers. Yet not all heavy drinkers are alcoholics, because they do not all meet the criterion of tolerance, or needing greater amounts of alcohol to achieve the same level of intoxication, and/or other criteria.

Early Initiation of Drinking

Men ages 21 and older are more likely than women to report taking their first drink before age 15, or 24 percent of males versus 13 percent of females, according to SAMHSA. The early initiation of drinking is linked to an increased risk for problems with alcohol dependence. For example, those who started using alcohol before age 15 are more than five times more likely to report past year alcohol dependence as adults than those who first used alcohol at age 21 or older (16 percent for the early users compared to 3 percent for the first use as legal users).

Army Study Comparing Men and Women

In the study by Lande et al., the researchers compared drinking behaviors among 666 male soldiers compared to 307 female soldiers. Many of the soldiers reported responsible drinking, but there were problem behaviors, and in many cases, the male drinking behavior was more extreme. For example, looking at *moderate* drinkers, who consumed 0–2 drinks per week, 59.8 percent of the males fit this category versus the greater percentage of 70.4 percent of the females.

In considering those who consumed 13 or more drinks per week, 5.1 percent of the males fit this category versus 2.9 percent of the females. A greater number of men (20.7 percent) reported interpersonal conflicts as a result of alcohol consumption, compared to 12.6 percent of the women. About twice as many males reported driving while intoxicated (11.7 percent) compared to the female soldiers (5.8 percent). About twice as many men reported that alcohol made them be late or miss work (11.7 percent), compared to the women (6.1 percent).

Said the researchers, "Men reported more alcohol-related acts of aggression as compared with women. Women more frequently than men reported doing something that later caused feelings of regret."

Antisocial Personality Disorder among Men

Men with antisocial personality disorder (ASPD) are, by definition, more likely to get into trouble than other men. Yet antisocial personality disorder itself is considered by many experts to be inherited. A study of the interrelationships between ASPD, major depression, alcohol dependence, and marijuana dependence was reported by Qiang Fu and colleagues in 2002 in the *Archives of General Psychiatry*. The researchers drew their subjects from The Vietnam Era Twin Registry, a registry of 5,150 male twins who served on active duty during the Vietnam War. They included 1,868 monozygotic twins (identical twins) and 1,492 dizygotic (non-identical twins).

The researchers identified a lifetime risk for ASPD (69 percent), major depression (40 percent), alcohol dependence (56 percent), and marijuana dependence (50 percent) among the subjects. However, after they controlled for the genetic effects of ASPD, the partial correlations that were originally found for depression with alcohol dependence and with marijuana dependence no longer held. Instead, said the researchers, "The shared genetic risk between MD [major depression] and both AD [alcohol dependence] and MJD [marijuana dependence] was largely explained by genetic effects on ASPD, which in turn was associated with increased risk of each of the other disorders." In other words, it was the ASPD which was the driving force in

leading to alcohol dependence, as well as depression and marijuana dependence.

Concluded the researchers, "The results of the present study confirm that, at least in men, genetic effects on risk for ASPD are a major determinant of risk of substance dependence. Because of the strong comorbidity between ASPD and MD, failure to control for ASPD may have led to an overstatement of the importance of MD in the inheritance of AD and MJD."

Stress and Men

In the study by Dawson and colleagues, the respondents were asked about 12 different stressful events that may have occurred to them in the past twelve months. The events fell into four key categories, including health-related stress (the serious illness of oneself or someone close or the death of someone close); social stress (divorce/breakup; change of job responsibilities, problems with a friend or neighbor, etc.); job stress (sustained unemployment or job loss); and legal stress (criminal victimization of oneself or a family member; self or family member's trouble with police or major financial crisis). The researchers found that health-related stress was the most common among respondents, reported by 48.3 percent, followed by social stress (43.9 percent), legal stress (20.5 percent), and job-related stress (12.7 percent).

According to the researchers, "Drinkers who experienced six or more stressful events had an average daily volume of ethanol intake and a frequency of heavy drinking that were more than thrice [three times] those of drinkers with no stressful events, and their usual and largest quantities consumed were about twice as high." Added the researchers, "With each additional stressor reported, average daily ethanol intake increased by 14% (a factor of 1.14) for men and by 8% (a factor of 1.08) for women." The number of heavy drinking days increased with each additional stressor by 24 percent for men and by 13 percent for women.

Drinking Men Harmed by Others Men who are intoxicated are at risk for becoming victims of physical aggression and violence. Researchers such as Leonard et al. in *Aggressive Behavior* have found that drunken men are more likely to be injured in a barroom brawl than are intoxicated women; 30

percent of severe injuries received by men in bars are due to assaults by intoxicated men, compared to 22 percent received by drunken women who are in bars.

The researchers also found that the more alcohol that a man consumes in a bar, the more likely he is to become severely injured by the perpetrator of the barroom violence. Interestingly, the more intoxicated the male perpetrator of the barroom violence becomes, the *less* likely it is that the victim is to be severely injured, probably because of worse reflexes and the fact that it is generally easier to avoid a very intoxicated person. (Of course, any injury is problematic.)

Inmates and Drinking The Bureau of Justice Statistics of the U.S. Department of Justice published a report in 2005 on substance abuse and dependence of 444,534 predominantly male jail inmates in the United States in 2002. It found that a third (34.9 percent) of male inmates said that they had been drinking alcohol when they committed their conviction offense. In addition, of individuals convicted of violent offenses, even greater percentages were drinking when they committed their crime; for example, 41.6 percent were using alcohol when they committed homicide, while 39.7 percent were drinking when they committed assault. These percentages were greater than the percentages of inmates using drugs when they committed their offenses.

Among jail inmates, 34.9 percent of the male convicts said they were using alcohol at the time of the offense compared to 22.2 percent of the female convicts. The highest rate of drinking was seen among white inmates. An estimated 50.3 percent of the males met the criteria for abuse or dependence on alcohol, compared to 39.2 percent of the female inmates.

Interestingly, the female convicts were *more* likely than the males to be using drugs at the time of their offense, or 34.4 percent of the female convicts, compared to 28.0 percent of the male prisoners. In addition, the females were more likely to meet the criteria for drug abuse or dependence or 61.3 percent for females, compared to the 54.4 percent of the male inmates who meet the criteria for drug abuse and dependence. See Table 4 for more information.

Intimate Partner Violence Men who engage in drinking, and particularly in heavy drinking, have an increased risk of engaging in intimate partner violence. In a study published in 2005 in the *Psychology of Addictive Behaviors* by Christopher M. Murphy and colleagues, the researchers interviewed 40 alcoholic men and their relationship partners about conflicts in physical or psychological aggression that occurred. They found that the amount of alcohol consumed by 72 percent of the men in the prior 12 hours was significant in the causes of violent physical abuse. In addition, 64 percent of the men said that they had engaged in heavy drinking, or drinking six or more drinks.

With regard to the time when physical aggression was exhibited, the largest percentage was violent between 5 P.M. and midnight. The researchers noted that their findings demonstrated that alcohol consumption was associated with a risk for physically aggressive conflict among some alcoholic men.

In another study by C. Eckhardt and reported in the *Journal of Consulting and Clinical Psychology* in 2007, the author studied 46 maritally violent and 56 maritally nonviolent men to determine how alcohol affected them when their anger was aroused in simulated or imagined marital conflicts. Eckhardt found that men with a history of marital violence were significantly more aggressive in their verbalization and had high levels of anger. Said Eckhardt, "Thus, alcohol may exert proximal effects on abusive behavior among individuals already prone to respond to conflict with increased anger."

Child Abuse and Drinking A study of the risk factors and injuries in child physical abuse from 2003 to 2007 in Finland, reported by T. Hulme and colleagues, was published in the *European Journal of Pediatric Surgery* in 2008. The researchers analyzed 48 cases of physical abuse among babies and toddlers, a crime most people would consider heinous. The researchers found that the usual perpetrator was the father or stepfather of the child, and parental risk factors were alcohol and drug abuse. Among the children who were abused, those who exhibited some behaviors increased their risk for abuse, such as overactivity and crying.

When men abuse women but not their children, their abuse can still affect children; for example,

TABLE 4
ALCOHOL OR DRUG USE AT TIME OF OFFENSE AMONG CONVICTED JAIL INMATES,
BY TYPE OF OFFENSE, BY SELECTED CHARACTERISTICS, 2002

Characteristic	Estimated number of inmates	Percent of convicted jail inmates			
		Using at the time of offense		Meeting dependence or abuse criteria	
		Alcohol	Drugs	Alcohol	Drugs
All inmates	444,534	33.4	28.8	49.0	55.3
Gender					
Male	391,809	34.9	28.0	50.3	54.4
Female	52,725	22.2	34.4	39.2	61.3
Race/Hispanic origin					
White	168,613	38.5	33.2	58.6	62.2
Black	172,186	29.3	27.3	42.7	53.9
Hispanic	80,157	30.1	23.8	41.8	45.0
Other	22,308	36.9	24.1	52.6	50.2
Age					
24 or younger	129,726	24.2	31.5	45.5	60.7
25–34	142,174	33.3	31.0	51.6	56.5
35–44	118,680	40.1	28.5	52.3	55.6
45–54	45,445	40.9	19.3	44.2	41.8
55 or older	8,509	40.5	5.5	38.5	16.4

Source: Karberg, Jennifer C., and Doris J. James. "Substance Dependence, Abuse, and Treatment of Jail Inmates, 2002." *Bureau of Justice Statistics Special Report.* Office of Justice Programs, July 2005, page 6.

in a study by Cecilia Casanueva and colleagues and reported in *Child Abuse & Neglect* in 2009, the researchers studied women investigated for maltreatment. They found that if the mothers had been physically abused by their partner, they were more than twice as likely to abuse their children (29 percent) than the mothers who were not abused (14 percent). In addition, reports of physical abuse to children occurred twice as fast by the mothers who experienced abuse compared to the mothers who had not suffered partner abuse.

In another study by Deborah Gibbs and colleagues and reported in *Child Maltreatment* in 2008, the researchers looked at substantiated incidents of maltreatment perpetrated by soldiers in the Army from 2000 to 2004. There were 464 male offenders and 57 female offenders. The researchers found that 13 percent of the offenders were abusing alcohol or illicit drugs at the time of the incident. In addition, the level of substance abuse was higher

for male offenders than for female; for example, 88.9 percent of the male abusers were using alcohol or drugs at the time of the incident, compared to 10.9 percent of the female abusers. The researchers also noted that the incidence of child abuse among the soldiers was significantly lower than among the general public, and when substances were abused, it was primarily alcohol that was used rather than illicit substances.

See also AGGRESSIVE BEHAVIOR AND ALCOHOL; ALCOHOL AND OTHER DRUGS; CHILD ABUSE AND NEGLECT; EXCESSIVE DRINKING AND HEALTH CONSEQUENCES; EXCESSIVE DRINKING AND NEGATIVE SOCIAL CONSEQUENCES.

Caetano, Raul, M.D., et al. "Alcohol-Related Intimate Partner Violence among White, Black, and Hispanic Couples in the United States." *Alcohol Research & Health* 25, no. 1 (2001): 58–65.

Casanueva, Cecilia, Sandra L. Martin, and Desmond K. Runyan. "Repeated Reports for Child Maltreatment among Intimate Partner Violence Victims: Findings from the National Survey of Child and Adolescent Well-Being." *Child Abuse & Neglect* 33, no. 2 (2009): 84–93.

Dawson, Deborah A., Bridget F. Grant, and W. June Ruan. "The Association between Stress and Drinking: Modifying Effects of Gender and Vulnerability." *Alcohol & Alcoholism* 40, no. 5 (2005): 453–460.

Eckhardt, C. "Effects of Alcohol Intoxication on Anger Experience and Expression among Partner Assaultive Men." *Journal of Consulting Clinical Psychology* 75, no. 1 (2007): 61–71.

Gibbs, Deborah A., et al. "Child Maltreatment and Substance Abuse among U.S. Army Soldiers." *Child Maltreatment* 13, no. 3 (2008): 259–268.

Hulme, T., et al. "Risk Factors for Physical Child Abuse in Infants and Toddlers." *European Journal of Pediatric Surgery* 18, no. 6 (2008): 387–391.

Karberg, Jennifer C., and Doris J. James. "Substance Dependence, Abuse, and Treatment of Jail Inmates, 2002. *Bureau of Justice Statistics Special Report.* Office of Justice Programs, July 2005.

Lande, R. Gregory, et al. "Gender Differences and Alcohol Use in the U.S. Army." *Journal of the American Osteopathic Association* 107, no. 9 (2007): 401–407.

Leonard, K. E., R. L. Collins, and B. M. Quigley. "Alcohol Consumption and the Occurrence and Severity of Aggression: An Event-based Analysis of Male to Male Barroom Violence." *Aggressive Behavior* 29, no. 4 (2003): 346–365.

Murphy, Christopher M., et al. "Alcohol Consumption and Intimate Partner Violence by Alcoholic Men: Comparing Violent and Nonviolent Conflicts." *Psychology of Addictive Behaviors* 19, no. 1 (2005): 35–42.

Office of Applied Studies. "Gender Differences in Alcohol Use and Alcohol Dependence or Abuse: 2004 and 2005." *NSDUH Report.* Substance Abuse and Mental Health Services Administration, August 2, 2007.

———. "Substance Abuse and Dependence among Women." *NSDUH Report.* Substance Abuse and Mental Health Services Administration, August 5, 2005.

Streppel, Marinette, et al. "Long-term Wine Consumption is Related to Cardiovascular Mortality and Life Expectancy Independently." *Journal of Epidemiology and Community Health* (2009): 534–540.

alcohol and other drugs   The abuse of or dependence on alcohol along with the use of illicit drugs or the misuse of prescribed drugs. In addition, many individuals who abuse or are dependent on alcohol are also addicted to the nicotine in tobacco products. In fact, the most common comorbid addiction with alcohol is nicotine, and up to 80 percent of individuals with alcohol dependence are also smokers. The death rate from smoking is very high (about 400,000 deaths per year), as are the numbers who die from alcoholism (about 100,000 deaths per year). It is important to treat both alcohol dependence and nicotine dependence, although until recently, most rehabilitative facilities ignored nicotine addiction. (See SMOKING AND ALCOHOL.)

According to Mark S. Gold, M.D., and Kimberly Frost-Pineda in their article in the *Journal of Dual Diagnosis* in 2004, "There may be a number of reasons that the two [alcohol and nicotine] are used together, including (1) either could produce changes to the brain's intrinsic rewarding system in a way that promotes the use of the other, (2) the combination of tobacco and alcohol could result in a new compound as in the case when alcohol and cocaine are combined, and/or (3) the two may be used in combination to counteract the negative effects of each other; for example, the nicotine in cigarettes can produce stress and anxiety which is counteracted by alcohol." The authors say that alcohol and nicotine together may also activate the brain reward system more effectively than either drug alone.

In their article on comorbid alcoholism and cigarette addiction in the *Journal of Addictive Diseases,* Norman S. Miller, M.D., and Mark S. Gold, M.D., noted that cigarettes and alcohol act together to cause some cancers, such as cancer of the head and neck. The authors said, "The mortality from cigarette smoking and alcohol addiction is high. The combination of nicotine and alcohol use is common. The contributions to mortality from nicotine and alcohol are independent and additive depending on the associated cause of death. The recent documentation of increased mortality from tobacco smoking in otherwise abstinent alcoholics is important for clinicians to use to advise treated alcoholic patients with continued nicotine addition."

In an article in the *Journal of Addictive Diseases* in 2005, Joanne A. Byars et al. write that NALTREXONE (a medication that is also used to treat alcohol dependence) combined with nicotine replacement therapy has been used successfully to improve smoking cessation rates. It is particularly effective in women.

About two-thirds of alcoholics have abused drugs other than nicotine. Individuals who abuse both alcohol and other drugs are at a high risk for experiencing dangerous MEDICATION INTERACTIONS; for example, the person who combines alcohol with BENZODIAZEPINES is at risk for suffering a fatal overdose.

According to the National Institute on Alcohol Abuse and Alcoholism (NIAAA), one study showed that of 248 alcoholics seeking treatment, 64 percent had met the criteria for a drug use disorder (drug abuse or drug addiction) at some time in their lives. The NIAAA also reports that individuals with an alcohol use disorder (alcohol abuse or dependence) have an increased risk for a dependence on other substances. In addition, they are more likely than those without an alcohol use disorder to have a psychiatric disorder, and they also are more likely to attempt SUICIDE.

Based on the National Epidemiologic Survey on Alcohol Abuse and Related Conditions (NESARC), an estimated 1.1 percent of individuals in the United States meet the criteria for having both an alcohol use disorder and a drug use disorder; however, people who are addicted to drugs are more likely to have an alcohol use disorder than are people with alcoholism to have a drug use disorder. Individuals ages 18–24 have the greatest risk for having both an alcohol use disorder and a drug use disorder.

According to Albert J. Arias, M.D., and Henry R. Kranzler, M.D., in their article for *Alcohol Research & Health* in 2008, those patients with both alcohol and drug issues generally have a greater severity of substance abuse than patients with either an alcohol use disorder or a drug abuse disorder alone. Interestingly, people with both an alcohol and drug abuse problem are more likely to seek treatment than are those with only an alcohol or drug abuse problem.

Demographics of Those Who Abuse Alcohol and Other Drugs

Other Demographic Factors The NESARC revealed other salient factors; for example, those individuals with the lowest incomes were most likely to use both alcohol and other drugs (65.4 percent), while those with higher educations were the most likely to abuse both substances (48.4 percent). Individuals with both alcohol and drug use disorders were more likely to have a PERSONALITY DISORDER, a mood disorder, or an ANXIETY DISORDER than individuals with neither an alcohol nor a drug use disorder.

Although males predominate among those who abuse alcohol and/or drugs, the percentage was most pronounced (73.9 percent) among those who had both an alcohol and a drug use disorder, compared to 26.1 percent among females with both disorders. In addition, it should be noted that those who were never married are the most likely to have both an alcohol and drug use disorder (63.2 percent). See Table 1 for further information.

College Students Who Abuse Alcohol and Prescription Drugs The abuse of prescription drugs is a major problem among men and women with an alcohol use disorder. According to researchers at the University of Michigan, people who drink in college are 18 times more likely to abuse prescription drugs than people who do not drink. According to the researchers, those COLLEGE STUDENTS who consumed alcohol and prescription drugs at the same time had an increased risk for having an ALCOHOLIC BLACKOUT as well as for engaging in risky behaviors, such as unplanned sex or drunk driving.

The prescription drugs most likely to be combined with alcohol are opiates such as acetaminophen with codeine (Tylenol 3), acetaminophen and hydrodocone (Vicodin), acetaminophen and oxycodone (Percocet), and timed release oxycodone (OxyContin), as well as antianxiety medications such as lorazepam (Ativan), diazepam (Valium), and alprazolam (Xanax). In addition, some college students combine alcohol with sleep remedies, such as zolpidem (Ambien), triazolam (Halcion), or temazepam (Restoril).

Said Dr. James Colliver, formerly of the National Institute of Drug Administration (NIDA), "The problem is that many people think that, because prescription drugs have been tested and approved by the Food and Drug Administration, they are always safe to use; but they are safe only when used under the direction of a physician for the purpose for which they are prescribed."

Intentional Simultaneous Uses of Alcohol and Drugs

According to Christopher S. Martin in his article on alcohol and other drug use, people who use both alcohol and other drugs may do so intentionally, with the goal of producing an additive effect of the substances. For example, some people purposely use alcohol in concert with cocaine to internally produce cocaethylene, a psychoactive compound. According to Bachaar Arnaout, M.D., and Ismene L. Petrakis, M.D., in their article on alcohol and other drugs for *Alcohol Research & Health* in 2008, it is possible that alcohol may enhance the pleasurable effects of cocaine and thus cause a greater increase in the heart rate that is seen with either substance alone.

Others use drugs to offset or reduce the effects of the other drug; for example, they may take sedatives to enable themselves to sleep after a cocaine binge.

Martin says that the most common drug used simultaneously with alcohol is marijuana, and as many as 11 percent of males and 4 percent of females over age 12 have used both drugs simultaneously.

Some individuals intentionally use two or more illicit substances along with alcohol. In one study by Martin in 1996, 25 percent of the subjects had consumed alcohol and two illicit drugs about once a week, and 10 percent had used alcohol with three or more illicit drugs on occasion.

Combining Alcohol and Drugs Can Be Very Dangerous According to Martin, commenting on simultaneous drug and alcohol use, "The majority of deaths attributed to heroin overdose involve significant levels of other drugs such as alcohol or benzodiazepines; opiate levels appear to be similar in both fatal and non fatal overdoses. Similarly, about two-thirds of oxycodone-related deaths were found to involve the use of alcohol and/or other drugs. Finally, fatalities and injuries reported to be 'alcohol-related' often involve other drug use."

Psychiatric Comorbidities Are High

Researchers have also found that people with both alcohol and other drug use disorders have a high risk for PSYCHIATRIC COMORBIDITIES. These are the psychiatric problems that accompany the substance disorder, such as DEPRESSION or an anxiety disorder, among many possible psychiatric diagnoses. In addition, these individuals are more likely to attempt suicide and to have serious health problems. They also have an elevated risk for personality disorders, as seen from Table 1.

Hiding Their Drug Use

Patients may fail to report or they may underreport their drug use to their physicians. According to Arnaout and Petrakis, patients are more likely and willing to report their use of lawful drugs such as alcohol and nicotine than they are to admit to the use of illegal drugs such as heroin. Patients may fear that if the doctor considers them drug addicts, they will not receive good medical care. They may also fear that the doctor will tell their families about the drug use and may not realize that doctors are usually bound by laws of medical confidentiality (with the exception of patients who confess to committing acts of child abuse and other exceptions).

Rarely, patients may purposely overstate their drug use because they are undertreated for severely painful conditions, and consequently, they are seeking a prescription for a medication such as methadone or buprenophine to adequately treat their severe pain. These are medications that are used to treat drug addicts but they are also opiates and thus, they can act as pain relievers as well.

Some Medications Treat Both Alcohol and Drug Abuse

According to Arias and Kranzler, some medications are effective at treating both alcoholism and some drug use disorders; for example, DISULFIRAM (Antabuse) is effective at treating alcohol dependence and may also help those with cocaine abuse or addiction. Topiramate, an antiseizure drug, may also help those with both alcohol and cocaine abuse, although it is an off-label treatment for both disorders. Another medication, baclofen, has been used to treat both alcohol and cocaine dependence. Naltrexone has been used to treat both alcohol and opioid dependence, as has disulfiram. Sometimes methadone is used to treat both alcohol and opioid dependence.

According to Arias and Kranzler, "For patients with alcohol and cocaine dependence, disulfiram

TABLE 1
PERCENT DISTRIBUTIONS OF SELECTED DEMOGRAPHIC CHARACTERISTICS AND PSYCHIATRIC DISORDERS
AMONG RESPONDENTS WITH ALCOHOL AND ANY DRUG USE DISORDERS COMPARED TO THOSE
WITH NO ALCOHOL OR DRUG USE DISORDERS, PERCENTAGE

Demographic Characteristic/ Psychiatric Disorder	Alcohol Use Disorder Only (n = 2,903)	Any Drug Use Disorder Only (n = 353)	Alcohol and Any Drug Use Disorder (n = 424)	No Alcohol or Drug Use Disorder (n = 39,413)
Sex				
Male	69.4	60.1	73.9	45.7
Female	30.6	39.9	26.1	54.3
Race/ethnicity				
White	75.8	68.5	68.5	70.6
Black	8.7	15.8	11.5	11.2
Native American	2.5	3.3	6.8	2.0
Asian/Pacific Islander	2.3	3.6	2.6	4.6
Hispanic	10.8	8.9	11.0	11.7
Age (years)				
18–29	38.3	47.8	65.0	19.7
30–44	37.0	33.8	25.9	30.4
45–64	21.6	15.9	9.1	32.3
65 and older	3.2	2.6	0.1	17.6
Marital status				
Married/living as if married	47.7	45.0	20.2	63.4
Widowed/separated/divorced	16.7	12.8	16.6	17.6
Never married	35.6	42.2	63.2	19.0
Education level				
Less than high school	12.2	18.3	18.2	15.9
High school diploma/GED	27.9	38.1	33.3	29.3
Some college or higher	59.8	43.6	48.4	54.8
Personal income (U.S. $)				
0–19,999	39.3	66.1	65.4	47.5
20,000–34,999	25.8	18.7	23.1	22.4
35,000–69,999	25.5	11.3	9.7	21.9
$70,000 or greater	9.4	4.0	1.8	8.2
Urbanicity				
Urban	79.6	84.3	78.4	80.3
Rural	20.4	15.7	21.6	19.7
Geographic region				
Northeast	17.8	21.1	20.5	19.8
Midwest	29.4	20.5	25.7	22.6
South	31.1	27.5	24.7	35.8
West	21.8	31.0	29.2	21.8
Any personality disorder?				
Yes	25.3	44.0	50.8	13.2
No	74.7	56.0	49.2	86.8
Any past-year independent mood disorder?				
Yes	16.4	27.5	35.3	8.1
No	83.6	72.5	64.7	91.9
Any past-year independent anxiety disorder?				
Yes	15.6	24.0	26.5	10.4
No	84.4	76.0	73.5	89.6

Adapted from: Stinson, Frederick, et al. "Comorbidity between DSM-IV Alcohol and Specific Drug Use Disorders in the United States: Results from the National Epidemiologic Survey on Alcohol and Related Conditions." *Alcohol Research & Health* 29, no. 2 (2006): 100.

has better empirical support than any other medication. Less compelling evidence exists for the use of either naltrexone or topiramate, but these also should be considered for treatment of these co-occurring disorders." The authors also said that alcohol-dependent patients who are on methadone maintenance may find that the methadone also helps them with their drinking problem.

The authors add, "Treatment planning for patients with AODUDs [alcohol and other drug use disorders] should include medical and psychiatric evaluations and integrated treatment to address co-occurring substance use and psychiatric disorders. Given the burden of psychopathology, patients with AODUDs often may require a higher level of care (e.g., inpatient rehabilitation, psychiatric partial hospital or intensive outpatient dual diagnosis programs) for initial stabilization."

See also ALCOHOL AND MEN; ALCOHOL AND WOMEN; ALCOHOLISM/ALCOHOL DEPENDENCE.

Arias, Albert J., M.D., and Henry R. Kranzler, M.D. "Treatment of Co-Occurring Alcohol and Other Drug Use Disorders." *Alcohol Research & Health* 31, no. 2 (2008): 155–166.

Arnaout, Bachaar, M.D., and Ismene L. Petrakis, M.D. "Diagnosing Co-Morbid Drug Use in Patients with Alcohol Use Disorders." *Alcohol Research & Health* 31, no. 2 (2008): 148–154.

Ashton, Elizabeth. "Alcohol Abuse Makes Prescription Drug Abuse More Likely: Research Findings." NIDA Notes 21, no. 5 (March 2008). Available online. URL: http://www.drugabuse.gov/NIDA_notes/NNvol12N5/alcohol.html. Accessed March 22, 2009.

Byars, Joanne A., et al. "Naltrexone Augments the Effects of Nicotine Replacement Therapy in Female Smokers." *Journal of Addictive Diseases* 24, no. 2 (2005): 49–60.

Gold, Mark S., M.D., and Kimberly Frost-Pineda. "Substance Abuse and Psychiatric Dual Disorders: Focus on Tobacco." *Journal of Dual Diagnosis* 1, no. 1 (2004): 15–36.

Martin, Christopher. "Timing of Alcohol and Other Drug Use." *Alcohol Research & Health* 31, no. 2 (2008): 96–99.

Martin, Christopher, et al. "Polydrug Use in an Inpatient Treatment Sample of Problem Drinkers." *Alcoholism: Clinical and Experimental Research* 20, no. 3 (1996): 413–417.

Miller, Norman S., M.D., and Mark S. Gold, M.D. "Comorbid Cigarette and Alcohol Addiction: Epidemiology and Treatment." *Journal of Addictive Diseases* 17, no. 1 (1998): 55–66.

National Institute on Alcohol Abuse and Alcoholism. "Alcohol and Other Drugs." Alcohol Alert no. 76 (July 2008): 1–6.

Office of Applied Studies. "Concurrent Illicit Drug and Alcohol Use." *NSDUH Report.* Substance Abuse and Mental Health Services Administration, March 19, 2009: 1–4.

Stinson, Frederick, et al. "Comorbidity between DSM-IV Alcohol and Specific Drug Use Disorders in the United States: Results from the National Epidemiologic Survey on Alcohol and Related Conditions." *Alcohol Research & Health* 29, no. 2 (2006): 94–106.

alcohol and women   Whether a woman uses alcohol normally, abuses or binges on it, or becomes addicted to this substance, alcohol affects women differently from men. These differences become particularly problematic with alcohol dependence. The basic female metabolism, as well as the general body weight of most women, differs from that of the male metabolism and body weight. In addition, gastric alcohol dehydrogenase (ADH) levels in the stomach are about twice as high in men as in women, which means that men metabolize alcohol faster than women. As a result of their metabolic and weight differences, in general, women generally become intoxicated faster and at lower levels of alcohol consumption than men. In addition, although they generally drink much less than most men, some women develop a problem with alcohol abuse or alcohol dependence. BINGE DRINKING is also problematic among some women, especially younger women or those who are COLLEGE STUDENTS.

Women's alcohol-related health problems often develop significantly faster than among males. These health issues also cause greater impairment more quickly than among males, a problem that some researchers refer to as "telescoping." For example, female alcoholics progress to alcoholic liver disease and heart disease at a much more rapid pace than male alcoholics. Women who drink also have an increased risk for the development of some cancers, according to Naomi E. Allen and colleagues in their article in the *Journal of the National Cancer Institute* in 2009. This risk is sometimes present even with a moderate intake of alcohol, and the risk escalates further with higher levels of drinking.

Says Susan Nolen-Hoeksema in her analysis of gender studies on alcohol, published in *Clinical Psychology Review* in 2004, "Evidence regarding gender differences in the consequences of alcohol consumption suggests that women suffer alcohol-related physical illnesses at lower levels of exposure to alcohol than men, and heavy alcohol use is associated with several reproductive problems in women."

In addition, although male trauma patients frequently wind up in the hospital due to alcohol-related problems, female trauma patients have even greater rates of physical and psychological harm connected to alcohol, according to researchers.

Some experts believe that although men generally have higher rates of alcoholism than women, the gender gap is apparently closing, which is also known as the convergence hypothesis. In their chapter on women, girls, and alcohol in *Women & Addiction: A Comprehensive Handbook,* authors Sherry H. Stewart, Dubravka Gavric, and Pamela Collins discuss possible reasons why women are apparently "catching up" to men in terms of alcohol use and alcohol disorders as well as the health problems that accompany alcohol abuse and alcoholism. The authors say that it is possible that many women have been drinking to excess in the past, but that they have been hiding this fact, because of the severe past stigmatization against females drinking. The authors say, "In other words, due to a general relaxation of sex roles and reduced stigmatization in more recent years, evidence for convergence may be based on a decrease in under-reporting among women, rather than on an actual increase in women's drinking."

It is also possible that more women *are* drinking heavily now than in the past, because some stigmatization toward female drinking continues. According to the authors, "In general, heavy drinking is viewed much more negatively when it occurs in women as opposed to men. Such stigmatization has several implications. On the one hand, it may serve as a protective factor that prevents women from engaging in heavy drinking and thus protects them against the development of alcohol-related problems. On the other hand, it may cause women to conceal their drinking behavior and prevent them from receiving treatment until their alcohol-related problems have become quite severe."

The authors write, "In summary, studies from around the world provide quite consistent evidence of gender convergence and suggest that this convergence appears particularly pronounced among younger women (i.e., women born since the advent of the women's movement). In fact, in recent years, several alarming trends in female adolescent alcohol use have emerged. Recent findings indicate an increased rate of alcohol involvement among adolescent girls, with a decline in the age of girls' first use, higher rates of alcohol use initiation, and an increased involvement of adolescent girls in alcohol-related crime. Such findings suggest the need for further attention to monitoring trends in females' drinking behavior and to developing targeted prevention programming for younger women."

According to the National Institute on Alcohol Abuse and Alcoholism (NIAAA), of those women who drink, an estimated 13 percent are heavy drinkers who consume more than seven drinks per week. Heavy drinking often leads to serious problems; for example, according to federal surveillance studies, teenage girls who are heavy drinkers are five times more likely to have sex than girls who do *not* drink. In addition hard-drinking teenage girls are one-third *less* likely to use contraception than other teenage girls who have sex. As a result, these female drinkers have a greater risk for unplanned pregnancies and for contracting sexually transmitted diseases. Females who abuse, binge, or are dependent on alcohol also face increased risks for victimization and abuse by others.

Childhood issues often deeply impact women who abuse or are dependent on alcohol; for example, women who were abused as children are about twice as likely to abuse alcohol in adulthood compared to females who were not abused in childhood. In fact, the more adverse events that a woman has experienced in childhood (such as child abuse, growing up in a family in which a family member is in prison, or a family member is an alcohol or drug abuser), the more likely that she is to abuse or become dependent on alcohol in adulthood.

Another major factor that affects drinking is peer pressure, which looms particularly large among teenage girls. Girls in middle school who say that their peers pressure them to drink are about twice as likely to consume alcohol as girls who experience no such pressure. For example, J. G. Barber and colleagues reported in 1999 in *Children and Youth Services Review* that if a girl has friends who smoke and drink, the girl has a seven times greater risk for consuming alcohol; the same situation among boys incurs a three times greater risk.

There are also protective factors against the development of alcohol use disorders, such as having parents who do not drink, living in a supportive environment, and participating in religious activities.

PSYCHIATRIC COMORBIDITIES are common among women who abuse or depend on alcohol; for example, some studies have found that about half of women with eating disorders are either alcohol abusers or alcoholics. The converse is also true, and women with alcohol use disorders have a higher rate of eating disorders than other women, particularly among those with bulimia nervosa or binge eating. Other common substances that women use with alcohol are cigarettes, caffeinated drinks, and amphetamine-related drugs such as Ritalin (psychostimulants).

Women who abuse or depend on alcohol are also significantly more likely than others to be depressed. Say Stewart et al., "Even after accounting for the higher prevalence of depression among women, women with alcohol use disorders are significantly more likely to experience a comorbid depression than men with alcohol use disorders."

In addition, women are more likely to have a depression that is independent of their alcoholism, while men are more likely to have an alcohol-induced depression. According to Stewart and colleagues, "The higher rates of independent depression among women with alcohol use disorders may have important clinical implications for at least two reasons. First, independent depression may be linked with greater severity of alcohol problems and with more difficulties during the alcoholism treatment process. For example, some studies have linked independent depression with more frequent alcohol abuse relapses and with more suicide attempts than alcohol-induced depression. And recent findings from our research group show that

for women with alcohol problems compared to men with alcohol problems, independent depression is associated with a more complex clinical presentation (e.g., more comorbid anxiety disorders) as well as more severe substance use problems. Second, by definition, independent depression is not expected to remit with alcohol abstinence. Thus women with co-occurring depression are more likely than men with co-occurring depression to require treatment services that specifically address their depression either concurrently or sequentially with their alcoholism treatment."

According to Stewart et al., there is also a high comorbidity of alcohol use disorders and borderline personality disorder among women. (Borderline personality disorder is the most common PERSONALITY DISORDER diagnosed in women.)

Some personality disorders are looked down upon, even by mental health professionals. Say Lisa A. Burckell and Shelly McMain in their chapter in *Women & Addiction* on concurrent personality disorders and substance abuse disorders in women, "Personality diagnoses—widely regarded as psychiatry's stepchildren—are also one of the most stigmatized of mental disorders." They conclude that as a result, women with both personality disorders and substance abuse disorders are less likely to seek treatment or remain in treatment.

Some women who abuse or depend on alcohol may have higher levels of impulsivity and substance use than most women, which may be yet another factor in the development of their alcohol abuse or dependence.

Women sometimes misconstrue men's attitudes toward drinking to their detriment, based on a 2009 study in the *Psychology of Addictive Behaviors* by Joseph W. La Brie and colleagues. In this study among college students, female students significantly overestimated the amount of alcohol that men approved of among their females friends, dates, and romantic partners. In addition, this misperception of the women affected their own drinking levels.

According to the authors, analyses of female perceptions "showed that a large percentage of women mistakenly believe that males want them to drink to risky levels. This is particularly the case within the friendship and sexual contexts, where additional analyses showed that 26.1% of women stated that men would most likely want to be friends with a woman who drinks 5 or more drinks, and 16.7% stated that men would be the most sexually attracted to the same. Both estimates are nearly double men's actual preference for that behavior."

Drinking heavily can be dangerous for women of all ages; for example, women who drink heavily are more likely to be in danger from physical and sexual assaults than others, particularly in the case of young women in college. Drinking females are also more likely than nondrinking women to suffer from sexual assaults and rapes. (See EXCESSIVE DRINKING AND NEGATIVE SOCIAL CONSEQUENCES.)

Sometimes older women have a late onset of drinking, largely due to loneliness and the deaths of spouses, friends, and others, as well as health problems. This behavior may escalate to alcohol dependence.

Drinking during pregnancy may cause potential severe risks in women's offspring, such as FETAL ALCOHOL SYNDROME. In addition, women who are breastfeeding should not drink because even small amounts of alcohol can be transmitted in the breast milk. Despite this, many women drink during pregnancy as well as when they are recent mothers.

Indicators of Alcohol Abuse or Alcoholism in Women

Possible indications that a woman is an alcohol abuser include the following behaviors, according to the NIAAA:

- missing work or skipping child care responsibilities because of drinking
- drinking in dangerous situations, such as before or while driving a vehicle
- being arrested for driving while under the influence of alcohol or for hurting someone while drunk
- continuing to drink despite the fact that there are alcohol-related tensions with friends and family members

Possible indications that a woman may be an alcoholic include the following signs, according to the NIAAA:

- a strong compulsion, or craving, to drink
- the inability to stop drinking once the person has started
- signs of physical dependence when the woman does not drink, such as nausea, sweating, shakiness, and anxiety
- tolerance, or the need for increasing amounts of alcohol in order to experience the euphoric feelings associated with drinking

Health Risks for Women Who Drink

Researchers have found an increased risk for some health problems among women who are alcoholics compared to male alcoholics, such as an increased risk for breast cancer and a more rapid onset to liver and heart disease and other diseases. According to Stewart et al., alcoholic women are more likely to suffer from gastrointestinal hemorrhage, malnutrition, obesity, anemia, hypertension, ulcers, and cardiovascular diseases. Some of these conditions are discussed below.

Risks for Cancer Research has demonstrated that as little as one alcoholic drink per day significantly increases the risk for the development of breast CANCER in women, and this is especially true in women who are postmenopausal and/or who have a history of breast cancer in their family. The risk for breast cancer is escalated further if a postmenopausal woman drinks alcohol and she also takes hormonal replacement medications.

In the Million Women Study in the United Kingdom, which followed about 1.3 million women, Naomi E. Allen and colleagues reported in the *Journal of the National Cancer Institute* in 2009 that they found that even moderate alcohol consumption significantly increased the risk of some cancers in women, such as cancer of the breast, esophagus, larynx, liver, and rectum.

Drinking beyond the level of moderate drinking further escalates the risk for the development of cancer in women. Said the researchers, "For every additional drink regularly consumed per day, the increased incidence up to age 75 years per 1000 for women in developed countries is estimated to be about 11 for breast cancer, 1 for cancers of the oral cavity and pharynx, 1 for cancer of the rectum, and 0.7 each for cancers of the esophagus, larynx and liver, giving a total excess of about 15 cancers per 1,000 women up to age 75." Clearly, increasing one's drinking level is particularly dangerous for women with a history of breast cancer in their family.

Alcoholic Liver Disease Studies have shown that women develop alcoholic hepatitis and CIRRHOSIS of the liver after shorter periods of heavy drinking than men. About twice as many men die of cirrhosis than women, because many more men are heavy drinkers than women. But women develop cirrhosis earlier at any level of alcohol consumption than men do. This may be because estrogen increases the liver's susceptibility to damage from alcohol. Genetic factors may also be implicated, or the cause may be the generally smaller liver size of women. Other factors that are yet to be discovered may also be implicated.

A Risk for Alcoholic Cardiomyopathy and Myopathy in Women Based on a study that included 50 alcoholic women without health symptoms, 100 alcoholic men without symptoms, and 50 female nonalcoholic controls, researchers found that although the female alcoholics in their study had consumed only about 60 percent of the amount of alcohol used by male alcoholics, their risk for cardiomyopathy (problems with heart muscles) as well as myopathy (problems with other muscles in the body) were the same among female alcoholics as the risk seen among male alcoholics. A. Urbano-Marquez and colleagues reported on the study, conducted in Spain, in the *Journal of the American Medical Association* in 1995.

Strength was assessed with a treadmill exercise electrocardiogram, an echocardiogram, a radionuclide cardiac angiography, and with a muscle biopsy. The researchers concluded that female alcoholics were significantly more sensitive to the toxic effects of alcohol on striated muscle than were male alcoholics.

Hospital Patients with Alcohol-Related Problems Among HOSPITAL PATIENTS, most patients who arrive at hospitals and trauma centers with alcohol-related injuries are men. According to research published in *The Journal of Trauma* in 2000 from Larry M. Gentilello, M.D. and colleagues, however, female alcoholics who go to trauma centers are just as severely impaired and have greater evidence of

alcohol-related physical and psychological harm. For example, the researchers found that 14.1 percent of the women reported physical abuse in the past 30 days compared to 2.5 percent of the men. Even more disturbing, 32.1 percent of the women reported recent sexual abuse compared to 5.9 percent of the men. The researchers also found that the alcoholic female trauma patients were more likely than the men to have liver dysfunction.

Heavy Drinking and Osteoporosis Moderate drinking may decrease the risk for osteoporosis (see MODERATE DRINKING AND HEALTH BENEFITS) among women, but conversely, heavy drinking significantly escalates the risk. Many women who drink also smoke. The combination of alcohol and nicotine further increases the risk of fractures and osteoporosis in this group.

Risky Sexual Behavior and STDs Women who binge drink may have a greater risk for developing sexually transmitted diseases (STDs). In a study of recent alcohol use and sexual behaviors by Heidi E. Hutton and colleagues and published in 2008 in *Alcoholism: Clinical and Experimental Research,* the researchers found that the rates of binge drinking among all 671 patients who were tested for STDs was high, or 30 percent of the women and 42 percent of the men. (These are people who went to a clinic to be tested; hence, they knew that they were at risk for STDs.) The researchers found that among women, binge drinking was significantly associated with engaging in risky sexual behaviors and receiving a diagnosis of STD; for example, gonorrhea was almost five times higher among the female binge drinkers compared to female abstainers. The rate of risky sexual behaviors and STDs was also high among men, but it did not differ according to their use of alcohol.

The researchers found that some risky sexual behaviors among women increased with greater use of alcohol. Anal sex is a risky behavior because condoms are rarely used and the anus is receptive to bacteria. In the study, anal sex among women increased at a linear rate among women based on their alcohol use. No alcohol use was associated with an 11.1 percent rate of anal sex, while women who used alcohol without binging had an anal sex rate of 15.6 percent. Among women who binged on alcohol, the rate of anal sex increased to 33.3

percent or three times the rate of women who did not drink and more than twice the rate of women who drank but did not binge.

An estimated 40.5 percent of women who binge drank had multiple sexual partners compared to those who abstained from alcohol, who had a rate of 16.87 percent. Said the researchers, "Among women, binge drinking is uniquely associated with risky sexual behaviors and an STD diagnosis. Our findings support the need to routinely screen for binge drinking as part of standard clinical care in STD clinics, particularly among women." They added, "Developing gender-specific interventions that focus on binge drinking and certain risky sexual behaviors may improve overall health outcomes in this population."

Female Hormonal Issues and Drinking Even moderate drinking among adolescents may affect their growth, and heavy drinking is more likely to cause growth problems. In addition, alcohol abuse and alcohol dependence disrupt menstrual cycles among women of all ages and can lead to infertility or spontaneous abortion (sudden and unplanned death of the fetus). Heavy drinking can cause irregular or missing menstrual cycles as well as painful menstruation. Chronic heavy drinking may cause an early onset of menopause.

Women who drink heavily often have menstrual and reproductive problems. The use of alcohol, including a mild to moderate use, can disrupt the onset of female puberty, and it may also impair adolescent growth and the health of the bones. After the onset of puberty, alcohol can affect normal reproductive functions, such as with disrupting the monthly menstrual cycle. Subsequent to menopause, alcohol can significantly increase the risk for the development of osteoporosis in older women.

Psychiatric Comorbidities in Women with Alcohol Disorders

Women who are alcohol abusers or alcohol dependent have a high risk of psychiatric comorbidities, including DEPRESSION, BIPOLAR DISORDER, personality disorders, anxiety disorders, and eating disorders.

Depression When comparing women who have alcohol use disorders (alcohol abuse or alcoholism) as well as those with drug disorders, researchers Monica L. Zilberman, M.D., and col-

leagues reported their findings of an analysis of studies in the *Canadian Journal of Psychiatry* in 2003. The researchers reported that women had higher rates of psychiatric comorbidities than men, especially in terms of diagnoses of anxiety disorders and mood disorders.

They also found that when there was a comorbid diagnosis of depression along with substance abuse, depression was more often the primary diagnosis in women, while among men depression was more frequently a diagnosis that was secondary to substance abuse. In addition, the researchers found that women with depression apparently responded better to antidepressants in the category of selective serotonin reuptake inhibitors (SSRIs), while depressed men seemed to respond better to tricyclic antidepressants.

The researchers also found that women with depression and an alcohol use disorder had a better outcome than women with only one disorder; however, the opposite was true for men, who did better when they had no comorbidities.

Bipolar Disorder Women with bipolar disorder have an increased risk for developing alcohol dependence. Diane Snow, Tonia Smith, and Susan Branham reported in their discussion of women with bipolar disorder who use alcohol and other drugs, published in 2009 in the *Journal of Addictions Nursing*, "Since women with bipolar disorder are at an extraordinarily high risk for alcoholism, it is recommended that mental health practitioners routinely assess alcohol and substance use in this group."

Personality Disorders and Disruptive Behavioral Disorders ANTISOCIAL PERSONALITY DISORDER is a psychiatric disorder that is directly associated with an increased risk for alcohol abuse and alcoholism in both men and women. Female prisoners (who have a greater risk than other women of a diagnosis of antisocial personality disorder) also often have a much greater risk for alcohol dependence than does the average law-abiding citizen. The authors of *Women Under the Influence*, published by the National Center on Addiction and Substance Abuse at Columbia University (CASA) in 2006, also noted that women with a childhood history of CONDUCT DISORDER are almost five times more likely to have alcohol dependence in adulthood than other women. In contrast, boys with conduct disorder have about twice the risk for alcohol dependence in adulthood as compared to boys without conduct disorder.

The authors speculated that this may be because conduct disorder is rarely diagnosed in girls; consequently, those outlying girls who have conduct disorder may experience more peer rejection than others, and they may also be more likely to associate with others who exhibit problematic behavior.

Anxiety Disorders In their chapter on women and alcohol, Stewart et al. said that women with any anxiety disorder have about twice the risk of women without anxiety disorder of a comorbid alcohol diagnosis, which is not a finding among men. Many researchers have noted the high risk of anxiety disorders among alcoholic women. (See ANXIETY DISORDERS.)

Eating Disorders The risks of eating disorders are increased among alcoholic women. Those who engage in binge eating and drinking often report problems with a loss of control as well as with using alcohol or food to help them cope with stress and deal with emotional issues. According to G. Terence Wilson in his chapter on eating disorders and addictive disorders in *Eating Disorders and Obesity*, alcoholics with eating disorders are generally younger than alcoholics without eating disorders. In addition, often the eating disorder comes first, which causes some researchers to believe that an eating disorder is preceding risk for alcoholism.

Recommends Wilson, "Given the association between eating disorders and psychoactive substance abuse, women seeking treatment for eating disorders should be routinely screened for the presence of substance abuse. Similarly, women in treatment primarily for substance abuse problems should be assessed for disturbances in eating. In cases where eating and substance abuse disorders co-occur, the latter [the substance abuse] should generally be treated first. Once the substance abuse problem is under control, attention can then be directed to the eating problem. If the alcohol or drug abuse is not severe, it may be possible to treat the two problems simultaneously."

Genetic and Environmental Issues

In considering genetic factors that are related to alcohol dependence, genetics appears to play a stronger role among males than females; however, some studies indicate that genetics may also play a major role in females. A study by Mimy Y. Eng, Marc A. Schuckit, and Tom L. Smith that was reported in 2005 in *Drug and Alcohol Dependence* compared 25 women with a family history positive for alcohol dependence with 25 women with no family history of dependence.

They sought to determine whether the "family history positives" had a lower response to alcohol than the women without a family history of alcohol dependence. Past research has indicated that individuals who become intoxicated more slowly than others may have an increased risk for substance abuse. In this study, the researchers found that, in fact, the family history positives *did* have a lower rate of intoxication. Said the researchers, "The results suggest that, similar to sons of alcoholics, a low LR [level of response] to alcohol might also be characteristic of daughters of alcoholics."

Family issues are relevant to drinking that occurs among teenagers as well as women. For example, sometimes drinking starts in adolescence because teenagers feel (or know) that their parents approve of drinking.

Say the authors of *Women Under the Influence*, "Whenever parents don't clearly communicate anti-substance-use messages to their children, they put their children at increased risk for substance use; this is especially true for drinking. Because drinking is a regular part of most adults' lives and many see it as a normal rite of passage for teens, many parents inadvertently encourage their daughters' drinking by being too lenient and permissive. For example, 18 percent of teens (25% of 15 to 17 year olds) report having attended a party in the past two years at which parents purchased alcohol for them or served alcohol to them."

Women Who Drink Heavily Risk Assault

Studies have shown that women who drink heavily, particularly those who are college students, have an increased risk for being raped. In a study reported by M. Mohler-Kuo and colleagues in the *Journal of Studies in Alcohol* in 2004, the researchers randomly sampled thousands of college women and found that 4.7 percent reported having been raped. Among those who were raped, 72 percent said that they had been raped while they were intoxicated.

The researchers found that the college women who were most at risk for rape had the following characteristics:

- under age 21
- white
- lived in sorority houses
- drank heavily in high school
- attended colleges with high rates of binge drinking
- used illegal drugs

Older Women and Alcoholism

Older women have physical risk factors that make them susceptible to harm from heavy alcohol consumption. For example, an age-related decrease in lean muscle mass makes them more vulnerable to the negative effects of alcohol. In addition, older women have a greater response to prescription drugs, and as a result, combining alcohol with drugs is especially dangerous for older women.

According to Frederic C. Blow and Kristen Lawton Barry in their 2003 article for the NIAAA, "Older women are more likely than older men to receive prescriptions for benzodiazepines in particular, and therefore more likely to be faced with problems related to the interaction of these medications with alcohol." According to Blow and Barry, from 1 to 8 percent of older women misuse alcohol.

Yet older women with alcohol dependence are less likely to be diagnosed than alcoholic older men. Because doctors do not expect to see alcohol abuse or dependence in older women, they, therefore, often do not see it, even when it exists. Blow and Barry recommend that everyone age 60 and older be screened for both alcohol and prescription drug abuse on an annual basis.

Some symptoms and signs of alcohol misuse in older women may include the following indicators that are listed below. (Note that not all older women with these signs and symptoms are alcohol abusers. There are many health problems that can cause these signs and symptoms, and alcohol misuse is only one factor that should be considered.)

- depression, mood swings
- poor hygiene
- an increased tolerance to alcohol or medications
- falls, bruises, burns
- seizures with no known causes
- headaches
- social isolation
- incontinence
- poor nutrition
- memory loss
- disorientation

Experts at NIAAA report that excessive drinking may increase the risk for Alzheimer's disease, especially since women appear to be more vulnerable than men to alcohol-related brain damage.

Drinking among Pregnant Women and Recent Mothers

According to the Substance Abuse and Mental Health Services Administration (SAMHSA), data from 2006–07 indicates that although drinking rates were lower among pregnant women than in past years, nearly 16 percent of pregnant females ages 15–17 years old used alcohol in the past month and consumed an average of 24 drinks in the month. These rates have not changed significantly since 2002, despite attempts to make the public aware of the severe risks of drinking during pregnancy. (See Table 1 for further information.)

College Graduates Who Drink During Pregnancy
Surprisingly, some women who drink during their pregnancy are college graduates with incomes at or exceeding $75,000. For example, 15.8 percent of pregnant college graduates drink during pregnancy, the highest rate of all educational levels. However, as can be seen from Table 1, it should also be noted that 69.7 percent of college graduates drink when they are *not* pregnant, so clearly there is some "cutting back" during pregnancy. Disturbingly, more than half, or 53.7 percent of recent mothers who are college graduates, consume alcohol; again, this is the highest percentage of all educational categories.

Yet it should also be noted that the research shows that college graduate females drink the

TABLE 1
PERCENTAGES OF PAST MONTH ALCOHOL USE AMONG WOMEN AGES 15–44 YEARS,
BY PREGNANCY STATUS AND DEMOGRAPHIC CHARACTERISTICS: 2006 AND 2007

Demographic Characteristic	Pregnant	Recent Mothers	Nonpregnant, Not Recent Mothers
Age			
15 to 17	15.8	26.8	25.3
18 to 25	9.8	41.2	62.2
26 to 44	12.5	42.9	55.7
Race/Ethnicity			
White	14.5	52.1	61.1
Black	15.7	31.9	44.6
Hispanic	4.1	22.9	41.6
Education Status			
Less than high school	8.9	28.1	37.7
High school graduates	8.3	35.7	51.8
Some college	11.7	45.6	60.9
College graduates	15.8	53.7	69.7
Income			
Less than $20,000	11.7	30.9	47.3
$20,000 to $49,999	9.2	38.3	50.7
$50,000 to $74,999	9.5	47.1	55.2
$75,000 or Higher	16.3	54.4	62.2

Source: Substance Abuse and Mental Health Services Administration. "Alcohol Use among Pregnant Women and Recent Mothers: 2006 to 2007." *NSDUH Report.* September 11, 2008. Page 3.

fewest number of drinks when educational statuses are compared as shown in Table 2; for example, they drank an average of 1.6 drinks per month when pregnant, compared to those with less than a high school education, who drank an average of 4.5 drinks, which was the highest reported level. Again, experts report that *any* level of alcohol consumption during pregnancy is potentially dangerous for the fetus.

Protective Factors against Drinking In women of all ages, some protective factors decrease the odds of alcohol abuse and alcoholism; for example, if their parents did not drink, then female adults are less likely to drink. If a partner does not drink, the woman is less likely to drink. When her friends are nondrinkers or moderate drinkers, a woman is less likely to abuse or depend on alcohol.

According to data from *Women Under the Influence*, women who are religious are significantly less likely to have a problem with drinking than are women who say that they are not religious. For example, about 91 percent of women who identify themselves as not religious consume alcohol and about 45 percent are current smokers. This is in stark contrast to those who say that they are Catholic (64 percent drink and 25 percent smoke) or Protestant (52 percent drink and 21 percent smoke). (See RELIGION.)

See also ALCOHOL AND MEN; ALCOHOL AND OTHER DRUGS; ALCOHOLISM/ALCOHOL DEPENDENCE AND ALCOHOL ABUSE; CHILD ABUSE AND NEGLECT; EXCESSIVE DRINKING AND HEALTH CONSEQUENCES; TREATMENT; VIOLENCE.

Allen, Naomi E., et al. "Moderate Alcohol Intake and Cancer Incidence in Women." *Journal of the National Cancer Institute* 101, no. 5 (2009): 296–305.

Barber, J. G., et al. "Intrapersonal versus Peer Group Predictors of Adolescent Drug Use." *Children and Youth Services Review* 21, no. 7 (1999): 565–579.

Blow, Frederic C., and Kristen Lawton Barry. "Use and Misuse of Alcohol among Older Women." Bethesda, Md.: National Institute on Alcohol Abuse and Alcohol-

TABLE 2
AVERAGE NUMBER OF ALCOHOLIC DRINKS CONSUMED PER DAY ON THE DAYS THAT ALCOHOL
WAS USED IN THE PAST MONTH AMONG PAST MONTH FEMALE ALCOHOL USERS AGES 15 TO 44 YEARS,
BY PREGNANCY STATUS AND DEMOGRAPHIC CHARACTERISTICS: 2006–2007

Demographic Characteristic	Pregnant	Recent Mothers	Nonpregnant, Not Recent Mothers
Age			
15 to 17	3.6	Not available	4.1
18 to 25	3.6	3.4	3.6
26 to 44	1.7	2.0	2.6
Race/Ethnicity			
White	1.9	2.6	3.0
Black	3.1	1.9	2.5
Hispanic	4.6	2.5	3.1
Education Status			
Less than high school	4.5	3.5	4.1
High school graduates	2.6	2.9	3.4
Some college	2.1	2.7	3.0
College graduates	1.6	1.7	2.2
Income			
Less than $20,000	3.7	3.1	3.7
$20,000 to $49,999	2.2	2.8	3.2
$50,000 to $74,999	2.3	2.0	2.8
$75,000 or Higher	1.6	2.1	2.5

Source: Substance Abuse and Mental Health Services Administration. "Alcohol Use among Pregnant Women and Recent Mothers: 2006 to 2007."
NSDUH Report. September 11, 2008. Page 4.

ism, 2003. Available online. URL: http://pubs.niaaa.
nih.gov/publications/arh26-4/308-315.htm. Accessed
March 20, 2009.

Burckell, Lisa A., and Shelley McMain. "Concurrent Personality Disorders and Substance Use Disorders in Women." In *Women & Addiction: A Comprehensive Handbook,* edited by Kathleen T. Brady, Sudie E. Back, and Shelly F. Greenfield, 269–285. New York: The Guilford Press, 2009.

Eng, Mimy Y., Marc A. Schuckit, and Tom L. Smith. "The Level of Response to Alcohol in Daughters of Alcoholics and Controls." *Drug and Alcohol Dependence* 79, no. 1 (2005): 83–93.

Gentilello, L. M., et al. "Alcohol Problems in Women Admitted to a Level I Trauma Center: A Gender-Based Comparison." *The Journal of Trauma: Injury, Infection, and Critical Care* 48, no. 1 (2000): 108–114.

Hutton, Heidi E., et al. "The Relationship between Recent Alcohol Use and Sexual Behaviors: Gender Differences Among Sexually Transmitted Diseases Clinic Patients." *Alcoholism: Clinical and Experimental Research* 32, no. 11 (2008): 2,008–2,015.

LaBrie, Joseph W., et al. "What Men Want: The Role of Reflective Opposite-Sex Normative Preferences in Alcohol Use among College Women." *Psychology of Addictive Behaviors* 23, no. 1 (2009): 157–162.

Mohler-Kuo, M., et al. "Correlates of Rape While Intoxicated in a National Sample of College Women." *Journal of Studies on Alcohol* 65, no. 1 (2004): 37–45.

National Center on Addiction and Substance Abuse at Columbia University. *Women Under the Influence.* Baltimore, Md.: Johns Hopkins University Press, 2006.

National Institute on Alcohol Abuse and Alcoholism. "Alcohol—An Important Women's Health Issue." *Alcohol Alert* no. 62 (July 2004): 1–6.

———. *Alcohol: A Women's Issue.* Bethesda, Md.: National Institutes of Health, 2008.

Nolen-Hoeksema, Susan. "Gender Differences in Risk Factors and Consequences for Alcohol Use and Problems." *Clinical Psychology Review* 24, no. 8 (2004): 981–1,010.

Register, Thomas D., et al. "Health Issues in Postmenopausal Women Who Drink." *Alcohol Research & Health* 26, no. 4 (2002): 299–307.

Urbano-Marquez, A., et al. "The Greater Risk of Alcoholic Cardiomyopathy and Myopathy in Women Compared with Men." *Journal of the American Medical Association* 274, no. 2 (1995): 149–154.

Snow, Diane, et al. "Women with Bipolar Disorder Who Use Alcohol and Other Drugs." *Journal of Addictions Nursing* 19 (2008): 55–60.

Stewart, Sherry H., Dubravka Gavric, and Pamela Collins. "Women, Girls, and Alcohol." In *Women & Addiction: A Comprehensive Handbook,* edited by Kathleen T. Brady, Sudie E. Back, and Shelly F. Greenfield, 341–359. New York: The Guilford Press, 2009.

Wilson, G. Terence. "Eating Disorders and Addictive Disorders." In *Eating Disorders and Obesity: A Comprehensive Handbook,* 2nd ed., edited by Christopher G. Fairburn and Kelly D. Brownell, 199–203. New York: Guilford Press, 2002.

Zilberman, Monica L., M.D., et al. "Substance Use Disorders: Sex Differences and Psychiatric Comorbidities." *Canadian Journal of Psychiatry* 48, no. 1 (2003): 5–15.

alcohol-containing mouthwash   See CANCER.

alcohol flushing response   A response to alcohol that is present among more than a third (about 36 percent) of East Asians, such as individuals who are Japanese, Korean, and Chinese. It is an inherited deficiency in the aldehyde dehydrogenase 2 (ALDH2) enzymes. If alcohol is consumed by individuals with this deficiency, it causes facial reddening, nausea, and rapid heartbeat. For some people, drinking alcohol causes a response similar to the response alcoholics in treatment with DISULFIRAM would experience if they consumed alcohol. This is because these individuals cannot metabolize aldehyde dehydrogenase into ACETALDEHYDE. Worldwide, there are an estimated 540 million individuals who are deficient in ALDH2 and who would exhibit alcohol flushing response if they drank any alcohol.

Many people with alcohol flushing response do not drink at all, which may be why drinking rates are generally lower among Asians; however, if the response is not severe, some will consume alcohol anyway. This is a dangerous choice because an ALDH2 deficiency combined with even moderate drinking causes an increased risk for esophageal CANCER (or more specifically, squamous cell car-

cinoma in the esophagus) according to Philip J. Brooks and colleagues in their 2009 article in *PLoS Medicine.* This is an extremely severe and often fatal cancer of the food tube. According to the authors, if Japanese male heavy or moderate drinkers with the ALDH2 deficiency changed to drank only lightly, then more than half (53 percent) of esophageal squamous cell carcinomas could be prevented.

Patients of Asian ancestry should tell their doctors if they experience the alcohol flushing response. Doctors should also ask patients of Asian ancestry if they experience alcohol flushing response if they drink and explain to them the importance of avoiding alcohol if they do have such a response.

Patients can also receive the ethanol patch test, described by Brooks et al., in which a patch of 0.1 ml of 70 percent ethanol is placed onto a 15 × 15 mm lint pad placed on an adhesive tape. The tape is then placed on the patient's upper arm for 10–15 minutes to see if redness occurs in the area.

Brooks and his colleagues are also concerned about COLLEGE STUDENTS with alcohol flushing response who drink. They say, "There are many East Asians now living in Western societies, particularly at universities and in metropolitan areas. A subpopulation of special concern is ALDH2-deficient university students who may face peer pressure for heavy drinking and binge drinking. Furthermore, anecdotal evidence indicates that some young people view the facial flushing response as a cosmetic problem and use antihistamines in an effort to blunt the flushing while continuing to drink alcohol. This practice is expected to increase the likelihood of developing esophageal cancer."

See also GENETICS AND ALCOHOL.

Brooks, Philip J., et al. "The Alcohol Flushing Response: An Unrecognized Risk Factor for Esophageal Cancer from Alcohol Consumption." *PLoS Medicine* 6, no. 2 (2009): 258–263.

alcoholic blackouts   Periods of a lack of cognitive awareness and a subsequent form of amnesia that are caused by extreme alcohol intoxication. During this time the individual may be moving about, speaking to others, and performing other actions;

for example, the individual in the course of a blackout may engage in unprotected sex with others and some individuals even drive their cars while in an alcoholic blackout state. The National Institute on Alcohol Abuse and Alcoholism (NIAAA) said in 2004 in *Alcohol Alert* that when large quantities of alcohol are consumed very quickly, particularly on an empty stomach, this circumstance can create an alcoholic blackout. Alcoholic blackouts were first identified by E. M. Jellinek in his studies on individuals with alcoholism in the 1940s, based on a survey of members of Alcoholics Anonymous.

The BLOOD ALCOHOL CONCENTRATION level of the person who is in a blackout state is estimated to be between 0.25 and 0.29, or about three times the legal definition of intoxication (0.08) in most states. There is no loss of physical consciousness during a blackout, which may last for minutes, hours, or even for several days. The individual later remembers little or nothing that occurred during the blackout period, nor will he or she recall these events at a later time. The occurrence of an alcoholic blackout is an indicator of alcohol abuse and is also a risk indicator for alcohol dependence.

According to researcher Aaron White in his article for *Alcohol Research & Health* in 2003, the following actions happen to the brain during an alcoholic blackout. "Alcohol disrupts activity in the hippocampus via several routes—directly, through effects on hippocampal circuitry, and indirectly, by interfering with interactions between the hippocampus and other brain regions. The impact of alcohol on the frontal lobes remains poorly understood, but probably plays an important role in alcohol-induced memory impairments."

Research on college students by White revealed that blackouts can also occur to social drinkers and are not limited solely to alcoholics. White and his colleagues surveyed 772 college undergraduates, asking such questions as, "Have you ever awoken after a night of drinking not able to remember things that you did or places that you went?" The results: 51 percent of students who ever consumed alcohol said they had blacked out at some point and 40 percent said that they had had a blackout in the year before the survey. Of those students who reported drinking in the two weeks before the survey, 9.4 percent said that they had blacked

out at some point during that time. Both men and women reported experiencing about the same number of blackouts.

Blackouts are also associated with BINGE DRINKING, which is defined as drinking five or more drinks in two hours for men or consuming four or more drinks within two hours for women. Because college students are at risk for binge drinking, they also have an increased risk for experiencing blackouts.

ADDICTIVE PERSONALITY; ALCOHOL AND ALCOHOL USE; ALCOHOLIC PSYCHOSIS; ALCOHOLISM/ALCOHOL DEPENDENCE AND ALCOHOL ABUSE; ALCOHOL POISONING; COLLEGE STUDENTS; EXCESSIVE DRINKING AND HEALTH CONSEQUENCES; UNDERAGE DRINKING.

National Institute on Alcohol Abuse and Alcoholism. "Alcohol's Damaging Effects on the Brain." *Alcohol Alert* 63 (October 2004): 1–7.

White, Aaron M. "What Happened? Alcohol, Memory Blackouts, and the Brain." *Alcohol Research & Health* 27, no. 2 (2003): 186–196.

White, A. M., D. W. Jamieson-Drake, and H. S. Swartzwelder. "Prevalence and Correlates of Alcohol-induced Blackouts among College Students: Results of an E-mail Survey." *Journal of American College Health* 51, no. 3 (2002): 117–131.

alcoholic hepatitis See HEPATITIS; LIVER DISEASES, ALCOHOLIC.

alcoholic liver disease See HEPATITIS; LIVER DISEASES, ALCOHOLIC.

alcoholic psychosis Severe mental illness that is caused by alcohol dependence. According to the National Institute for Alcohol Abuse and Alcoholism (NIAAA), in 2005, for the first time the number of cases of alcoholic psychoses surpassed the number of cases of alcohol dependence syndrome in hospital discharge diagnoses, and this pattern continued in 2006, the latest information available as of this writing. The NIAAA reported that more than a third (34.5 percent) of principal alcohol diagnoses were for alcoholic psychosis, followed by alcohol dependence syndrome (29.5 percent),

CIRRHOSIS of the liver (27.0 percent), and nondependent abuse of alcohol (9.1 percent). There were an estimated 430,000 hospital discharges in the United States for individuals ages 15 and older with a principal (first-listed) alcohol-related diagnosis in 2006. In addition, there were 1.7 million discharges in which any diagnosis was related to alcohol.

The NIAAA reported that the following diagnostic classifications were included under the umbrella of alcoholic psychoses: alcohol withdrawal delirium; alcohol amnesic syndrome; other alcoholic dementia; alcohol withdrawal hallucinosis; idiosyncratic alcohol intoxication; alcoholic jealousy; other specified alcoholic psychosis; unspecified alcoholic psychosis. Diagnoses that were classified under the umbrella of alcohol dependence syndrome included the following: acute alcoholic intoxication; other and unspecified alcohol dependence; pellagra; alcoholic polyneuropathy; alcoholic cardiomyopathy; and alcoholic gastritis.

According to the NIAAA, the average length of hospital stay for alcoholic psychosis was 4.7 days. In contrast, the average stay for alcoholic cirrhosis was 5.4 days, and it was 4.7 days for alcohol dependence syndrome. The average stay for nondependent abuse of alcohol was 2.2 days.

See also BIPOLAR DISORDER; DELIRIUM TREMENS; PSYCHIATRIC COMORBIDITIES; SCHIZOPHRENIA; TREATMENT; WERNICKE-KORSAKOFF SYNDROME.

Chen, Chiung M., and Hsiao-ye Yi. *Surveillance Report #84: Trends in Alcohol-Related Morbidity among Short-Stay Community Hospital Discharges, United States, 1979–2006.* National Institute on Alcohol Abuse and Alcoholism. Rockville, Md.: National Institutes of Health, August 2008.

alcoholic steatosis See EXCESSIVE DRINKING AND HEALTH CONSEQUENCES; LIVER DISEASES, ALCOHOLIC.

alcoholism/alcohol dependence and alcohol abuse Alcohol is the most commonly abused drug in the United States by adolescents, college students, young adults, and many other adults. Its excesses can cause a lifetime of devastation for those who do not seek treatment and recovery as well as for their families. In addition, alcohol abuse and dependence are harmful to those around them, such as those who are injured or even killed in drunken car crashes or assaults.

Important Basic Statistics

According to the National Epidemiologic Survey on Alcohol and Related Conditions (NESARC) data for 2001–02, an estimated 4.7 percent of the U.S. population ages 18 years and older fit the criteria over 12 months for alcohol abuse disorder, and 3.8 percent meet the criteria for alcohol dependence. (This means that over the course of one year, these percentages of individuals would be diagnosed with alcohol abuse or alcoholism.) In addition, the lifetime rates (of ever having these disorders) were 17.8 percent for alcohol abuse and 12.5 percent for alcohol dependence.

Extrapolating to 2010 by translating the percentage data into terms of the U.S. population ages 18 and older into the projected U.S. Census population for 2010 (when there will be an estimated 235,016,000 people in the United States ages 18 years and older), and assuming that percentages of those with alcohol use disorders (alcohol abuse and dependence together) remain about the same, this then means that an estimated 11,045,752 people will have a 12-month alcohol abuse diagnosis in 2010 and an estimated 8,930,608 will have a 12-month alcohol dependence—for a total of 19,976,360, or nearly 20 million people, with alcohol use disorders.

It also means that an estimated 41,832,848 will have a lifetime alcohol abuse diagnosis and an estimated 29,377,000 will have a lifetime diagnosis of alcoholism in 2010 for a total of about 71.2 million people with alcohol use disorders. (See Table 1.)

Considering Terminology

To fully comprehend the key issues surrounding alcoholism and alcohol abuse, it is helpful to understand some basic terminology; for example, as mentioned, alcohol abuse and alcoholism are together known as *alcohol use disorders* by the American Psychiatric Association. Yet the phrase "substance abuse" is also frequently used and it is often unclear as to what substance is meant. Sometimes "substance abuse" is used to denote either or both alcohol abuse and alcohol dependence; this

TABLE 1
ESTIMATED NUMBERS OF INDIVIDUALS WITH 12-MONTH AND LIFETIME ALCOHOL USE DISORDERS,
BASED ON NESARC DATA AND THE PROJECTED U.S. POPULATION IN 2010

Characteristic	12-Month, Estimated Numbers			Lifetime, Estimated Numbers		
	Alcohol Use Disorder	Alcohol Abuse	Alcohol Dependence	Alcohol Use Disorder	Alcohol Abuse	Alcohol Dependence
Total	19,976,360	11,045,752	8,930,608	71,209,848	41,832,848	29,377,000

Source: NESARC data for 2001–02 was used and generalized to the 2010 population, based on U.S. Census estimated figures: U.S. Census Bureau. See Table 3 for percentage of totals that were used to extrapolate this data.

term is also used to connote abuse or dependence on alcohol that is combined with abuse and/or dependence on illicit drugs. (And sometimes substance abuse refers only to illicit drug use.) Many people assume that the phrase "substance abuse" refers to marijuana abuse or cocaine addiction, and although it is true that it *may* refer to these behaviors, the individual using the term could be alluding to alcohol abuse alone. As a result, when the term "substance abuse" is used, it is best to ascertain what type of substances are being considered and also whether abuse or addiction (dependence) is being discussed.

Alcohol dependence is itself another important term and it refers to the same behavior as defined by the word *alcoholism:* an addictive use of alcohol. In 1849, Magnus Huss, a Swedish physician, first used the term *alcoholism* in *Alcoholismus Chronicus.* According to Virginia Berridge and Sarah Mars in their article for the *Journal of Epidemiology and Public Health* in 2003, the term *dependence* was first used by the World Health Organization in 1964 as a word to replace both *addiction* and *habituation.* Today, many experts prefer the term *alcohol dependence* to the word alcoholism, which they regard as pejorative.

The Impact of Alcohol Use Disorders

The impact of alcohol abuse and alcoholism extends far beyond the bounds of terminology and semantics; for example, alcoholism could be called "sad fluffy disease" and its effects would be no less damaging to the lives of those who are harmed by this problematic behavior. Alcohol use disorders also have a profound impact on society that extends well beyond their effect on individuals who abuse or depend on alcohol.

For example, a family of nondrinkers may regard themselves as living in a safe and secure environment, but their world can come crashing down instantly when a spouse or a child is injured or killed by a drunken driver or when the family is robbed and assaulted by someone who is high on alcohol and drugs. The family is traumatized, and the criminal justice system and possibly the media become involved. The average family in the neighboring area feels less safe, even though they are not directly affected.

Or the situation may be more mundane, as when a nondrinking family allows their teenage daughter to attend a party where they know that another teen's parents will be present. What they might never imagine is that the other girl's parents will not only condone UNDERAGE DRINKING but will actually serve alcohol to the girls who come to their home, somehow perceiving this behavior as enlightened. It might seem rude to an adolescent girl to not drink at such a gathering, and so the girl takes her first drink at age 14 or 15, rapidly becoming intoxicated, and then ill. After a few such parties, drinking may start to seem cool or normal to the teenager, and by the time her parents finally realize to their horror what is going on at these parties, it is hard to slam the door shut on this new peer-accepted behavior. Study after study shows that teenage drinking that starts early, before age 14 or 15, increases the risk for alcohol dependence in adulthood.

Sometimes drinking occurs in the child's family, where one or both parents may drink until they pass out, leaving their children, including sometimes very small children, to wander about and fend for themselves. It is not rare to hear on the news about a toddler discovered wandering near an interstate highway or the train tracks. No one had reported the child as missing because the parents were too intoxicated to realize or care that the child was gone. The child welfare authorities may then become involved to perform an investigation and follow-up visits, and the court system subsequently also becomes involved, with all the costs borne by the taxpayers.

Parental bad behavior stemming from alcohol use sometimes extends into physical abuse and sexual abuse, as when parents ignore or are unaware of sexual harm perpetrated by their boyfriends or others on their children. CHILD ABUSE AND NEGLECT represent serious social problems that are directly tied to alcoholism and alcohol abuse, as well as to the combined abuse of ALCOHOL AND OTHER DRUGS.

Of course, not everyone who consumes alcohol drinks to excess. In the United States and other countries, many people use alcohol sparingly. Such individuals drink alcohol in moderation, and they may enjoy enhanced health benefits as a result of their limited drinking. About one glass of wine or beer per day for women and two glasses for men are considered moderate drinking. (See MODERATE DRINKING AND HEALTH BENEFITS.) However, others use alcohol to excess, and some use this substance illegally, such as minors who consume alcohol for the sole purpose of getting drunk.

Although alcohol abuse and alcoholism are two separate disorders, the alcohol abuser's drinking may escalate to the level of alcohol dependence. For this reason, it is best to identify alcohol abuse before that point is reached, so that the person can take actions to avoid the severe psychiatric and physical health problems that often accompany alcohol dependence. Often a physician who realizes that alcohol abuse is a problem will make a brief intervention, advising a patient to cut back on drinking to avoid health risks; for example, a person with hypertension could suffer a stroke or heart attack as a result of excessive drinking. Such interventions generally do not work with alcoholics, but they can be very effective among alcohol abusers.

Defining Alcohol Abuse and Alcohol Dependence

According to the National Institute on Alcohol Abuse and Alcoholism (NIAAA), a person is an alcohol abuser if he or she fits even one of the following criteria:

- fails to fulfill work, school, or home responsibilities, due to alcohol use

- drives a motor vehicle or operates dangerous equipment while under the influence of alcohol

- drinks despite family or personal relationship issues that are created or worsened by the excessive drinking

- has been arrested for an alcohol-related problem, such as assaulting another person while intoxicated or driving while under the influence of alcohol

The American Psychiatric Association defines alcohol abuse in the *Diagnostic and Statistical Manual of Mental Disorders, Fourth Edition, Text Revision (DSM-IV-TR)*. This definition of alcohol abuse includes the person who uses alcohol on a recurrent basis and is also one who has failed to fulfill important family, school, or work requirements. In addition, the person has experienced legal problems on more than one occasion as a direct result of alcohol consumption.

The four essential elements of alcoholism, or alcohol dependence, according to the NIAAA, are:

1. An overwhelming craving or need to drink
2. A loss of control and an inability to stop drinking once the person has started drinking
3. Physical dependence on alcohol, such that the individual exhibits such withdrawal symptoms as anxiety, nausea, shakiness, and sweating if they stop drinking
4. Tolerance or the need to drink greater amounts of alcohol in order to achieve the same level of intoxication

In general, individuals are defined as alcohol-dependent when they meet three or more of the following criteria:

1. Addictive behavior: The individual spends much time getting, using, or recovering from the effects of alcohol.
2. Lack of control: The individual uses alcohol more often than he or she intends to and/or cannot set limits on alcohol use.
3. Tolerance: The person needs to use an increasing amount of alcohol to achieve the desired state of intoxication or notices that the same amount of

alcohol has less effect than in the past. In this case, the person has developed a *tolerance* to alcohol.

4. Unable to stop: The person cannot cut back or stop using alcohol even when he or she tries to do so on their own.

5. Health problems: The person continues to use alcohol although its use is causing a problem with mental or physical health. For example, the person continues to use alcohol despite the development of an ulcer that is exacerbated by drinking.

6. Social losses: The person has cut back or eliminated participation in activities formerly considered important because of alcohol use.

7. Withdrawal: The individual experiences withdrawal symptoms if he or she fails to use alcohol, such as insomnia, trembling hands, or muscle cramps.

Demographics of Alcoholics in the United States

A report on data from the 2001–02 National Epidemiologic Survey on Alcohol and Related Conditions (NESARC) by Deborah A. Dawson and colleagues revealed demographic features and other data on individuals with alcohol dependence based on a sample of more than 43,000 individuals nationwide.

According to an analysis of the NESARC data, the majority of alcoholics are younger than age 45 and predominately male. The largest percentage (78.9 percent) are white, and 60 percent have attended or completed college. (However, as seen in Table 3, where NATIVE AMERICANS are included, it is clear that of all races and ethnicities, Native Americans have the greatest risk for alcohol abuse and dependence.)

The broad majority of alcoholics have a family history of alcoholism. Only about a third have *not* used illicit drugs. In addition, more than half (54.0 percent) have had a mood or anxiety disorder. See Table 2 for more details on alcoholics. Note that Table 3 provides details on individuals with both alcohol abuse and alcohol dependence. As can be seen from Table 3, Asians have the lowest rates of alcohol use disorders. This may be due in part because of the ALCOHOL FLUSHING RESPONSE inherited by some Asians, which causes an extremely red face if they drink any alcohol. Some Asians also have a more severe response to alcohol, and drinking causes nausea and vomiting. (See GENETICS AND ALCOHOL.)

TABLE 2
PERCENTAGE DISTRIBUTION OF U.S. ADULTS AGES 18 AND OLDER WITH PRIOR TO PAST-YEAR ALCOHOL DEPENDENCE, BY SELECTED CHARACTERISTICS

Characteristics	Number	Percentage Distribution
Ages 18–29	1,081	26.6
Ages 30–44	1,763	39.6
Age 45 and older	1,578	33.8
Gender		
Male	2,782	67.5
Female	1,640	32.5
Race/Ethnicity		
White, non-Hispanic	3,027	78.9
Black, non-Hispanic	566	7.1
Other, non-Hispanic	210	5.7
Hispanic	619	8.3
Education		
Less than high school graduate	591	12.3
High school graduate	1,192	27.7
Attended/completed college	2,639	60.0
Marital Status		
Married	2,096	56.6
Not married	2,326	43.5
Family History of Alcoholism		
A family history of alcoholism	3,381	76.5
No family history of alcoholism	1,041	23.5
Number of lifetime dependence symptoms		
3–9 lifetime dependence symptoms	1,354	29.5
10–14 lifetime dependence symptoms	1,468	33.4
15–19 lifetime dependence symptoms	740	17.6
20+ lifetime dependence symptoms	860	19.4
Tobacco Use		
Ever used tobacco	3,274	74.2
Never used tobacco	1,148	25.8
Use of illicit drugs		
Any dependent use of illicit drugs	658	14.7
Any nondependent use of illicit drugs	2,059	47.5
Never used illicit drugs	1,705	37.8
Lifetime diagnosis of mood/anxiety disorder		
Any lifetime mood/anxiety disorder	2,442	54.0
No lifetime mood/anxiety disorder	1,980	46.0
Personality disorder diagnoses		
Any lifetime personality disorder	1,542	34.5
No lifetime personality disorder	2,880	65.5
Total	4,422	100.0

Adapted from: Dawson, Deborah A., et al. "Recovery from *DSM-IV* Alcohol Dependence: United States, 2001–2002." *Alcohol Research & Health* 29, no. 2 (2006). Page 135.

TABLE 3
PREVALENCE OF 12-MONTH AND LIFETIME DSM-IV ALCOHOL USE DISORDERS
BY SOCIODEMOGRAPHIC CHARACTERISTICS

	12-Month, %			Lifetime, %		
	Alcohol Use Disorder (n=3,327)	Alcohol Abuse (n=1,843	Alcohol Dependence (n=1,484)	Alcohol Use Disorder (n=11,843)	Alcohol Abuse (n=7,062)	Alcohol Dependence (n=4,781)
Characteristic						
Total	8.5	4.7	3.8	30.3	17.8	12.5
Sex						
Male	12.4	6.9	5.4	42.0	24.6	17.4
Female	4.9	2.6	2.3	19.5	11.5	8.0
Race/ethnicity						
White	8.9	5.1	3.8	34.1	20.3	13.8
Black	6.9	3.3	3.6	20.6	12.2	8.4
Native American	12.1	5.8	6.4	43.0	22.9	20.1
Asian	4.5	2.1	2.4	11.6	5.6	6.0
Hispanic	7.9	4.0	4.0	21.0	11.5	9.5
Age, years						
18–29	16.2	7.0	9.2	30.1	12.8	17.3
30–44	9.7	6.0	3.8	36.7	21.4	15.4
45–64	5.4	3.5	1.9	31.4	20.4	11.0
65 and older	1.5	1.2	0.2	16.1	12.7	3.4
Marital status						
Married/cohabiting	6.1	4.0	2.1	30.4	19.5	10.9
Widowed/separated/divorced	8.1	4.4	3.7	28.8	16.5	12.3
Never married	15.9	6.9	9.0	31.2	14.0	17.2
Education						
Less than high school	7.0	3.1	4.0	23.7	13.5	10.2
High school	8.3	4.5	3.7	28.2	16.3	11.9
Some college or higher	9.0	5.2	3.8	33.2	19.8	13.4
Personal income, $						
0–19,999	7.6	3.2	4.5	23.9	12.6	11.3
20,000–34,999	9.5	5.5	4.0	32.3	18.6	13.8
35,000–69,999	9.0	6.2	2.9	37.8	23.7	14.1
$70,000 or more	8.8	6.6	2.2	41.4	30.0	11.4
Urbanicity						
Urban	8.4	4.6	3.8	29.6	17.4	12.2
Rural	8.8	4.8	4.0	33.3	19.4	13.8
Region						
Northeast	7.8	4.3	3.5	27.1	16.6	10.6
Midwest	10.6	5.9	4.6	35.3	20.7	15.0
South	7.3	4.2	3.1	27.0	16.7	10.3
West	8.8	4.5	4.3	32.6	17.6	15.1

Adapted from: the table "Prevalences of 12-Month and Lifetime DSM-IV Alcohol Use Disorders by Sociodemographic Characteristics" in the article by Deborah S. Hasin et al. "Prevalence, Correlates, Disability, and Comorbidity of DSM-IV Alcohol Abuse and Dependence in the United States: Results from the National Epidemiologic Survey on Alcohol and Related Conditions." *Archives of General Psychiatry* 64, no. 7 (2007): Page 833. [Permission pending.]

As also can be seen from Table 3, in considering marital status, never-married individuals had the highest rate of a 12-month alcohol dependence, or 9.0 percent. In sharp contrast, the rate for widowed/separated/divorced individuals was 3.7 percent and the rate for those who were currently married or cohabiting was 2.1 percent.

Predictive Factors in Childhood and Adolescence for Adult Alcohol Abuse or Dependence

Some factors are predictive for the development of alcohol use disorders, and the more of these factors that are present, the higher the risk for alcohol abuse or dependence. However, the risk is never 100 percent. Some people with no known risk factors become alcoholics while others with many risk factors do not become dependent on alcohol. The most recent research indicates that many risk factors lie within the events of childhood and adolescence, and key risk factors are the following:

- Early drinking (before age 14 or 15) is a risk factor for alcoholism in adulthood, increasing the risk for alcohol dependence by five times.

- Antisocial behavior in preadolescent children (hurting animals, destroying property, theft, and other problematic behaviors) is predictive for alcohol use disorders in adolescence.

- The presence of other traits, such as a high rate of novelty-seeking and impulsivity, is predictive of alcoholism.

- genetic risks: Individuals whose biological parents are alcoholics have an increased risk for alcohol use disorders.

- peer influences

- adverse events in childhood

- individuals who smoke

- low response to the effects of alcohol

Early Drinking Many studies have demonstrated that drinking before age 14 or 15 increases the risk for alcoholism in adulthood by up to five times. In addition, drinking increases the risk for serious accidents and many other problems among adolescents. Studies also indicate that many children *are* drinking at young ages, as young as age 10 or younger. For example, data from the National

TABLE 4
PERCENT DISTRIBUTION OF AGE FIRST HAD A DRINK OF ALCOHOL, AMONG THOSE WHO DRANK ALCOHOL, BY SELECTED CHARACTERISTICS

Characteristic	10 years or younger	11–12 years	13–14 years	15–17 years
Total	18.5	18.4	34.5	28.5
Gender				
Male	23.5	18.1	33.5	24.9
Female	13.4	18.8	35.6	32.2
Race/ethnicity				
Mexican American	15.4	19.6	36.4	28.6
Non-Hispanic white	18.0	17.2	35.2	29.5
Non-Hispanic black	20.6	21.2	29.5	28.6
Poverty status *				
PIR less than 1	22.1	16.7	31.9	29.4
PIR 1 to less than 2	19.9	27.1	31.9	21.1
PIR 2 or greater	17.1	15.1	37.0	30.9

* Poverty status levels are based on poverty income ratio (PIR): the ratio of the family's income to the poverty threshold (U.S. Census Bureau). PIR less than 1: family income is below the poverty threshold; PIR 1 to less than 2: family income is one to less than two times the poverty threshold; and PIR 2 or greater: family income is two or more times the poverty threshold.
Source: Fryar, Cheryl D., et al. "Smoking, Alcohol Use, and Illicit Drug Use Reported by Adolescents Aged 12–17 Years: United States, 1999–2004." *National Health Statistics Reports* 15, May 20, 2009. Hyattsville, Md.: National Center for Health Statistics. Page 13.

Health Statistics for the period 1999–2004 reveals that of those who started drinking in childhood or adolescence, 23.5 percent of boys took their first drink at age 10 or younger. Females who started drinking at age 10 or younger had a lower rate, but one that is still alarming: 13.4 percent. See Table 4 for further information.

In a comprehensive analysis of the effects of early drinking by Ralph W. Hingson and Wenxing Zha, published in *Pediatrics* in 2009, the researchers interviewed thousands of adults ages 18 and older from a sample of more than 43,000 adults in 2001–02. They then reinterviewed about 35,000 of these same subjects from 2004 to 2005 to further determine the rate of early drinking related to alcohol abuse and alcohol dependence, as well as some of the consequences of the age at which drinking started, such as driving while intoxicated or unintentionally harming themselves or others between the time of the two surveys.

The researchers found a significant relationship between early drinking and alcohol dependence; for example, those who started drinking at or before age 14 had an adult alcohol dependence rate of 14 percent. Those who started drinking at age 15–16 had a lower adult alcoholism rate of 9 percent. Among those who delayed drinking until they were age 19 or older, the alcoholism rate in adulthood was 3 percent. The researchers also found that those who began drinking early were more likely to drive under the influence of alcohol in adulthood; for example, 21 percent of those who

started drinking before age 16 admitted to drinking while intoxicated compared to 7 percent who started drinking at or after age 21. See Table 5 for more information.

The researchers also found that those who began drinking early had a higher rate of unintentionally injuring themselves or others than those who began drinking later; for example, among those who started drinking at age 14 or younger, 5.8 percent had accidentally injured themselves and 2.2 percent had unintentionally injured others. The rates were significantly lower among those who delayed drinking until age 21 or thereafter, or less than 1 percent. (See Table 6.) Thus, early drinking clearly had a long-term impact on the adults that these early drinkers later became.

Childhood Antisocial Behavior In their article on childhood antisocial behavior leading to adolescent alcohol use disorders, published in 2002 in *Alcohol Research & Health*, Duncan B. Clark, M.D., and colleagues discussed early antisocial behaviors such as aggression toward people and animals, the destruction of property, deceitfulness, and theft, as well as related childhood mental disorders such as conduct disorder and oppositional defiant disorder. The authors wrote, "Childhood antisocial behaviors are a central element in the development pathway leading to adolescent alcohol abuse or dependence."

Conduct disorder (CD) is a psychiatric diagnosis of a child who exhibits such behavior as bullying or threatening others, initiating physical fights, and

TABLE 5
ALCOHOL USE DISORDERS, HEAVY DRINKING, AND RISKS AFTER DRINKING,
ACCORDING TO AGE OF DRINKING ONSET

Age of Drinking Onset, years	n (%)	Alcohol Dependence, %	Alcohol Abuse, %	Drank ≥5 Drinks at Least Weekly, %	Drank ≥5 Drinks Less than Weekly, %	Drove Under the Influence of Alcohol, %	Put Self in Risk Situation After Drinking, %
≤ 14	2,092 (7)	14	12	23	30	21	9
15–16	4,096 (14)	9	15	20	32	21	7
17–18	8,519 (28)	5	11	14	27	14	3
19–20	4,360 (15)	3	8	11	21	11	2
≥ 21	10,926 (36)	3	5	7	15	7	1

Source: Hingson, Ralph W., and Wenxing Zha. "Age of Drinking Onset, Alcohol Use Disorders, Frequent Heavy Drinking, and Unintentionally Injuring Oneself and Others After Drinking." *Pediatrics* 123, no. 6 (2009). Page 1,480. Reproduced with permission from Pediatrics, vol. 123, no. 6. Copyright © 2009 by the American Academy of Pediatrics (AAP).

TABLE 6
INJURIES TO SELF OR ANOTHER UNDER THE INFLUENCE OF ALCOHOL, ACCORDING TO AGE OF DRINKING ONSET

Age of Drinking Onset, years	Unintentionally Injured Self, %	Unintentionally Injured Another Person, %
≤14	5.8	2.2
15–16	4.0	0.8
17–18	2.2	0.5
19–20	1.6	0.5
≥ 21	0.7	0.2

Source: Hingson, Ralph W., and Wenxing Zha. "Age of Drinking Onset, Alcohol Use Disorders, Frequent Heavy Drinking, and Unintentionally Injuring Oneself and Others After Drinking." *Pediatrics* 123, no. 6 (2009). Page 1,480. Reproduced with permission from Pediatrics, vol. 123, no. 6. Copyright © 2009 by the American Academy of Pediatrics (AAP).

forcing someone into sexual acts. The child with conduct disorder may purposely set fires with the aim of causing harm and/or destroying property. He or she may break into homes and steal items. Such children are often truant from school.

Oppositional defiant disorder (ODD) is a less severe disorder, although it is still a problematic diagnosis. The child with ODD often loses his or her temper, frequently defies adult rules, and displays anger and even vindictiveness toward others.

It is difficult for most adults to wrap their minds around a preadolescent child who exhibits such behaviors, but sadly, such children do exist in society. Often they grow up to an adult diagnosis of antisocial personality disorder, and they also have an increased risk for alcohol dependence. If identified early on, some reports indicate that behavior modification programs and the learning of social skills may help the child with ODD or CD. Some studies have also found that such programs delay the use of regular alcohol, first marijuana use, and the first police arrest.

Adolescents with diagnoses of CD or ODD generally do poorly in treatment programs for adolescents with alcohol use disorders, apparently because of their inherent antisocial tendencies. According to Clark et al., "For patients with co-occurring antisocial behaviors and AUDs [alcohol use disorders], behavioral treatments may be more effective when the interventions target multiple domains, including the individual, family, and peers. Interventions using this strategy, such as the Multisystemic Treatment approach, have been shown to improve outcome compared with less intensive approaches. For example, in a clinical adolescent sample, the Multisystemic Treatment approach reduced both drug use and antisocial behavior."

Other Traits Children and adolescents who have a high rate of novelty seeking as well as a low rate of inhibition and a high rate of impulsivity are more likely to abuse alcohol (and drugs) than others. This may be a factor in problematic substance abuse among individuals with ATTENTION-DEFICIT/HYPERACTIVITY DISORDER (ADHD) that is not identified or treated.

According to an overview of psychosocial processes published in *Alcohol Research & Health* in 2004/2005, studies have found relationships between alcohol use issues and behavioral under-control, rebelliousness, low self-constraint, and low harm avoidance. Some researchers have found high levels of impulsivity and externalizing (acting out) behaviors among the adolescent children of alcoholics. In 1997, A. Caspi and colleagues reported in the *Journal of Personality and Social Psychology* that the traits of aggression, alienation, low harm avoidance, low social closeness, and low control at age 18 were predictive for alcohol dependence by age 21.

Genetic Risks Children whose parent or parents are alcoholics have a four times greater risk of alcoholism in adulthood than children without alcoholic parents. This is true even if the child was adopted by nondrinking individuals but when a biological parent was an alcoholic. (See ADOPTION AND TWIN STUDIES.) This has been perceived as primarily a problem for males, but some studies have found that the daughters of alcoholic mothers are at risk for alcoholism as well.

In a study of childhood risk factors that were related to the initiation of alcohol use and the progression to alcohol dependence, researchers Carolyn E. Sartor and colleagues studied 1,269 subjects who were the children of twins from the Vietnam Era Twin Registry; 46.2 percent were the children of alcoholic fathers. The researchers, reporting their findings in *Addiction* in 2006, found that among the subjects for whom the first drink occurred at an average age of 15.7 years, of those who became alcoholics, at an average age of 19.1 years, the only risk factor that predicted both early drinking and alcoholism was conduct disorder. Since conduct disorder is considered heritable, there is an apparent underlying genetic basis.

The genetic risk for alcoholism may be combined with the environmental risk, if the biological child of an alcoholic observes this behavior as he or she grows up. Children and adolescents who grow up in a family in which parents are heavy drinkers or alcoholics may believe that drinking is normal, and children of alcoholics have an increased risk for alcohol abuse and alcoholism. However, sometimes children of alcoholics are nondrinkers and actively avoid alcohol in response to the behavior of their parents, whom they do not wish to emulate.

Peer Influences Although peer influences are the most influential in adolescence and young adulthood, in many cases peers continue to exert their negative (or positive) influence on individuals throughout life. For example, if a 40-year-old man has friends who are all heavy drinkers, it is more difficult for such an individual to give up drinking.

Adverse Events in Childhood The Adverse Childhood Experiences (ACE) study, a collaboration between the Centers for Disease Control and Prevention (CDC) and the Kaiser Permanente Health Appraisal Clinic in San Diego, California, analyzed childhood risk factors in more than 17,000 adults. The study concentrated on such areas as childhood abuse and neglect as well as household dysfunction (a mother who was treated violently, or the presence of household substance abuse, household mental illness, an incarcerated family member, or parental separation or divorce). Nearly two-thirds of the participants reported at least one adverse childhood event, and about 20 percent reported three or more such events. This

data was reported by Jennifer S. Middlebrooks and Natalie C. Audage in *The Effects of Childhood Stress on Health Across the Lifespan* in 2008.

The researchers found that the more ACEs that a child experienced, the more likely he or she was to have serious problems in adulthood, such as alcoholism or alcohol abuse, depression, suicide attempts, unintended pregnancies, and suffering from intimate partner violence. ACEs were also linked to risky behaviors in adolescence, such as suicide attempts, early initiation of smoking, and illicit drug use.

The researchers found that men and women who reported childhood sexual abuse had an increased risk for marrying an alcoholic. (About 25 percent of the women and 16 percent of the men reported childhood sexual abuse.) The more frequently the adults witnessed intimate partner violence in childhood, the more likely in adulthood they were to report alcoholism, as well as illicit drug use and depression. Participants with high ACE scores were also at a greater risk for becoming alcoholics as well as for marrying an alcoholic.

Individuals Who Smoke Smoking is linked to drinking and may in fact potentiate drinking. Many people start smoking at an early age, and for some individuals, this also increases the probability of early drinking.

Rebecca Gilbertson and colleagues wrote in their 2008 article for *Alcohol Research & Health,* "Whereas alcohol dependence is associated with subtle, yet significant cognitive dysfunction, acute nicotine is known to enhance cognition, particularly processes associated with vigilance and attentional aspects of working memory. Given the opposing effects, it follows that acute nicotine may serve to compensate for deficits associated with alcohol dependence. If so, the strong association between the use of the two substances may not lie entirely in the reward systems or shared genetic risks but also in their functional interaction."

Low Response to the Effects of Alcohol Some individuals have a low response to the effects of alcohol. It takes longer for the negative (and positive) effects of alcohol to affect them. Such individuals have an increased risk for alcohol use disorders. In a study of 297 individuals drawn from the long-term San Diego Prospective Study, researchers Ryan S. Trim, Marc A. Schuckit, and Tom L. Smith reported on the subjects' low sensitivity to alcohol as well as their family history of alcohol use disorders (AUDs), the age of drinking onset, and other factors. They reported on their findings in *Alcoholism: Clinical and Experimental Research* in 2009. The researchers analyzed their subjects' response in terms of self-reports as well as their body sway/standing steadiness and their cortisol blood levels from before drinking to 60 minutes after drinking.

The researchers found that low response (LR) to alcohol was a unique risk factor increasing the odds for AUDs, irrespective of other risk factors, such as the family history and age of drinking onset. According to the researchers, "These data provide prospective evidence that the LR to alcohol is a unique risk factor for alcohol-related problems, and not simply a reflection or 'marker' for a broader range of risk factors which influence adulthood."

Of those individuals who were diagnosed with an AUD, 69 percent were diagnosed before age 30; however, the researchers noted that 6 percent of the subjects were newly diagnosed after age 40. The researchers noted that these individuals could represent a "relatively understudied high-risk population deserving of further clinical attention."

Earlier studies by Schuckit and Smith in 2000 found that the sons of alcoholic fathers consistently rate themselves lower than the sons of nonalcoholic fathers on drug effect, sleepiness, drunkenness, and dizziness after drinking alcohol. A decreased sensitivity to alcohol is thus a predictive measure for males at increased risk for alcoholism. Other research by Schuckit has indicated that Native Americans have a low level of response as well as an increased risk for alcoholism.

Risk Factors in Young Adulthood and Adulthood

In addition to the risk factors for future alcohol abuse and dependence that stem from childhood and adolescence, there are also risk factors for drinking in young adulthood and adulthood. The major ones include the following:

- gender
- college student status

- the presence of other psychiatric problems
- severe losses, such as the death of a spouse to an older person

Gender In general, men are about twice as likely to abuse or become dependent on alcohol as women. Men are also significantly more likely to engage in BINGE DRINKING than women. This does not mean that women are free from the effects of alcohol; research has indicated that female alcoholics progress to severe liver disease more rapidly than male alcoholics. They are also at an increased risk for breast cancer and other diseases. (See ALCOHOL AND WOMEN; ALCOHOL AND MEN.)

College Students Heavy drinking is a major problem among COLLEGE STUDENTS, according to the National Institute on Alcohol Abuse and Alcoholism (NIAAA). The NIAAA reports that four of every five college students drink, including 60 percent of underage students ages 18 to 20 years old. In addition, more than 40 percent of college students of all ages engage in binge drinking at least once in the past two weeks. Some studies have shown that college students are more likely to drink heavily on days when football games are held, largely because of the social context associated with the game rather than the actual game itself.

According to data from the 2007 Monitoring the Future survey, about two-thirds (66.6 percent) of college students have used alcohol in the past 30 days, compared to 44.4 percent of high school seniors and the larger figure of 69.5 percent of young adults. Daily drinking is even more of a problem. In 2007, 4.3 percent of college students reported drinking every day, compared to the lower figure of 3.1 percent of high school seniors and the higher figure of 5.6 percent of young adults ages 19–28 years. (See Table 7.)

However, binge drinking is a worse problem among college students than their noncollege peers; for example, in 2007, 41.1 percent of college students reported binge drinking, compared to 25.9 percent of high school seniors and 37.8 percent of their young adult peers.

In fact, this pattern of heavier binge drinking among college students compared to their young adult peers has held since 1998. (See Table 8.) Note that female college students who engage in binge

TABLE 7
TRENDS IN 30-DAY PREVALENCE OF DAILY USE OF ALCOHOL AMONG 12TH GRADERS, COLLEGE STUDENTS, AND YOUNG ADULTS (AGES 19–28), 1998–2007, BY PERCENT, UNITED STATES

	1998	1999	2000	2001	2002	2003	2004	2005	2006	2007
12th Grade	3.4	2.9	3.6	3.5	3.2	2.8	3.1	3.0	3.1	3.1
College Students	3.9	4.5	3.6	4.7	5.0	4.3	3.7	4.6	4.8	4.3
Young Adults	4.0	4.8	4.1	4.4	4.7	5.1	4.5	5.2	5.4	5.6

Source: Adapted from Johnston, Lloyd D., et al. *Monitoring the Future: National Survey Results on Drug Use, 1975–2007. Volume II. College Students and Adults Age 19–45.* Bethesda, Md.: National Institute on Drug Abuse, 2008. Page 53.

drinking and heavy drinking have an increased risk for sexual assault. (See EXCESSIVE DRINKING AND NEGATIVE SOCIAL CONSEQUENCES.)

Interestingly, some female college students are drinking heavily to attract men, yet men have reported that they do not want or expect women to drink as much as men. According to researchers Joseph LaBrie and colleagues in their study reported in the *Psychology of Addictive Behaviors* in 2009, the researchers found that 71 percent of the women overestimated the men's preference for women drinking by about 1.5 drinks. In addition, 26 percent of the women said that men would wish to be friends with women who drink five or more drinks and 16 percent thought that men would be sexually attracted to women who drank five or more drinks. (This is binge-drinking behavior.) But these estimates were about double what men said they preferred. As a result, some women are drinking to excess to please men, but they are achieving the opposite result from their intention.

Psychiatric Comorbidities   The presence of some PSYCHIATRIC COMORBIDITIES significantly increases the risk for alcoholism, particularly ANTISOCIAL PERSONALITY DISORDER, BIPOLAR DISORDER, and ANXIETY DISORDERS such as panic disorder. (However, it is often unclear whether the psychiatric disorders stem from or cause alcoholism.)

Some individuals have a greater risk for alcohol dependence than others, such as individuals with chronic DEPRESSION, bipolar disorder, disruptive behaviors disorders such as CONDUCT DISORDER or oppositional defiant disorder, or PERSONALITY DISORDERS. In addition, individuals with some IMPULSE CONTROL DISORDERS, such as PATHOLOGICAL GAMBLING, are at risk for alcohol dependence.

It is also true that psychotic individuals, who cannot identify what is real from what is false, have an increased risk for alcoholism or alcohol abuse, particularly those with SCHIZOPHRENIA or a psychotic mania caused by bipolar disorder. Some research indicates that such individuals have an increased risk for physical violence, especially when they are under the influence of alcohol.

Severe Losses or Traumas   Although most ELDERLY people do not have alcohol use disorders, the risk increases for some, especially older women. Experts believe this is because of severe losses they have incurred, such as the loss of a long-term partner and/or friends they have relied upon for years. When an older person suddenly begins to exhibit behavior of confusion and an increased number of

TABLE 8
TRENDS IN BINGE DRINKING (5+ DRINKS IN A ROW IN THE LAST TWO WEEKS) AMONG 12TH GRADERS, COLLEGE STUDENTS, AND YOUNG ADULTS (AGES 19–28), 1998–2007, UNITED STATES

	1998	1999	2000	2001	2002	2003	2004	2005	2006	2007
Twelfth Graders	31.5	30.8	30.0	29.7	28.6	27.9	29.2	27.1	25.4	25.9
College Students	38.9	40.0	39.3	40.9	40.1	38.5	41.7	40.1	40.2	41.1
Young Adults	34.1	35.8	34.7	35.9	35.9	35.8	37.1	37.0	37.6	37.8

Source: Adapted from Johnston, Lloyd D., et al. *Monitoring the Future: National Survey Results on Drug Use, 1975–2007. Volume II. College Students and Adults Age 19–45.* Bethesda, Md.: National Institute on Drug Abuse, 2008. Page 53.

falls, it may not mean the person has Alzheimer's disease; it could be that alcohol excess is the underlying cause.

Identifying Alcohol Abuse or Dependence

Individuals who are alcohol abusers or even who are alcoholics often fail to recognize that they have a problem. Family members may complain to them about their behavior, or they may lose their jobs because of too frequent absences due to hangovers or other alcohol-related issues. Despite this, they may still deny that alcohol has a hold over them. This is why organizations such as Alcoholics Anonymous (AA) are so helpful; they not only help the individual face the fact that alcohol *is* a problem in his or her life, but they offer plans to overcome its effects. The difficulty can come in persuading an individual to attend an AA meeting.

Screening Instruments The primary means that physicians use to identify possible problematic alcohol use are the CAGE, the AUDIT, or the AUDIT-C tests. There are also some intervention instruments used specifically with pregnant women. (See PREGNANCY.) With the CAGE questionnaire, there are four questions:

1. Have you ever felt you should *C*ut down on your drinking?
2. Have people *A*nnoyed you by criticizing your drinking?
3. Have you ever felt bad or *G*uilty about your drinking?
4. Have you ever had a drink first thing in the morning to steady your nerves or get rid of a hangover (*E*ye-opener)?

Researchers have found that if the patient responds no to all four questions, the probability of alcoholism is 7 percent. If the patient answers yes to one question, the probability of alcohol dependence is 46 percent. Two affirmative responses indicate an alcoholic probability of 72 percent. Three yeses means that there is an alcoholic probability of 88 percent. If the patient responds yes to all four questions, the probability of alcohol dependence is 98 percent.

The Alcohol Use Disorders Identification Test (AUDIT) is a 10-item questionnaire. The AUDIT-C is a shorter version with only three questions and thus is often preferred, because it is quick and easy to administer during the course of a patient encounter. These instruments screen for heavy drinking as well as alcohol dependence. The questions on the AUDIT-C are:

1. How often did you have a drink containing alcohol in the past year?
2. How many drinks did you have on a typical day when you were drinking in the past year?
3. How often did you have six or more drinks on one occasion in the past year?

The Michigan Alcohol Screening Test (MAST) is a 24-item test used to assess drinking levels as well as already-experienced adverse consequences from drinking.

Another questionnaire that may be used with adolescents is the CRAFFT questionnaire. This questionnaire includes the following items on both alcohol and drugs:

- Have you ever ridden in a *C*ar driven by someone (including yourself) who was "high" or had been using alcohol or drugs?
- Do you ever use alcohol or drugs to *R*elax, feel better about yourself, or fit in?
- Do you ever use alcohol or drugs while you are by yourself, *A*lone?
- Do you ever *F*orget things you did while using alcohol or drugs?
- Does your family or *F*riends tell you that you should cut down on your drinking or drug use?
- Have you ever gotten into *T*rouble while you were using alcohol or drugs?

Laboratory Tests for Possible Alcohol Abuse or Dependence

When a driver is stopped for possibly violating state laws on intoxication, a police officer may administer basic field sobriety tests (such as having a person close his or her eyes and then touch the nose) as well as a breath test. The person may also be taken for a blood test to check the BLOOD ALCOHOL CONCENTRATION.

In daily life, if physicians suspect that an individual has issues with alcohol, they may check for the blood levels of alcohol, which will be elevated in the event of alcohol abuse or dependence. The carbohydrate-deficient transferrin (CDT) test is a reliable test for alcohol dependence, which can still show past alcohol use even after weeks of abstinence. Test results are generally available within four hours. The CDT is often used in combination with a screening test such as the gamma-glutamyl transferse (GGT) test.

Other tests for chronic alcohol dependence and abuse include:

- cholesterol
- alkaline phosphatase
- serum transferring
- uric acid
- serum glutamic oxaloacetic transaminase (SGOT)
- lactic dehydrogenase (LDH)
- mean corpuscular volume (MCV)
- triglycerides
- blood alcohol concentration (BAC)

The Effects of Alcoholism and Alcohol Abuse on the Individual

The person who has a diagnosable problem with alcohol incurs many negative consequences. In general, the more severe the alcoholism, the greater the consequences; however, a person who is an alcohol abuser may also develop health problems as well as lose out on a potential promotion or even get fired from a job because of alcohol abuse.

Of course, not all problems related to alcohol are caused by those with diagnosable alcohol use disorders. Individuals who binge drink may not meet the criteria for either alcohol abuse or alcoholism, but they may cause severe harm to themselves and others by their alcohol binges. Their drinking may result in physical injuries and possibly death, as well as harm to others from drunken assaults, car crashes, and other incidents that likely would not have occurred had the person not been under the influence of alcohol. For example, half of those who die in traffic crashes involving drunk drivers who are under age 21 are people other than the drunken driver. The point is that all problems associated with alcohol can-

not be laid at the feet of those with a diagnosable alcohol use disorder.

Health Effects   The health effects on the alcoholic impact virtually every system of the body. Female alcoholics have a greater risk for breast cancer, and both male and female alcoholics have a greater risk for many forms of CANCER. In addition, alcoholics of both genders have an increased risk for liver disease, up to and including CIRRHOSIS, which cannot be treated and which requires a liver transplant to sustain life. Women have a more rapid progression to liver cirrhosis than men, although the reason for this is unknown. There are many other health risks, such as the risk for PANCREATITIS, gastrointestinal disorders, vitamin deficiencies, and more. (See EXCESSIVE DRINKING AND HEALTH CONSEQUENCES.)

The Effects of Alcoholism and Alcohol Abuse on Others

An individual's alcohol abuse or alcoholism significantly affects his or her family members. Alcohol use disorders also affect fellow workers if the individual is employed. In addition, society at large is affected by drunk driving and alcohol-related violence.

The Family   Two common phenomena in families with untreated alcoholics are CODEPENDENCY and PARENTIFICATION. A codependent person makes excuses for the heavy drinker or alcoholic, justifying even unjustifiable behavior. Codependent people are emotionally needy and perceive themselves as very important to the alcoholic person. According to the authors of *Family Matters: Substance Abuse and the American Family*, "Codependents are characterized by a constant need for approval from others, difficulty in adapting to change, feeling overly responsible for the feelings and behaviors of others, indecisiveness, martyrdom, making excuses for the addict, denying problems, perpetuating crises, and losing a sense of self."

When parentification occurs, a child assumes the role of an adult, often a role the child is not prepared to handle. Because there is no one else to act like an adult, the child attempts to be the grownup. Say the authors of *Family Matters*, "Parentification can have profound effects on children, contributing to substance use, emotional distress and problem behaviors such as inappropriate sexual behaviors and conduct problems."

Violent Behavior AGGRESSIVE BEHAVIOR and acts of VIOLENCE occur more frequently among those who are impaired by alcohol than among sober individuals. A significant percentage of convicted criminals in prison report that their crimes were committed while they were drinking alcohol. Intimate partner violence is more common among individuals who are alcoholics, and often their victims are partners who have also been drinking.

The Workplace When a person abuses alcohol or is dependent on it, at least part of the time, he or she is usually a slacker on the job, which means that other people may do their work and/or "cover" for the person who is unable to perform job responsibilities. Others may also fail to cover for the alcoholic at work or may perform a poor job out of resentment. On the surface, this may seem minor; however, if the products being made are medications, cars, or other items in which safety is paramount, the issue becomes much more significant.

Drunk Driving and Society and Research One major cause of concern is that intoxicated individuals may cause an accident while DRIVING UNDER THE INFLUENCE of alcohol. In a study of aggressive young adult drivers by Loretta S. Malta, Edward B. Blanchard, and Brian M. Freidenberg, published in 2005 in *Behaviour Research and Therapy*, the researchers found that aggressive drivers were also very angry drivers. In addition, they found a significant number of subjects with substance abuse problems, primarily alcohol abuse or alcohol dependence.

The aggressive drivers were about three times more likely to drive while drunk compared to the nonaggressive drivers, and nearly a third of the aggressive drivers had psychiatric diagnoses of alcohol abuse or dependence, compared to none of the nonaggressive drivers. Alcohol is known to increase an individual's level of aggressive behavior.

According to the National Highway Traffic Safety Administration (NHTSA), 12,998 people died as a result of alcohol-related motor vehicle crashes in 2007 in the United States, or 31.7 percent of all traffic fatalities. Most alcohol-related fatalities were caused by individuals whose blood alcohol level

exceeded 0.08 percent, according to the NHTSA. Most impaired drivers involved in fatal crashes in 2007 were male (about 83 percent). Many alcohol-impaired drivers also failed to wear their seat belts; for example, in 2007, nearly two-thirds (62 percent) of drivers involved in fatal crashes were wearing their seat belts, but only 34 percent of alcohol-impaired drivers wore their seat belts.

Not everyone involved in a car crash with a drunk driver died; many are severely injured, some with lifelong injuries incurred in the crash, such as brain damage, lost limbs, and so forth. Even among those who recover completely from a severe accident, the effect of a car crash is devastating to most people and can lead to such anxiety disorders as POSTTRAUMATIC STRESS DISORDER. They may be traumatized further by having to testify in court against the drunk driver, who may marshal his friends and an attorney to defend him or her and offer a myriad of excuses for the behavior, as well as extensive promises that it will never happen again.

Although not all who are convicted of driving while under the influence (DWI) of alcohol (also known as driving while intoxicated, as well as other terms) are alcoholics or even fit the criteria of alcohol abuse, many do fit the criteria, particularly if they are repeat offenders. In a study of individuals convicted of at least one DWI in New Mexico by Lawrence M. Scheier, Sandra C. Lapham, and Janet C'DeBaca, published in 2008 in *Substance Use & Misuse*, the researchers analyzed the subjects' cognitive motivations to drink (the thinking processes that preceded the act of drinking) using various psychological scales and measures.

Interestingly, the researchers found that 61.7 percent of the 552 males and 70.1 percent of the 701 females met the criteria of a lifetime diagnosis of alcoholism, and in addition, 23.9 percent of the males and 21.3 percent of the females met the criteria for alcohol abuse. Only 14.4 percent of the males and 8.6 percent of the females had no alcohol diagnosis. The researchers also found that 6.8 percent of the females and 11.0 percent of the males had at least one DWI and less than 1 percent of the females and 2.3 percent of the males had three or more DWIs.

The subjects also reported their drinking patterns to the researchers; for example, 16 percent said that they binged with alcohol, drinking for several days and stopping drinking, repeating this pattern. About 25 percent said that they drank every day, and 46 percent said that they had been drunk many times. Clearly, alcohol was a major influence in most of these subjects' lives.

The researchers found that cognitive cues were significant in the subjects' deciding to drink and discussed the likely internal thought processes. These cognitive factors combine to propel the person toward (or away from) drinking. According to the researchers, "One component represents the decision to spend time with friends, which can hold its own intrinsic motivation. A second component deals with the expectancy that drinking is pleasurable, can heighten certain sensations (e.g., relaxation and tension reduction), and thus constitutes its own positive reward structure (positive expectancy). A third and perhaps decisive cue may regard availability of financial resources to purchase alcoholic beverages (with the money received on payday serving as an incentive). A fourth situational factor may reflect relief from work-related stress."

The researchers found that situational cues (such as being criticized by someone, passing by a liquor store, or being out with friends who decided to stop by a bar) had the most significant effect on harmful alcohol use, followed by the individual's own drinking urges and triggers and expectancies about drinking.

Treating Alcoholism and Alcohol Abuse

Only about 24 percent of those with alcohol abuse or alcohol dependence ever seek any TREATMENT. The rest continue on with their abuse or dependence on alcohol, many erroneously believing that they can "stop whenever I want to." They tell themselves that they just never want to stop.

Most Alcoholics Deny or Refuse Treatment One key reason for this refusal to obtain treatment is DENIAL that any problem exists. Most alcoholics are very adept at finding reasons for virtually any problems caused by their alcoholism. Another reason for refusing treatment, according to Hugh Myrick, M.D., in his article on alcohol dependence for *Medscape Psychiatry & Mental Health*, is that drinkers perceive a substantial level of pub-

lic stigma surrounding alcoholism. They believe (and often rightly so) that their physicians will view them negatively if they know that they are alcoholics.

When Treatment Is Received Sometimes alcoholics do receive treatment, either because they choose to receive treatment or (more likely) a court or another agency such as the EMPLOYEE ASSISTANCE PROGRAM in their company compels them to seek treatment. For example, among IMPAIRED PHYSICIANS who are alcoholics, many are required by their states or professional organizations to seek treatment or they will lose their medical licenses. Interestingly, treatment programs for physicians have an extremely high success rate and the broad majority of doctors do not return to drinking, an atypical response compared to other drinkers. This may be because physicians are highly motivated compared to others, or it may be because the programs that they enter are far superior to other programs; many other factors may also be in play. Some experts have suggested that since such programs are so successful, they should be studied further to see which elements of these programs could be used or adapted into programs for nonphysician alcoholics.

Treatment Options and Outlook Alcoholism is treated by expert physicians on either an inpatient or outpatient basis. Treatment often includes medications such as NALTREXONE, DISULFIRAM, and acamprosate, as well as psychotherapy. Mutual aid groups such as Alcoholics Anonymous or Women for Sobriety are also very important in helping the individual remain abstinent and in providing support when relapses occur. Relapses are considered common among alcoholics.

Probably the most effective method of "treatment" is regular attendance at meetings of Alcoholics Anonymous (AA). AA meetings are almost universally available in every city, many times a day and for free. This group's aim is to help individuals attain and maintain sobriety, and it is not affiliated with any religious groups, government organizations, or any other agencies. It is run solely by members. AA was founded in 1935 by two alcoholics (Bill W. and Dr. Bob) and since then has helped countless alcoholics (in the millions) turn their lives around.

The philosophy of AA is embedded in its 12-step program, which has also been adapted by other groups, such as Narcotics Anonymous, Cocaine Anonymous, Gamblers Anonymous, Overeaters Anonymous, Debtors Anonymous, and Sex and Love Addicts Anonymous. Going through the 12 steps is sometimes referred to by members as "working the program." This is in contrast with the fellowship offered by AA, including a chance to meet and socialize with other alcoholics and learn how they have overcome their problems. Some meetings are open to anyone, while others are for beginners, discussion, and other topics. Some meetings are closed.

A study by Maria E. Pagano and colleagues on predictors of participation in AA-related helping of other alcoholics subsequent to treatment admission for alcoholism, published in the *Journal of Studies on Alcohol and Drugs* in 2009, found that the number of meetings attended, the number of steps worked, and the length of sobriety was predictive for helping others. Those who had a sponsor in AA were about twice as likely to start helping others. In addition, prior to helping, participants reported higher levels of depressive symptoms, so helping others lowered depressive symptoms.

In AA, new members choose a home group where they will attend meetings. They are also given a sponsor who will help them with the difficulties of ending drinking and working through the steps.

The first step (Step One) addresses the issue of denial among most alcoholics. With this step, the individual admits powerlessness over alcohol and that life has become unmanageable. Step Two involves accepting that there is a power greater than oneself. This step (and several others) has caused some people to label AA as a religious organization, but that is not the purported goal of the second step. Rather, it is to offer hope that the individual can attain sobriety, but that he or she needs help to achieve this goal. The third step (which some also perceive as religiously oriented) is the resolution of the individual to turn his or her will and life to God as understood by them. Those who do not believe in God can reframe this concept as accepting and loving the life force within themselves.

Other steps involve making a searching personal inventory of their own failings, a step which almost inevitably generates guilt, shame, and grief, and which a sponsor must help the person work through, and then admitting to others the nature of past wrongs; asking God (or the life force) to remove these failings from the person; making a list of people who have been wronged and seeking to make amends to them for past misdeeds and others. The last step involves carrying the message to other alcoholics.

One rare problem with AA is that some individuals take needed psychiatric medications under the control of a physician; however, if this use is revealed to the group, sometimes members will urge the individual to stop taking medications that are sleep remedies or tranquilizers or medications for ADHD, because they may mistakenly perceive such medications as bad, since these type of medications are sometimes abused. As a result, it may be best to limit the mention of such drugs to only the group leader or one's own individual sponsor.

Health Issues Associated with Treatment   Long-term alcoholics may have serious health problems that need to be addressed in conjunction with their treatment. In the most severe cases, the individual may be malnourished, having depended mostly or even solely on alcohol for nutrition. As a result, he or she likely has multiple vitamin and mineral deficiencies.

Withdrawal from Alcohol and Its Treatment   Withdrawing from alcohol has some effect on the alcoholic, although the effects may not be as severe as many people believe. Many people assume that the long-term alcoholic who suddenly stops drinking will inevitably lurch into the throes of DELIRIUM TREMENS (DTs), a life-threatening state that includes hallucinations and other severe bodily reactions that require emergency medical treatment. However, although there are physical and psychological effects when someone addicted to alcohol abruptly stops drinking (for whatever reason, voluntary or involuntary), in most cases these effects can be controlled and limited with medications, such as BENZODIAZEPINES. The primary problem with alcoholism does not lie with the side effects of a sudden cessation of drinking but rather with the risk of relapsing to drinking once a person stops.

Some of the common effects of withdrawal from alcohol may include headache, nausea, and vomiting, as well as rapid heartbeat, elevated blood pressure, excessive sweating, and shaking. Emotional symptoms of withdrawal include agitation, anxiety, irritability, and sleep disturbances, as well as a reported feeling of aching all over, which may indicate a reduced pain threshold sensitivity. Most of these symptoms abate within days, although the psychological distress may continue for an extended period, especially depressive symptoms or anhedonia (the inability to experience pleasure), and they are factors in relapse.

Some researchers believe that repeated instances of withdrawal from alcohol may lead to more severe and more persistent symptoms from withdrawal, thus increasing the risk for relapse. Howard C. Becker in his 2008 article for *Alcohol Research & Health* on withdrawal and relapses writes, "Furthermore, multiple withdrawal episodes provide repeated opportunities for alcohol-dependent individuals to experience the negative reinforcing properties of alcohol—that is to associate alcohol consumption with the amelioration of the negative consequences (e.g., withdrawal-related malaise) experienced during attempts at abstinence. This association not only may serve as a powerful motivational force that increases relapse vulnerability, but also favors escalation of alcohol drinking and sustained levels of potentially harmful drinking. Thus for many dependent individuals, repeated withdrawal experiences may be especially relevant in shaping motivation to seek alcohol and engage in excessive drinking behavior."

What to Do When an Alcoholic Refuses Help

Experts advise that family members can and should take action when an alcoholic family member refuses to acknowledge that he or she has a problem with alcohol and thus, also refuses to obtain any assistance. It is not necessary to wait until the person hits "rock bottom" to take action. The NIAAA recommends the following steps:

- Stop covering up for the alcoholic. Let him or her suffer the consequences of drinking. For example, if the alcoholic has a hangover and asks the spouse to call in "sick" for him, he or she should refuse. If the alcoholic person passes out on the floor of the living room (assuming that there is no apparent physical injury), let the person wake up there and do not try to move him or her to bed.

- Time the intervention. The best time to talk to an alcoholic about the problem is after it is readily apparent that there is a problem, such as shortly after the person has an accident or a serious family argument caused by drinking.

- Provide specific examples. Rather than simply saying that the drinking makes a family member upset, explain how or why it caused distress; for example, because the family member was worried the person would be killed in a car crash and/or harm others because of driving while intoxicated.

- Describe consequences the family member will face. The family member should tell the drinker that if he or she refuses to get help for the alcohol abuse or alcoholism, then certain consequences will occur. These consequences should be actions that the family member is willing to carry out and may include a broad array of actions, such as moving out of the home, refusing to go with the person to any social events if alcohol will be served, or other actions.

- Find out what help is available in the community. Virtually all communities have nearby chapters of Alcoholics Anonymous. Many communities also have chapters of Al-Anon, which is an organization for family members suffering from the results of their relative's drinking.

- Ask others to help. A friend who is a recovering alcoholic or another person who has some familiarity with alcoholism may be willing to talk to the alcoholic and urge him/her to seek treatment.

- Consider an intervention: Some family members and friends join together to confront an alcoholic as a group and urge him or her to seek help. Such an intervention should be guided with the help of a health-care professional who is knowledgeable and experienced with such interventions. If the individual is willing to seek help, it should be available immediately; hence, it must be set up ahead of time.

Alcohol and Other Drugs

Many people who abuse or depend on alcohol also use other substances such as marijuana, cocaine, amphetamines, and other drugs, including misused prescription drugs, such as painkillers or sedatives. In addition, an estimated 80 percent of alcoholics are also smokers. (See SMOKING AND ALCOHOL.) For those individuals who both smoke and use tobacco, the risk for developing throat and mouth cancer is 38 times higher than nondrinkers and nonsmokers. Some research indicates that smoking can increase the level of drinking in some smokers. According to the NIAAA, there is a mutual craving for nicotine and alcohol, and consequently, one substance can potentiate the action of the other.

In addition to the dangers involved in using illicit substances or misusing prescription drugs, when such substances are combined with alcohol, the risks are often increased exponentially. For example, when a person uses both cocaine and alcohol at the same time, the body forms a substance known as cocaethylene, which can cause overdoses as well as harm the heart, the brain, and other organs.

Alcohol and Nicotine Dependence

One reason why many alcoholics do not stop smoking lies within treatment centers. Often treatment centers do not encourage alcoholics to stop smoking. In fact, they may offer "smoke breaks" as privileges for good behavior. Experts report that often staff members themselves are nicotine-dependent, making them less inclined to help alcoholic patients give up smoking. The staff may also believe that smoking is a minor addiction compared to alcohol dependence. They may also believe that if individuals who have undergone treatment are urged to stop smoking, they may relapse to drinking again. Some AA groups may also condone smoking.

Yet according to the NIAAA, research tends to show the opposite is true: that quitting smoking is *less* likely to cause a relapse to drinking than continuing to smoke. However, even experts who support smoking cessation assistance for alcoholics do not agree on the best timing for such a program to occur; for example, whether it should occur concurrently with treatment for alcoholism or soon thereafter or at another time.

Alcohol and Cocaine

One combination of alcohol and drugs that is abused by some individuals is cocaine and alcohol. Alcohol is sedating and cocaine is stimulating, and for some people, the two drugs in concert provide what they seek. Most alcoholics are not cocaine addicts, but many people addicted to cocaine also abuse or are dependent upon alcohol.

Relapsing to Drinking

Little data is available on those who relapse, but the National Epidemiological Survey on Alcohol and Related Conditions (NESARC) studied 1,772 people ages 18 and over who had apparently recovered from their alcohol use disorder. Over the course of three years, 26 percent exhibited symptoms of alcohol abuse and another 5 percent were dependent on alcohol. Thus, nearly a third had relapsed from their apparent recovery from alcoholism. Further research is needed on specifics of behaviors that predispose a recovered alcoholic to relapsing.

A Rapid Progression to Alcoholism

Although for most people it takes years to become an alcoholic, a small percentage of people who start drinking become rapidly dependent on alcohol within about a year or two. For example, according to a report published in 2008 by the Office of Applied Studies office of the Substance Abuse and Mental Health Services Administration (SAMHSA), of those who reported beginning drinking alcohol within 13 to 24 months prior to the survey interview, 3.2 percent had become dependent on alcohol in the past year.

See also AGE AND ALCOHOL; ALCOHOL AND ALCOHOL USE; ALCOHOLISM MUTUAL AID SOCIETIES; STAGES OF CHANGE.

Alling, C. "Revealing Alcohol Abuse: To Ask or to Test?" *Alcoholism: Clinical and Experimental Research* 29, no. 7 (2005): 1,257–1,263.

American Psychiatric Association. *Diagnostic and Statistical Manual of Mental Disorders.* 4th Edition. Text Revision. *(DSM-IV-TR),* 197. Washington, D.C.: American Psychiatric Association, 2000.

Becker, Howard C. "Alcohol Dependence, Withdrawal, and Relapse." *Alcohol Research & Health* 31, no. 4 (2008): 348–361.

Berridge, Virginia and Sarah Mars. "History of Addictions." *Journal of Epidemiology and Public Health* 58, no. 9 (2003): 747–750.

Blanco, Carlos, M.D., et al. "Mental Health of College Students and Their Non-College-Attending Peers: Results from the National Epidemiologic Study on Alcohol and Related Conditions." *Archives of General Psychiatry* 65, no. 12 (2008): 1,429–1,437.

Caetano, Raul, M.D. "NESARC Findings on Alcohol Abuse and Dependence." *Alcohol Research & Health* 29, no. 2 (2006): 152–155.

Caspi, Avshalom, et al. "Personality Differences Predict Health-Risk Behaviors in Young Adulthood: Evidence from a Longitudinal Study." *Journal of Personality and Social Psychology* 73, no. 5 (1997): 1,052–1,063.

Center for Substance Abuse Treatment. *Detoxification and Substance Abuse Treatment.* Treatment Improvement Protocol (TIP) Series 45. Rockville, Md.: Substance Abuse and Mental Health Services Administration, 2006.

Clark, Duncan B., M.D., Michael Vanyukov, and Jack Cornelius, M.D. "Childhood Antisocial Behavior and Adolescent Alcohol Use Disorders." *Alcohol Research & Health* 26, no. 2 (2002): 109–115.

Dawson, Deborah A., et al. "Recovery from DSM-IV Alcohol Dependence: United States, 2001–2002." *Alcohol Research & Health* 29, no. 2 (2006): 131–142.

"Environmental and Contextual Considerations." *Alcohol Research & Health* 28, no. 3 (2004/2005): 155–162.

Gilbertson, Rebecca, Robert Prather, and Sara Jo Nixon. "The Role of Selected Factors in the Development and Consequences of Alcohol Dependence." *Alcohol Research & Health* 31, no. 4 (2008): 389–399.

Gilpin, Nicholas, and George F. Koob. "Neurobiology of Alcohol Dependence: Focus on Motivational Mechanisms." *Alcohol Research & Health* 31, no. 3 (2008): 185–194.

Gold, Mark S., M.D., and Mark D. Aronson, M.D. "Treatment of Alcohol Abuse and Dependence." *UptoDate.* Available to subscribers online. Accessed March 13, 2009.

Hasin, Deborah S., et al. "Prevalence, Correlates, Disability, and Comorbidity of DSM-IV Alcohol Abuse and Dependence in the United States: Results from the National Epidemiologic Survey on Alcohol and Related Conditions." *Archives of General Psychiatry* 64, no. 7 (2007): 830–842.

Hester, Reid K., and Joseph H. Miller. "Computer-based Tools for Diagnosis and Treatment of Alcohol Problems." *Alcohol Research & Health* 29, no. 1 (2006): 36–40.

Grant, Bridget F., et al. "The 12-Month Prevalence and Trends in DSM-IV Alcohol Abuse and Dependence: United States, 1991–1992 and 2001–2002." *Alcohol Research & Health* 29, no. 2 (2006): 79–91.

Hingson, R. W., T. Heeren and M. R. Winter. "Age at Drinking Onset and Alcohol Dependence: Age at Onset, Duration, and Severity." *Archives of Pediatric and Adolescent Medicine* 160, no. 7 (July 2006): 739–746.

Hingson, Ralph W., and Wenxing Zha. "Age of Drinking Onset, Alcohol Use Disorders, Frequent Heavy Drinking, and Unintentionally Injuring Oneself and Others After Drinking." *Pediatrics* 123, no. 6 (2009): 1,477–1,484.

Johnston, Lloyd D., et al. *Monitoring the Future: National Survey Results on Drug Use, 1975–2007. Volume II. College Students and Adults Age 19–45.* Bethesda, Md.: National Institute on Drug Abuse, 2008.

Malta, Loretta S., Edward B. Blanchard, and Brian M. Freidenberg. "Psychiatric and Behavioral Problems in Aggressive Drivers." *Behaviour Research and Therapy* 43, no. 11 (2005): 1,467–1,484.

Middlebrooks, Jennifer S., and Natalie C. Audage. *The Effects of Childhood Stress on Health Across the Lifespan.* Atlanta, Ga.: Centers for Disease Control and Prevention, National Center for Injury Prevention and Control, 2008.

Myrick, Hugh, M.D. "Diagnosis of Alcohol Dependence." *Medscape Psychiatry & Mental Health.* Available online to subscribers. URL: http://cme.medscape.com/viewarticle/543758_print. Accessed May 8, 2009.

National Center on Addiction and Substance Abuse at Columbia University. *Family Matters: Substance Abuse and the American Family.* New York: National Center on Addiction and Substance Abuse at Columbia University, March 2005.

National Highway Transportation Safety Administration. *Traffic Safety Facts: Repeat Intoxicated Driver Laws.* January 2008.

National Institute on Alcohol Abuse and Alcoholism. *FAQ for the General Public.* February 2007. Available online. URL: http://www.niaaa.nih.gov/FAQs/Genderal-English/default.htm. Accessed April 23, 2009.

Pagano, Maria E., et al. "Predictors of Initial AA-Related Helping: Findings from Project MATCH." *Journal of Studies on Alcohol and Drugs* 70, no. 1 (2009): 117–125.

Pettinati, Helen M., et al. "A Double Blind, Placebo-Controlled Trial that Combines Disulfiram and Naltrexone for Treating Co-Occurring Cocaine and Alcohol Dependence." *Addictive Behaviors* 33, no. 5 (2008): 651–667.

Poikolainen, Kari. "Risk Factors for Alcohol Dependence: A Case-Control Study." *Alcohol & Alcoholism* 35, no. 2 (2000): 190–196.

Sartor, Carolyn E., et al. "The Role of Childhood Risk Factors in Initiation of Alcohol Use and Progression to Alcohol Dependence." *Addiction* 102, no. 2 (2006): 216–225.

Scheier, Lawrence M., Sandra C. Lapham, and Janet C'De Baca. "Cognitive Predictors of Alcohol Involvement and Alcohol Consumption-Related Consequences in a Sample of Drunk-Driving Offenders." *Substance Use & Misuse* 43, no. 14 (2008): 2,089–2,115.

Schuckit, M. A., and T. L. Smith. "The Relationships of a Family History of Alcohol Dependence, a Low Level of Response to Alcohol and Six Domains of Life Functioning to the Development of Alcohol Use Disorders." *Journal of Studies on Alcohol* 61, no. 6 (2000): 827–835.

"The Scope of the Problem." *Alcohol Research & Health* 28, no. 2 (2004/2005): 111–120.

Trim, Ryan S., Marc A. Schuckit, and Tom L. Smith. "The Relationships of the Level of Response to Alcohol and Additional Characteristics to Alcohol Use Disorders Across Adulthood: A Discrete-Time Survival Analysis." *Alcoholism: Clinical and Experimental Research* 33, no. 9 (2009): 1–9.

alcoholism mutual aid societies Organizations that seek to help individuals who are dependent on alcohol. According to William L. White in his 2001 article in *Alcoholism Treatment Quarterly*, the first abstinence-based mutual aid societies were formed by NATIVE AMERICANS in the 1750s, nearly 100 years before the Washingtonian Revival, a successful 19th century alcoholism mutual aid society. According to White, "Wagomend, an Assinsink Munsee, and Papoonan, a Unami Delaware, exhorted their tribes to denounce rum and return to their cultural traditions. Wagomend hosted quarterly meetings where walking, singing, dancing and cathartic weeping were used to support the personal and cultural rejection of alcohol." White says that the early Native American abstinence societies perceived recovery from alcohol as vital to the very survival of their Native American life. Today the most famous and successful example of an alcoholism mutual aid society is Alcoholics Anonymous (AA). This organization promotes complete ABSTINENCE from all forms of alcohol and offers members an opportunity to learn from the experiences of others as well as to help others who are at risk for resuming drinking. Individuals designated as "sponsors" assist the new member to resist the urges pulling him or her toward using alcohol again.

Sometimes individuals believe that they are the only people who have felt dependent on alcohol or who experienced certain emotions or fears. Through AA and other groups, these individuals learn that they are not alone and that many others have experienced the same feelings, fears, and issues. This knowledge helps with abstinence as well as with recovery from relapses to drinking.

Founded in 1935 by surgeon Robert Smith and stock analyst William Wilson, Alcoholics Anonymous is a global organization that continues as a highly effective self-help organization that aids many alcohol-dependent individuals. Spinoff organizations have also developed to treat individuals addicted to narcotics in general, to cocaine in particular, and to other substances. In addition, Al-Anon is an international organization for the self-help benefit of spouses, partners, or other family members of an alcoholic. It helps them to face their own DENIAL about the problem and also to cease enabling the alcoholic in his or her alcoholic behavior.

According to the Substance Abuse and Mental Health Services Administration (SAMHSA), about 5 million people ages 12 and older attended self-help groups in 2006 or 2007 because of problems with alcohol and/or drugs. About 45 percent attended a mutual aid group because of a problem with alcohol only, while 21.8 attended a group for illicit drug use only. A third of all those attending mutual aid self-help groups attended because of an involvement in both alcohol and illicit drugs.

Most attendees (66.1 percent) were male, and the largest age grouping was ages 26 to 49 years (57.4 percent). Self-help attendees were primarily white (67.7 percent), and the majority lived in a large metropolitan area (55.6 percent). Most had a family income of less than $50,000 (68.1 percent).

Research reported by Rudolf H. Moos, Bernice S. Moos, and Christine Timko in 2006 based on 461 individuals with alcohol use disorders (50 percent of whom were female) found that women were more likely than men to participate in both treatment and Alcoholics Anonymous sessions, and they also had better alcohol-related outcomes than men. Women also had greater reductions in their levels of DEPRESSION and avoidance coping subsequent to their participation in AA. However, the researchers also found that in the cases of both women and men, more dependence symptoms, more drinking problems, a heavier alcohol use, and a greater reliance on alcohol to reduce tension were all predictive of a lower probability of a stable remission.

Another finding was that close relationships with friends was a greater factor with the recovery of women compared to recovery among men. According to the researchers, "With respect to gender differences, self-efficacy and a larger circle of supportive friends were the most important predictors of stable remission for women, whereas more overall social resources and less depression, chronic stressors, and reliance on avoidance coping and drinking to cope predicted a higher likelihood of stable remission for men. Enhanced self-confidence and support from close relationships with friends may be especially important factors in recovery for women, whereas men appear to need a broader array of social resources from both family members and friends, along with skills that enable them to reduce their reliance on avoidance coping."

In another study by Moos and Moos, the researchers compared previously untreated individuals with alcoholism at baseline, one year, three years, eight years, and 16 years later. They found that individuals who received 27 weeks or more of treatment in the first year after seeking help had better alcohol-related outcomes than those who were not treated in the first year. They also found that those who participated in AA for at least 27 weeks had better outcomes at the 16-year point. There were 461 subjects at the 16-year point.

In the first year, 59.2 percent received professional treatment for at least 20 weeks, and 58.4 percent participated in AA meetings. In the second and third years, 36.2 percent were in treatment and 38.2 percent participated in treatment. The individuals who attended AA had better social functioning than the nonattenders.

The researchers said, "Part of the association between AA attendance and better social functioning, which reflects the composition of the social network, likely is a direct function of participation in AA. In fact, for some individuals, involvement with a circle of abstinent friends may reflect a turning point that enables them to address their

problems, build their coping skills, and establish more supportive social resources. Participation in a mutual support group may enhance and amplify these changes in life context and coping to promote better long-term outcomes."

See also ALCOHOL AND ALCOHOL USE; ALCOHOLISM/ ALCOHOL DEPENDENCE AND ALCOHOL ABUSE; DISULFIRAM; IMPAIRED PHYSICIANS; NALTREXONE; TREATMENT.

Moos, Rudolf H., and Bernice S. Moos. "Participation in Treatment and Alcoholics Anonymous: A 16-Year Follow-up of Initially Untreated Individuals." *Journal of Clinical Psychology* 62, no. 6 (2006): 735–750.

Moos, Rudolf H., Bernice S. Moos, and Christine Timko. "Gender, Treatment and Self-Help in Remission from Alcohol Use Disorders." *Clinical Medicine & Research* 4, no. 3 (2006): 163–174.

Office of Applied Studies. "Participation in Self-Help Groups for Alcohol and Illicit Drug Use: 2006 and 2007." *The NSDUH Report.* November 13, 2008, pp. 1–4.

White, William L. "Pre-A.A. Alcoholic Mutual Aid Societies." *Alcoholism Treatment Quarterly* 19, no. 2 (2001): 1–21.

alcohol poisoning   Excessive drinking over a brief period to the point that the body is unable to metabolize the alcohol rapidly enough, and the body is at risk for severe harm. This harmful level of drinking also suppresses the gag reflex that prevents choking, and thus the individual could choke to death on his or her own vomit. Clearly, alcohol poisoning is a very dangerous situation which can lead to death if the person is not treated by a physician within a short period of time, because the liver cannot metabolize an excessive level of alcohol rapidly enough. Even if the person survives, he or she may suffer from irreversible brain damage. If an individual may have succumbed to alcohol poisoning, it is very important to contact emergency services as soon as possible by calling 911.

An individual's blood alcohol level can continue to rise even if he or she has passed out from drinking. As a result, it should not be assumed that a person can just "sleep it off" after very heavy drinking.

In an analysis of accidental deaths caused by alcohol poisoning, reported by Yoon et al., 317 deaths per year were attributed to alcohol poisoning with an additional 1,076 in which alcohol poisoning was a contributing factor, for a total of 1,393 deaths per year from alcohol poisoning. Males represented 80 percent of these deaths. The researchers also found that alcohol poisoning was a contributing cause of death for 10 underlying causes of deaths, including alcohol poisoning by other drugs, accidental poisoning by analgesics and other drugs, and other causes. (See Table 1.)

The BLOOD ALCOHOL CONCENTRATION of the person with alcohol poisoning may be as high as 0.4, which is five times the legal limit of 0.08 for operating a motor vehicle in the United States. Some cases of alcohol poisoning occur on college campuses, where BINGE DRINKING may occur.

Symptoms and Diagnostic Path

Symptoms of alcohol poisoning may include the following:

- mental confusion, stupor, coma, or the person cannot be roused

- vomiting

- seizures

- slowed breathing (less than eight breaths per minute)

- irregular breathing (10 seconds or more between breaths)

- hypothermia (low body temperature), signified by bluish skin color and/or paleness

The person with possible alcohol poisoning needs immediate medical attention. The medical professional needs to be alerted that the individual has consumed an extreme amount of alcohol. Untreated cases of alcohol poisoning can lead to the following outcomes:

- The victim chokes to death on his or her own vomit.

- The breathing slows, becomes irregular, or stops.

- The heart beats irregularly or it stops altogether.

TABLE 1
TOP TEN UNDERLYING CAUSES OF DEATHS FOR WHICH ACCIDENTAL ALCOHOL POISONING WAS CODED AS A CONTRIBUTING CAUSE OF DEATH, UNITED STATES, 1996–1998

Rank	Underlying Causes of Death	Number of Deaths 1996–1998	Yearly Average Number of Deaths, 1996–1998	Percent
1	Accidental poisoning by other drugs	1,258	419	39.0
2	Accidental poisoning by analgesics, antipyretics and anti-rheumatics	1,154	385	35.7
3	Accidental poisoning by other drugs acting on central and autonomic nervous systems	310	103	9.6
4	Accidental poisoning by tranquilizers	76	25	2.4
5	Accidental poisoning by other psychotropic agents	70	23	2.2
6	Diseases of the circulatory system	57	19	1.8
7	Suicide and self-inflicted injury	47	16	1.5
8	Accidental drowning and submersion	45	15	1.4
9	Motor vehicle traffic and non-traffic accidents	38	13	1.2
10	Other external causes of accidents, injuries, and poisoning	28	9	0.9
	Subtotal*	3,083	1,027	95.7
	Total	3,229	1,076	100.0

*Subtotal figures are totals for the top ten underlying causes of death for which alcohol poisoning was coded as the contributing cause of death.
 Total figures include all deaths in which alcohol poisoning was given as a contributing cause.
Adapted from Yoon, Young-Hee, et al. "Accidental Alcohol Poisoning Mortality in the United States, 1996–1998." *Alcohol Research & Health* 27, no. 1 (2003): 113.

- The body temperature drops dangerously low (hypothermia).
- Hypoglycemia (too little blood sugar) leads to seizures.
- Untreated severe dehydration from vomiting can cause seizures, permanent brain damage, or death.

Treatment Options and Outlook

Medical treatment may include intravenous fluids to prevent dehydration, as well as monitoring of the airways to watch for breathing problems.

Risk Factors and Preventive Measures

The highest rates of alcohol poisoning are seen among Hispanic and black males, based on data from Young-Hee Yoon and colleagues for 1996–98. Those who were at the greatest risk for alcohol poisoning were males between the ages of 35 and 54 years. Only 2 percent of the deaths from alcohol poisoning were among underage drinkers. The rate of alcohol poisoning deaths was lower among married compared to unmarried people (including divorced, widowed, or never-married individuals). The researchers also found that in the broad majority of cases (90 percent), other drugs in addition to alcohol were present.

To avoid alcohol poisoning, excessive drinking should be avoided.

See also ACETALDEHYDE; ADOLESCENTS AND DRINKING; ALCOHOL AND ALCOHOL USE; ALCOHOL AND MEN; ALCOHOL AND OTHER DRUGS; ALCOHOL AND WOMEN; ALCOHOLIC BLACKOUTS; COLLEGE STUDENTS; EMERGENCY TREATMENT; EXCESSIVE DRINKING AND HEALTH CONSEQUENCES; EXCESSIVE DRINKING AND NEGATIVE SOCIAL CONSEQUENCES; TREATMENT; UNDERAGE DRINKING.

Yoon, Young-Hee, et al. "Accidental Alcohol Poisoning Mortality in the United States, 1996–1998." *Alcohol Research & Health* 27, no. 1 (2003): 110–118.

Antabuse   See DISULFIRAM; TREATMENT.

antidepressants   Medications that are used to treat clinical DEPRESSION. Individuals with other disorders sometimes may also be treated with antidepressants; for example, many individuals with ANXIETY DISORDERS, ATTENTION-DEFICIT/HYPERACTIVITY DISORDER (ADHD), or BIPOLAR DISORDER may also have a depressive disorder. In addition, sometimes individuals with ADHD who are *not* depressed are treated off-label for their ADHD symptoms with atypical antidepressants, such as bupropion (Wellbutrin, Wellbutrin XL).

Many individuals who either abuse or are dependent on alcohol have an underlying problem with untreated major depression. They may wrongly assume that the lowering of inhibitions that is caused by intoxication with alcohol will make them feel better; however, alcohol itself is a depressant, and thus, it cannot free people from an inherent depression. Once a person develops a dependence on alcohol, even if he or she is diagnosed and treated for major depression, this will not invariably mean that the alcoholism itself will abate. It is an independent behavior that must be challenged by the individual, with the help of counselors, physicians, medications, 12-step groups such as Alcoholics Anonymous, and other proven strategies.

There are several different categories of antidepressants, including tricyclics, such as desipramine (Norpramin) and imipramine; selective serotonin reuptake inhibitors (SSRIs), such as fluoxetine (Prozac) or sertraline (Zoloft); and serotonin norepinephrine reuptake inhibitors (SNRIs), such as venlafaxine (Effexor, Effexor XR) and duloxetine (Cymbalta). Monoamine oxidase inhibitors are another class of antidepressants, but they are infrequently prescribed today because of the extremely strict dietary rules that must be followed and that are difficult for most people to comply with.

As with all medications, antidepressants may cause side effects. Some antidepressants often cause weight gain, particularly mirtazapine (Remeron). Paroxetine (Paxil) may also cause weight gain. Weight gain is less likely with bupropion (Wellbutrin, Wellbutrin XL), and some people who take bupropion may lose two to three pounds, according to the Agency for Healthcare Research and Quality. Some antidepressants may cause nausea and vomiting, particularly venlafaxine (Effexor, Effexor XR). Another side effect of some antidepressants may be the loss of sexual desire or other sexual problems. This side effect is the most common among those taking parox-etine (Paxil), and it is the least common among those taking bupropion. Diarrhea is another com-mon side effect of some antidepressants, and it is the most common among those taking sertraline (Zoloft).

In individuals younger than age 25, taking anti-depressants may sometimes increase the risk for SUICIDE, particularly when the individual first starts taking the drug. It should never be assumed that the risk for suicide has abated the day a person starts taking antidepressants. Instead, the risk may temporarily increase.

In most cases, individuals taking antidepres-sants should not stop taking them abruptly. It is also wise to consult with a physician first about whether antidepressants should be tapered off. Some antidepressants may cause flu-like symptoms if they are suddenly stopped, particularly such anti-depressants as paroxetine (Paxil) and venlafaxine (Effexor). In contrast, fluoxetine (Prozac) is the least likely to cause flu-like symptoms when the medication is stopped abruptly.

Rarely, individuals may obtain an excess of sero-tonin as a result of antidepressants or other drugs that they take, a condition that is referred to as serotonin syndrome. Medications which may some-times increase serotonin to excessive levels include some antidepressants, some migraine headache drugs (particularly triptan medications, such as Imitrex and Amerge), some herbal remedies (such as St. John's Wort), some over-the-counter medi-cations that contain dextromethorphan (a cough remedy), and some prescribed pain killers (such as the narcotic meperidine [Demerol]). Symptoms of serotonin syndrome include hallucinations, confu-sion, fever, rapid heartbeat, vomiting, and loss of coordination.

See also IMPULSE CONTROL DISORDERS; MEDICA-TIONS INTERACTIONS WITH ALCOHOL; PERSONALITY DIS-ORDERS; PSYCHIATRIC COMORBIDITIES; SCHIZOPHRENIA; TREATMENT.

Robinson, Sandra, et al. *Antidepressant Medicines: A Guide for Adults with Depression.* Washington, D.C.: Agency for Healthcare Research and Quality, 2007.

antisocial personality disorder/antisocial behavior

A psychiatric disorder that is characterized by a lack of empathy, insensitivity, lack of regard for the rights of others, and that includes committing criminal acts and sometimes violent acts as well. In the past, a person with this behavior was referred to as a sociopath. The antisocial person often sees his or her victims as stupid or even comical, and although he or she lacks empathy, the antisocial person may be very adept at manipulating the emotions of others in order to obtain whatever gains are sought.

Antisocial behavior includes such acts as bur-glary, assault, and even rape or murder, although most people with antisocial personality disorder commit lesser crimes. Some individuals who are politicians or businessmen have antisocial person-ality disorder (ASPD). Many people incarcerated in prison have antisocial personality disorder, and they are there so that others are protected from them; however, some people with ASPD have never been arrested or incarcerated. Alcohol abuse and ALCOHOLISM/ALCOHOL DEPENDENCE are common among those with antisocial personality disorder.

A study of college students and their noncollege peers, reported in 2008 by Carlos Blanco and col-leagues in the *Archives of General Psychiatry*, revealed that 4.7 percent of college students had antisocial personality disorder, as did 8.5 percent of their noncollege peers. Thus, it is clear that it is not only individuals in jail or prison who have antiso-cial personality disorder, although the percentage among non-incarcerated individuals with this diag-nosis is much lower than among individuals who have been convicted of crimes and are in jail.

Symptoms and Diagnostic Path

Antisocial personality disorder is diagnosed by a person's acts rather than their feelings; for example, DEPRESSION is characterized by extreme sadness and feelings of worthlessness (among other symptoms), but antisocial personality disorder is diagnosed by criminal acts that are unaccompanied by remorse. Often antisocial personality disorder in the adult was preceded by ATTENTION-DEFICIT/HYPERACTIV-ITY DISORDER, CONDUCT DISORDER, or oppositional defiant disorder in the child or adolescent. Some individuals with antisocial personality disorder had both attention-deficit/hyperactivity disorder and either conduct disorder or oppositional defiant disorder as children.

Treatment Options and Outlook

Antisocial personality disorder is difficult for mental health professionals to treat, although accompanying disorders, such as alcohol dependence, depression, and other accompanying disorders, are treatable with medication and therapy. Often individuals with antisocial personality disorder do not think there is anything wrong with them, and thus, they receive treatment only if they are compelled to, for example, as part of a criminal sentence.

Risk Factors and Preventive Measures

There is an apparent genetic risk for antisocial personality disorder, but there are no known preventive measures against the development of this disorder. Men are more likely to have ASPD than women.

See also AGGRESSIVE BEHAVIOR AND ALCOHOL; ALCOHOL AND MEN; ALCOHOL AND OTHER DRUGS; ANXIETY DISORDERS; BIPOLAR DISORDER; COLLEGE STUDENTS; GENETICS AND ALCOHOL; IMPULSE CONTROL DISORDERS; PERSONALITY DISORDERS; PSYCHIATRIC COMORBIDITIES; SCHIZOPHRENIA.

Blanco, Carlos, M.D., et al. "Mental Health of College Students and Their Non-College-Attending Peers: Results from the National Epidemiologic Study on Alcohol and Related Conditions." *Archives of General Psychiatry* 65, no. 12 (2008): 1,429–1,437.

anxiety disorders A category of serious yet common psychiatric disorders that cause a level of personal distress significant to impair an individual's life at work and at home. Anxiety disorders as defined by the American Psychiatric Association include generalized anxiety disorder, panic disorder, posttraumatic stress disorder (PTSD), obsessive-compulsive disorder (OCD), specific phobia, and social phobia. Some anxiety disorders seriously impede treatment for ALCOHOLISM; for example, the person with untreated social phobia may find it difficult or impossible to attend group therapy or sessions at Alcoholics Anonymous. Many people suffer from more than one type of anxiety disorder as well as from other problems, such as alcohol abuse or alcoholism.

Sometimes anxiety can be triggered by giving up drinking, and sometimes alcohol can cause symptoms that resemble anxiety disorders. In addition, high dosages of other substances such as caffeine can mimic the symptoms of panic disorder. Sudie E. Back and Kathleen T. Brady, M.D., reported in their article in 2008 in *Psychiatric Annals* on anxiety disorders with comorbid substance use disorders, writing, "The best way to differentiate substance-induced, transient symptoms of anxiety from anxiety disorders that warrant treatment is through observation of symptoms during a period of abstinence."

They add, "A family history of anxiety disorder, the onset of anxiety symptoms before the onset of the SUD [substance use disorder], and sustained anxiety symptoms during lengthy periods of abstinence all suggest an anxiety disorder that will need to be addressed with specific treatment."

An estimated 18 percent of Americans suffer from an anxiety disorder at some point in their lives according to the National Institute on Mental Health (NIMH). In a survey of 956 primary care patients by Krut Kroenke, M.D., and colleagues and published in 2007 in the *Annals of Internal Medicine,* the researchers found that 19.5 percent had at least one anxiety disorder. The largest percentage, or 8.6 percent, had posttraumatic stress disorder, followed by generalized anxiety disorder (7.6 percent), panic disorder (6.8 percent), and social anxiety disorder (6.2 percent). Kroenke et al. also reported that 41 percent of the patients with an anxiety disorder were not currently receiving treatment.

The researchers also found that self-reported disability days (sick days) were significantly higher among those with anxiety disorders; for example, among patients with no anxiety disorders, individuals took off an average 5.7 days in the past three months. For those with one anxiety disorder, individuals had 11.2 sick days. Individuals with two anxiety disorders had 13.2 sick days and those with three or four anxiety disorders had 30.6 sick days. Clearly, those with more anxiety disorders likely find it difficult or impossible to hold a job or accomplish tasks at home.

The person with GENERALIZED ANXIETY DISORDER (GAD) is constantly worried, with little reason for this chronic worrying. Others may reassure them that everything will be all right but they continue to ruminate about problems they have or even possible problems that they or others might have. The person with GAD is consumed with this worry, which affects their ability to function normally and even to sleep.

PANIC DISORDER is another anxiety disorder. The person with panic disorder often believes that he or she is having a heart attack because of a racing heart and a feeling of imminent doom. Often they seek help from the nearest hospital emergency room. If no cardiac causes are found, they may be diagnosed with panic disorder by the emergency room physician.

Another common anxiety disorder is POST-TRAUMATIC STRESS DISORDER (PTSD). This disorder is caused by a traumatic event, such as a violent attack (such as a rape or severe beating), or by combat experience. The person with PTSD often has terrifying flashbacks when he or she reexperiences the trauma in the mind, just as if it were happening all over again.

OBSESSIVE-COMPULSIVE DISORDER (OCD) is an anxiety disorder in which the individual has recurrent thoughts that they cannot block, as well as a compulsion to perform illogical acts, such as frequently washing their hands or counting items. The person may leave the house and then worry that he or she did not lock the door, having to return to check that the door is actually locked. Then the individual may leave and wonder if the door was "really" locked. Individuals with OCD usually know that their thoughts and behaviors are irrational, but they cannot stop them without treatment.

Some individuals suffer from a SPECIFIC PHOBIA, such as a fear of ants or a fear of tunnels. Virtually anything can become a specific phobia for an individual. When a person has a specific phobia, they actively seek to avoid the feared object. In some cases, avoidance is relatively easy; for example, if a person fears snakes and lives in Alaska, it is unlikely he or she will encounter snakes, just as a person who lives in Florida and fears polar bears is unlikely to encounter the feared object. But sometimes the specific phobia is about a common object, which makes life much more difficult for the person unless he or she receives treatment.

SOCIAL PHOBIA is another form of anxiety disorder, in which the individual is extremely uncomfortable around others, lest they judge him or her harshly. This anxiety disorder can severely limit the ability to deal with others and affect the person at work as well as in social situations. Such individuals generally avoid social contact as much as possible unless they receive treatment.

See also ALCOHOL AND MEN; ALCOHOL AND WOMEN; ALCOHOLIC PSYCHOSIS; ANTISOCIAL PERSONALITY DISORDER/ANTISOCIAL BEHAVIOR; ATTENTION-DEFICIT/HYPERACTIVITY DISORDER; BIPOLAR DISORDER; COLLEGE STUDENTS; CONDUCT DISORDER; DEPRESSION; EXCESSIVE DRINKING AND HEALTH CONSEQUENCES; EXCESSIVE DRINKING AND NEGATIVE SOCIAL CONSEQUENCES; IMPULSE CONTROL DISORDERS; PERSONALITY DISORDERS; PSYCHIATRIC COMORBIDITIES; SCHIZOPHRENIA; TREATMENT.

Back, Sudie E., and Kathleen T. Brady, M.D. "Anxiety Disorders with Comorbid Substance Use Disorders: Diagnostic and Treatment Considerations." *Psychiatric Annals* 38, no. 11 (2008): 724–729.

Barlow, David H. "Anxiety Disorders, Comorbid Substance Abuse, and Benzodiazepine Discontinuation: Implications for Treatment." In *Treatment of Drug-Dependent Individuals with* Comorbid Mental Disorders, edited by Lisa Simon Onken, Jack D. Blaine, M.D., Sandra Genser, M.D., and Arthur MacNeill Horton, 33–51. Rockville, Md.: National Institute on Drug Abuse, 1997.

Blanco, Carlos, M.D., et al. "Mental Health of College Students and Their Non-College-Attending Peers: Results from the National Epidemiologic Study on Alcohol and Related Conditions." *Archives of General Psychiatry* 65, no. 12 (2008): 1,429–1,437.

Doctor, Ronald, Ada Kahn, and Christine Adamec. *The Encyclopedia of Phobias, Fears and Anxiety Disorders.* 3rd ed. New York: Facts On File, Inc., 2008.

Doctor, Ronald, and Frank Shirimoto. *Encyclopedia of Traumatic Stress Disorders.* In press. New York: Facts On File, Inc., 2009.

Grant, Bridget F., et al. "Prevalence and Co-Occurrence of Substance Use Disorders and Independent Mood and Anxiety Disorders: Results from the National Epidemiologic Survey on Alcohol and Related Conditions." *Alcohol Research & Health* 29, no. 2 (2006): 107–120.

Kroenke, Kurt, M.D., et al. "Anxiety Disorders in Primary Care: Prevalence, Impairment, Comorbidity, and Detection." *Annals of Internal Medicine* 146, no. 5 (2007): 317–325.

attention-deficit/hyperactivity disorder (ADHD)

A developmental disorder that occurs in children, adolescents, and adults, and which is characterized by severe impulsivity and hyperactivity or extreme inattentiveness. There is also a combined form of ADHD in which the individual has features of impulsivity, inattentiveness, and hyperactivity. It is estimated that about 8 percent of all children and 4 percent of all adults in the United States have ADHD. In many cases, the symptoms of ADHD are untreated because the disorder has not been diagnosed. Boys are more than twice as likely to be diagnosed with ADHD than are girls; however, it is unclear if this much greater level of diagnosis is because more boys actually have ADHD than girls or if it is instead due to a gender bias in diagnosis or there is some other cause. (See Table 1 for demographic information on children with ADHD.)

Often, ADHD presents very differently in adults with the disorder than in children and adolescents; for example, hyperactive children and even some adolescents may be very physically active, while hyperactive adults have generally learned to control their motor hyperactivity. They are more likely to squirm about while sitting or they may talk very rapidly. (Often ADHD is misdiagnosed in adults as bipolar disorder.)

ADHD is generally treated with stimulants, although some nonstimulants such as atomoxetine (Strattera) or antidepressants or other medications are also used, particularly if the physician fears the potential abuse of stimulants (as is more likely to occur with adolescents and young adults).

Many studies have shown a link between ADHD and an increased risk for alcohol abuse. Ronald C. Kessler and his colleagues reported higher rates of drug and alcohol abuse and dependence among individuals with ADHD compared to those without ADHD in the National Comorbidity Survey Replication, reported in the *American Journal of Psychiatry* in 2006. For example, 5.6 percent of the respondents (ages 18–44 years) without ADHD had a substance

TABLE 1

PERCENTAGE OF DIAGNOSED ATTENTION-DEFICIT/ HYPERACTIVITY DISORDER (ADHD) AMONG CHILDREN AGES 6–17 YEARS, BY SELECTED CHARACTERISTICS

Selected Characteristic	Percent with ADHD
Total	8.4
Gender	
Boys	11.8
Girls	4.8
Age	
6–11 years	7.1
12–17 years	9.6
Birthweight	
Low (less than 2,500 grams)	11.7
Not low (2,500 grams or more)	8.1
Race and ethnicity	
Non-Hispanic white	9.8
Non-Hispanic black	8.6
Hispanic	5.3
Family structure	
Mother only	11.2
Mother and father	7.1
Health insurance coverage at interview	
Uninsured	5.7
Medicaid	11.6
Private	7.7
Mother's education	
Less than high school graduate	6.4
High school graduate or GED	9.2
Some college	9.5
Bachelor's degree or more	6.5

Source: Adapted from Pastor, P. N., and C. A. Reuben. *Diagnosed Attention Deficit Hyperactivity Disorder and Learning Disability: United States, 2004–2006.* Hyattsville, Md.: National Center for Health Statistics. Vital Health Stat 10 (237), 2008. Page 10.

use disorder, while the rate was 15.2 percent for those adults with ADHD. With regard to alcohol abuse or dependence alone, Kessler found that 5.9 percent of adults with ADHD were alcohol abusers, compared to 2.4 percent of non-ADHD adults. He also found a rate of 5.8 percent of alcohol dependence (alcoholism) among adults with ADHD, compared to a rate of 2.0 percent among non-ADHD subjects. As a result, alcohol abuse and dependence is more than twice as prevalent in adults with ADHD compared to adults who do not have ADHD.

Some studies such as by Mannuzza et al. have shown that when children with ADHD are prescribed methylphenidate, they may have a reduced risk for substance abuse in adulthood; however, other studies, such as by Biederman et al., have found neither an increased or decreased risk for substance abuse in adulthood among those who were prescribed stimulants for their ADHD in childhood. The one area of agreement appears to be that taking stimulants for ADHD in childhood does not increase the risk for substance abuse in adulthood, as was feared by some parents and others.

Among those adolescents and young adults with ADHD who divert or misuse their prescription stimulants, Wilens et al. found that the majority (80 percent) also had conduct disorder or a substance use disorder.

Symptoms and Diagnostic Path

ADHD is characterized by inattentiveness and distractibility. Many children with ADHD are also hyperactive and very impulsive. The adolescent or adult with ADHD may exhibit some or all of the following behaviors:

- acting without thinking (impulsivity)
- failing to consider the consequences of actions (impulsivity)
- daydreaming (inattentiveness)
- distractibility—moving from one task to another without completing any tasks (inattentiveness)
- constantly moving about or (as with an adult) motion while sitting, jiggling a leg or moving about (hyperactivity)

Among children and adolescents, ADHD is diagnosed by their behavior and through various psychiatric instruments that check for indicators of ADHD. In addition, the reports of parents are considered, as well as information from teachers, such as report card evaluations. Among adults, ADHD is generally diagnosed by the physician's observations of the individual's behavior and self-reports of behavior, as well as by retrospective reports of childhood behavior, such as comments from teachers in old report cards. Sometimes spouses of adults who may have ADHD are also interviewed by physicians to help determine if the adult exhibits symptoms at home.

There are also rating scales that help physicians to determine if an adult patient has ADHD, such as the Adult ADHD Self-Report Scale (ASRS), a six-item test available online at http://www.med.nyu.edu/psych/psychiatrist/adhd.html. Other scales for ADHD include the Brown Attention-Deficit Disorder (ADD) Rating Scale for Adults, the Conners' Adult ADHD Rating Scales, and the Copeland Symptom Checklist for Adult Attention Deficit Disorders.

Adults with ADHD may also complain of frequently losing items and having problems with being on time or completing important tasks.

Treatment Options and Outlook

ADHD is usually treated with short-acting or long-acting stimulant medications, such as methylphenidate (Ritalin, Ritalin-LA, Concerta) or with amphetamines. Nonstimulant medications are also available, such as atomoxetine (Strattera), which is approved by the Food and Drug Administration (FDA) for the treatment of ADHD. In 2008, Concerta was approved for the treatment of adult ADHD, as was Vyvanse, a long-acting form of amphetamine. In general, long-acting medications are recommended for children or adults with ADHD because medication compliance is a serious problem. In addition, children who must receive their medication from the school nurse during the day report experiencing embarrassment and teasing from their peers.

If the individual is at risk for substance abuse or he or she is currently a substance abuser, physicians generally avoid prescribing stimulants; instead, they use atomoxetine or another medication, such as the atypical antidepressant bupropion (Wellbutrin, Wellbutrin XL). Bupropion is not approved by the FDA to treat ADHD, but it can be prescribed off-label by physicians and often is used in this manner. In some cases, the stimulant modafinil (Provigil) is used to treat ADHD in an off-label manner. Modafinil is a scheduled drug (controlled by the Drug Enforcement Administration) that is used to treat narcolepsy, and it is a lower-level stimulant. Amphetamines and methylphenidate are Schedule II drugs, and modafinil is a Schedule IV drug, because it has a lower abuse potential. However, it should not be prescribed to an individual with an alcohol use disorder.

Some children and adults with ADHD benefit from psychotherapy as well as from individual coaching, which provides the individual with targeted advice on how to change and improve behavior. Individual psychotherapy may also be helpful.

Issues of Medication Noncompliance Many parents are opposed to giving stimulant medication to their children with ADHD, largely because of their fear of stimulant drugs and because of fears that are actively generated by such groups as Scientologists, who are opposed to all psychiatric drugs but have particularly lobbied against medications for ADHD. (In past years, Scientologists lobbied against antidepressants, but many Americans believe that it is important to treat depression with medications. However, they are much less sure about if or how ADHD should be treated.)

As a result, research indicates that only about half of children and adolescents diagnosed with ADHD are taking medications for their symptoms, according to Visser, Lesesne, and Perou in their article for *Pediatrics* on national estimates and factors associated with medication treatment, based on data from the National Survey of Children's Health in 2003. Factors increasing the probability of receiving current treatment were being white, under age 13, having English spoken in the home as the primary language, having a health-care contact in the past year, and reported psychological difficulties.

It is unknown how many adults with ADHD take medication for their disorder, but since many adults with ADHD are undiagnosed, it is unlikely to be the large majority. Even among those who are diagnosed with ADHD and are prescribed medication for the disorder, there is often a problem with medication compliance (following the doctor's orders regarding taking medication).

Risk Factors and Preventive Measures

There is a genetic risk for ADHD, and there are no known preventive measures against its development. However, the treatment of ADHD in childhood may be protective against many of the consequences of ADHD or its co-existing conditions (comorbidities),

such as substance abuse. In addition, treatment may be protective against other consequences, such as the higher rate of problematic consequences such as injuries that are found among individuals with ADHD compared to their non-ADHD peers. It is likely that many of these injuries stemmed from impulsive acts, and if the impulsivity of an individual is restrained or better controlled, then his or her safety outlook will improve.

See also ALCOHOLIC PSYCHOSIS; ANTISOCIAL PERSONALITY DISORDER/ANTISOCIAL BEHAVIOR; ANXIETY DISORDERS; BIPOLAR DISORDER; CONDUCT DISORDER; DEPRESSION; IMPULSE CONTROL DISORDERS; PERSONALITY DISORDERS; PSYCHIATRIC COMORBIDITIES; SCHIZOPHRENIA.

Biederman, Joseph, Michael C. Monuteaux, Thomas Spencer, et al. "Stimulant Therapy and Risk for Subsequent Substance Use Disorders in Male Adults with ADHD: A Naturalistic Controlled 10-year Follow-up Study." *American Journal of Psychiatry* 165, no. 5 (2008): 597–603.

Kessler, Ronald C., et al. "The Prevalence and Correlates of Adult ADHD in the United States: Results from the National Comorbidity Survey Replication." *American Journal of Psychiatry* 163 (April 2006): 716–723.

Mannuzza, Salvatore, Rachel G. Klein, Nhan L. Truong, et al. "Age of Methylphenidate Treatment Initiation in Children with ADHD and Later Substance Abuse: Prospective Follow-up into Adulthood." *American Journal of Psychiatry* 165, no. 5 (2008): 604–609.

Pastor, P. N., and C. A. Reuben. *Diagnosed Attention Deficit Hyperactivity Disorder and Learning Disability: United States, 2004–2006.* Vital Health Statistics 10, no. 237. Hyattsville, Md.: National Center for Health Statistics, 2008.

Visser, Susanna N., Catherine A. Lesesne, and Ruth Perou. "National Estimates and Factors Associated with Medication Treatment for Childhood Attention-Deficit/Hyperactivity Disorder." *Pediatrics* 119, Supp. (2007): S99–S106.

Wilens, Timothy E., M.D., Martin Gignac, M.D., Allison, Swezey, et al. "Characteristics of Adolescents and Young Adults with ADHD Who Divert or Misuse Their Prescribed Medications." *Journal of the American Academy of Child Adolescence & Psychiatry* 45, no. 4 (2006): 408–414.

avoidant personality disorder See PERSONALITY DISORDERS.

barbiturates Sedating medications that are derived from barbituric acid and which are sometimes used to treat individuals who are undergoing detoxification from alcohol, in order to decrease the side effects that are associated with ending alcohol use. Barbiturates are also sometimes used to treat insomnia. In addition, they can be used as a surgical anesthetic. Barbiturates should never be combined with alcohol, because this combination can be fatal.

Most barbiturates are Schedule III drugs, as classified by the Drug Enforcement Administration (DEA), because they have a risk for abuse and dependence. (Schedule I drugs are illegal drugs such as heroin and marijuana, and Schedule II drugs are drugs that carry a higher risk of dependence than barbiturates, such as oxycodone.)

There are about 12 different barbiturates that may be prescribed in the United States. Barbiturates are classified into ultra-short-acting, short-acting, intermediate-acting, and long-acting drugs. Ultra-short barbiturates act within about one minute of injection of the drug into the body. Examples of ultra-short-acting barbiturates include methohexital (Brevital), thiamyl (Surital), and thiopental (Pentothal).

Examples of short-acting or intermediate-acting barbiturates are amobarbital (Amytal), pentobarbital (Nembutal), and secobarbital (Seconal). These drugs are all Schedule II drugs controlled by the Drug Enforcement Administration because of their risk for dependence. There are also short-acting or intermediate-acting barbiturates that are Schedule III drugs, denoting a lower risk for dependence than with Schedule II drugs. Drugs in this category include butalbital (Fiornal, Fiorcet), butabarbital (Butisol), and aprobarbital (Alurate).

Several long-acting barbiturates are Schedule IV drugs, with a lower risk for drug dependence than Schedule II or Schedule III drugs. Examples of barbiturates in this category include phenobarbital (Luminal) and mephobarbital (Mebareal). These drugs do not take effect for about an hour, but their effects may last for as long as 12 hours.

If a person is addicted to barbiturates, withdrawal can be very distressing for the individual, and may include hallucinations, an elevated body temperature, and seizures. Withdrawal from barbiturates is said to be similar to that of withdrawal from alcohol dependence.

See also ALCOHOL AND OTHER DRUGS; DELIRIUM TREMENS; MEDICATION INTERACTIONS WITH ALCOHOL; TREATMENT.

benzodiazepines Central nervous system depressant medications that are prescribed to treat anxiety and ANXIETY DISORDERS. They are sometimes also used to treat short-term insomnia. Benzodiazepines are sometimes used to ease the symptoms of alcohol withdrawal.

Benzodiazepines should never be combined with alcohol, because the combination of alcohol and benzodiazepines is very dangerous and potentially lethal. Some individuals may suffer from an accidental overdose and may die from using alcohol and drugs. Some individuals combine alcohol and benzodiazepine purposely in order to commit SUICIDE.

The first benzodiazepines were introduced in the early 1960s. They were chlordiazepoxide hydrochloride (Librium) and diazepam (Valium). They were considered a safe alternative to barbiturates at that time; however, in the 1970s, physicians and others realized that benzodiazepines carried the risk of addiction. At its peak sales year in 1973, there were annual sales of $230 million of diazepam.

Benzodiazepines are now scheduled drugs, as classified by the Drug Enforcement Administration (DEA), because of their potential risk for drug abuse and dependence.

Benzodiazepines that are approved by the Food and Drug Administration (FDA) as of this writing include chlordiazepoxide (Librium), diazepam (Valium), alprazolam (Xanax, Xanax XR), triazolam (Halcion), lorazepam (Ativan), clonazepam (Klonopin), and oxazepam (Serax). Some benzodiazepines are used as sleep remedies, including such drugs as eszopiclone (Lunesta), zaleplon (Sonata), and zolpidem (Ambien). Some benzodiazepines such as alprazolam have a short-acting and high potency formulation, which increases the risk for abuse.

See also ALCOHOL AND OTHER DRUGS; ALCOHOLIC PSYCHOSIS; BARBITURATES; BIPOLAR DISORDER; PSYCHIATRIC COMORBIDITIES; SCHIZOPHRENIA; TREATMENT.

binge drinking   Very heavy drinking that occurs over a short period. According to the Substance Abuse and Mental Health Services Administration (SAMHSA), for men, binge drinking is specifically defined as the consumption of five or more drinks on the same occasion, either at the same time or within a few hours of each other and on at least one day in the past 30 days. For women, binge drinking is defined as the consumption of four or more drinks on the same occasion, at the same time or within a few hours of each other and at least once in the past 30 days. It should be noted, however, that some researchers do not differentiate between male and female subjects in their definition of binge drinking, and when no gender differentiation is made, a parameter of five or more drinks at least once in the past 30 days for both males and females is generally used.

Binge drinking is sometimes referred to as heavy episodic drinking. It always increases the blood alcohol level of the individual to .08 percent or greater, a rate at which it is illegal to drive in every state in the United States.

Binge drinking increases the risk of AGGRESSIVE BEHAVIOR by the binger, as well as the risk for exhibiting dangerously impulsive behavior. It also increases health risks; binge drinkers have an increased risk for both heart attacks and strokes. In addition, they also have an elevated risk for

injuries and death. Some studies have shown that binge drinkers are more likely to cause car fatalities and injuries than alcoholics.

The Centers for Disease Control and Prevention (CDC) estimate that about 15 percent of the total population in the United States engaged in binge drinking in 2007. According to the Office of Justice Programs at the U.S. Department of Justice, those who are frequent binge drinkers represent only about 7 percent of the population, but they drink nearly half (45 percent) of all the alcohol that is consumed in the United States.

Despite the many problems that binge drinking generates among binge drinkers (and others), the CDC says that more than 90 percent of them do *not* meet the criteria for alcohol dependence. As a result, some people conclude that binge drinking is not really a serious problem, since most binge drinkers are not alcoholics. But the first binge a person goes on may be the one that ends his or her life, or the life of another person, in a car crash or other type of accident. Binge drinking is also a risk factor for strokes. (See EXCESSIVE DRINKING AND HEALTH CONSEQUENCES.)

Age and Gender of Bingers

Binge drinking may occur among people of all ages, from adolescents (or children who are pre-adolescents) to young adults, as well as among individuals who are older alcoholics. In fact, some research has shown that when significant numbers of adults in a state are binge drinkers, this is predictive for COLLEGE STUDENTS in that state to binge drink. In general, men who binge average about 12.5 binge drinking episodes per year according to the CDC, while female bingers average about 2.7 binge drinking episodes annually.

Binge drinking most commonly occurs among young adults ages 18–25 years. It is generally a worse problem among males than females, although some research has found that female college students mistakenly believe that heavy drinking is attractive to male college students. (See ALCOHOL AND WOMEN.)

According to research by Timberlake and colleagues and reported in *Alcoholism: Clinical and Experimental Research* in 2007, most individuals are *less* likely to be binge drinkers before they attend college but then they are *more* likely to binge drink after they start attending college. This is believed to be at least partly due to the intense peer pressure to drink in college, particularly among members of fraternities and sororities. College athletes also have a high risk of binge drinking, whether they are male or female athletes.

Binge drinking is a problem among some members of the military service, particularly males and particularly those in the Marines. Some experts believe that heavy drinking and binging is part of the engrained culture of military life. (See MILITARY VETERANS/COMBAT AND ACTIVE DUTY MILITARY.)

Adolescents who were abused or neglected as children have a significantly higher rate of binge drinking than do those who were not abused or neglected. (See CHILD ABUSE AND NEGLECT.)

Problem Behaviors among Teens Who Binge Researchers have identified problematic behavioral patterns among adolescents who engage in binge drinking. For example, according to J. W. Miller and colleagues in their article in *Pediatrics* in 2007, of all the high school students drawn from the 2003 National Youth Risk Behavior Survey, about 45 percent had consumed alcohol in the past 30 days, including 29 percent who binge drank and 16 percent who drank alcohol but who did not binge drink. The researchers found that binge-drinking rates were similar among girls and boys. Binge drinkers in high school were more likely than both nondrinkers and current drinkers to perform poorly in school and to be involved in high risk behaviors, such as riding in a car with a driver who had been drinking, using illicit drugs, and being sexually active.

Possible Negative Consequences among Adult Bingers In their article for the *Journal of the American Medical Association* in 2003, Timothy S. Naimi, M.D., and colleagues point out that binge drinking is associated with many health risks. Say the authors, "Adverse health effects specifically associated with binge drinking include unintentional injuries (e.g., motor vehicle crashes, falls, drowning, hypothermia, and burns), suicide, sudden infant death syndrome, alcohol poisoning, hypertension, acute myocardial infarction [heart attack], gastritis, pancreatitis, sexually transmitted disease, meningitis, and poor control of diabetes."

The researchers found that an estimated 1 billion or more episodes of binge drinking had occurred each year from 1993 to 2001. The highest rates of binge drinking centered among young adults, as well as among males and heavy drinkers.

Surprisingly, however, the researchers found that about half of the binge drinking episodes occurred among people who were normally moderate drinkers. Said the authors, "Our finding that there are almost as many binge drinking episodes among moderate drinkers as heavy drinkers has been noted in other countries, and is largely because there are more moderate drinkers than heavy drinkers in the general population. However, these findings also emphasize why it is important to assess binge alcohol use independent of average daily alcohol consumption, and underscores why binge drinking is a key indicator of alcohol abuse among both moderate and heavy drinkers."

Beer: The Bingers' Choice

According to a study by Naimi et al., reported in 2007, the beverage of choice for most binge drinkers is beer, and in their survey of 14,150 adult binge drinkers, 74.4 percent consumed only beer or mostly beer. The researchers also reported that beer was the most common type of alcohol consumed by individuals at risk for causing or incurring harm caused by intoxication. They speculated that the lower excise taxes on beer as well as marketing practices and other factors may have influenced the selection of beer as the favorite option for the binge drinking population.

Research: Binge Drinking in North Dakota

Several interesting findings were made in a study of binge drinking among residents of North Dakota from 2004–05, based on a sample of 7,055 adults ages 18 years and older and published by the Centers for Disease Control and Prevention (CDC) in *Preventing Chronic Disease.* According to the researchers, North Dakota was chosen for the study because it consistently has one of the highest rates of binge drinking in the United States. (It is unknown, however, if residents of other states with high rates of binge-drinking resemble the binge-drinking residents of North Dakota.)

The researchers found that 19.8 percent of all adults in their sample reported binge drinking at least once in the past 30 days. In considering the age of binge drinkers, individuals ages 21–35 years had the highest rate of binge drinking (35.2 percent) and individuals ages 50 and older had the lowest (7.9 percent). Males had nearly three times the rate of binge drinking as females, or 29.1 percent for males compared to 10.6 percent for females. Binge drinking was heavy among all income levels.

Because of the unusual racial makeup of North Dakota compared to many other states, races in the North Dakota study were divided into White, American Indian and Alaska Natives, and "Other." Among these categories, American Indians and Alaska Natives had the highest rate of binge drinking, or 22.7 percent, while Whites were close behind, at 19.98 percent. Individuals classified as other races had a binge-drinking rate of 10.0 per-

cent. (See Table 1.) In considering marital status, cohabiting couples had the highest binge-drinking rate (52.9 percent), and widowed individuals had the lowest rate (2.9 percent).

In considering categories of occupations, the highest prevalence of binge drinking was found among farm or ranch employees (45.3 percent) and the lowest prevalence among health care workers (13.2 percent). People out of work for more than a year had a higher binge drinking rate (19.1 percent) than people who were out of work for less than a year (13.7 percent). See Table 1 and Table 2 for more comparative information.

More than a third of the binge-drinking workers (37.6 percent) reported having had three or more binge drinking occasions in the past 30 days.

TABLE 1
PREVALENCE OF BINGE DRINKING [a] AMONG NORTH DAKOTA ADULTS,
BY SELECTED CHARACTERISTICS, 2004–2005

Characteristic	Employed [b, c]		Nonemployed [c, d]		All adults [c]	
	Population Estimate	Binge Drinking %	Population Estimate	Binge Drinking %	Population Estimate	Binge Drinking %
Age group						
18–20	13,019	28.8	14,614	24.4	27,632	26.5
21–35	105,830	36.0	27,423	31.9	133,252	35.2
36–49	108,104	22.2	13,221	9.5	121,325	20.8
≥50	98,336	12.7	99,331	3.2	197,667	7.9
Sex						
Male	179,701	32.9	59,167	17.2	238,868	29.1
Female	146,623	13.2	96,898	6.9	243,521	10.6
Race						
White	311,491	24.1	142,102	10.6	453,593	19.9
American Indian/ Alaska Native	8,697	28.4	10,005	17.8	18,702	22.7
Other	5,414	14.3	2,711	1.2	8,125	10.0
Marital Status						
Married	222,555	19.2	83,879	6.2	306,433	15.6
Divorced	24,839	26.1	9,050	10.8	33,888	22.0
Widowed	7,021	5.1	28,051	1.7	35,072	2.4
Separated	2,112	20.9	794	14.5	2,906	19.1
Never married	58,540	38.6	31,143	28.1	89,683	35.0
Member of an unmarried couple	10,370	54.4	2,745	47.0	13,115	52.9

Characteristic	Employed [b, c]		Nonemployed [c, d]		All adults [c]	
	Population Estimate	Binge Drinking %	Population Estimate	Binge Drinking %	Population Estimate	Binge Drinking %
Income, $						
<25,000	54,699	27.0	56,971	12.6	111,670	19.6
25,000–49,999	114,363	27.0	42,601	8.1	156,964	21.9
≥50,000	128,645	22.5	23,650	11.6	152,295	20.8
Education						
Less than college	104,662	27.2	75,513	6.8	180,175	18.7
Some or more college	221,415	22.6	80,119	14.6	301,534	20.4
Employment Status						
Employed for wages	267,110	23.5	0	n/a	267,110	23.5
Self-employed	59,213	26.4	0	n/a	59,213	26.4
Out of work (<1 year)	0	n/a	4,296	13.7	4,296	13.7
Out of work (>1 year)	0	n/a	8,097	19.1	8,097	19.1
Homemaker	0	n/a	29,884	4.5	29,884	4.5
Student	0	n/a	28,350	34.7	28,350	34.7
Retired	0	n/a	72,532	3.5	72,532	3.5
Unable to work	0	n/a	11,417	7.2	11,417	7.2
Total	326,323	24.1	154,396	10.8	480,719	19.8

Source: Adapted from Jarman, Dwayne W., et al. "Binge Drinking and Occupation, North Dakota, 2004–2005." *Preventing Chronic Disease* 4, no. 4 (2007), pages 8–9.
[a] Binge drinking was defined as having consumed five or more drinks on one or more occasions during the previous 30 days.
[b] Employed is defined as working for wages or being self-employed.
[c] Represents prevalence of binge drinkers by group with the selected characteristic; therefore, percentages do not total 100.
[d] Nonemployed is defined as one of the following: out of work for more than 1 year, out of work for less than 1 year, a homemaker, a student, retired, or unable to work.

TABLE 2
PREVALENCE OF BINGE DRINKING [a] AMONG NORTH DAKOTA WORKERS [b]
BY OCCUPATIONAL CATEGORY, 2004–2005

Occupational Category	Population Estimate, N [c]	Proportion of Workers	Prevalence of Binge Drinking
Farm or ranch employee	3,484	1.1	45.3
Food or drink server	12,208	4.0	33.4
Farm or ranch owner	26,381	8.6	32.5
Manufacturing	26,033	8.4	28.0
Other occupation	104,230	33.8	26.4
Wholesale or retail sales	30,431	9.9	23.8
Financial sales	12,340	4.0	18.6
State government employee	27,965	9.1	17.6
Other government employee	26,317	8.5	21.5
Health care	39,148	12.7	13.2

Source: Adapted from Jarman, Dwayne W., et al. "Binge Drinking and Occupation, North Dakota, 2004–2005." *Preventing Chronic Disease* 4, no. 4 (2007), page 10.
[a] Binge drinking was defined as having consumed five or more drinks on one or more occasions during the previous 30 days.
[b] Workers was defined as all respondents employed in one of the nine occupational categories or the "other" occupation category.
[c] Indicates the total weighted population estimate of all North Dakota adults employed in the selected occupational category.

See also ADOLESCENTS AND DRINKING; AGE AND ALCOHOL; ALCOHOL AND MEN; ALCOHOLIC BLACKOUTS; ALCOHOLIC PSYCHOSIS; ALCOHOL POISONING; DRIVING UNDER THE INFLUENCE/DRIVING WHILE INTOXICATED; NATIVE AMERICANS; OCCUPATIONS; TREATMENT; UNDERAGE DRINKING; VIOLENCE.

Jarman, Dwayne W., et al. "Binge Drinking and Occupation, North Dakota, 2004–2005." *Preventing Chronic Disease* 4, no. 4 (2007): 1–11.

Miller, J. W., et al. "Binge Drinking and Associated Health Risk Behaviors Among High School Students." *Pediatrics* 119, no. 1 (2007): 76–85.

Naimi, Timothy S., M.D., et al. "Binge Drinking Among U.S. Adults." *Journal of the American Medical Association* 289, no. 13 (2003): 70–75.

Naimi, T. S., et al. "What Do Binge Drinkers Drink? Implications for Alcohol Control Policy." *American Journal of Preventive Medicine* 33, no. 3 (2007): 188–193.

Timberlake, D. S., et al. "College Attendance and Its Effects on Drinking Behaviors in a Longitudinal Study of Adolescents." *Alcoholism: Clinical and Experimental Research* 31, no. 6 (2007): 1,020–1,030.

bipolar disorder A severe psychiatric disorder that is often characterized by periods of mania and feelings of euphoria that alternate with periods of clinical DEPRESSION, sometimes also called manic-depression. These mood changes make it difficult for individuals with bipolar disorder to work or function in society. Some people with bipolar disorder may experience a psychotic mania, or a time when they believe that they have magical powers, or they imagine that they are celebrities or people with whom celebrities would wish to associate. In her book on bipolar disorder, *An Unquiet Mind: A Memoir of Moods and Madness,* psychiatrist Kay Redfield Jamison writes firsthand about the terrors, spending sprees, violence, and even her own attempted suicide, providing considerable insight to this condition. Individuals with bipolar disorder are at high risk for both alcohol abuse and ALCOHOLISM. Francis Mark Mondimore, M.D., author of *Bipolar Disorder,* says that bipolar disorder makes patients more vulnerable to alcoholism and drug abuse. "Perhaps the easiest-to-understand model for the observed link between bipolar disorder and alcoholism and drug abuse is the idea that the mood changes of bipolar disorder propel people into situations they would otherwise be able to avoid and cause them to do things they otherwise wouldn't do." He also says that in the worst case scenario "the mood disorder and the substance-abuse disorder start feeding on each other, and a vicious cycle of mood symptoms, increased substance abuse, and even more severe mood fluctuations take over until it's impossible to separate one problem from the other."

There are two primary forms of bipolar disorder, including bipolar I and bipolar II. Bipolar I is the more severe form of the disorder, and it is the most commonly known form. Bipolar I disorder is characterized by very low depressed states and extremely agitated manic states, and it is considered a severe mental illness. In contrast, bipolar II disorder is characterized by depression that alternates with hypomania, or a mania that is less extreme than that experienced by those with bipolar I disorder. There is also a form of bipolar disorder called cyclothymia, which is characterized by depression and hypomania that alternate with normal mood states. All forms of bipolar disorder can be difficult to diagnose, and as a result, the patient may not receive the correct diagnosis for years. About 2.6 percent of the population in the United States, or an estimated 5.7 million Americans, has bipolar disorder, and most of those have bipolar I disorder.

In the manic stage of bipolar I disorder, the person may make dangerous and impulsive choices. In contrast, while in the depressed state, the person may have difficulty making any choices. It can be hard for the lay person (and sometimes even for the psychiatrist) to differentiate between the hyperactivity of attention-deficit/hyperactivity disorder (ADHD) and the mania of bipolar disorder; however, the hyperactive person with ADHD is consistently hyperactive, while the person with bipolar disorder is inconsistently manic. In another example, the person with ADHD may impulsively purchase items that he or she can ill afford, while the person with bipolar disorder may drive to Atlantic City or Las Vegas and bet every cent on the color red. The intervals between the mania and the depression may be brief or lengthy, depending on the patient. Patients with short periods between intervals are said to experience "rapid cycling."

Large studies such as the Epidemiological Catchment Area Study (ECA) have documented that the majority (about 60 percent) of those with bipolar disorder also have a substance abuse disorder. Alternatively, data from the National Epidemiologic Survey on Alcohol and Related Conditions (NESARC) indicated that about 40 percent of those with an alcohol use disorder had a mood disorder. (Mood disorders primarily refer to depression and bipolar disorder.)

Researchers have also found that patients with both bipolar disorder and alcoholism are about twice as likely to commit SUICIDE as are bipolar patients without alcohol dependence. In addition, individuals with bipolar disorders who have substance use disorders have an increased risk for psychiatric hospitalization.

Research has also demonstrated that individuals with alcoholism/alcohol dependence have an elevated risk for other psychiatric disorders as well, and the odds ratio is very high for an alcoholic person to have bipolar disorder. For example, according to research by Petrakis et al. that was published in *Alcohol Research & Health* in 2002, an alcoholic person was 6.3 times more likely to have bipolar disorder than a person who was not an alcoholic. This is the highest risk ratio when comparing the risks for alcoholics to have bipolar disorder, major depressive disorder, anxiety disorders, or schizophrenia. (See Table 1.)

According to research by Timothy E. Wilens, M.D., and colleagues and published in *Drug and Alcohol Dependence* in 2008, the risk for a substance abuse disorder (alcohol or drug abuse or dependence) is extremely high among adolescents with bipolar disorder, and it is the bipolar disorder, rather than CONDUCT DISORDER, that is the driving force toward the development of a substance abuse problem. The relationship is so strong, according to Wilens et al., that all substance-abusing youth who exhibit a mood instability should also be evaluated for the possible presence of bipolar disorder.

Among 105 adolescents with bipolar disorder with an average age of 13.6 years, 70 percent of whom were male, Wilens found a 23 percent prevalence of alcohol abuse and a 22 percent prevalence of drug abuse. In the control group of 98 teenagers without bipolar disorder, 3 percent had

TABLE 1
ODDS RATIO FOR SERIOUS PSYCHIATRIC DISORDERS IN PEOPLE WITH ALCOHOL DEPENDENCE (ALCOHOLISM)

Comorbid Disorder	Odds Ratio
Major depressive disorder	3.6
Bipolar disorder	6.3
Generalized anxiety disorder	4.6
Panic disorder	1.7
Posttraumatic stress disorder	2.2
Schizophrenia	3.8

Adapted from Petrakis, Ismene L., M.D., et al. "Comorbidity of Alcoholism and Psychiatric Disorders." *Alcohol Research & Health* 26, no. 2 (2002): 82.

an alcohol abuse problem and only 1 percent had a drug abuse problem.

In an article for *Psychosomatic Medicine,* Dr. Krishnan stated that medical disorders are common with bipolar disorder; however, often it can be difficult to determine whether the disorder is comorbid (accompanying the bipolar disorder independently) or whether it was a consequence of treatment. Sometimes it may be both; for example, treatment may exacerbate an existing psychiatric disorder. According to Krishnan, bipolar men are about twice as likely as bipolar women to have an alcohol use disorder (alcohol abuse or dependence), but at the same time, bipolar women are about four times more likely than women without bipolar disorder to have an alcohol use disorder.

Some evidence indicates that severe childhood abuse may be implicated in some cases of bipolar disorder. In a retrospective study of 100 adults with bipolar disorder, severe childhood abuse was identified in about half the patients, based on a study by Jessica L. Garno and her colleagues and published in the *British Journal of Psychiatry* in 2005. Severe abuse in childhood among the subjects was also correlated with an earlier onset of the bipolar disease. The researchers also found that severe emotional abuse was linked to a lifetime substance misuse as well as past-year rapid cycling.

The overwhelming proportion of those with bipolar disorder also suffer from anxiety disorders. The National Comorbidity Survey showed that 92 percent of those who had bipolar I disorder (the more severe form of bipolar disorder) also had ever had an anxiety disorder, particularly SOCIAL PHOBIA (47.2 percent) and POSTTRAUMATIC STRESS DISORDER (38.8 percent). This group included subjects aged 55 and older.

In a study of elderly noninstitutionalized subjects with bipolar disorder, reported in the *American Journal of Psychiatry* in 2006 by Benjamin I. Goldstein, M.D., and colleagues, the researchers evaluated comorbid conditions in 84 subjects. They found a 12-month rate of alcohol use disorders in more than a third (38.1 percent) of the subjects. They also found other disorders in more frequency than among other elderly subjects without bipolar disorder; for example, the 12-month rate of PANIC DISORDER was 11.9 percent while the 12-month rate of GENERALIZED ANXIETY DISORDER was 9.5 percent. However, the researchers did find that the elderly people with bipolar disorder had lower rates of alcohol use disorders than younger individuals with bipolar disorder. Elderly men had a greater risk for a diagnosis of alcohol dependence, while elderly women with bipolar disorder had a greater risk for a diagnosis of panic disorder.

Said the researchers, "Taken together, these findings provide confirmatory evidence that bipolar disorder in old age remains a severe illness frequently characterized by comorbid disorders with their attendant burden and risk."

In a study of 2,963 military veterans who were diagnosed with bipolar disorder, reported by Jennifer C. Hoblyn, M.D., and colleagues in *Psychiatric Services* in 2009, the researchers found that 20 percent of the patients had been hospitalized in a psychiatric facility in the past year. The researchers found that the patients with both an alcohol abuse disorder and polysubstance dependence (an addiction to multiple drugs) had a 100 percent risk of hospitalization. However, this risk decreased to 52 percent if the patient was not separated from a partner. In contrast, if there was no alcohol abuse disorder or polysubstance dependence present in the bipolar patients and they were not separated from their partners, the risk for rehospitalization among these patients was a much lower 12 percent.

Symptoms and Diagnostic Path

Individuals with bipolar disorder are often not diagnosed or they are misdiagnosed for years. They may exhibit the following symptoms when in a manic state:

- speaking in a very rapid speech that is hard or impossible for others to understand
- expressing grandiose and wild ideas
- exhibiting promiscuity and hypersexuality
- having extreme irritability
- having unusual energy and restlessness
- having racing thoughts and jumping from one idea to another
- needing little sleep
- abusing drugs, such as alcohol, cocaine, or sleep remedies
- exhibiting aggressive or intrusive behavior

The following are symptoms of a depressed state:

- sad or anxious mood
- hopeless or helpless feelings
- feelings of worthlessness or guilt
- a lack of interest in activities that were once enjoyed
- a decreased energy level
- trouble concentrating or making decisions
- either sleeping too much or not enough
- a change in appetite, causing an unintended weight loss or gain
- chronic pain that is unexplained by disease or injury
- thoughts of suicide or suicide attempts (Expressed ideas of suicide should always be taken seriously.)

Treatment Options and Outlook

Bipolar disorder is primarily treated with medications, although psychotherapy is sometimes used as well. The key drugs that are used to treat bipolar disorder are known as mood stabilizers, which are used to "even out" the highs and lows of bipolar disorder. The two most prominently used drugs are lithium and valproate (Depakote, Depakene).

Some patients (particularly those with bipolar I disorder) say that they do not like taking their medication because their former periods of euphoria are no longer present. Thus, medication compliance may be difficult to achieve. In addition, another negative factor is that if the patient does take lithium, it can cause an extreme weight gain of up to 100 pounds. Weight gain may also occur with valproate. According to the National Institute of Mental Health (NIMH), the thyroid levels of the bipolar patient should be monitored, because patients with bipolar disorder may develop hypothyroidism or hyperthyroidism. Treatment with lithium may also cause a need for thyroid supplementation.

Anticonvulsants are sometimes used to treat bipolar disorder, such as topiramate (Topamax), gabapentin (Neurontin), and lamotrigine (Lamictal). Anticonvulsants may also be combined with lithium, if recommended by the physician. More recently, some doctors have treated patients with bipolar disorder with NALTREXONE, which is a drug that is often used to treat alcohol dependence. Thus, if the individual has both bipolar disorder and alcohol dependence, naltrexone may help with both disorders.

Sometimes patients with bipolar disorder experience psychotic symptoms. Patients with psychotic symptoms may be treated with atypical antipsychotics, such as olanzapine (Zyprexa), risperidone (Risperdal) or aripiprazole (Abilify). However, patients taking atypical antipsychotics have an increased risk for developing type 2 diabetes or metabolic syndrome. Patients with bipolar disorder who have insomnia may be treated with benzodiazepines, such as lorazepam (Ativan) or clonazepam (Klonopin). Sometimes sleep remedies such as zolpidem (Ambien) are used to treat insomnia.

If medication and therapy are ineffective, sometimes electroconvulsive therapy (ECT), or electrical shocks, are used to treat the person. The amount of electrical current used is far less than what was used in years past and is considered safe.

Risk Factors and Preventive Measures

A family history of bipolar disorder increases the risk for an individual's developing bipolar disorder. There are no preventive measures for avoiding the development of bipolar disorder, but if it is diagnosed, it is very important that the disorder be treated.

See also ALCOHOL AND WOMEN; ALCOHOLIC PSYCHOSIS; ANTISOCIAL PERSONALITY DISORDER/ANTISOCIAL BEHAVIOR; ANXIETY DISORDERS; ATTENTION-DEFICIT/HYPERACTIVITY DISORDER; COLLEGE STUDENTS; PERSONALITY DISORDERS; PSYCHIATRIC COMORBIDITIES; SCHIZOPHRENIA.

Garno, Jessica L., et al. "Impact of Childhood Abuse on the Clinical Course of Bipolar Disorder." *British Journal of Psychiatry* 186 (2005): 121–125.

Goldstein, Benjamin, M.D., Nathan Herrmann, M.D., and Kenneth I. Shulman, M.D. "Comorbidity in Bipolar Disorder among the Elderly: Results from an Epidemiological Community Sample." *American Journal of Psychiatry* 163, no. 2 (2006): 319–321.

Hirschfeld, Robert, M.D., and Lana A. Vornik. "Bipolar Disorder—Costs and Comorbidity." *American Journal of Managed Care* 11, no. 3, Supp. (2005): S85–S90.

Hoblyn, Jennifer C., M.D., et al. "Substance Use Disorders as Risk Factors for Psychiatric Hospitalization in Bipolar Disorder." *Psychiatric Services* 60, no. 1 (January 2009): 50–55.

Krishnan, K. Ranga Rama. "Psychiatric and Medical Comorbidities of Bipolar Disorder." *Psychosomatic Medicine* 67 (2005): 1–8.

Mondimore, Francis Mark, M.D. *Bipolar Disorder: A Guide for Patients and Families.* Baltimore, Md. 1999.

Petrakis, Ismene L., M.D., et al. "Comorbidity of Alcoholism and Psychiatric Disorders." *Alcohol Research & Health* 26, no. 2 (2002): 81–89.

Sonne, Susan C., and Kathleen T. Brady, M.D. "Bipolar Disorder and Alcoholism." *Alcohol Research & Health* 26, no. 2 (2002): 103–108.

Verduin, Marcia L., M.D., Bryan K. Tolliver, M.D., and Kathleen T. Brady, M.D. "Substance Abuse and Bipolar Disorder." *Medscape Psychiatry and Mental Health* 10, no. 2 (2005). Available online to subscribers. URL: http://www.medscape.com/viewarticle/515954. Accessed February 24, 2009.

Wilens, Timothy E., M.D., et al. "Further Evidence of an Association between Adolescent Bipolar Disorder with Smoking and Substance Use Disorders: A Controlled Study." *Drug and Alcohol Dependence* 95, no. 3 (2008): 188–198.

blood alcohol concentration (BAC) The amount of alcohol in the blood as a percentage, and also a measure that is used to determine whether a

TABLE 1
APPROXIMATE BLOOD ALCOHOL PERCENTAGE AMONG FEMALES, BY NUMBER OF DRINKS AND BODY WEIGHT

Number of Drinks	Body Weight in Pounds								
	90	100	120	140	160	180	200	220	240
0	.00.	.00	.00	.00	.00	.00	.00	.00	.00
1	.05	.05	.04	.03	.03	.03	.02	.02	.02
2	.10	.09	.08	.07	.06	.05	.05	.04	.04
3	.15	.14	.11	.11	.09	.08	.07	.06	.06
4	.20	.18	.15	.13	.11	.10	.09	.08	.08
5	.25	.23	.19	.16	.14	.13	.11	.10	.09
6	.30	.27	.23	.19	.17	.15	.14	.12	.11
7	.35	.32	.27	.23	.20	.18	.16	.14	.13
8	.40	.36	.30	.26	.23	.20	.18	.17	.15
9	.45	.41	.34	.29	.26	.23	.20	.19	.17
10	.51	.45	.38	.32	.28	.25	.23	.21	.19

Source: Adapted from Substance Abuse and Mental Health Services Administration (SAMHSA), "Alcohol Impairment Chart." Available online. URL: http://pathwayscourses.samhsa.gov/aaap/aaap_2_pg4_pop1.htm. Accessed July 27, 2008.

person who has been driving a vehicle is legally intoxicated. A blood alcohol level of 0.10 percent is equivalent to 0.10 grams of alcohol per 100 milliliters of blood. A drink contains .54 ounces of alcohol. This is equivalent to one shot of distilled spirits, one five-ounce glass of wine, or one 12-ounce beer.

Blood alcohol concentration can be measured with a breath test machine or by testing the individual's blood or urine. If a driver refuses to take a BAC test when asked to do so by a police officer, this may constitute a presumption of guilt of driving while over the legal intoxication limits.

Body weight also affects blood alcohol concentration. In addition, women become impaired more quickly than men, because their bodies contain more water. For example, in general, a woman who weighs 140 pounds has a blood alcohol level of .07 after only two drinks (nearly the legal level of intoxication, or .08 percent). In contrast, a man who weighs 140 pounds has a blood alcohol level of .05 after two drinks. (See Tables 1 and 2.)

TABLE 2
APPROXIMATE BLOOD ALCOHOL PERCENTAGE AMONG MALES, BY NUMBER OF DRINKS AND BODY WEIGHT

Drinks	Body Weight in Pounds							
	100	120	140	160	180	200	220	240
0	.00	.00	.00	.00	.00	.00	.00	.00
1	.04	.03	.03	.02	.02	.02	.02	.02
2	.09	.06	.05	.05	.04	.04	.03	.03
3	.11	.09	.08	.07	.06	.06	.05	.05
4	.15	.12	.11	.09	.08	.08	.07	.06
5	.19	.16	.13	.12	.11	.09	.09	.08
6	.23	.19	.16	.14	.13	.11	.10	.09
7	.26	.25	.21	.19	.17	.15	.14	.13
8	.30	.25	.21	.19	.17	.15	.14	.13
9	.34	.28	.24	.21	.19	.17	.15	.14
10	.38	.31	.27	.23	.21	.19	.17	.16

Source: Adapted from Substance Abuse and Mental Health Services Administration (SAMHSA), "Alcohol Impairment Chart." Available online. URL: http://pathwayscourses.samhsa.gov/aaap/aaap_2_pg4_pop1.htm. Accessed July 27, 2008.

Blood alcohol concentrations that exceed .40 percent may be present in individuals who have consumed alcohol very quickly and they are at risk for ALCOHOL POISONING, a medical emergency.

If the individual's blood alcohol level is over 0.08 percent, then he or she is considered above the level of legal intoxication in all states in the United States. According to the National Highway Transportation Safety Administration, some judgment loss occurs at 0.02 percent BAC. (See Table 3.)

Elevated BAC Increases the Risk for Accidents

Higher blood alcohol levels are also associated with a greater risk for car crashes and also for other types of accidents. For example, among those who are ages 16–20 years old, the risk of being killed in a single-car crash increases by five times if the BAC of the driver is between 0.02 and 0.048. The risk further increases markedly at greater BAC levels, and if the driver aged 16–20 has a BAC of 0.15 or greater, the risk of being killed in a car crash increases by 15,560 times.

According to an article by Ralph Hingson and Michael Winter for *Alcohol Research & Health* in 2003, car crashes related to alcohol abuse are more likely to occur at night and on weekends. In considering the blood alcohol levels of individuals, among those with any alcohol in their blood, the risk of

TABLE 3
EFFECTS ON DRIVING AT DIFFERENT LEVELS OF BLOOD ALCOHOL CONCENTRATION

Blood Alcohol Concentration (BAC)	Typical Effects	Predictable Effects on Driving
.02%	• Some loss of judgment • Relaxation • Slight body warmth • Altered mood	• Decline in visual functions (rapid tracking of a moving target) • Decline in ability to perform two tasks at the same time (divided attention)
.05%	• Exaggerated behavior • May have loss of small-muscle control (such as focusing eyes) • Impaired judgment • Usually good feeling • Lowered alertness • Release of inhibition	• Reduced coordination • Reduced ability to track moving objects • Difficulty steering • Reduced response to emergency driving situations
.08%	• Muscle coordination becomes poor (balance, speech, vision, reaction time, and hearing) • Harder to detect danger • Judgment, self-control, reasoning, and memory are impaired	• Concentration impaired • Short-term memory loss may occur • Speed control impaired • Reduced information processing capability (such as signal detection, visual search) • Impaired perception
.10%	• Clear deterioration of reaction time and control • Slurred speech, poor coordination, and slowed thinking	• Reduced ability to maintain lane position and brake appropriately
.15%	• Far less muscle control than normal • Vomiting may occur (unless this level is reached slowly or a person has developed a tolerance for alcohol) • Major loss of balance	• Substantial impairment in vehicle control, attention to driving task, and in necessary visual and auditory information processing

Source: Adapted from National Highway Transportation Safety Administration, "The ABCs of BAC." Available online. URL: http://www.nhtsa.dot.gov/people/injury/alcohol/stopimpaired/ABCsBACWeb/page2.htm. Accessed July 27, 2008.

TABLE 4
FATAL CAR CRASHES BY DAY OF THE WEEK AND BLOOD ALCOHOL LEVEL (BAC), 2002 (IN PERCENT)

	Blood alcohol level				
	0.00%	0.01–0.07%	0.08–0.14%	0.15%+	0.01%+
Monday	14	10	9	9	9
Tuesday	14	11	9	9	9
Wednesday	15	10	11	9	10
Thursday	14	12	12	11	11
Friday	16	17	16	15	16
Saturday	14	22	24	25	24
Sunday	13	18	20	21	21

Source: Hingson, Ralph, and Michael Winter, "Epidemiology and Consequences of Drinking and Driving," *Alcohol Research & Health* 27, no. 1 (2003), page 65.

a fatal crash was highest on Saturday, followed by Sunday. For example, among those with a blood alcohol level of 0.08–0.14 percent, based on 4,204 fatal crashes, 24 percent of the individuals who were killed died on Saturday and 20 percent died on Sunday. Among people with no alcohol in their blood, the fatal crashes are fairly evenly dispersed throughout the week. (See Table 4.)

In another study of blood alcohol levels, the researchers looked at the BACs of individuals in Ireland who died from either accidents or suicides. The researchers studied data from 129 deaths in 2001 and 2002. They found that the majority (76 percent) of the deceased were males. In the largest percentage of cases (42.6 percent), the individuals died from car crashes, followed by suicides (24.0 percent), substance misuse (9.3 percent), house fires (8.5 percent), and other causes (15.5 percent).

Of the 93.5 percent of subjects for whom BAC was available, more than half (55.5 percent) had alcohol in their bloodstream. Those who were younger than age 30 were more likely to have had alcohol in their blood at the time of their deaths. There was generally a high level of BACs for individuals who died from injuries or suicide.

See also ALCOHOL AND ALCOHOL USE; ALCOHOLISM/ALCOHOL DEPENDENCE AND ALCOHOL ABUSE; BINGE DRINKING; DRIVING UNDER THE INFLUENCE/DRIVING WHILE INTOXICATED.

Bedford, D., A. O'Farrell, and F. Howell. "Blood Alcohol Levels in Persons Who Died from Accidents and Suicide." *Irish Medical Journal* 99, no. 3 (2006): 80–83.
Hingson, Ralph, and Michael Winter. "Epidemiology and Consequences of Drinking and Driving." *Alcohol Research & Health* 27, no. 1 (2003): 63–78.

borderline personality disorder See PERSONALITY DISORDERS.

brief intervention See INTERVENTION, BRIEF.

Campral See TREATMENT.

cancer Cancer is a malignant tumor, and once present, cancer cells will continue to proliferate throughout the body unless the cancer is treated with surgery, radiation, chemotherapy, or other forms of therapy or combined therapies. There are many different types of cancer, often named for the part of the body in which they originate, such as breast cancer, colon cancer, lung cancer, and so on. Specific treatment options differ by type of cancer. Some individuals with advanced cancer join clinical studies so that they may have a chance to undergo treatment with leading edge therapies.

Alcoholism or alcohol abuse increases the risk for the development of some forms of cancer, particularly oral cancer, breast cancer, and cancers of the digestive system, such as cancer of the esophagus, liver, colon, and rectum. Some researchers have speculated that ACETALDEHYDE is one of the primary cancer-causing substances that increases the risk for cancer among those who are alcohol-dependent. Acetaldehyde is a toxic byproduct of the body metabolizing alcohol. Many heavy drinkers also smoke, and SMOKING that is combined with excessive drinking increases the cancer risk in an individual by an estimated 50 times, according to researchers Helmut K. Seitz and Peter Becker in their article for *Alcohol Research & Health* in 2007.

In general, according to the National Cancer Institute (NCI), there are risk factors for all forms of cancer, including age (with older age being a greater risk for most forms of cancer), tobacco use, the use of alcohol, a family history of cancer, a poor diet, overweight and obesity, and a lack of physical activity. Some hormones increase the risk for some forms of cancer; for example, estrogen increases the risk for breast cancer, which is why hormone replacement therapy for more than a year or two is a bad idea for most menopausal women.

There are also apparent gender differences in how alcohol triggers the development of cancer; for example, moderate drinking (an average of one drink per day) compared to no drinking among females *increased* the risk for some forms of cancer, such as breast cancer, anal cancer, and liver cancer, and each additional drink per day further increased the risk for the development of these cancers, based on research with about 1.3 million women in England and published in the *Journal of the National Cancer Institute* in 2009. Interestingly, the researchers also found that moderate drinking was associated with a *lower* risk for thyroid cancer among women, as well as a lower rate of non-Hodgkin's lymphoma and renal cell carcinoma (kidney cancer).

In another study by Lee et al. published in the *Journal of the National Cancer Institute* in 2007, researchers found that moderate drinking decreased the risk for kidney cancer among both men and women. However, breast cancer and colorectal cancer are far more common forms of cancer, while thyroid cancer and kidney cancer appear much less frequently; thus, the benefits of moderate drinking and avoidance of some forms of cancer are mitigated by the increased risks for developing a more common form of cancer.

Many forms of cancer, such as colorectal cancer and breast cancer, appear to have a strong genetic component. However, there are also environmentally induced risks for cancer, such as chronic alcohol abuse and ALCOHOLISM/ALCOHOL DEPENDENCE. In their article in *Pharmaceutical Research* in 2008, authors Preetha Anand et al. contend that 90 to 95 percent of all cases of cancer are rooted in lifestyle choices, such as the excessive use of alcohol, as well as smoking, physical inactivity, and obesity. As a result, lifestyle choices can act as either risk factors toward the development of cancer or conversely, they may act as protective factors against its development.

General Signs of All Forms of Cancer

There are some general indicators that a person may have cancer, and anyone with these signs should report them to a physician. Of course each type of cancer has its own particular signs and symptoms as well. The seven general signs of a possible cancer are:

1. An unintentional or unexplained weight loss
2. An obvious change in the color or the appearance of a mole or a wart
3. A change in bowel habits
4. A lump in the breast or elsewhere
5. A cut or sore that does not heal
6. A discharge that is unusual or unusual bleeding
7. Chronic difficulty with swallowing or hoarseness

Note that the presence of one or more of these signs does *not* prove that a person has cancer. Instead, these signs are indicators that should be reported to a physician for further evaluation. According to the National Cancer Institute (NCI), in addition to the signs already mentioned, any of the following symptoms should also be reported to the physician:

- a cough that does not go away
- a new mole or a change in an existing mole
- discomfort that appears after eating
- chronic fatigue and tiredness with no apparent cause

Important Facts to Keep in Mind about Cancer

According to the NCI, everyone should be aware of basic facts about cancer in general. First, cancer is not caused by an injury, such as a bump. Second, cancer is not contagious, although when a person is infected with some viruses, such as viral hepatitis, the risk for cancer may increase. It is also important to understand that even if a person

has one or more risk factors for cancer (such as a family history, heavy consumption of alcohol, and obesity), this does not mean that an individual will invariably develop cancer. Instead, it means that the odds are increased but they are still not 100 percent.

The NCI says that the key risk for developing cancer is age, and most forms of cancers occur in people ages 65 years and older. Next there are environmental risk factors; for example, refraining from the use of tobacco is an excellent idea, because its use is considered the most preventable cause of death. People who smoke are significantly more likely than others to develop lung cancer as well as cancer of the mouth, bladder, esophagus, kidney, throat, stomach, and pancreas.

Some viruses and bacteria increase the risk for cancer, including infection with the human papillomavirus (the main cause of cervical cancer); infection with hepatitis B and C (which can develop into liver cancer after years); and infection with *helicobacter pylori,* a stomach bacterium that can lead to stomach ulcers as well as to stomach cancer. People infected with the human immunodeficiency virus (HIV) are also at an increased risk for the development of lymphoma and leukemia.

According to the NCI, two drinks per day for years can increase the risk for cancer of the breast, mouth, throat, esophagus, larynx, and liver. If the person also smokes, the risks for cancer are elevated even further.

Questions to Ask About All Forms of Cancer

If cancer is diagnosed, the NCI recommends that patients ask their physicians the following questions before any treatment starts:

- What is my diagnosis?
- Has the cancer spread? If so, to where? What is the stage of the disease?
- What is the goal of treatment? What are my treatment choices? Which do you recommend for me and why?
- What are the expected benefits of each type of treatment?
- What are the risks and possible side effects of each treatment? How can side effects be managed?

- Will infertility result from treatment? If so, can anything be done about it? Should I consider storing sperm or eggs?

- What can I do to prepare for treatment?

- How often will I have treatments? How long will the treatment last?

- Will I have to change my normal activities? If so, for how long?

- What is the treatment likely to cost? Will my insurance cover the costs?

- What new treatments are under study? Would a clinical trial be appropriate for me?

All Types of Cancer

In considering all forms of cancer (cancers of the digestive system as well as every other form of cancer), the National Cancer Institute estimated that 745,180 men and 692,000 women (for a total of 1,437,180 adults) were diagnosed with cancer in the United States in 2008. More than a half million people, or 565,650 adults, died of some form of cancer in 2008. The median age at diagnosis for all cancer sites was 67 years. (Median is a statistical measure that means that half the people diagnosed with cancer in 2008 were younger than 67 and half were older—it is a middle point and not an average.) Alcohol dependence increases the risk for many forms of cancer.

Cancer of all types is most prominently found among black males, followed by white males. As can be seen from Table 1, the largest incidence (new cases) of cancer in the period 2001–05 was found among black men, or 651.5 per 100,000

men. As a result, it is particularly important for black men to be screened for cancer, especially if they have health risk factors, such as a family history of cancer. Gender is also a factor and in general, all men have a greater risk for cancer than all women. For example, after black men, the next highest incidence for all forms of cancer was found among white males, or 551.4 per 100,000 men.

A study of the prevalence of colon polyps that were detected by colonoscopy among black and white patients who had no symptoms, reported in 2008 in the *Journal of the American Medical Association*, revealed that both black men and black women who had colonoscopies had a significantly higher rate of having large polyps compared to white men and women. (Polyps may be precancerous and are removed by the physician during a colonoscopy.) In addition, in this study, black adults older than age 60 had a higher risk of having larger polyps than older white adults.

The researchers found that 7.7 percent of the 422 black patients and 6.2 percent of the population of 4,964 patients had one or more colon polyps that were larger than 9 mm. They stated, "In summary, we find that asymptomatic black men and women undergoing colonoscopy screening are more likely to have 1 or more polyps sized more than 9 mm compared with white individuals. The differences were especially striking among women. These findings emphasize the importance of encouraging all black men and women to be screened. We found that black women younger than 50 years have similar rates of polyps sized more than 9 mm compared with white men aged 50 to 59 years."

TABLE 1
INCIDENCE OF ALL FORMS OF CANCER BY RACE AND GENDER, UNITED STATES, 2001–2005

Race/Ethnicity	Male	Female
All races	549.3 per 100,000 men	411.0 per 100,000 women
White	551.4 per 100,000 men	423.6 per 100,000 women
Black	651.5 per 100,000 men	398.9 per 100,000 women
Asian/Pacific Islander	354.0 per 100,000 men	287.8 per 100,000 women
American Indian/Alaska Native	336.6 per 100,000 men	296.4 per 100,000 women
Hispanic	419.4 per 100,000 men	317.8 per 100,000 women

Source: Adapted from Ries, L. A. G., et al., eds. Surveillance Epidemiology and End Results, Cancer of the Liver and Intrahepatic Duct. *SEER Cancer Statistics Review, 1975–2005.* Bethesda, Md.: National Cancer Institute. Available online. URL: http://seer.cancer.gov/csr/1975_2005/. Based on November 2007 SEER submission, posted to the SEER Web site, 2008. Downloaded February 1, 2009.

The researchers recommended further study for these findings.

Screening for Cancer

The symptoms of cancer depend on the type of cancer that is present, and for some forms of cancer, often there are no symptoms until the cancer is in an advanced stage. However, some cancers can be screened for, and physicians routinely do screen for these forms; for example, doctors screen for colorectal cancer and breast cancer, particularly among at-risk individuals, such as those older than age 50 or those with a family history of colon cancer or breast cancer.

Screening for colorectal cancer is performed with a rectal examination and with a colonoscopy, a procedure in which the patient takes medications to thoroughly clean out the bowel beforehand. At the time of the procedure, the patient is sedated and the colonoscope is inserted through the rectum and into the colon, while the physician checks on a screen for abnormalities. A biopsy is taken if there is any evidence of cancer, and the pathologist analyzes the removed tissue.

If the physician finds precancerous polyps (growths) that are present in the colon during the colonoscopic examination, he or she will remove them and they will be biopsied for cancer. Many patients forego the colonoscopy because they do not like the necessary bowel-cleansing preparation that occurs prior to the procedure; however, it is a minor and temporary inconvenience that saves lives.

Physicians screen adult women for breast cancer with mammography, a special type of X-ray of the breast, as well as through direct examination of the breasts performed by physicians and by the patient herself. If a lump is found, it is then biopsied to determine if cancer is present. Some women find the physical examination of their breasts embarrassing, and they may find the mammogram uncomfortable. Again, these are minor and temporary risks that save lives.

Dentists screen for oral cancer during regular checkups and if abnormalities are noted, they recommend that the patient seek urgent medical care.

There are no routinely performed screening tests for other forms of cancer whose risks are increased by excessive alcohol consumption, such as liver cancer or esophageal cancer, although physicians may choose to screen individuals who are at risk for such cancer because of their alcohol dependence. Screening is performed with an endoscopy, and patients who are at risk for liver cancer may be screened with a special type of endoscopy in which the physician inserts a tiny camera into the digestive system.

With any screening, the patient is responsible for complying with the doctor's recommendations for further screening, laboratory tests, and other preventive or treatment procedures. If the patient fails to follow the doctor's recommendation—for example, if he or she fails to comply with a recommendation to obtain a colonoscopy or a mammogram—then an existing cancer can continue to grow and metastasize (spread) to other parts of the body.

Cancer Risks Are Increased by Alcohol Abuse and Alcoholism

Some forms of cancer are directly affected by excessive chronic drinking as well as alcohol dependence. This includes breast cancer and many forms of digestive cancers, such as colorectal cancer, esophageal cancer, liver cancer, oral cancer, pancreatic cancer, and stomach cancer. Often, liver cancer develops as a result of liver cirrhosis that was caused by excessive alcohol use. In the case of chronic alcohol abuse and dependence, it is believed that various factors may be implicated, particularly acetaldehyde.

According to Seitz and Becker, "Acetaldehyde itself is a cancer-causing substance in experimental animals and reacts with DNA to form cancer-promoting compounds. In addition, highly reactive, oxygen-containing molecules that are generated during certain pathways of alcohol metabolism can damage the DNA, thus also inducing tumor development. Together with other factors related to chronic alcohol consumption, these metabolism-related factors may increase tumor risk in chronic heavy drinkers."

According to Seitz and Becker, the greatest cancer risk with alcohol-associated cancer is with cancer of the upper aerodigestive tract, which includes the area of the oral cavity, voice box, and esophagus. In addition, heavy drinking (which means drinking more than five or six drinks per day) that is also combined with smoking increases the risk for developing these forms of cancer by an astonishing 50 times.

Claudio Pelucchi and colleagues reported in 2006 that the combination of alcohol and tobacco increases the risk for oral cancer and esophageal cancer as well as liver cancer; however, with oral and esophageal cancer, the tobacco and alcohol together work to increase the risk of cancer synergistically. In contrast, alcohol and tobacco use are independent risk factors for the developing of liver cancer.

Considering Types of Cancer Related to Alcohol Abuse/Alcoholism

Some forms of cancer are strongly linked to alcohol abuse and dependence.

Breast Cancer After lung cancer, breast cancer is the most common form of cancer contracted by women in the United States. According to the National Cancer Institute, 182,460 women were diagnosed with breast cancer in 2008 and 40,480 women died of breast cancer in that year. The median age at diagnosis for breast cancer was 61 years, based on data from the Surveillance Epidemiology and End Results (SEER) research from the National Cancer Institute for the period 2001–05. (Some few men are also diagnosed with breast cancer each year, but the disease is rare among men.)

According to the American Cancer Society, alcohol consumption is directly associated with an increased risk for breast cancer, and just 2 drinks per day increases the breast cancer risk by 21 percent among women. It does not matter which type of alcohol is consumed: any type of alcohol that is consumed on a regular basis elevates a woman's risk for developing breast cancer. As a result, decreasing alcohol consumption to only one drink per day (or drinking no alcohol) will decrease the risk for developing breast cancer.

In considering racial and ethnic differences, white women have the greatest risk of a breast cancer diagnosis, or 130.6 women per 100,000 white women, compared to the next highest of 117.5 black women per 100,000 women. However, although they have a lower rate of breast cancer diagnosis, black women are more likely to die from breast cancer than individuals of other races or ethnicities; for example, the death rate for black women was 33.5 per 100,000 women, compared to 24.4 per 100,000 white women based on SEER data. Researchers have debated for years, and will continue to debate, the possible reasons for this racial disparity in deaths from breast cancer and other forms of cancer. Some experts believe that the cause is a diagnosis later in the stage of cancer, while others blame lifestyle factors. Still others believe that blacks generally receive poorer quality health care than whites.

There is some good news with regard to breast cancer. The Women's Health Initiative (WHI) clinical trial has shown that the number of cases in breast cancer is on the decline, and some experts attribute this decrease to fewer women using hormone replacement therapy.

Shumin M. Zhang and colleagues analyzed data from the Women's Health Study (1992–2004) and they found a modest but significant increase in breast cancer among those women who had a higher alcohol consumption than others. The women who were evaluated drank 30 grams or more of alcohol per day; other studies have shown that women who are heavier drinkers have an even further increased risk for breast cancer. The risk for cancer also appeared linked to whether the women who drank were also taking hormonal replacement therapy (HRT)—alcohol and HRT together increased the risk.

Other risk factors for breast cancer in addition to alcohol consumption and HRT are age (the risks for breast cancer increase as a woman gets older), genetic factors (women with BRCA1 and BRCA2 have an increased risk for breast cancer), and some personal factors, such as having a menstrual cycle before the age of 12 or going through a natural menopause after age 55. Other risk factors include obesity, the use of birth control pills, having no children or having a first child after age 35, and having dense breasts. Having close family members (such as a mother or a sister) who have had breast cancer is another risk factor.

Symptoms of breast cancer may include a lump in the breast, a natural (non-cosmetic) change in the shape or size of the breast, and a discharge from the nipple. Mammography and breast self-examination, as well as examination by the physician, can help screen women for breast cancer. If breast cancer is found, the treatment may include lumpectomy (removal of the breast lump only), mastectomy (removal of the entire breast), radiation, chemotherapy, and hormone therapy.

Colorectal Cancer Symptoms of colorectal cancer may include blood in the feces as well as diarrhea or constipation, unintentional weight loss, and stools that are narrower than normal for a person. Many people have no symptoms in the early stages of colorectal cancer, which is why regular checkups are important, including digital rectal examinations performed by the physician, as well as colonoscopies on a schedule as recommended by a physician. A gastroenterologist knows which groups are most at risk for colorectal cancer, by age, gender, race, and so forth and will order the appropriate tests to screen his or her patients. Colorectal cancer represented 8 percent of all adult male cancer deaths in 2008 and 9 percent of all adult female cancer deaths, according to the American Cancer Society.

According to data from the Surveillance Epidemiology and End Results (SEER), based on a compilation of data for the period 2001–05, it was estimated that 77,250 men and 71,560 women were diagnosed with colorectal cancer in 2008 in the United States, and that 49,960 adults died of colorectal cancer in 2008. (See Table 2.) The median age at death from colorectal cancer was 75 years. The overall five-year survival rate for 1996–2004 was 64.4 percent. The five-year survival rate by gender and race among those with colorectal cancer was 65.4 percent for white males, 65.2

percent for white females, 55.5 percent for black females, and 54.7 percent for black males.

Esophageal Cancer Esophageal cancer may present with such signs and symptoms as difficulty with swallowing, unintentional weight loss, a chronic cough, and chronic hoarseness. An estimated 148,810 people (77,250 men and 71,560 women) were diagnosed with esophageal cancer in 2008. Males, particularly black males, have the highest risk of developing this form of cancer. The average age at the point of diagnosis was 71 years over the period 2001–05. The median age of death was 75 years. According to SEER data, the five-year survival rate, using data from 1996–2004, was 64.4 percent, including 65.4 percent for white males, 65.2 percent for white females, 54.7 percent for black males, and 55.5 percent for black females.

Some studies have found that moderate drinking of red wine is protective against the development of esophageal cancer.

Liver Cancer (Hepatocellular Carcinoma) Individuals who are heavy drinkers are more likely to have liver diseases such as CIRRHOSIS, which is itself a risk factor for the development of liver cancer. They may also have viral hepatitis, such as hepatitis B or C, which are both risk factors for liver cancer. The use of both tobacco and alcohol increases the risk for liver cancer. The prognosis for survival from liver cancer is poor as of this writing, because the disease is usually not diagnosed until the late stages.

In considering cancer of the liver and the intrahepatic duct, it was estimated that 15,190 adult males and 6,180 adult females were diagnosed

TABLE 2
INCIDENCE RATES OF COLORECTAL CANCER BY RACE AND GENDER, 2001–2005, UNITED STATES

Race/Ethnicity	Male	Female
All races	59.2 per 100,000 men	43.8 per 100,000 women
White	58.9 per 100,000 men	43.2 per 100,000 women
Black	71.2 per 100,000 men	54.5 per 100,000 women
Asian/Pacific Islander	48.0 per 100,000 men	35.4 per 100,000 women
American Indian/Alaska Native	46.0 per 100,000 men	41.2 per 100,000 women
Hispanic	47.3 per 100,000 men	32.8 per 100,000 women

Source: Adapted from Ries, L. A. G., et al., eds. Surveillance Epidemiology and End Results, Cancer of the Liver and Intrahepatic Duct. *SEER Cancer Statistics Review, 1975–2005.* Bethesda, Md.: National Cancer Institute. Available online. URL: http://seer.cancer.gov/csr/1975_2005/. Based on November 2007 SEER submission, posted to the SEER Web site, 2008. Downloaded February 1, 2009.

TABLE 3
INCIDENT RATES OF LIVER CANCER BY RACE AND GENDER, 2001–2005, UNITED STATES

Race/Ethnicity	Male	Female
All Races	9.9 per 100,000 men	3.5 per 100,000 women
White	8.2 per 100,000 men	2.9 per 100,000 women
Black	13.2 per 100,000 men	4.0 per 100,000 women
Asian/Pacific Islander	21.7 per 100,000 men	8.3 per 100,000 women
American Indian/Alaska Native	14.4 per 100,000 men	6.3 per 100,000 women
Hispanic	15.0 per 100,000 men	5.8 per 100,000 women

Source: Adapted from Ries, L.A.G., et al., eds. Surveillance Epidemiology and End Results, Cancer of the Liver and Intrahepatic Duct. *SEER Cancer Statistics Review, 1975–2005.* Bethesda, Md.: National Cancer Institute. Available online. URL: http://seer.cancer.gov/csr/1975_2005/. Based on November 2007 SEER submission, posted to the SEER Web site, 2008. Downloaded February 1, 2009.

in 2008, and 18,410 people died of these cancers in 2008. In contrast to other forms of cancer, the highest rates of incidence are found among Asian/Pacific Islanders, American Indians/Alaska Natives, and Hispanics. (See Table 3.)

The average age at the diagnosis of liver cancer was 65 years old for the period 2001–05. The median age at death was 70 years. The survival rates were poor, or an average of 11.7 percent who survived. Survival rates were as follows: 12.3 percent for white women, 11.0 percent for white men, 7.9 percent for black men, and 7.7 percent for black women. (The survival rates for Asians and other high risk groups are unknown.)

Oral Cancer Some symptoms of oral cancer include difficulty with chewing and swallowing, numbness in the tongue or other parts of the mouth, a sore or irritation in the mouth, lip, or throat, and difficulty moving the jaw or tongue. According to the National Institute of Dental and Craniofacial Research, 75 percent of oral cancers are related to the use of tobacco and/or alcohol. It is most prevalent among those older than 40 years and is twice as common among men as women.

Cancer of the oral cavity and pharynx was diagnosed in 35,310 adults in 2008, according to the National Cancer Institute. The incidence of oral cancer was highest among blacks, followed by whites. Looking at all individuals who were diagnosed with oral cancer, more than half of them survived for five or more years: the overall five-year survival rate for the period 1996–2004 was 59.7 percent. Black men had the lowest five-year survival rate, or 36.1 percent, followed by 52.1 per-

cent for black women. Among whites, nearly two-thirds survived for five or more years; the five-year survival rate was 61.0 percent for white males and 62.9 percent for white females.

Alcohol consumption increases the risk for oral cancer. In fact, in a study reported by M. J. McCullough and C. S. Farah in the *Australian Dental Journal* in 2008, the two researchers reported that a review of literature on alcohol-containing mouthwashes and oral cancer indicates that these mouthwashes increase the risk for the development of oral cancer and should be avoided over the long-term. Some research has indicated that daily use of alcohol-containing mouthwash is linked to the development of oral cancer. The authors also support restricting mouthwashes for adults by prescription use only and for short periods.

Pancreatic Cancer Cancer of the pancreas is a rare cancer that is often diagnosed in a late stage because it has few or no symptoms in its early stages. It is a cancer with a poor prognosis, as with liver cancer. Often the first symptom is jaundice, which indicates that an advanced cancer is present. According to data from the National Cancer Institute, an estimated 37,680 adults, including 18,770 men and 18,910 women, were diagnosed with pancreatic cancer in 2008. The median age at diagnosis was 72 years.

The incidence of pancreatic cancer was highest among black males, followed by black females; the rate for black males for the period 2001–05 was 16.2 per 100,000 men, and the rate for black females was 14.3 per 100,000 women. The lowest rates of pancreatic cancer were found among Asian and Pacific Islander and American Indian/Alaska Native females, which groups each had a rate of 8.2 per 100,000 women.

The overall five-year survival rate from pancreatic cancer was a very low 5.1 percent for all races and genders, based on SEER data for the period 1996–2004. Considering black and white races and genders, the five-year survival rates were as follows: 5.4 percent for black women, 5.1 percent for white men, 4.9 percent for white women, and only 3.6 percent for black men.

Stomach Cancer Signs and symptoms of stomach cancer may include mild nausea, a loss of appetite, heartburn, and a bloated feeling after eating. If the cancer is more advanced, symptoms may include an unintentional weight loss, stomach pain, jaundice, a buildup of fluid in the abdomen (ascites), blood in the stool, and difficulty swallowing.

According to SEER data from the National Cancer Institute, 13,190 men and 8,310 women (for a total of 21,500 adults) in the United States were diagnosed with stomach cancer in 2008. An estimated 10,880 adults died of stomach cancer in 2008. The incidence of stomach cancer was highest among male and female Asians and Pacific Islanders, or 18.6 per 100,000 men and 10.5 per 100,000 women. This rate was much higher than the rate for all races of 11.3 per 100,000 men and 5.5 per 100,000 women.

The overall five-year survival rate from stomach cancer, using data for the period 1996–2004, was 24.7 percent.

Treating Cancer

The treatment of cancer depends on whether it has already metastasized (spread) to other parts of the body when it is diagnosed and also depends on how advanced the cancer is when it is identified. Whenever possible, a biopsy of the cancerous tissue is taken and a pathologist examines the biopsied tissue to determine these factors, also referred to as staging the cancer. If the cancer is in its early stage and it is still localized (it has not spread), often surgery or radiation therapy may be used to treat the patient. If the cancer *has* spread beyond the local area, the patient may need chemotherapy to try to contain the spread from going any further. Treat-

ment may be given even if the patient's life can no longer be saved; for example, radiation therapy is sometimes given in cases of advanced cancer to decrease the pain, such as when the cancer has spread to the bones.

Preventing Cancer

Preventive measures against the development of cancer include immediate treatment for any existing alcohol dependence. In addition, lifestyle changes are very important as well; for example, if the individual smokes, he or she should stop smoking immediately so that the risk for cancer will start to drop. Alcohol-containing mouthwashes should be avoided unless they are specifically recommended by dentists or physicians. Regular medical checkups should be undergone so that the physician can recommend any needed diagnostic tests as well as provide treatment if a form of cancer is identified.

Sometimes people who are physically fit, eat nutritious diets, do not drink alcohol or smoke cigarettes, and who seem to exemplify the way that one should live develop cancer anyway. This does not mean that because some healthy people develop cancer, there is no reason to live in a healthy manner. What it means is that healthy people have a much lower risk of developing most cancers, but the risk is not zero. (They may have a family history of cancer or have genetic risk factors for cancer.) Despite this fact, it is still advisable to take actions to prevent against cancer, such as having regular physical examinations and complying with the doctor's recommendations.

See also ALCOHOL AND MEN; ALCOHOL AND WOMEN; EXCESSIVE DRINKING AND HEALTH CONSEQUENCES; MODERATE DRINKING AND HEALTH BENEFITS.

Allen, Naomi, et al. "Moderate Alcohol Intake and Cancer Incidence in Women." *Journal of the National Cancer Institute* 101, no. 5 (2009): 296–305.

Anand, Preetha, et al. "Cancer is a Preventable Disease that Requires Major Lifestyle Changes." *Pharmaceutical Research* 29, no. 9 (2008): 2,097–2,116.

Baan, Robert, et al. "Carcinogenicity of Alcoholic Beverages." *Lancet* 8, no. 4 (2007): 292–293.

Lee, Jung Eun, et al. "Alcohol Intake and Renal Cell Cancer in a Pooled Analysis of 12 Prospective Studies." *Journal of the National Cancer Institute* 99, no. 10 (2007): 801–810.

Lieberman, David A., M.D., et al. "Prevalence of Colon Polyps Detected by Colonoscopy Screening in Asymptomatic Black and White Patients." *Journal of the American Medical Association* 300, no. 12 (2008): 1,417–1,422.

McCullough, M. J. and C. S. Farah. "The Role of Alcohol in Oral Carcinogenesis with Particular Reference to Alcohol-Containing Mouthwashes." *Australian Dental Journal* 53, no. 4 (2008): 302–305.

Pelucchi, Claudio, et al. "Cancer Risk Associated with Alcohol and Tobacco Use: Focus on Upper Aerodigestive Tract and Liver." *Alcohol Research & Health* 29, no. 3 (2006): 193–198.

Ries, L. A. G., et al., eds. Surveillance Epidemiology and End Results, Cancer of the Liver and Intrahepatic Duct. *SEER Cancer Statistics Review, 1975–2005.* Bethesda, Md.: National Cancer Institute. Available online. URL: http://seer.cancer.gov/csr/1975_2005/. Based on November 2007 SEER submission, posted to the SEER Web site, 2008. Downloaded February 1, 2009.

Seitz, Helmut K., M.D., and Peter Becker, M.D. "Alcohol Metabolism and Cancer Risk." *Alcohol Research & Health* 30, no. 1 (2007): 38–47.

Virnig, Beth A., et al. "A Matter of Race: Early-versus Late-stage Cancer Diagnosis." *Health Affairs* 28, no. 1 (January/February 2009): 160–168.

Zhang, Shumin M., et al. "Alcohol Consumption and Breast Cancer Risk in the Women's Health Study." *American Journal of Epidemiology* 165, no. 6 (2007): 667–676.

child abuse and neglect *Abuse* generally refers to the commission of physical or sexual abuse (or emotional abuse) against a child or adolescent, while *neglect* refers to the omission or failure to provide necessary care or sustenance, such as the failure to provide basic food and shelter or the failure to seek medical attention (medical neglect) for a child. Abandonment is a form of neglect. More infants and small children die of neglect than of abuse; babies and toddlers need food, shelter, and medical care in order to survive. Alcohol abuse and dependence increases the risk for child abuse and neglect. In addition, experiencing childhood abuse as well as the alcoholism of at least one parent increases the risk for alcohol dependence in adulthood. According to the Substance Abuse and Mental Health Services Administration, in 2007, about 7.3 million minor children (10.3 percent of all children) in the United States lived with a parent who abused or who was dependent on alcohol. The National Institute on Alcohol Abuse and Alcoholism (NIAAA) estimates that the abuse of alcohol is a factor in 30 percent of all child abuse cases.

Such childhood abuse often also affects the adult that the child grows into, making him or her more likely to become dependent on alcohol as well as to suffer a multitude of other consequences. For example, some children suffer from multiple forms of maltreatment, and when they become adolescents or adults, they are at greater risk for alcohol abuse and binge drinking than those who were not abused or neglected. In a study published in *Addictive Behaviors* in 2009, researchers Sunny Hyucksun Shin and colleagues found that adolescents ages 12–21 with a sexual abuse history had more than double the risk of BINGE DRINKING compared to those with no history of maltreatment. In addition, adolescents who had been both physically abused and neglected in childhood had a 1.3 times greater risk for binge drinking than those who were not maltreated.

According to the U.S. Department of Health and Human Services in their annual report on child maltreatment published in 2008, about 905,000 children were abused or neglected in 2006, and 1,530 children died from abuse or neglect. Children who were younger (children under age four have the greatest risk for severe injury or death from abuse or neglect), white or of mixed race, who had disabilities, and whose caregivers abused alcohol were more likely to be re-reported for maltreatment and for their abuse or neglect to be substantiated by caseworkers.

An estimated 5 million parents in the United States who abused alcohol had at least one child younger than age 18 living in the household in 2002, according to the Substance Abuse and Mental Health Services Administration in 2004.

When abused and neglected children grow up, they have an increased risk for abusing or neglecting their own children, as well as an elevated risk for alcohol dependence, drug abuse, DEPRESSION, obesity, SUICIDE, SMOKING, and other serious health problems. (However, it should not be assumed that abused children who grow up always abuse their own children; this is not true.)

Substance-abusing Fathers vs. Non-substance-abusing Fathers

A study of children in three groups looked at 40 children with fathers who were alcoholics, 40 with fathers who were addicted to drugs, and 40 with non-substance-abusing fathers. As reported by Michelle L. Kelley and William Fals-Stewart in the *Journal of the American Academy of Child & Adolescent Psychiatry* in 2004, the study found significant differences. For example, 25 percent of the children of alcoholic fathers had a psychiatric diagnosis, compared to 53 percent of the children of drug-using fathers and 10 percent of the non-substance-abusing fathers. They also found a depression rate among the children of 13 percent among those with alcoholic fathers, 38 percent among those with drug-abusing fathers, and only 3 percent among those with fathers who were not dependent on substances.

The Alcohol and Drug Use Continuum

The use of alcohol as well as its abuse and dependence have important implications regarding the care of minor children, and child welfare workers know to consider these factors. Table 1 from the Substance Abuse and Mental Health Services Administration provides key examples of the social use of alcohol (and drugs) and its potential harmful effects on children as well as the abuse of alcohol and the dependence on alcohol and its possible adverse effects on children.

The Adverse Childhood Experiences Study

A study of Adverse Childhood Experiences (ACEs), drawn from thousands of adults, revealed that of those adults who reported abuse as children, the most common ACEs were physical abuse in childhood (28 percent) or alcohol or substance abuse by a family member during childhood (27 percent). Other ACEs were

- suffering recurrent emotional abuse in childhood
- experiencing sexual abuse
- witnessing violence against their mothers during childhood

- losing a biological parent in childhood for any reason
- living with someone with a mental illness
- living in a household in which a member was in jail or prison

The consequences of adverse childhood experiences were more common among females; the researchers found that, with the exception of those who were physically abused in childhood, females had a greater prevalence of ACEs than males. Females also had a higher number of ACEs; for example, 4 percent of the women had experienced four or more ACEs, compared to 2 percent of the males.

The researchers found that adults with a past history of ACEs were more likely to abuse alcohol and/or drugs in adulthood. Adults with ACEs were also more likely than those who had not had adverse childhood events to

- abuse their own children
- commit suicide
- contract sexually transmitted diseases
- have unintended pregnancies

Researchers also found that the risk for alcoholism in adulthood was increased among those who experienced ACEs. In addition, the risk for experiencing all eight categories of ACEs was significantly greater among the adults who reported parental alcohol abuse.

According to Robert F. Anda, M.D., and colleagues in their 2002 article in *Psychiatric Services,* "Improved recognition and treatment of alcoholism in adults and tandem family interventions to reduce the burden of adverse childhood experienced in alcoholic households would probably decrease the long-term risk of alcoholism, depression, and other adverse effects of trauma observed among adult children of alcoholics."

See also AGE AND ALCOHOL; AGGRESSIVE BEHAVIOR AND ALCOHOL; ALCOHOL AND MEN; ALCOHOL AND WOMEN; ALCOHOLISM/ALCOHOL DEPENDENCE AND ALCOHOL ABUSE; EXCESSIVE DRINKING AND NEGATIVE SOCIAL CONSEQUENCES; FAMILIES AND ALCOHOL; PSYCHIATRIC COMORBIDITIES; UNDERAGE DRINKING.

TABLE 1
PARENTAL ALCOHOL AND DRUG USE CONTINUUM AND EXAMPLES OF POTENTIAL RISKS TO CHILDREN

Alcohol and Drug Use Continuum	Examples of Potential Risks to Children
Use of alcohol or drugs to socialize and feel effects; use may not appear abusive and may not lead to dependence; however the circumstances under which a parent uses can put children at risk of harm.	Use during pregnancy can harm the fetus
Abuse of alcohol or drugs includes at least one of these factors in the last 12 months: • Recurrent substance use resulting in failure to fulfill obligations at work, home, or school • Recurrent substance use in situations that are physically hazardous • Recurrent substance-related legal problems • Continued substance use despite having persistent or recurrent social or interpersonal problems caused by or exacerbated by the substance	• Driving with children in the car while under the influence • Children may be left in unsafe care—with an inappropriate caretaker or unattended—while parent is partying • Parent may neglect or sporadically address the children's needs for regular meals, clothing, and cleanliness • Even when the parent is in the home, the parent's alcohol or drug use may leave children unsupervised • Behavior toward children may be inconsistent, such as a pattern of violence, then remorse
Dependence, also known as addiction, is a pattern of use that results in three or more of the following symptoms in a 12-month period: • Tolerance—needing more of the alcohol or drug to get "high" • Withdrawal—physical symptoms when alcohol or other drugs are not used, such as tremors, nausea, sweating, and shakiness • Substance is taken in larger amounts and over a longer period than intended • Persistent desire or unsuccessful efforts to cut down or control substance use • A great deal of time is spent in activities related to obtaining the substance, use of the substance, or recovering from its effects • Important social, occupational, or recreational activities are given up or reduced because of substance use • Substance use is continued despite knowledge of persistent or recurrent physical or psychological problems caused or exacerbated by the substance	• Funds are used to buy alcohol or other drugs, while other necessities, such as buying food, are neglected • A parent may not be able to think logically or make rational decisions regarding children's needs or care • A parent may not be able to prioritize children's needs over his or her own need for the substance

Adapted from: Breshears, E. M., S. Yeh, and N. K. Young. *Understanding Substance Abuse and Facilitating Recovery: A Guide for Child Welfare Workers.* Rockville, Md.: Substance Abuse and Mental Health Services Administration, 2004. Page 3.

Anda, Robert F., M.D., et al. "Adverse Childhood Experiences, Alcoholic Parents, and Later Risk of Alcoholism and Depression." *Psychiatric Services* 53, no. 8 (August 2002): 1,001–1,009.

Bagnardi, Vincenzo, et al. "Alcohol Consumption and the Risk of Cancer: A Meta-Analysis." *Alcohol Research & Health* 25, no. 4 (2001): 263–270.

Breshears, E. M., S. Yeh, and N. K. Young. *Understanding Substance Abuse and Facilitating Recovery: A Guide for*

Child Welfare Workers. Rockville, Md.: Substance Abuse and Mental Health Services Administration, 2004.

Clark, Duncan B., et al. "Physical and Sexual Abuse, Depression and Alcohol Use Disorders in Adolescents: Onsets and Outcomes." *Drug and Alcohol Dependence* 69, no. 1 (2003): 51–60.

Clark, Robin E., and Judith Freeman Clark, with Christine Adamec. *The Encyclopedia of Child Abuse.* 3rd ed. New York: Facts On File, Inc., 2006.

Edwards, Valerie J., et al. "Relationship between Multiple Forms of Childhood Maltreatment and Adult Mental Health in Community Respondents: Results from the Adverse Childhood Experiences Study." *American Journal of Psychiatry* 160, no. 8 (August 2003): 1,453–1,460.

Kelley, Michelle L., and William Fals-Stewart. "Psychiatric Disorders of Children Living with Drug-Abusing, Alcohol-Abusing, and Non-Substance-Abusing Fathers." *Journal of the American Academy of Child & Adolescent Psychiatry* 43, no. 5 (May 2004): 621–628.

Shun, Sunny Hyucksun, Erika M. Edwards, and Timothy Heeren. "Child Abuse and Neglect: Relations to Adolescent Binge Drinking in the National Longitudinal Study of Adolescent Health (Add Health) Study." *Addictive Behaviors* 34, no. 3 (2009): 277–280.

Substance Abuse and Mental Health Services Administration. "Children Living with Substance-Dependent or Substance-Abusing Parents: 2002 to 2007." The NSDUH Report (April 16, 2009): 1–4.

U.S. Department of Health and Human Services, Administration on Children, Youth and Families. *Child Maltreatment 2006.* Washington, D.C.: U.S. Government Printing Office, 2008.

cirrhosis   A serious disease that is characterized by severe liver damage, scarring, and inflammation of the liver, often caused by excessive drinking that has occurred over the course of many years. Individuals with cirrhosis are at an increased risk for the development of liver CANCER, a disease with a poor prognosis as of this writing, because it is usually not diagnosed until the late stage.

According to a report on liver cirrhosis deaths in the United States by Young-Hee Yoon and Hsiao-ye Yee, published in 2008 by the National Institute on Alcohol Abuse and Alcoholism, liver cirrhosis was the 12th leading cause of death in the United States in 2005, with 28,175 deaths, or 621 more than in 2004. Also according to this report, the death rate from alcohol-related cirrhosis increased by 2.3 percent from 2004 to 2005, and nearly half (45.9 percent) of all liver cirrhosis deaths were alcohol-related.

The largest percentages of deaths occurred among those ages 65 and older; for example, nearly a third, or 29.7 percent of all deaths per 100,000 population in the age group of 75–84 years, died from cirrhosis, and 20 percent of the deaths were to individuals 85 years and older. Among those who were ages 65–74, 27.8 percent of the deaths per 100,000 population were from liver cirrhosis.

Some adults with alcoholic cirrhosis also contract a viral form of hepatitis, such as hepatitis B or hepatitis C, which further damages their livers. However, according to Alice Yang and colleagues, chronic alcoholic hepatitis (CAH) is the most common cause of hospital admissions among individuals with alcohol-related liver or pancreatic complications. CAH also has the highest rate of deaths. If individuals give up drinking before they reach a point of no return and when the liver is still able to recover, this is the best outcome for the patient. However, determining that particular point for any individual is impossible.

Yang et al. say that in general, CAH is preceded by acute PANCREATITIS, chronic pancreatitis, acute alcoholic hepatitis, and chronic alcoholic hepatitis with cirrhosis.

Symptoms and Diagnostic Path

In the early stages of alcoholic cirrhosis, there are few or no symptoms, and liver function tests of the blood may show normal values. When symptoms develop, they may include the following:

- fatigue

- nausea

- jaundice (yellowing of the skin and of the whites of the eyes, caused by a buildup of bilirubin)

- an increased sensitivity to prescribed or over-the-counter drugs that are metabolized by the liver, such as acetaminophen (Tylenol)

- ascites (fluid buildup in the abdomen)

- an altered mental state (hepatic encephalopathy)

Imaging tests may show damage to the liver, and patients with advanced cirrhosis will have abnormal liver function laboratory values.

Treatment Options and Outlook

Patients with alcoholic cirrhosis need hospitalization both to stabilize them and to enforce their ABSTINENCE from alcohol, as well as to treat their withdrawal symptoms, such as extreme vomiting, hallucinations, and other symptoms that are caused by DELIRIUM TREMENS. (By itself, delirium tremens is a cause for hospitalization. When combined with alcoholic cirrhosis, hospitalization becomes even more crucial.)

There is no cure for alcoholic cirrhosis other than a liver transplant, thus the prognosis is poor in advanced cases of the disease. Patients may receive a partial liver transplant from a donor; however, they must stop all consumption of alcohol or they will destroy the new liver tissue as well. Medical facilities may evaluate whether a patient who needs a liver is likely to stop drinking and stay off alcohol before approving a liver transplantation. It may be difficult to impossible to obtain a nonrelative donor when the patient's own liver has been destroyed by ALCOHOLISM.

Risk Factors and Preventive Measures

Race represents one risk factor for suffering death from alcoholic liver cirrhosis. Among all races in the United States, white Hispanic males have the highest rate of cirrhosis deaths, and according to the 2008 report from the National Institute on Alcohol Abuse and Alcoholism (NIAAA), the age-adjusted rate from all cirrhosis for white Hispanic males was 1.8 times the rate for white non-Hispanic and black non-Hispanic males. Among females, the rate for white Hispanic females was 1.4 times the rate for white non-Hispanic females and was 1.7 times the rate for black non-Hispanic females.

Female alcoholics often develop alcoholic liver disease including cirrhosis at a more rapid rate than male alcoholics; however, there are many more male alcoholics, and thus the death rate from cirrhosis is higher among males who are alcohol dependent.

The best preventive measure against alcoholic cirrhosis is to avoid excessive drinking or to have alcohol dependence treated if it has already begun.

See also ALCOHOL AND ALCOHOL USE; ALCOHOL AND WOMEN; ALCOHOLIC PSYCHOSIS; EXCESSIVE DRINKING AND HEALTH CONSEQUENCES; HEPATITIS; LIVER DISEASE, ALCOHOLIC; TREATMENT.

National Institute on Alcohol Abuse and Alcoholism. "Alcoholic Liver Disease." *Alcohol Alert* 64 (January 2005): 1–5.
Yang, Alice L., et al. "Epidemiology of Alcohol-Related Liver and Pancreatic Disease in the United States." *Archives of Internal Medicine* 168, no. 6 (March 24, 2008): 649–656.
Yoon, Young-Hee, and Hsiao-ye Yi. *Surveillance Report #83: Liver Cirrhosis Mortality in the United States, 1970–2005.* National Institute on Alcohol Abuse and Alcoholism. Baltimore, Md.: National Institutes of Health, August 2008.

codependency Refers to an unhealthy relationship that occurs between the alcoholic person and other individuals, such as spouses or partners, siblings, adult children, and others who seek to prevent the consequences of excessive drinking from acting upon the alcoholic. For example, the codependent partner of an alcoholic individual may call his or her employer to report that the person is "sick," perhaps with the "flu," when in fact, the alcoholic person actually has a hangover from the effects of heavy drinking. The excuse-making behavior is sometime referred to as enabling the alcoholic.

The codependent person usually feels very strongly that he or she is helping the alcoholic, and that nobody truly understands him or her, but the converse is actually true. As long as the alcoholic person does not have to face the consequences of his or her actions, the more likely it is that the drinking will continue to occur.

Individuals who are involved in a codependent relationship in which they suffer as a result of the alcoholic person's actions (and their reactions and acquiescence to the alcoholism) are called enablers. These are individuals who will call a spouse's employer to say that he or she is "too sick" to go to work, when the fact is that the person is too hungover to be able to perform on the job.

Often enablers feel they are the only people who truly love and understand the alcohol-dependent person, and they also believe that the alcoholic really needs them. They will sometimes go to great lengths to do what they consider helping the alcoholic, including neglecting the needs of themselves or their children. For example, if the alcoholic person is physically or verbally abusive to the children when intoxicated, the enabler will excuse such behavior. Sometimes the state social services department informs the enabler that she (or occasionally he) must leave the alcoholic in order to retain custody of the children. For the enabler, the choice is often the alcoholic rather than the children, who will then be sent to other relatives or to the state foster care system.

This behavior is believed to be counteractive to actually helping the alcoholic, who needs to suffer some consequences in order to make the choice to change his or her behavior.

The enabler may perceive him or herself as very virtuous and may also believe that others cannot possibly understand the alcoholic person or love him or her as much as does the enabler. There is a certain power attached to the role of an enabler who helps the alcoholic continue his or her behavior, although it is often not apparent to others. For example, should the alcoholic overcome ALCOHOLISM, he or she may no longer need the enabler. In any case, this is the underlying common fear of the enabling person.

See also ALCOHOL AND MEN; ALCOHOL AND WOMEN; ALCOHOL MUTUAL AID SOCIETIES; DENIAL; ENABLERS; FAMILIES AND ALCOHOL; STAGES OF CHANGE; TREATMENT.

college students   Individuals attending secondary institutions. Often when individuals go away to college and to a new environment, they confront new behaviors among their peers. One of these behaviors may be excessive drinking or BINGE DRINKING, or drinking five or more drinks on one occasion in the past two weeks. New students may experience severe peer pressure to drink and may feel like they must drink to excess in order to be accepted by other students and make friends.

Serious Consequences from Alcohol Excesses

An estimated 1,700 college students ages 18–24 years die every year from alcohol-related causes, including car crashes, according to the National Institute on Alcohol Abuse and Alcoholism (NIAAA). About half of them are underage drinkers, younger than age 21. In addition, about 599,000 students ages 18–24 are accidentally injured while under the influence of alcohol (and about half of them are under age 21). Assaults are also a common problem among drinking college students; for example, each year an estimated 696,000 students ages 18–24 are assaulted by another student who has been drinking.

Sexual abuse is another problem on the college campus that is related to alcohol misuse and abuse. More than 97,000 students are sexually assaulted or date-raped every year. About half of them are under age 21. Unsafe sex is a serious issue among those college students who drink to excess, and studies indicate that about 400,000 students per year have had unprotected sex while drinking. The possible consequences of unsafe sex are unplanned pregnancies and the contracting of sexually transmitted diseases. About 100,000 students, ages 18–24 years, have said that they were too intoxicated to be sure whether or not they actually gave consent to sex.

College students who drink are at risk for receiving poor grades, and an estimated 25 percent of all college students miss classes, do poorly, or fail examinations and receive overall bad grades as a result of their drinking.

Vandalism is another issue among college students who drink, and an estimated 11 percent of college student drinkers say that they damaged the property of others while they were drinking.

Heavy drinking is also associated with a greater number of emergency room visits, and SUICIDE is an increased risk among those students who are heavy drinkers.

Drinking as a Cultural Issue

According to the NIAAA, drinking is deeply engrained in the culture of many colleges. For example, some students attempt to drink 21 shots in the first hour after they reach their 21st birthday, and this practice has resulted in ALCOHOL POISONING. The body simply cannot metabolize that much alcohol that fast.

It should also be noted that heavy drinking and binge drinking is a problem among college students in other countries, according to Karam et al. in their study for *Current Opinion in Psychiatry,* published in 2007. They found that students in Europe, South America, New Zealand, and Australia also evinced heavy drinking. In addition, the researchers found similar risk factors toward and protective factors against problem drinking as have been found in the United States. For example, risk factors favoring heavy drinking in college included male gender, higher family education, and higher socioeconomic status as risk factors. Even greater risk factors toward alcohol issues, however, were the excessive use of alcohol by the students' peers and/or their families.

In contrast, protective factors against excessive drinking were a belief in God, participating in religious practices, and having peers and/or family members who opposed heavy drinking.

College Students vs. Their Noncollege Peers

College students are heavier drinkers by several percentage points than are their same-age peers who are not in college. A study by Carlos Blanco and colleagues, published in 2008 in the *Archives of General Psychiatry* revealed that college students had a greater risk for alcohol abuse and alcohol dependence than did their noncollege peers. For example, of the 2,188 college student subjects, 20.4 percent had any alcohol use disorder, compared to 17 percent of their noncollege peers. Of those with alcohol abuse, 7.9 percent of the college students had this problem, compared to 6.8 percent of their noncollege peers. Even more disturbing was that the researchers found that 12.5 percent of the college students were alcoholics, compared to 10.2 percent of their noncollege peers.

Injuries among Drinking College Students

In their study for the *Annual Review of Public Health* in 2005, Ralph Hingson and colleagues studied college students ages 18–24 years old in both 1998 and 2001 for alcohol-related unintentional injury deaths and other health problems. They found that alcohol-related deaths from injuries increased from about 1,600 in 1998 to 1,700 in 2001, an increase of 6 percent. The researchers also found that the percentage of students who reported driving while under the influence of alcohol increased from 2.3 million students in 1998 to 2.8 million in 2001, or an increase from 26.5 percent of the students to nearly a third (31.4 percent). This is a disturbingly high increase.

The researchers also found that in both the years that were studied, about 500,000 students were unintentionally injured because of their alcohol use, and 600,000 students were either hit or assaulted by another student who was drinking.

The researchers concluded, "The magnitude of problems posed by excessive drinking among college students should stimulate both improved measurement of these problems and efforts to reduce them. We believe every unnatural death in the United States should be tested for alcohol."

Alcohol and Sexual Assaults and Victimization

Another problem that college students, particularly females, may face is alcohol-related sexual assaults. Sexual assault may include anything from unwanted kissing to completed sexual intercourse. Yet the female may question whether it is acceptable to report such an assault, believing that it may be her "fault" because maybe she was intoxicated or perhaps she did not make it clear enough that she did not wish to have sex. She may wrongly feel that if she strives hard to remain alert (although she is consuming alcohol), she will be able to resist sexual advances. The drinking female college student may also reproach herself for her appearance, dress, companions, and many other aspects of the unwanted sexual encounter. She may also tell herself that she is smart enough to have known better and that it is her fault when an assault occurred.

According to Antonia Abbey in a 2002 article in the *Journal of Studies on Alcohol Supplement* on college students who are sexually assaulted, at least half of all these sexual assaults are associated with alcohol use, including either alcohol that was used by the victim or used by the perpetrator or by both. Because white students are more likely to drink to excess, they are also more likely to be sexually assaulted than individuals of other races. Most sexual assaults are perpetrated by someone that the victim already knows, such as her date (the majority of assaults are on females, although males can also be sexually assaulted). Often the assault occurs in a familiar environment, such as in the dormitory room or at the home of the man or woman.

Abbey says that it is a mistake to assume that alcohol alone somehow causes a sexual assault to occur without the control of the perpetrator. Instead, she says, "The causal direction could be the opposite; men may consciously or unconsciously drink alcohol prior to committing sexual assault to have an excuse for their behavior. Alternatively, other variables may simultaneously cause both alcohol consumption and sexual assault. For example, personality traits, such as impulsivity, or peer group norms may lead some men both to drink heavily and to commit sexual assault."

Abbey says that what alcohol does do, however, is to impede effective communication about an individual's sexual intent and to increase the risk for misperceptions about intent. It also increases a biased view of what the other person desires sexually. Men may later justify their behavior by saying they could not control themselves because of their heavy alcohol intake. Abbey says that such men may believe that being intoxicated "caused them to initially misperceive their partner's degree of sexual interest and later allowed them to feel comfortable using force when the women's lack of consent finally became clear to them. These date rapists did not see themselves as 'real' criminals because real criminals used weapons to assault strangers."

Another related issue is that sometimes men, including male college students, perceive that women who drink heavily are sexually promiscuous, and thus it is acceptable to be sexually aggressive with such women. Men may also encourage women to drink so that they can make it easier to obtain their sexual favors. Drinking games in college have been linked to sexual victimization. Peer norms are another factor in sexual assaults in college. Some men give unknowing women punch spiked with alcohol in order to cause their intoxication and to provide them with an easier means to a sexual assault, and this behavior may be considered acceptable by their peers.

Psychiatric Disorders among College Students and Drinking

Research released in 2008 revealed that greater than expected percentages of college students suffered from serious psychiatric issues such as alcohol abuse and dependence. Carlos Blanco and his colleagues published their research in the *Archives of General Psychiatry*. Their study showed that college students had a significantly greater risk for developing a problem with alcohol abuse and alcohol dependence than their noncollege peers.

Of the 2,188 college students who were surveyed, about 8 percent of them had a problem with alcohol abuse. Even more disturbingly, about 13 percent of the students were alcoholics. In contrast, about 7 percent of the 2,904 noncollege students of the same age had a problem with alcohol abuse, and 10 percent of this group were alcoholics. Thus, the college students had a higher rate of alcohol use disorders than their noncollege peers.

A Movement to Lower the Drinking Age

Some individuals seek to consider a lowering of the drinking age, saying that it is unreasonable to allow people to vote or enlist in the military but not consume alcohol. At the forefront of this group is the Amethyst Initiative, a Washington, D.C.–based organization of about 100 college presidents nationwide that was formed in 2008. They acknowledge that binge drinking is a problem on campus but believe that limiting the drinking age to 21 years and above is not the solution. In contrast, groups such as Mothers Against Drunk Driving (MADD) are very opposed to any decrease in the drinking age, believing that it would only increase the problem of heavy drinking among young people.

See also AGE AND ALCOHOL; AGGRESSIVE BEHAVIOR AND ALCOHOL; ALCOHOL AND MEN; ALCOHOL AND WOMEN; ALCOHOLISM/ALCOHOL DEPENDENCE AND ALCOHOL ABUSE; ALCOHOL POISONING; ANXIETY DISORDERS; ATTENTION-DEFICIT/HYPERACTIVITY DISORDER; BIPOLAR DISORDER; CONDUCT DISORDER; DEPRESSION; DRIVING UNDER THE INFLUENCE/DRIVING WHILE INTOXICATED; EXCESSIVE DRINKING AND HEALTH CONSEQUENCES; EXCESSIVE DRINKING AND NEGATIVE SOCIAL CONSEQUENCES; IMPULSE CONTROL DISORDERS; PERSONALITY DISORDERS; PSYCHIATRIC COMORBIDITIES; TREATMENT; UNDERAGE DRINKING.

Abbey, Antonia. "Alcohol-Related Sexual Assault: A Common Problem among College Students." *Journal of Studies on Alcohol Supplement* 14 (2002): 118–128.
Blanco, Carlos, M.D., et al. "Mental Health of College Students and Their Non-College-Attending Peers: Results

from the National Epidemiologic Study on Alcohol and Related Conditions." *Archives of General Psychiatry* 65, no. 12 (2008): 1,429–1,437.

Hingson, Ralph, Timothy Heeren, Michael R. Winter, and Henry Wechsler. "Early Age of First Drunkenness as a Factor in College Students' Unplanned and Unprotected Sex Attributable to Drinking," *Pediatrics* 111, no. 1 (2003): 34–41.

———. "Magnitude of Alcohol-Related Mortality and Morbidity among U.S. College Students Ages 18–24: Changes from 1998 to 2001." *Annual Review of Public Health* 26 (2005): 259–279.

Karam, E., K. Kypri, and M. Salamoun. "Alcohol Use among College Students: An International Perspective." *Current Opinion in Psychiatry* 20, no. 3 (2007): 213–221.

LaBrie, Joseph W., et al. "What Men Want: The Role of Reflective Opposite-Sex Normative Preferences in Alcohol Use Among College Women." *Psychology of Addictive Behaviors* 23, no. 1 (2009): 157–162.

National Institute on Alcohol Abuse and Alcoholism National Advisory Council on Alcohol Abuse and Alcoholism Task Force on College Drinking. *High-Risk Drinking in College: What We Know and What We Need to Learn.* Bethesda, Md.: National Institutes of Health, April 2002.

O'Connor, Roisin M., Sherry H. Stewart, and Margo C. Watt. "Distinguishing BAS Risk for University Students' Drinking, Smoking, and Gambling Behaviors." *Personality and Individual Differences* 46, no. 4 (2009): 514–519.

conduct disorder A disruptive behavior disorder that is diagnosed in some children and adolescents and which is characterized by lying, cheating, stealing, harming the property of others, and generally disrespecting other people. Some individuals with conduct disorder (CD) are also violent toward others. In the past, this behavior may have been referred to as juvenile delinquency. In a study of COLLEGE STUDENTS versus their noncollege peers by Carlos Blancos, M.D., and colleagues and reported in the *Archives of General Psychiatry* in 2008, conduct disorder was about twice as common among the noncollege young adults; 2.3 percent of the noncollege peers had conduct disorder, compared to 1.2 percent of the college students.

Individuals with conduct disorder have a markedly increased risk for both alcohol abuse and ALCOHOLISM/ALCOHOL DEPENDENCE, in part because drinking may be perceived as thumbing the nose at moral conventions. In addition, drinking may also occur because the individual with conduct disorder is frequently depressed and may seek to blot out feelings of depression or anger, as well as a periodic awareness that breaks through defenses of his or her own culpability in the problems faced. Other underlying genetic issues may be a factor as well. (See GENETICS AND ALCOHOL; PSYCHIATRIC COMORBIDITIES.)

When the individual reaches adulthood, if the behavior continues, he or she may be diagnosed with ANTISOCIAL PERSONALITY DISORDER, which is itself another risk factor for alcoholism.

Symptoms and Diagnostic Path

The individual with conduct disorder commits crimes, such as property damage or burglaries. Often he or she is contemptuous of other individuals, and the person with conduct disorder frequently blames others for problems that the individual has actually created himself or herself. Another common symptom of CD is that the individual often feels and exhibits anger or even rage toward others for their real or imagined minor offenses (or for no offenses at all). Conduct disorder is diagnosed by psychiatrists based on the individual's recent past acts as well as what he or she says to the doctor.

Treatment Options and Outlook

It is very difficult to treat conduct disorder, because the child or adolescent is often highly resistant to any treatment. The treatment is also complicated by the fact that often other accompanying disorders are present along with conduct disorder, such as ATTENTION-DEFICIT/HYPERACTIVITY DISORDER (ADHD). In some cases, treatment of the ADHD may improve the symptoms of conduct disorder, but there is no guarantee that this will happen. If the person with conduct disorder is a child who is still living at home, it is very important for the therapist to engage the parents, who may benefit from learning new and effective techniques to help them better control the child's behavior, as well as to minimize the negative effect of the child's behavior upon them.

Risk Factors and Preventive Measures

Individuals with attention-deficit/hyperactivity disorder have an increased risk for developing conduct disorder, particularly if they were previously diagnosed with oppositional defiant disorder (ODD). ODD is characterized by the chronic refusal to comply with the wishes of parents and other authority figures and by constant arguing, but it is not considered to be as serious a disorder as conduct disorder. In general, males are more likely to be diagnosed with conduct disorder than females.

There are no known preventive measures against conduct disorder, but when symptoms occur, they should not be ignored. Instead, the assistance of an experienced child or adolescent psychiatrist should be sought. If the child with conduct disorder also has an alcohol use disorder, this problem should be treated as well.

See also AGGRESSIVE BEHAVIOR AND ALCOHOL; ALCOHOLIC PSYCHOSIS; ANXIETY DISORDERS; BIPOLAR DISORDER; DEPRESSION; EXCESSIVE DRINKING AND NEGATIVE SOCIAL CONSEQUENCES; IMPULSE CONTROL DISORDERS; PERSONALITY DISORDERS; SCHIZOPHRENIA.

Blanco, Carlos, M.D., et al. "Mental Health of College Students and Their Non-College-Attending Peers: Results from the National Epidemiologic Study on Alcohol and Related Conditions." *Archives of General Psychiatry* 65, no. 12 (2008): 1,429–1,437.

delirium tremens A dangerous condition caused by the sudden withdrawal from alcohol in a long-term alcoholic and which may also occur with the abuse of and sudden withdrawal from benzodiazepine medications. In general, the person who suffers from delirium tremens is an extreme alcoholic who may consume up to a fifth of distilled spirits daily until for some reason, he or she suddenly stops drinking. If the person is not a benzodiazepine abuser, BENZODIAZEPINES are sometimes used to calm the agitated symptoms of individuals with delirium tremens. Delirium tremens is sometimes referred to as the "DTs."

People with delirium tremens should not be left unattended or untreated, as sometimes occurs in a prison or another institutional environment (or by family members at home), who may assume that he or she will simply "get over" it or "sleep it off." Without treatment the individual may die or suffer from coma and brain damage caused by seizures if he or she survives. Thus, the individual needs to be treated urgently as an inpatient in a hospital.

Symptoms and Diagnostic Path

Most physicians and some lay people can recognize the symptoms of delirium tremens, which may include the following:

- severe tremor
- hallucinations (auditory and visual)
- confusion
- severe perspiration
- nausea and vomiting
- insomnia
- fever
- seizures

Treatment Options and Outlook

The individual with delirium tremens should be treated as a hospital inpatient, for his or her own safety. If the individual is treated by medical professionals, often recovery occurs. However, the condition may recur if the person resumes heavy drinking and then subsequently withdraws suddenly from alcohol use. Detoxification from alcohol should be a tapering process done in a hospital environment.

Risk Factors and Preventive Measures

Individuals who are very heavy alcohol and/or benzodiazepine consumers have the greatest risks for developing delirium tremens. The best way to avoid delirium tremens is to avoid heavy drinking or to withdraw from heavy drinking with the help of medical professionals.

See EXCESSIVE DRINKING AND HEALTH CONSEQUENCES; TREATMENT; WERNICKE-KORSAKOFF SYNDROME.

denial The refusal to accept that a serious problem is present in oneself or another person, such as the refusal of an individual to accept that he or she or someone else that the individual cares about has a problem with alcohol abuse or ALCOHOLISM/ ALCOHOL DEPENDENCE. Sometimes the denial that there is a problem occurs on the part of others in the family, such as a spouse or partner or even an adult child who denies a parent's problem with alcohol, although it is readily apparent to others. Even when the victim receives severe beatings or other negative consequences at the hands of the alcoholic, these victims may still deny that a problem with alcohol is present. The person who is in denial that a problem exists may also be complicit in helping the alcoholic to deny his or her own symptoms, which often occurs in a relationship that is characterized by CODEPENDENCY. This is also known as enabling behavior.

Denial is a very powerful defense mechanism, which is commonly used by individuals who either cannot or will not face the reality of their dangerous situation. As long as the denial continues on the part of the alcoholic, he or she will not seek treatment, and the behavior will continue or may even escalate. Because denial is so paramount an issue in alcohol dependence, it is also the first of twelve steps as outlined by Alcoholics Anonymous: "We admitted we were powerless over alcohol—that our lives had become unmanageable." Individuals with denial would benefit by attending meetings of Al-Anon, a sister organization of Alcoholics Anonymous for the families of individuals with alcoholism; however, often their denial prevents them from attending such meetings.

See also ALCOHOLISM MUTUAL AID SOCIETIES; ENABLERS.

dependent personality disorder   See PERSONALITY DISORDERS.

depression   Clinical symptoms of extreme sadness and distress which may also be accompanied by suicidal tendencies, attempted SUICIDE, or completed suicide. Depression is *not* a temporary sad mood but is instead a much more severe and longstanding problem. Many famous people have suffered from depression, such as President Abraham Lincoln and numerous other political figures, authors, and celebrities, as well as many average individuals from all walks of life and careers. Many people in the United States realize that depression is a common and serious problem, and depression does not carry the social stigma still associated with other psychiatric illnesses, such as ANXIETY DISORDERS, BIPOLAR DISORDER, and SCHIZOPHRENIA.

The symptoms of depression may be mimicked by some medical disorders such as hypothyroidism, vitamin deficiency, CANCER, multiple sclerosis, substance abuse, or other medical problems. Thus, the individual needs to be medically screened for other possible health disorders. The individual also needs to report if he or she just stopped taking a stimulant medication or other medication, which may also cause symptoms of depression.

Depression is a problem in the United States as well as worldwide. It can seriously affect an individual's physical health as well as his or her mental health. According to Saba Moussavi and colleagues in their article on depression in *Lancet* in 2007, depression is frequently comorbid (present at the same time) with other medical problems, and this comorbidity often worsens their outcomes. For example, the authors found that depression was often comorbid with such serious medical problems as angina, diabetes, arthritis, and asthma, based on the observations of more than 245,000 individuals worldwide and their health with and without depression. In this World Health Organization–funded research study, the researchers also found that the physical health of those with the diseases studied was significantly worse when they also had depression. This was particularly true in the case of individuals who had diabetes combined with depression.

Many individuals with clinical depression drink alcohol to excess; however, alcohol is a depressant, and eventually the temporary euphoria that may come with drinking becomes a feeling of hopelessness and helplessness. It is also true that chronic drinking may itself lead to depression. Sometimes it appears to be a "chicken and egg" question as to which came first, the excessive drinking or the depression. Some experts argue that depression often leads to drinking, while other experts offer evidence that drinking may trigger depression. According to the National Institute of Mental Health (NIMH), people with ALCOHOLISM suffer from major depression at about twice the rate of people who are not alcoholics.

A surprisingly large number of high school students report feeling "sad or hopeless," according to the Centers for Disease Control and Prevention (CDC), or 35.8 percent who said that they had felt this way every day for two or more weeks in a row, to the extent that they stopped doing some of their usual activities. This may be a factor in the relatively high rates of adolescent drinking that occur in the United States. Such feelings of depression were reportedly the highest among Hispanic females (42.3 percent), followed by white females (34.6 percent) and black females (34.5 percent). This rate of depression among various races and ethnicities generally tracks the rates of drinking and BINGE DRINKING among adolescents by race and ethnicity.

Among male high school students, researchers found that Hispanic males were the most depressed (30.4 percent), followed by black males (24.0 percent) and white males (17.8 percent). The CDC also reports that 15.9 percent of Hispanic high school students have seriously considered attempting suicide, followed by 14.0 percent of white students, and then by 13.2 percent of black high school students. In addition, 12.8 percent of Hispanic students had made a suicide plan, followed by 10.8 percent of white students, and 9.5 percent of black high school students.

Important note: Any person who says that he or she is thinking about suicide and/or has made a plan to commit suicide is in urgent need of mental health assistance similar to how a person who has or may have just had a heart attack, stroke, or other life-threatening occurrence needs urgent medical care. The individual may need to be hospitalized with or without his or her permission, which is permissible (for short periods) in each state if the person is a threat to himself/herself and/or to others.

In a study of college students and their non-college peers by Carlos Blanco, M.D., et al., and reported in 2008 in the *Archives of General Psychiatry,* the college student subjects had about the same rate of major depressive disorder, or 7.0 percent, compared to the 6.7 percent rate for their noncollege peers. However, the college students had a significantly higher rate of alcohol abuse and alcohol dependence. (See COLLEGE STUDENTS.)

Depression may also co-occur along with many other psychiatric disorders, such as PERSONALITY DISORDERS, ANTISOCIAL PERSONALITY DISORDER, schizophrenia, ATTENTION-DEFICIT/HYPERACTIVITY DISORDER, bipolar disorder, and others. The more psychiatric disorders that a person has, the more likely that he or she also has a problem with alcohol abuse or dependence. In addition, the more psychiatric disorders that a person has, the more

likely that the person is clinically depressed. (See PSYCHIATRIC COMORBIDITIES.)

Symptoms and Diagnostic Path

Most physicians are familiar with the symptoms and diagnosis of depression. Some common symptoms include:

- a significant weight loss or weight gain
- insomnia or excessive sleeping
- restlessness or irritability
- a failure to enjoy or to participate in activities that were formerly pleasurable for the individual
- feelings of hopelessness and helplessness
- the mention to others that life is not worth living
- persistent physical symptoms such as chronic headaches, stomach aches, or other chronic pain that does not respond to treatment
- decreased energy and fatigue
- feelings of worthlessness and guilt
- discussion of a wish for death or a plan to die (this symptom should be reported to emergency authorities)

Treatment Options and Outlook

Depression is treated with ANTIDEPRESSANTS and psychotherapy. If the person has a psychotic form of depression, antipsychotic medications are also prescribed. There are several key categories of antidepressants, including tricyclics, selective serotonin reuptake inhibitors (SSRIs), and serotonin norepinephrine reuptake inhibitors (SNRIs). In addition, atypical antidepressants such as bupropion (Wellbutrin, Wellbutrin XL) are sometimes prescribed to treat depression. Sometimes a person may need more than one type of antidepressant to control a clinical depression.

Many doctors recommend therapy and an antidepressant rather than one form of treatment alone. When an antidepressant is chosen, the doctor considers the patient's past medical history, and if he or she has responded well to a particular antidepressant in the past, then that medication is usually chosen again. If the patient has not taken antidepressants before, but a close family member has responded well to a particular antidepressant, the physician may elect to prescribe this medication. If there is no personal or family history of treatment with antidepressants, many doctors choose to prescribe a medication in the selective serotonin reuptake inhibitor (SSRI) class, because they are rarely abused and are often effective. Some doctors choose bupropion (Wellbutrin, Wellbutrin XL), an atypical antidepressant, because it affects the person's dopamine levels (improving mood), and it is also an effective medication for smokers and alcohol abusers. Doctors also consider symptoms that the patient has; for example, if the patient has severe insomnia, the physician may prescribe an antidepressant with sedative action, such as a tricyclic medication.

Cognitive-behavioral therapy (CBT) is often used to treat depression. This therapy evolved from the theories of Aaron Beck and Albert Ellis, who both developed similar therapies at about the same time in the mid-20th century. With CBT, the therapist (often a psychologist or a social worker) identifies the key illogical premises in a person's underlying thinking and then teaches the individual to challenge these premises in his or her own mind. For example, one common irrational thought is, "My family is angry at me. I am worthless." In fact, the family may *be* angry at the individual because of the chaotic life an alcoholic can create for others, but this does not automatically mean that the person is then "worthless." There are many different underlying irrational premises that individuals with alcohol dependence may believe that can be challenged by therapists trained in CBT.

Many primary care practitioners treat depression, but psychiatrists are the most knowledgeable physicians with regard to its symptoms and how to treat it effectively. However, many individuals fear seeing a psychiatrist, believing (wrongly) that psychiatrists treat only the severely mentally ill. They may also fear that they will be stigmatized by seeing a psychiatrist. Because many people see their internists or general practitioners for many different medical problems, they are less fearful of potential stigma from seeking treatment there.

It is important for the prescribing physician to be aware of the individual's drinking habits in order to ensure that there will be no medication interactions between the antidepressant and alcohol. In general, it is best to avoid alcohol altogether when taking prescribed psychiatric medications.

Risk Factors and Preventive Measures

There is a genetic risk for depression, and if one biological family member has clinical depression, then others in the family are also at risk. In general, women have a higher risk for depression than men. Distressing life circumstances can trigger a depression, such as the death of a loved one, the loss of a job, a divorce, and other forms of harm that befall an individual or others whom he or she cares about. Sometimes, however, there is no apparent cause of a depression in the person's life, and to others, the person's life appears to be going well or even very well. Depression cannot be prevented because life circumstances and genetic inheritances are not controllable factors.

See also ALCOHOL AND MEN; ALCOHOL AND WOMEN; ALCOHOLIC PSYCHOSIS; CHILD ABUSE AND NEGLECT; CONDUCT DISORDER; IMPULSE CONTROL DISORDERS.

Blanco, Carlos, M.D., et al. "Mental Health of College Students and Their Non-College-Attending Peers: Results from the National Epidemiologic Study on Alcohol and Related Conditions." *Archives of General Psychiatry* 65, no. 12 (2008): 1,429–1,437.

Burns, Lucy, and Maree Teesson. "Alcohol Use Disorders Comorbid with Anxiety, Depression and Drug Use Disorders: Findings from the Australian National Survey of Mental Health and Well Being." *Drug and Alcohol Dependence* 68, no. 3 (2002): 299–307.

Centers for Disease Control and Prevention. Youth Risk Behavior Surveillance—United States, 2007. *Morbidity and Mortality Weekly Report* 57, no. SS-4 (June 6, 2008).

Grant, Bridget F., et al. "Prevalence and Co-Occurrence of Substance Use Disorders and Independent Mood and Anxiety Disorders: Results from the National Epidemiologic Survey on Alcohol and Related Conditions." *Alcohol Research & Health* 29, no. 2 (2006): 107–120.

Moussavi, Saba, et al. "Depression, Chronic Diseases, and Decrements in Health: Results from the World Health Surveys." *Lancet* 370, no. 9,590 (2007): 851–858.

detoxification See ALCOHOLISM/ALCOHOL DEPENDENCE AND ALCOHOL ABUSE.

disulfiram (Antabuse) An aversive drug that is taken orally (although it can also be injected) and that is used to treat individuals with ALCO-HOLISM/ALCOHOL DEPENDENCE. Disulfiram prevents the metabolizing of alcohol and consequently causes extreme vomiting if the person consumes any amount of alcohol, even in cooked foods or personal products that contain alcohol, such as mouthwash. Antabuse has been used since the late 1940s as a medication to treat alcoholism/alcohol dependence, although newer medications are also available, such as acamprosate (Campral) and NAL-TREXONE, and are approved by the Food and Drug Administration (FDA) for this purpose.

The drug was first used by Erik Jacobsen and Jens Hald in Denmark. Sometimes other drugs which cause similar severely nauseous reactions such as metronidazole, are used instead of disulfiram. The basis of the therapy is that the patient will develop a conditioned reflex so that he or she associates drinking with extreme vomiting and overall unpleasantness and develops an aversion to even the smell of alcohol.

This drug should not be used in patients with coronary artery disease or severe myocardial disease, nor should it be taken by people with a hypersensitivity to rubber derivatives, according to the National Institute on Alcohol Abuse and Alcoholism (NIAAA). It should also be used only with caution in patients with a history of psychosis as well as those with diabetes, epilepsy, hypothyroidism, and kidney disease. Patients taking this drug should wear a medical alert bracelet in the event of an emergency.

Some serious adverse reactions to disulfiram include peripheral neuropathy, psychotic reactions, and hepatoxicity (toxic reaction of the liver). More common side effects to this drug are experiencing a metallic aftertaste in the mouth, dermatitis, and short-term mild drowsiness. Antabuse reacts with blood thinners such as warfarin (Coumadin) as well as with metronidazole, isoniazid, phenytoin (Dilantin), and any nonprescription medication that contains any amount of alcohol. Before patients begin taking this drug, their liver function should be evaluated and it should continue to be monitored while the patient is taking the drug.

Patients taking disulfiram should call their doctors immediately if they notice any of the following warning signs of a dangerous reaction to the drug:

- yellowing of the skin or eyes
- darkened urine
- light-colored or grayish stools
- severe stomach pain
- numbness or tingling or pain in the hands or feet
- mood changes

Sometimes disulfiram is ordered by the court, and in such cases, individuals taking monitored disulfiram must go to a pharmacy and be administered the drug while the pharmacist watches. The reason for this oversight is to ensure that medication compliance occurs. In a study by Brandon K. Martin and colleagues on the adherence to court-ordered disulfiram, published in the *Journal of Substance Abuse Treatment* in 2004, the researchers studied 19 voluntary and 17 court-ordered patients taking disulfiram over 15 months. They found that treatment adherence was much higher in the court-ordered group, or 61.0 percent, compared to 18.2 percent for the voluntary subjects.

The researchers also found a direct and high association between medication compliance at three months and then compliance at 15 months. They also found an association for some subjects between compliance and the risk of jail time for those who failed to comply. People at risk for incarceration if they did not take the drug generally took the disulfiram.

Individuals taking disulfiram should be careful about topical products that contain alcohol, as well as orally ingested products. Even aftershave lotions, colognes, mouthwash, hand sanitizer and perfumes may cause a reaction. They may not lead to extreme nausea and vomiting but may cause other side effects, such as headache and skin itching.

In another study by Brandon Martin, Laura Mangum, and Thomas P. Beresford, M.D., on the use of court-ordered disulfiram with military veterans at Veterans Administration (VA) Medical Centers, reported in the *American Journal of Addictions* in 2005, the researchers did telephone interviews with 48 VA substance abuse clinics in 48 states. The responders reported a low usage of disulfiram. The general use was never/rarely: 63 percent; sometimes: 32 percent; and often: 5 percent. In contrast, court-ordered disulfiram was used never/rarely: 95 percent; sometimes: 3 percent; and often: 2 percent. Nationally, fewer than 1 percent of the veterans were using disulfiram, and the researchers suggested that the drug was underused for alcohol dependence, since it is well-known among experts that disulfiram is effective if taken as directed.

The researchers found that the lack of use centered on several explanations, including a misreading of the literature on disulfiram, based on early studies that did not adequately supervise patients. Another misunderstanding centered on a fear that the drug was unsafe, based on past cases in which excessively high dosages were administered to patients to purposely induce severe vomiting.

According to the researchers, "With substantial efficacy and safety data available in the literature, clinicians may wish to reconsider the use of supervised disulfiram. This seems especially relevant for clinicians working in DVA facilities where the severity and frequency of alcohol-use disorders is greater than in the private sector. Furthermore, new data demonstrating the ability of a court order to enhance adherence with supervised disulfiram therapy significantly indicate further use of this treatment option."

See also TREATMENT.

Martin, Brandon K., et al. "Adherence to Court-Ordered Disulfiram at Fifteen Months: A Naturalistic Study." *Journal of Substance Abuse Treatment* 26, no. 3 (2004): 233–236.

Martin, Brandon, Laura Mangum, and Thomas P. Beresford, M.D. "Use of Court-Ordered Supervised Disulfiram Therapy at DVA Medical Centers in the United States." *American Journal on Addictions* 14, no. 3 (2005): 208–212.

doctors with alcohol problems   See IMPAIRED PHYSICIANS; TREATMENT.

driving under the influence/driving while intoxicated (DUI/DWI)   Operating a motor vehicle while under the excessive influence of alcohol, which is a crime in every state in the United States. People can be arrested and charged with driving under the influence while driving an automobile, truck, motorcycle, or other registered vehicle, or even nonregistered vehicles or non–motor vehicle items. For example, a man in Oregon was arrested for DUI while driving an adult tricycle on the wrong side of a public road in mid-afternoon in 2008. In the same year, a Georgia man was arrested for DUI after it was reported that he was weaving on a boy's bicycle down a public road and fell off the bike. A man in Pennsylvania was arrested for DUI driving after he was apprehended driving an Amish buggy home at night from a carnival with no lights. He had reportedly drunk 12 beers and then attempted to drive home. He told police he was a "bad Amish." Others have received DUIs for driving drunk on horses, golf carts, lawnmowers, and many other types of vehicles. Some states use the term "driving under the influence" (DUI) while others use "driving while intoxicated" (DWI), or other terms such as "impaired driving," all of which refer to the driver being intoxicated with alcohol either at or beyond the legal blood alcohol level of 0.08 percent. According to author Sarah W. Tracy in her book *Alcoholism in America,* the first laws against driving under the influence were passed in New York in 1910, followed a year later by laws enacted in California. Today, all states in the United States criminalize driving with a blood alcohol level of 0.08 or greater, although penalties for violating the law vary from state to state. The blood alcohol level of 0.08 for each state was prompted by the federal government, which threatened to withhold federal funds from states that did not enact this change from prior state blood alcohol level limits that allowed a higher blood alcohol level for DUI.

In 2006, more than a million people in the United States were arrested for driving under the influence of alcohol. Driving while intoxicated must be measured and quantified in the United States; however, in other countries, such as Japan, intoxication may be determined by a person's visible behavior. It should also be noted that some people are able to drive at a 0.08 level, while others at a much lower level of intoxication are poor drivers because they miss random events and concentrate instead on keeping their car inside the lines on the road.

Although people may not admit that they have driven while drunk to their friends and family, some individuals have candidly admitted to researchers that they have engaged in this behavior. As a result, researchers have been able to make generalizations about drunken drivers; for example, men are more likely to drive in an intoxicated state than women. In addition, about a third of high school students have admitted to researchers that they knowingly rode in a car with a driver who had been drinking alcohol, based on research published in *Morbidity and Mortality Weekly Report* (MMWR) in 2008.

Alcohol-related motor vehicle crashes killed 12,998 people in 2007 in the United States, according to the National Highway Traffic Safety Administration (NHTSA). Most alcohol-related fatalities are committed by individuals whose blood alcohol level exceeded 0.08 percent, according to the NHTSA. BINGE DRINKING is also a major problem among many people who become involved in car accidents, particularly among younger individuals.

Driving under the influence of alcohol is usually measured by a breath test or the individual's blood alcohol level. In many states, a refusal to take one of these tests for alcohol levels constitutes an automatic admission of guilt.

In a Canadian survey of drivers that occurred in 2008, published in *Alcohol and Drug Use Among Drivers: British Columbia Roadside Survey, 2008,* researchers Douglas J. Beirness and Erin E. Beasley found that two-thirds of the drivers who were interviewed were males and that drivers of pickup trucks and sports utility vehicles (SUVs) were the most likely to have been drinking. SUV drivers were the most likely to be intoxicated. Most of the intoxicated people were male: Males represented 78.4 percent of all drunk drivers. The researchers found that alcohol use was most common during weekends and late evening hours and among drivers ages 19 to 24 and 25 to 34 years. In contrast, illicit drug use by drivers was evenly spread out throughout the day and night by all age groups in Canada.

The researchers also found that 10.4 percent of the Canadian drivers tested positive for one or more impairing substances other than alcohol, such as cannabis (marijuana) or cocaine. These two drugs were the two most commonly identified, in each case found in 4.6 percent of drivers. The researchers determined that of those drivers who tested positive for cannabis, 22 percent had also consumed alcohol, and half of these drivers had a blood alcohol level in excess of 0.08, an illegal level of intoxication for drivers.

Some studies have also shown that individuals who have been convicted of driving while under the influence of alcohol are significantly more likely to die in a future car crash than others who were charged with impaired driving. This research indicates that individuals who are convicted of driving while intoxicated should receive a comprehensive alcohol evaluation as well as compulsory treatment for alcohol abuse or dependence.

Today, penalties for driving while intoxicated vary from state to state, but most states exact some sort of penalty. In the past as recently as in the early 1980s, however, many individuals repeatedly drove while drunk and only minor penalties were imposed. The grassroots organization Mothers Against Drunk Driving (MADD) had a profound effect on the implementation of stricter penalties for those convicted of drunken driving in most states. MADD was founded by Candy Lightner, the parent of a 13-year-old child killed by a drunken driver, and Cindi Lamb, a mother whose five-month-old daughter was paralyzed by the crash caused by a drunken driver. Some experts believe, however, that current penalties are still not strict enough. Others believe that in the 21st century, MADD and related organizations have gone too far, emulating 19th-century organizations, such as the Woman's Christian Temperance Union.

Some drivers who are impaired with alcohol are also impaired with other substances, such as marijuana or misused prescription drugs, particularly BENZODIAZEPINES and narcotics. This combination is very risky for the driver as well as for others who are out on the road at the same time.

UNDERAGE DRINKING is also a serious problem. Some adolescents drive when they have been drinking alcohol. According to the Youth Risk Behavior Surveillance for the United States in 2007, published in 2008 in the *Morbidity and Mortality Weekly Report,* during the 30 days before the survey, 10.5 percent of high-school students nationwide said they had driven a car or other vehicle one or more times when they had been drinking alcohol. Males were more likely to drink before driving (12.8 percent) than females (8.1 percent).

To combat underage drinking while driving, at least in part, some states have instituted ZERO TOLERANCE policies, which means that any amount of alcohol in a driver under age 21 is illegal. Penalties for violation of this law vary among states. According to researchers such as L. Liang and J. Huang, zero tolerance policies are effective, especially in the case of reducing drinking among individuals who drink away from their homes.

Significant Percentages of Adult Drivers Admit to Driving While Intoxicated

Large numbers of individuals have candidly admitted to researchers that they have driven while under the influence of alcohol. In a report released by the Substance Abuse and Mental Health Services Administration (SAMHSA) in 2008, a nationwide report revealed that 15.1 percent of drivers ages 18 and older said that they drove while under the influence of alcohol in the past year. In some states, the rates were much higher, as in the high of 26.4 percent in Wisconsin, 24.9 percent in North Dakota, and 23.5 percent in Minnesota. (See Table 1.) These individuals were not necessarily arrested and prosecuted for driving under the influence; however, they did admit to SAMHSA that they drove while intoxicated.

It should also be noted that the states where individuals were the least likely to drive under the influence of alcohol were Utah (9.5 percent), West Virginia (10.1 percent), and North Carolina and Kentucky (both 10.4 percent).

TABLE 1
STATE ESTIMATES OF DRIVING UNDER THE INFLUENCE OF ALCOHOL AND ILLICIT DRUGS IN THE PAST YEAR AMONG CURRENT DRIVERS AGED 18 OR OLDER: AVERAGE OF 2004–2006

State	Percent
Wisconsin	26.4
North Dakota	24.9
Minnesota	23.5
Nebraska	22.9
South Dakota	21.6
Kansas	21.1
Massachusetts	20.5
Rhode Island	20.4
Montana	20.3
District of Columbia	19.1
Michigan	18.4
Wyoming	18.3
Missouri	18.0
Iowa	17.6
Hawaii	17.4
Connecticut	17.2
Colorado	17.0
New Hampshire	16.7
Illinois	16.5
Vermont	16.4
Louisiana	16.0
Nevada	15.9
Oregon	15.9
Texas	15.7
Ohio	15.7
Indiana	15.2
Arizona	14.9
Pennsylvania	14.8
South Carolina	14.7
Maryland	14.7
Washington	13.8
California	13.8
Delaware	13.7
Oklahoma	13.7
Alaska	13.7
Idaho	13.6
Virginia	13.6
New Mexico	13.5
Georgia	13.5
Florida	13.5
New York	13.0
Maine	12.4
Tennessee	12.4
Mississippi	11.9
Alabama	11.4
New Jersey	11.3
Arkansas	10.8
Kentucky	10.4
North Carolina	10.4
West Virginia	10.1
Utah	9.5

Source: Adapted from press release for State Estimates of Persons Aged 18 or Older Driving. Available online. URL: http://www.oas.samhsa.gov/2k8/stateDUI/press.htm. Accessed December 11, 2008.

Demographics of DWI

Based on data from 1991–92 and 2001–02, reported by Chou et al. in *Alcohol Research & Health* in 2006, young adults ages 18–29 years are significantly more likely to drive while they are intoxicated (about 5.3 percent) than those who are ages 30–44 years old (3.5 percent). Only about 1.9 percent of those who are ages 45–64 drive while intoxicated. Elderly individuals age 65 and older have the lowest rate of driving while intoxicated of all age groups, or less than 1 percent (0.2 percent).

In considering race and ethnicity, NATIVE AMERICANS had the highest rate of driving while intoxicated, or 4.1 percent, compared to other races, based on the data from Chou et al. Native Americans also have a higher rate of alcohol consumption in general. This rate was followed by whites (3.3 percent) and then Hispanic/Latinos (2.1 percent). See Table 2 for further information.

In considering single ages alone, from ages 18–29, the data from Chou et al. revealed that among males, individuals age 22 years (11.5 percent) and age 23 years (10.4) percent had the highest risk for drinking and driving. Among females, the highest risks for drinking and then driving were among those who were age 23 years (7.1 percent), followed by those who were age 21 years (5.7 percent).

In considering males and females together as a group, the greatest risk for drunken driving by age occurred among those who were age 23 (8.7 percent) and those who were age 22 (7.8 percent). The lowest risk for drunken driving occurred among males and females ages 65 years and older, or less than one percent (0.2 percent).

In another analysis by SAMHSA in their annual National Survey on Drug Use and Health, an estimated 3.14 million people in the United States ages 12 and older drove a vehicle while under the influence of alcohol in 2007, the most recent data as of this writing. Males age 12 or older were almost twice as likely as females to drive under the influence as females, or 16.6 percent of males compared to 9.0 percent of females.

Measuring Blood Alcohol Levels of Suspected Drunk Drivers

In nearly all states, police officers who suspect a driver is intoxicated may stop the driver and perform field sobriety tests to determine if the driver is drunk. These tests may include asking the driver to follow a flashlight with his or her eyes or walk a straight line. They may also ask the driver to take an alcohol breath test, which involves blowing into a balloon-like device that measures the alcohol content in the person's breath. There are also some noninvasive breath tests that police may administer, such as the passive alcohol sensor. In many states, refusal to submit to a breath test is tantamount to admitting guilt to intoxication while driving. This is sometimes referred to as "implied consent."

Binge Drinking and Driving Under the Influence

Often the alcohol-impaired driver is also a binge drinker. According to a study published in 2008 by Flowers et al., based on an analysis of alcohol-impaired (AI) driving among adults ages 18 and older in all 50 states, 84 percent of alcohol-impaired drivers were binge drinkers. Binge drinkers are men who consumed five or more drinks on at least one occasion in the past 30 days and women who consumed at least four or more drinks on at least one occasion in the past 30 days. Nearly half of all accidents involve people who are binge drinkers. (See ALCOHOL AND MEN and ALCOHOL AND WOMEN.) The researchers also found that binge drinkers were less likely than others to consistently wear their car seat belts, further increasing their risk for severe injury.

The researchers said, "Examples of effective interventions to reduce AI driving include lowering legal BACs [blood alcohol content], promptly suspending the licenses of people arrested for driving while impaired, sobriety checkpoints, alcohol ignition interlock programs for convicted AI driving offenders, and sustained public education and enforcement. In conclusion, efforts to reduce AI driving should focus on preventing excessive drinking behaviors—particularly binge drinking—that are so strongly associated with AI driving."

Minimum Drinking Ages

In 1984, the National Minimum Drinking Age Act was signed into law by President Ronald Reagan. This law required all states to enact laws making age 21 as the minimum legal drinking age in the state or risk losing federal highway funds. The federal government could not pass a national minimum

TABLE 2
TWELVE-MONTH PREVALENCE OF DRIVING AFTER DRINKING, BY AGE, SEX, AND RACE:
UNITED STATES, 2001–2002

Age (years)	Male		Female		Total	
	Percent	Population Estimate in Thousands	Percent	Population Estimate in Thousands	Percent	Population Estimate in Thousands
Total						
Total	4.4	4,388	1.5	1,585	2.9	5,973
18–29	7.8	1,759	2.9	659	5.3	2,418
30–44	5.2	1,653	1.8	598	3.5	2,251
45–64	3.0	929	0.9	301	1.9	1,231
65 and older	0.3	47	Not available	26	0.2	73
White						
Total	5.0	3,516	1.7	1,296	3.3	4,812
18–29	9.9	1,364	3.5	492	6.7	1,857
30–44	6.1	1,301	2.5	542	4.2	1,842
45–64	3.4	810	1.0	251	2.2	1,061
65 and older	0.3	41	Not available	11	0.2	52
Black						
Total	2.6	258	0.7	90	1.5	348
18–29	3.1	84	1.2	40	2.1	124
30–44	3.5	118	0.4	18	1.8	136
45–64	1.9	54	Not available	32	1.3	85
65 and older	Not available	2	0.0	0	0.1	2
Native American						
Total	5.9	124	2.4	56	4.1	180
18–29	Not available	32	Not available	18	5.8	50
30–44	9.9	69	Not available	11	5.5	80
45–64	Not available	19	Not available	12	2.0	31
65 and older	Not available	4	Not available	15	Not available	19
Asian						
Total	2.0	89	0.8	35	1.4	124
18–29	4.3	57	2.6	32	3.5	89
30–44	Not available	24	Not available	Not available	Not available	24
45–64	Not available	8	0.0	Not available	Not available	8
65 and older	0.0	0	0.0	0	0.0	0
Hispanic/Latino						
Total	3.3	402	0.9	107	2.1	509
18–29	5.0	222	2.0	76	3.6	298
30–44	3.1	141	0.6	24	1.9	165
45–64	1.5	39	Not available	7	0.9	45
65 and older	0.0	0	0.0	0	0.0	0

Adapted from: Chou, S. Patricia, et al. "Twelve-Month Prevalence and Changes in Driving After Drinking: United States, 1991–1992 and 2001–2002." *Alcohol Research & Health* 29, no. 2 (2006), page 146.

drinking age law by itself, because states are allowed to regulate alcohol, based on the 21st Amendment. However, the federal government *could* and did provide an incentive to pass the law, which was for states to continue receiving federal highway funds; for example, states without the minimum drinking age law of 21 would have lost 5 percent in federal highway funds by October 1, 1986 and would have lost 10 percent by October 1, 1987.

The federal law was challenged and was upheld by the U.S. Supreme Court in 1987 in *South Dakota v. Dole,* U.S. 203. Since 1988, all states and the District of Columbia have held age 21 as the minimum drinking age. Minimum drinking age laws have saved an estimated 26,333 lives from 1975 to 2007, according to the National Highway Traffic Safety Administration (NHTSA). (See graph.)

In addition, according to the National Institute on Alcohol Abuse and Alcoholism, research has shown that the minimum drinking age laws have decreased traffic crashes among those under age 21 as well as suicides and have also decreased the consumption of alcohol.

Deaths Caused by Excessive Alcohol Use

Drinking and driving combined are among the best predictors of motor vehicle deaths in the United

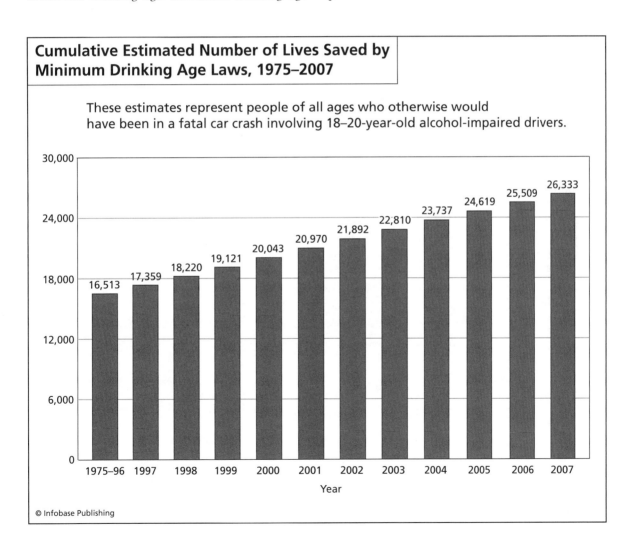

Cumulative Estimated Number of Lives Saved by Minimum Drinking Age Laws, 1975–2007

These estimates represent people of all ages who otherwise would have been in a fatal car crash involving 18–20-year-old alcohol-impaired drivers.

Year	Lives Saved
1975–96	16,513
1997	17,359
1998	18,220
1999	19,121
2000	20,043
2001	20,970
2002	21,892
2003	22,810
2004	23,737
2005	24,619
2006	25,509
2007	26,333

© Infobase Publishing

TABLE 3
FATALITIES, BY ROLE, IN CRASHES INVOLVING AT LEAST ONE DRIVER WITH A BAC OF .08 OR HIGHER, 2007

Role	Number	Percent of Total
Driver with BAC=.08+	8,644	66.5
Passenger Riding w. Driver with BAC=.08+	2,148	16.5
Subtotal	10,792	83.0
Occupants of Other Vehicles	1,433	11.0
Nonoccupants	773	5.9
Total Fatalities	12,998	100.0

Source: National Highway Traffic Safety Administration. "Alcohol-Impaired Driving." *Traffic Safety Facts*. 2007.

States and worldwide. According to the National Highway Traffic Safety Administration, alcohol was involved in 12,998 fatalities in 2007, and in two-thirds of all the cases (66.5 percent), it was the impaired driver who was killed. However, in other cases, passengers or occupants of other vehicles or individuals, such as pedestrians, who were not in cars were the ones who were killed. See Table 3 for further information.

The greater the blood alcohol level, the higher the risk of traffic fatalities, based on research by Ralph Hingson and Michael Winter, reported in *Alcohol Research & Health* in 2003. Many deaths from car crashes occur even with no alcohol involvement, as can be seen from Table 4. However, the death rates increase with an increasing blood alcohol level; for example, among those ages 21–29 years, less than

half (43 percent) died in car crashes when the driver or pedestrian who was involved in the crash had a zero blood alcohol level. The percent of deaths was 7 percent in this group when the BLOOD ALCOHOL CONCENTRATION (BAC) was 0.01–0.07 percent. This rate increased to 16 percent for a BAC of 0.08–0.14 percent and further increased to 34 percent for a BAC of 0.15 percent or greater. Clearly, alcohol was implicated in the deaths of these young adults.

Hingson and Winter have also reported that the top two driver behaviors contributing to fatal car crashes among individuals of all blood alcohol levels were:

1. the failure to keep in the lane or being run off the road
2. driving too fast for conditions

However, the percentage of deaths from these problematic behaviors also increases dramatically with higher blood alcohol levels. For example, when the blood alcohol level was zero, then 23 percent died from the failure to keep in their lane or being run off the road. But when the BAC was 0.15 percent or greater, this percentage was 58 percent, more than double the rate of no alcohol in the blood. (See Table 5.)

In another analysis, the Fatality and Analysis Reporting System (FARS) of the National Highway Traffic Safety Administration looked at drivers involved in fatal crashes and their BAC levels in 2007. Alcohol was not involved in the majority of

TABLE 4
TRAFFIC DEATHS BY AGE AND BLOOD ALCOHOL LEVEL, UNITED STATES, 2002

BAC *	Under age 16	Ages 16–20	Ages 21–29	Ages 30–45	Ages 46–64	Ages 65+
0.0%	77%	63%	43%	47%	62%	85%
0.01–0.07%	5%	7%	7%	6%	5%	3%
0.08–0.14%	7%	13%	16%	13%	9%	5%
0.15%+	11%	17%	34%	35%	24%	7%
All BACs	100%	100%	100%	100%	100%	100%
Percentage alcohol involved	23	37	57	53	38	15
Number of alcohol involved	573	2,329	4,595	5,682	3,192	971
Total of all fatalities	2,542	6,277	8,022	10,707	8,487	6,622

*BAC = the highest blood alcohol concentration of a driver or pedestrian involved in the crash
Source: Hingson, Ralph, and Michael Winter, "Epidemiology and Consequences of Drinking and Driving," *Alcohol Research & Health* 27, no. 1 (2003), page 64.

TABLE 5
DRIVER BEHAVIORS AND CHARACTERISTICS IN FATAL TRAFFIC CRASHES,
BY BLOOD ALCOHOL LEVEL (BAC), 2002 (IN PERCENT)

	Driver's BAC			
	0.00% (n = 43,141)	0.01–07% (n = 2,317)	0.08–0.14% (n = 42,274)	0.15%+ (n = 8,070)
Failure to keep in lane or run off road	23	43	49	58
Driving too fast for conditions	15	33	38	43
Failure to yield right of way	10	6	5	3
Inattentive	6	7	7	8
Failure to obey traffic signals	5	5	5	5
Operating in a reckless or erratic fashion	4	10	12	12
Overcorrecting	3	5	6	8
Driving wrong way	Less than 1%	Less than 1%	Less than 1%	Less than 1%
Operator inexperienced	Less than 1%	Less than 1%	Less than 1%	Less than 1%

Source: Hingson, Ralph, and Michael Winter, "Epidemiology and Consequences of Drinking and Driving," *Alcohol Research & Health* 27, no. 1 (2003), page 69.

fatal car crashes; for example, in 74 percent of car crashes nationwide, the BAC was zero. However, alcohol consumption in the driver was involved in 26 percent of all fatal car crashes in the United States in 2007. In addition, in that 26 percent when alcohol was involved, 22 percent of the cases involved a BAC of .08 percent or greater. Clearly, alcohol consumption above the legal limit is very dangerous and sometimes fatal.

There was considerable variation among states. For example, illegal alcohol use was involved in only 12 percent of the fatal crashes in Utah. In contrast, illegal alcohol use was involved in a high of 39 percent of drivers who died in North Dakota, followed by 32 percent in South Carolina, and 31 percent in Montana. (See Table 6.)

Often individuals who are impaired by alcohol fail to put on their seat belts, thus further increasing

TABLE 6
PERCENT OF DRIVERS INVOLVED IN FATAL CAR CRASHES BY STATE AND
BLOOD ALCOHOL CONCENTRATION OF THE DRIVER: 2007

	Blood Alcohol Concentration of the Driver		
	BAC = .00 (Percent involved in fatal crashes)	BAC = .01–.07 (Percent involved in fatal crashes	BAC = .08+
State			
Alabama	72	4	25
Alaska	73	4	23
Arizona	74	5	22
Arkansas	75	5	20
California	76	4	20
Colorado	76	3	21
Connecticut	70	5	25
Delaware	68	6	26
District of Columbia	70	8	22

(continues)

(continued)

	Blood Alcohol Concentration of the Driver		
	BAC = .00 (Percent involved in fatal crashes)	BAC = .01–.07 (Percent involved in fatal crashes	BAC = .08+
Florida	78	4	18
Georgia	79	3	18
Hawaii	64	12	25
Idaho	73	5	22
Illinois	72	5	24
Indiana	80	3	17
Iowa	79	4	17
Kansas	79	4	17
Kentucky	80	3	17
Louisiana	68	5	26
Maine	70	4	26
Maryland	76	5	20
Massachusetts	68	6	25
Michigan	78	4	18
Minnesota	78	3	19
Mississippi	72	3	25
Missouri	72	4	24
Montana	64	5	31
Nebraska	75	6	20
Nevada	74	5	21
New Hampshire	77	6	17
New Jersey	76	6	19
New Mexico	73	4	23
New York	75	5	20
North Carolina	76	3	20
North Dakota	56	5	39
Ohio	74	5	21
Oklahoma	78	3	19
Oregon	71	5	23
Pennsylvania	74	4	22
Rhode Island	61	10	29
South Carolina	64	5	32
South Dakota	71	5	24
Tennessee	74	3	22
Texas	69	5	27
Utah	85	3	12
Vermont	70	5	25
Virginia	72	5	23
Washington	72	5	23
West Virginia	72	4	24
Wisconsin	65	6	29
Wyoming	71	3	26
USA	74	4	22

Note: Percentages do not always add up to 100 percent because of rounding.
Adapted from the *FARS Encyclopedia: States-Alcohol.* Pages 2–3. Available online. URL: http://www-fars.nhtsa.dot.gov/States/StatesAlcohol.aspx.
Downloaded February 18, 2009.

their risk for severe injury or death. In their study in *Alcohol Research & Health*, researchers Hingson and Winter found that the more intoxicated that the individual in a fatal car crash was, the less likely that he or she was wearing a seat belt. For example, among individuals with a blood alcohol level of zero, 48 percent were belted. As the BAC increased, the percentage of drivers who used their seat belt decreased, and only 20 percent of fatally injured drivers with a BAC of 0.15 percent or greater were wearing their seat belts. (See Table 7.)

Of note, of the drivers who survived a car crash, individuals at all levels of intoxication (or no intoxication) who wore their seat belts had a higher survival rate compared to those drivers who were not wearing their seat belts. If the BAC level was zero and the driver was belted, the survival rate was 79 percent. However, if the driver was belted and had alcohol in his or her system, the survival level decreased at each greater range of alcohol, from 56 percent of belted survivors in the range of 0.01 percent to 0.07 percent to 43 percent of survivors among those whose BAC was 0.15 percent or greater.

Clearly, the intoxication of the drivers reduced their awareness of or the feeling of a necessity for wearing a seat belt, while at the same time increasing their risk for death in a car crash.

Subsequent Fatalities among Those Convicted of Drunken Driving

In a study conducted by Robert D. Brewer and colleagues, reported in 1994 in the *New England Journal of Medicine*, the researchers studied 1,648 drivers (called "case drivers") in North Carolina who had died in motor vehicle crashes from 1980 to 1989 and who had a blood alcohol concentration of at least 20 milligrams per deciliter. These drivers were compared to the 1,474 "control drivers" group, with lower blood alcohol levels at the time of death. The researchers looked at the driving records for each group for five years before the death to determine if there were any arrests for driving while impaired.

The researchers found that the deceased case drivers age 21 to 34 years old at the time of their deaths were 4.3 times more likely to have been arrested in the past for impaired driving than the control drivers. However, in considering the case drivers ages 35 years and older, they were 11.7 times more likely than the control drivers to have been arrested in the past for impaired driving.

The researchers found that most case drivers were male and that crashes in which most case drivers were killed occurred at night (from 6 P.M. to 6 A.M.) or on the weekend (Friday, from 6 P.M. to 6 A.M. on the following Monday.) They also found that 26.2 percent of the case drivers had one or more past arrests for impaired driving before their deaths, compared to 3.1 percent of the control drivers. According to the researchers,

If we consider arrest for driving while impaired to be a possible marker for problem drinking, the results of this study suggest that a history of problem drinking may be more common among younger drivers. This hypothesis is consistent with other studies that have reported an increased prevalence of problem drinking among younger persons, particularly those less than 30 years of age. However, our findings regarding the effect

TABLE 7
SEAT BELT USE BY DRIVERS IN FATAL CAR CRASHES, BY DRIVER'S BLOOD ALCOHOL LEVEL, 2002

	Driver's BAC			
	0.00% n (%)	0.01–0.07% n (%)	0.08–.14% n (%)	0.15%+ n (%)
Drivers in fatal crashes who survived the crash	25,287	986	1,704	1,861
Percent belted	(79)	(56)	(51)	(43)
Fatally injured drivers	14,685	995	1,973	5,412
Percent belted	(48)	(33)	(24)	(20)

Source: Hingson, Ralph, and Michael Winter, "Epidemiology and Consequences of Drinking and Driving," *Alcohol Research & Health* 27, no. 1 (2003), page 70.

of the length of time since the most recent arrest for driving while impaired on the association between prior arrests and alcohol-related deaths suggest that many of the older case drivers may have been alcoholics. Indeed alcoholism is most common among men 35 to 50 years of age. Taken together, these findings suggest that the differences we observed in the strength of the associations between alcohol-related deaths and prior arrests for drunk driving among drivers of different ages may be related to the natural history of alcoholism.

Penalties for Drunk Driving

In much of the 20th century, drivers who drove while they were impaired with alcohol received minimal or no fines or punishment, sometimes even when their driving caused the deaths or severe injuries of others, and even when they had received multiple drunk-driving convictions. For example, the drunk driver who struck and killed MADD founder Candy Lightner's daughter in 1980 while she was walking in a bike lane had been out of jail for only two days since his most recent drunk-driving charge. He had also been arrested three times before that for drunk driving. Five days after her daughter died, Lightner and her friends decided to create an organization to protect families against drunk drivers. In the case of Cindi Lamb, the drunk driver whose actions caused her infant daughter to become paralyzed in 1979 was also a repeat offender. Lamb established the first MADD chapter in Maryland. In 1980, MADD was incorporated as an organization in California. Lightner and Lamb held many press conferences.

The plight of these two mothers put a face on the carnage caused by drunk drivers and mobilized people nationwide to rally their state and federal legislators to impose much stricter penalties for those who drove while intoxicated with alcohol. In 2005, MADD further expanded their mission to combat underage drinking. Other organizations, such as Students Against Driving Drunk (SADD), have also had an impact in decreasing the number of drunken drivers.

The actions of MADD, SADD, and other groups have made a strong and discernible difference, according to research provided by the NHTSA for the period 1982 to 2005. For example, in 2005, 20 percent of drivers involved in fatal crashes had a blood alcohol level of 0.08 or greater, down considerably from 35 percent in 1982. This decrease is largely attributed to deterrents to drunken driving, such as fines, jail, required participation in treatment, social ostracization, and so forth.

In their analysis of MADD in a 2006 issue of *Traffic Injury Prevention,* researchers J. C. Fell and R. B. Voas say that since 1982, 312,549 lives have been saved due to a reduction in alcohol in fatal crashes. The authors concluded, "There is considerable evidence that MADD has made a difference in the United States regarding alcohol-impaired driving. MADD has contributed to the public's view that drunk driving is socially unacceptable. MADD has also played an important role in encouraging state legislatures to enact more effective impaired-driving laws and has been a prominent player in landmark federal legislation." (The authors are referring to the 0.08 BAC level, zero tolerance, and other laws.)

In many states, individuals who are found guilty of driving while intoxicated with alcohol must undergo some form of treatment and/or attendance at meetings such as those offered by Alcoholics Anonymous. They may also face jail, probation, and fines, depending on whether this is a first or subsequent conviction. In addition, if anyone is injured or killed as a result of the individual's drunk driving, the penalties may be more severe, such as higher fines and longer periods of incarceration. Often the individual will lose his or her driver's license for a given period.

Some states also require that if the individual who was convicted of drunk driving is allowed to drive, then he or she must pay for special ignition lock devices to be placed on their cars to measure any amount of alcohol consumed by the person. These devices are connected to the ignition system, so that if the individual does test positive for alcohol, then the vehicle will not start. If a person receives more convictions for driving while intoxicated, the penalties usually are higher and may involve a term in jail or even prison, depending on whether another person was injured or killed.

Considering Even Tougher Penalties
for Drunk Drivers

Some researchers believe that even stricter penalties should be imposed on drunk drivers than currently exist; for example, in his article for the *Rutgers Law Journal* in 2008, Michael J. Watson supports a federal law similar to those that oversee child sex abusers (such as Megan's law), arguing that drunken drivers are far more recidivistic than sex offenders. He calls the proposed federal law the Intoxicated Driving Eradication Act (IDEA), and says that, as with sex offenders, the law would require that the public be notified about drivers who have been convicted of driving while they were intoxicated. This might include compelling drunken drivers to use DWI license plates for up to five years. According to Watson, these proposed license plates, in addition to complying with all state requirements, would be white with a bright orange X on the length of the plate, to make them obvious and distinguishable to other drivers on the road.

Watson says that DUI offenders would be divided into two tiers, depending on the frequency and severity of their past record, and the worst offenders (those in Tier Two) would not be allowed to drive on the weekend, at night or in the early morning, or on holidays, which are the times when previous offenders are most likely to reoffend. In addition, the zero tolerance policy toward underage drinkers would be reduced to a BAC of .01 rather than .02.

Watson argues that the laws against sex offenders have been tested in many courts and held up, with regard to privacy rights, unusual punishment, and so forth. He urged such a law against drunk drivers be considered and said that "we cannot sit back and watch drunk drivers inflict injury and death upon our nation any longer."

High School Students Who Admit to Drinking Before Driving

Based on data from the Youth Risk Behavior Surveillance for the United States in 2007, white males (13.9 percent) and Hispanic males (13.0 percent) in high school were the most likely to report driving when they had been drinking alcohol. High-school seniors were the most likely to drive when they had been drinking (18.3 percent). When considering all states covered in the study, the median percentage of high-school students who drove when they had been drinking was 10.4 percent. As can be seen from the Table 8, in considering both males and females in 39 states, the highest percentage of students who reported driving while drinking alcohol were in

North Dakota (18.7 percent) and Montana (16.0 percent), and the lowest percentages were seen in Utah (4.7 percent) and New York (7.1 percent).

Zero Tolerance Laws among Underage Drinkers

The purpose of zero tolerance laws is to actively discourage individuals younger than age 21 from drinking and driving. A separate BAC law for minors was first initiated in some states in 1989, and Congress provided incentives for all states to pass such laws as well as penalties by withholding state federal highway funds if states did *not* pass such laws. As anticipated, all states passed zero tolerance laws by 1998. These laws required penalties for minors who drove with a BAC level of 0.02.

Some studies, such as by Voas et al. in 2003, have demonstrated that zero tolerance laws reduced the percentage of underage drinking fatalities in car crashes by 25 percent. According to Liang and Hung, zero tolerance has worked particularly well among one population: underage college students.

Repeat Offender Laws

Most states have passed laws providing for stricter penalties for individuals convicted of more than one drunk-driving offense. The federal government is requiring all states to pass such laws or lose federal highway funds, under Section 164 of title 23 of the United States Code. At a minimum, the state laws must include the following:

- a minimum one-year driver's license suspension for repeat intoxicated drivers
- the impoundment or immobilization of all motor vehicles of repeat intoxicated drivers for a specified period or the installation of an ignition interlock system for a specified period
- the mandatory assessment of the repeat intoxicated driver's degree of alcohol abuse and referral to treatment as deemed appropriate
- the establishment of a mandatory minimum sentence for repeat intoxicated drivers
  - not less than five days of imprisonment or 30 days of community service for a second offense
  - not less than 10 days of imprisonment or 60 days of community service for a third or subsequent offense

TABLE 8
PERCENTAGE OF HIGH SCHOOL STUDENTS WHO DROVE WHILE DRINKING ALCOHOL, UNITED STATES, 2007, BY GENDER AND BY STATE

State	Female	Male	Total
Alaska	7.8	11.3	9.7
Arizona	9.7	14.8	12.3
Arkansas	8.5	13.8	11.1
Connecticut	8.4	11.8	10.2
Delaware	9.2	11.5	10.4
Florida	8.8	11.2	10.0
Georgia	7.5	10.6	9.1
Hawaii	7.9	8.1	8.0
Idaho	12.1	15.2	13.8
Illinois	9.9	12.8	11.3
Indiana	8.6	15.0	11.9
Iowa	11.3	13.9	12.6
Kansas	13.7	16.9	15.3
Kentucky	6.4	10.0	8.4
Maine	6.5	11.1	8.8
Maryland	7.2	9.5	8.5
Massachusetts	9.4	11.7	10.6
Michigan	8.3	9.8	9.1
Mississippi	8.1	15.3	11.8
Missouri	12.1	13.3	12.8
Montana	14.9	17.0	16.0
Nevada	8.7	8.6	8.7
New Hampshire	10.0	13.7	11.9
New Mexico	11.5	13.4	12.5
New York	5.6	8.5	7.1
North Carolina	7.2	11.1	9.2
North Dakota	18.4	18.9	18.7
Ohio	7.9	10.9	9.5
Oklahoma	10.0	16.5	13.3
Rhode Island	7.4	12.3	9.8
South Carolina	8.3	11.2	9.9
South Dakota	13.2	12.9	13.0
Tennessee	6.4	10.6	8.5
Texas	10.8	18.5	14.7
Utah	3.5	5.8	4.7
Vermont	6.5	11.6	9.2
West Virginia	6.8	12.8	10.0
Wisconsin	11.9	16.5	14.3
Wyoming	14.1	16.8	15.6
Median	8.6	12.3	10.4

Source: Adapted from Centers for Disease Control and Prevention. "Youth Risk Behavior Surveillance—United States, 2007." *Morbidity and Mortality Weekly Report* 57, no. SS-4 (June 6, 2008), page 42.

Drivers Who Drink Alcohol and Abuse Other Substances

Many people who abuse alcohol also abuse other substances, including illicit drugs such as marijuana, methamphetamine, and heroin, as well as prescription drugs, particularly painkillers and sedatives. In a study by Eugene Schwikke, Maria Isabel Sampaio dos Santo, and Barry K. Logan, published in the *Journal of Forensic Sciences* in 2006, the researchers studied the blood alcohol results for 370 fatally injured drivers in Washington State. They found that alcohol was present in a concentration above 0.01 g/100 mL in 41 percent of the cases, and the average alcohol concentration was 0.17 g/100 mL. Of the cases positive for alcohol, 42 percent were also positive for one or more drugs.

They also found the presence of a significant percentage of other drugs in the fatally injured drivers, including such central nervous depressants as diazepam (Valium), hydrocodone, amitriptyline (Elavil), and other drugs, in 14.1 percent of the cases. Cannabinoids (marijuana) were present in 12.7 percent of the cases. Stimulants such as cocaine and amphetamines were present in 9.7 percent of the cases, and narcotic painkillers were present in 3.2 percent of the fatally injured drivers. Yet in many cases, law enforcement authorities concentrate on testing only for alcohol with a breath test or blood test. According to the researchers, "Combined drug and alcohol use is a very significant pattern in this population and is probably overlooked in DUI enforcement programs."

They added, "We strongly recommend that drug screening be applied more universally in serious traffic crimes cases so that combined drug and alcohol use can be identified, and the appropriate sanctions or treatment applied." They also recommended increased sentencing for vehicular homicide or assault after the use of illicit drugs.

In another study of drug and alcohol use among drivers admitted to a trauma center, published in 2005 in *Accident Analysis & Prevention*, researchers J. Michael Walsh and colleagues studied data on trauma center victims at a Level-1 trauma center. They found that two-thirds of the victims had been involved in car crashes. Blood and urine were tested on 168 of the car crash patients. It was determined that 108 of the 168 trauma patients were the drivers in the car accident. The researchers found that the abuse of alcohol and marijuana was the most common among male drivers under age 35.

The researchers said, "These data from a regional trauma center demonstrate that drug and alcohol use among motor vehicle crash victims is common. While alcohol use among crash victims is generally well known, the high prevalence of drug use is not widely recognized. In this study more than half of the MVC [motor vehicle crash] victims identified as driving a car when the accident occurred tested positive for drugs (50.9%). About one-third of those using drugs had also been drinking, but alcohol was detected in only 30.6% of the drivers. The synergistic effect of combining alcohol and other drugs makes it especially important to identify this group, both for clinical management at the trauma center and for subsequent substance abuse treatment."

They concluded, "It is clear that drug use among motor vehicle crash victims is common. The use of rapid point of collection devices to routinely test for commonly abused drugs could provide valuable epidemiological data to document the prevalence of drugged driving and serve as an efficient and timely way to identify substance abusers for treatment intervention."

See also AGE AND ALCOHOL; ALCOHOL AND ALCOHOL USE; ALCOHOLISM/ALCOHOL DEPENDENCE AND ALCOHOL ABUSE; ELDERLY AND DRINKING ISSUES; EMERGENCY TREATMENT; EXCESSIVE DRINKING AND HEALTH CONSEQUENCES; EXCESSIVE DRINKING AND NEGATIVE SOCIAL CONSEQUENCES.

Beirness, Douglas J., and Erin E. Beasley. *Alcohol and Drug Use Among Drivers: British Columbia Roadside Survey, 2008.* Canadian Centre on Substance Abuse: Ottawa, Ontario, 2009.

Brewer, Robert, et al. "The Risk of Dying in Alcohol-Related Automobile Crashes Among Habitual Drunk Drivers." *New England Journal of Medicine* 331, no. 8 (August 25, 1994): 513–517.

Centers for Disease Control and Prevention. Youth Risk Behavior Surveillance—United States, 2007. *Morbidity and Mortality Weekly Report* 57, no. SS-4 (June 6, 2008).

Chou, S. Patricia, et al. "Twelve-Month Prevalence and Changes in Driving After Drinking: United States, 1991–1992 and 2001–2002." *Alcohol Research & Health* 29, no. 2 (2006): 143–151.

Dang, Jennifer. National Highway Traffic Safety Administration. *Statistical Analysis of Alcohol-Related Driving Trends, 1982–2005.* Springfield, Va.: U.S. Department of Transportation, May 2008.

Dill, Patricia L., and Elisabeth Wells-Parker. "Court-Mandated Treatment for Convicted Drinking Drivers." *Alcohol Research & Health* 29, no. 1 (2006): 41–48.

Fell, James C., and Robert B. Voas. "Mothers Against Drunk Driving (MADD): The First 25 Years." *Traffic Injury Prevention* 7, no. 3 (2006): 195–212.

Flowers, Nicole T., et al. "Patterns of Alcohol Consumption and Alcohol-Impaired Driving in the United States." *Alcoholism: Clinical and Experimental Research* 31, no. 4 (2008): 639–644.

Hingson, Ralph, and Michael Winter. "Epidemiology and Consequences of Drinking and Driving." *Alcohol Research & Health* 27, no. 1 (2003): 63–78.

Liang, Lan, and Jidong Huang. "Go Out or Stay In? The Effects of Zero Tolerance Laws on Alcohol Use and Drinking and Driving Patterns Among College Students." *Health Economics* 17, no. 11 (2008): 1,261–1,275.

National Highway Traffic Safety Administration. "2007 Traffic Safety Annual Assessment—Highlights." *Traffic Safety Facts* (August 2008): 1–2.

Office of Applied Studies. "State Estimates of Persons Aged 18 or Older Driving Under the Influence of Alcohol or Illicit Drugs." *NSDUH Report* (April 17, 2008): 104.

Schwilke, Eugene W., Maria Isabel Sampaio dos Santos, and Barry K. Logran. "Changing Patterns of Drug and Alcohol Use in Fatally Injured Drivers in Washington State." *Journal of Forensic Sciences* 51, no. 5 (2006): 1,191–1,198.

Tracy, Sarah W. *Alcoholism in America: From Reconstruction to Prohibition.* Baltimore, Md.: Johns Hopkins University Press, 2005.

Toomey, Traci L. "American Beverage Licensees Attack Mothers Against Drunk Driving." *Addiction* 100, no. 10 (2005): 1,389–1,391.

TotalDUI. "DUI Lite—No Car Required!" Total DUI. Available online. URL: http://www.totaldui.com/news/celebrity-dui-spotlight/non-car-dui.aspx. Accessed August 31, 2009.

Voas, R. B., A. S. Tippetts, and J. C. Fell. "Assessing the Effectiveness of Minimum Legal Drinking Age and Zero Tolerance Laws in the United States." *Accident Analysis and Prevention* 35, no. 4 (2003): 579–587.

Watson, Michael. "Carnage on Our Nation's Highways: A Proposal for Applying the Statutory Scheme of Megan's Law to Drunk-Driving Legislation." *Rutgers Law Journal* 39 (2008): 459–527.

Walsh, J. Michael, et al. "Drug and Alcohol Use Among Drivers Admitted to a Level-1 Trauma Center." *Accident Analysis & Prevention* 37, no. 5 (2005): 894–901.

dual disorders   See ALCOHOL AND OTHER DRUGS.

E

elderly and drinking issues Individuals age 65 years and older and their problems with alcohol abuse and dependence as well as with problem drinking that does not rise to the level of alcohol abuse or dependence. Because aging slows down an older person's ability to metabolize alcohol, lower amounts of alcohol than the person may have consumed in the past can lead to intoxication. If an older person says that he or she feels "tipsy" with just a small amount of alcohol, he or she may be reporting the feeling accurately. Some elderly people with alcohol dependence may have had a long-term problem with ALCOHOLISM that continues into later life. In other cases, alcohol dependence or problematic alcohol use occurs late in life, often because of loneliness related to feelings of sadness over the loss of deceased loved ones, distress over medical problems, ANXIETY DISORDERS, DEPRESSION, and other psychiatric issues. According to Frederick C. Blow and Kristen Lawton Barry in their article for *Alcohol Research & Health* in 2002, when it occurs, the late onset form of alcoholism among the elderly is more likely to occur among elderly females than males.

In an article based on their study of unhealthy drinking patterns in older adults, reported in a 2008 issue of the *Journal of the American Geriatric Society,* Elizabeth Merrick and her colleagues say that unhealthy drinking is a problem among an estimated 9 percent of elderly Medicare beneficiaries, with a much higher prevalence in men (16 percent) than among women (4 percent). The researchers defined unhealthy drinking as the monthly use of more than 30 drinks a month or "episodic" drinking of four or more drinks on any one day in a typical month in the past year. The researchers believe that this unhealthy drinking problem among the elderly is often ignored in soci-

ety. According to the researchers, "Unhealthy use of alcohol by older adults is a serious problem and is underidentified and undertreated. Unhealthy alcohol use has been defined as encompassing risky use, problem drinking, and alcohol disorders including abuse and dependence."

Merrick's research revealed that heavy drinking among older people was associated with being white, being divorced, or being single. Having a higher education and income was also associated with unhealthy drinking. The researchers noted that elderly people were hospitalized for alcohol-related conditions at about the same level as older people who were hospitalized for heart attacks. It is also true that elderly individuals who drink to excess are more likely to fall because of intoxication. Because of their age, a fall is a serious risk, and older people who fall are at a greater risk for fractures than young individuals. In addition, hip fracture is a leading cause of death in older people in the United States. Alcohol abuse can worsen other conditions, such as hypertension. Because many older people take at least one or more medications, the use of alcohol increases the risk of a medication interaction.

In his article on alcohol use among the elderly with mental disorders for *Current Opinions in Psychiatry* in 2003, Greg Whelan says that heavy alcohol use is a risk factor for the development of dementia. This dementia may be caused by an interaction of alcohol with a serious deficiency of thiamine. Long-term alcoholism can also lead to a severe thiamine deficiency and a dementia-like disorder that is known as WERNICKE-KORSAKOFF SYNDROME.

Whelan also states that many studies indicate that alcohol abuse and dependence are lower among those who are elderly than among other age groups; however, Whelan hypothesizes that this finding actually may occur at least in part because researchers fail to ask older people about their alcohol consumption. (Thus, they are making an underlying assumption that older people do not drink.) In addition, researchers may mistakenly attribute problems that the elderly have to aging issues rather than to alcohol. Sometimes drunken behavior among elderly people may be misconstrued as Alzheimer's disease or another form of dementia by their caregivers or even by their physician. Whelan also notes that elderly individuals who are substance abusers often abuse BENZODIAZEPINES and have nutritional deficiencies of folate and thiamine.

Alcohol abuse is also associated with an increased risk for SUICIDE in the elderly, particularly among older men, but among elderly women as well.

Depression is associated with alcohol use as well as withdrawal from alcohol among elderly people. Says Whelan, "The occurrence of depression at the time of withdrawal from alcohol may be due to the effects of alcohol on the thyroid-pituitary-hypothalamic axis. This is highly relevant as the depression may lead to relapse."

Treating Alcohol Abusers

Care must be taken in treating the alcoholism or alcohol abuse of an older person. Many physicians are hesitant about treating elderly people because of an array of other serious and/or chronic health conditions the person may have and for which they are being treated. However, ending problem drinking while under the care of a physician is the best means of prolonging life.

The primary medications that are used to treat alcoholism are acamprosate (Campral), NALTREXONE (ReVia), or DISULFIRAM (Antabuse). Some individuals with alcohol dependence are admitted to detoxification facilities. However, many physicians are very hesitant to prescribe disulfiram to elderly people because of the copious vomiting it causes, even when very minute quantities of alcohol are consumed by accident (as with cooking sherry or wine that is present in food).

The alcohol-disulfiram reaction may also cause hypotension or tachycardia (rapid heartbeat), which can be extremely dangerous to an older person. It may also be dangerous to rapidly detoxify an older person, and insufficient research has been performed to guide health professionals. It is known that older people metabolize drugs at a different rate than younger people, and it can be difficult to ascertain the dosage of drug or the speed of detoxification which is safe.

Mutual aid self-help groups such as Alcoholics Anonymous may help older alcohol abusers, but sometimes transportation problems preclude them from attending meetings on a regular basis.

Complicating matters further, other family members may be reluctant or unwilling to admit that their parent or other elderly relative has an alcohol abuse or dependence problem and may assist their relative in resisting treatment, mistakenly believing that they are being loving or helpful. It is also true that sometimes more nefarious motives arise, and family members may hope that the relative's life ends soon, particularly if the older person has assets that could be passed on to their heirs after their death.

Drinking and Driving

Most older people do not drive when they are drunk; according to the Substance Abuse and Mental Health Services Administration (SAMHSA), an estimated 1.7 percent of individuals ages 65 and older drove their vehicles while intoxicated in 2006. (This is in sharp contrast to younger individuals ages 21–25 years old, or 27.3 percent of that age group who drove while they were intoxicated.) However, when the elderly person *does* drive while under the influence of alcohol, the combination of the alcohol and their inherently slowed reflexes caused by aging can exacerbate the risk for serious accidents and for causing harm to themselves and others. According to the U.S. Census Bureau, the older population ages 65 years and older had the second highest death rate from car crashes in 2000, following the highest rate, which occurred among those ages 15 to 24 years old.

See also AGE AND ALCOHOL; ALCOHOL AND MEN; ALCOHOL AND WOMEN; DELIRIUM TREMENS; EMERGENCY TREATMENT; EXCESSIVE DRINKING AND HEALTH CONSEQUENCES; EXCESSIVE DRINKING AND NEGATIVE SOCIAL CONSEQUENCES; TREATMENT.

Blow, Frederick C., and Kristen Lawton Barry. "Use and Misuse of Alcohol Among Older Women." *Alcohol Research & Health* 26, no. 4 (2002): 308–315.

Kandel, Joseph, M.D., and Christine Adamec. *The Encyclopedia of Elder Care.* New York: Facts On File, Inc., 2009.

Merrick, Elizabeth L., et al. "Unhealthy Drinking Patterns in Older Adults: Prevalence and Associated Characteristics." *Journal of the American Geriatric Society* 56, no. 2 (2008): 214–233.

Whelan, Greg. "A Much Neglected Risk Factor in Elderly Mental Disorders." *Current Opinions in Psychiatry* 16, no. 6 (2003): 609–614.

emergency treatment   Urgent care treatment that is received in a hospital emergency room or clinic. ALCOHOLISM/ALCOHOL DEPENDENCE AND ALCOHOL ABUSE, as well as BINGE DRINKING are a leading cause of injuries. Alcohol intoxication, even among individuals who are not alcoholics or binge drinkers, is a leading risk factor for injuries in the United States. Intoxicated patients who have been seriously injured also require considerably more care than nonintoxicated patients; for example, according to Ernest E. Moore in his article on alcohol and trauma care in 2005 in *Journal of Trauma, Injury, Infection and Critical Care,* the nonintoxicated patient who has been in a moderate car crash may need a chest X-ray, an abdominal examination, an ultrasound, a complete blood count, urinalysis, and a physical examination; however, in sharp contrast, the intoxicated patient often needs all of these tests and procedures, *plus* a spinal X-ray, a pelvic X-ray, and computed tomography (CT) scans of the head, chest, and abdomen.

Moore also says that intoxication approximately doubles the severity of a traumatic brain injury (TBI). In addition, alcohol is immunosuppressive, and thus, when the severely injured patient needs his or her immune system to work well more than ever, it is unable to cope with post-injury infections, acute respiratory distress syndrome, and multiple organ failure.

The Drug Abuse Warning Network (DAWN), a division of the Substance Abuse and Mental Health Services Administration, performs an annual estimate of the abuse of alcohol and other drugs among those patients admitted to emergency departments nationwide. In 2006, DAWN estimated that alcohol was used in combination with another drug in 450,817 cases nationwide in individuals ages 12 and older, including 284,425 males and 166,278 females (in some cases, gender was not recorded). An estimated 10 percent of emergency room visits involved alcohol and prescribed drugs, and 3 percent involved alcohol combined with pharmaceuticals and illicit drugs. In 12.5 percent of the cases of patients under the age of 21 who were treated at hospital emergency rooms, alcohol only was involved. See Table 1 for more information. (Cases in which alcohol alone was involved are reported only for individuals younger than age 21, since DAWN concentrates on

TABLE 1
DRUG MISUSE AND ABUSE IN EMERGENCY DEPARTMENT VISITS IN THE UNITED STATES BY TYPE OF DRUG INVOLVEMENT: 2006

Drug involvement	Estimated visits	% of visits
All types of drug misuse/abuse	**1,742,887**	**100 percent**
Illicit drugs only	536,554	7 percent
Alcohol only (age less than 21 years)	126,704	12.5 percent
Pharmaceuticals only	486,276	28 percent
Combinations		
Illicit drugs with alcohol	219,521	13 percent
Illicit drugs with pharmaceuticals	142,535	8 percent
Alcohol with pharmaceuticals	171,743	10 percent
Illicit drugs with alcohol and pharmaceuticals	59,553	3 percent

Adapted from Substance Abuse and Mental Health Services Administration. *Drug Abuse Warning Network, 2006: National Estimates of Drug-Related Emergency Department Visits.* DAWN Series D-30, DHHS Publication No. (SMA) 08-4339. Rockville, Md.: August 2008, page 18.

TABLE 2
DRUGS MOST FREQUENTLY REPORTED
WITH ALCOHOL: 2006

Drugs Reported with Alcohol	Estimated Visits
Cocaine only	101,588
Marijuana only	41,653
Cocaine and marijuana only	21,241
Heroin only	14,958
Cocaine and heroin only	10,628
Alprazolam (Xanax) only	8,007
Stimulants only	7,895

Adapted from Substance Abuse and Mental Health Services Administration. *Drug Abuse Warning Network, 2006: National Estimates of Drug-Related Emergency Department Visits.* DAWN Series D-30, DHHS Publication No. (SMA) 08-4339. Rockville, Md.: August 2008, page 29.

combined drug misuse. As a result, there are many alcohol-only cases of adults that are *not* reported in this data.)

When other drugs were involved with alcohol, the most common drug was cocaine, followed by marijuana. (See Table 2.)

In addition, according to the DAWN data, 30 percent of emergency department treatments involved SUICIDE attempts in which alcohol was the only drug involved.

Some doctors support screening trauma patients for possible alcohol abuse and alcoholism. According to Gentilello et al. in their article in *Annals of Surgery* on trauma patients that are treated in emergency departments and hospitals, nearly a third (27 percent) of emergency room patients are potential candidates for a brief alcohol intervention in which doctors determine if the patient may have an alcohol use disorder. (See HOSPITAL PATIENTS AND ALCOHOL-RELATED ADMISSIONS.)

Sometimes individuals who are dependent on alcohol and who suddenly stop consuming the drug develop DELIRIUM TREMENS, a potentially life-threatening condition which requires emergency treatment. Alcohol can lead to or cause car crashes, which cause the individual to require emergency medical treatment. It can also lead to burns and many other types of accidental injuries. Children who are seriously injured or abused are often harmed by an alcoholic parent or caregiver. (See CHILD ABUSE AND NEGLECT.)

Alcohol-related emergency room visits may be more common than realized by physicians and others; for example, in a study based on data from the National Hospital Ambulatory Medical Care Survey for 1992–2000, researchers Alden J. McDonald III and colleagues reported on their findings in *Archives of Internal Medicine* in 2004. They found that alcohol-related emergency department (ED) visits were three times higher than previously determined by doctors or by patient disclosures. The researchers recommended more frequent alcohol screening in emergency rooms.

See also AGE AND ALCOHOL; DRIVING UNDER THE INFLUENCE/DRIVING WHILE INTOXICATED; EXCESSIVE DRINKING AND HEALTH CONSEQUENCES; INTERVENTION, BRIEF.

Gentilello, Larry M., et al. "Alcohol Interventions for Trauma Patients Treated in Emergency Departments and Hospitals: A Cost-Benefit Analysis." *Annals of Surgery* 241, no. 4 (2005): 541–550.

McDonald, Alden J. III, Nan Wang, and Carlos A. Camargo Jr., M.D. "US Emergency Department Visits for Alcohol-Related Diseases and Injuries Between 1992 and 2000." *Archives of Internal Medicine* 164, no. 5 (2004): 531–537.

Moore, Ernest E., M.D. "Alcohol and Trauma: The Perfect Storm." *Journal of Trauma, Injury, Infection and Critical Care* 59 (2005): S53–S56.

Neuner, Bruno, et al. "Hazardous Alcohol Consumption and Sense of Coherence in Emergency Department Patients with Minor Trauma." *Drug and Alcohol Dependence* 82, no. 2 (2006): 143–150.

Substance Abuse and Mental Health Services Administration. *Drug Abuse Warning Network, 2006: National Estimates of Drug-Related Emergency Department Visits.* DAWN Series D-30, DHHS Publication No. (SMA) 08-4339. Rockville, Md.: August 2008.

employee assistance programs   Workplace programs provided or sponsored by corporations to help individuals with serious substance abuse and/ or psychiatric problems, so that individuals may continue to remain employed with the company. According to Elizabeth S. Levy Merrick and colleagues in their 2007 article for *Psychiatric Services,* about two-thirds (66 percent) of companies with 100 or more employees have an employee assistance program (EAP) and 90 percent of Fortune

500 corporations have EAP programs. In most cases, EAP programs address many issues including substance abuse, mental health problems, problems with balancing work and family issues, and other areas where problems arise.

In some cases, employees are referred by the supervisor to an EAP program, while more commonly, the employee seeks out help. Sometimes services are also extended to family members of the employee. Most EAP services are delivered away from the workplace and are contracted out to managed behavioral health care organizations. Confidentiality is guaranteed to the employee; however, as a practical matter, it is likely that the individual's supervisor will hear through the office grapevine that the individual has sought some assistance through EAP. Of course, if the supervisor has ordered the employee to seek help through EAP as a condition of employment, then it is even more likely that the supervisor will be aware of the assistance although he or she may not know what is specifically said between a therapist and a client.

Levy Merrick et al. said, "In the contemporary U.S. work environment, there is great interest in EAPs as a way of addressing substance use problems, which can be costly and detrimental to both individuals and their employers. EAPs are uniquely positioned to provide relatively barrier-free preventive services and screening, early identification, short-term counseling, referral to specialty treatment, and other behavioral health interventions for the privately insured population."

In their article on alcohol problems in the workplace for *Alcohol Research & Health*, Paul M. Roman and Terry C. Blum said that EAPs have a goal of preventing a loss of employment and assisting employed people to continue their careers. "EAPs can thus prevent both employer and the employee from suffering the costly consequences of the employee's job loss," according to the researchers.

Roman and Blum say that many employees seek out help from EAPs, while others are referred by a supervisor. An estimated 80 percent of referrals (including self-referrals) are informal, while 20 percent are formally referred by supervisors.

See also IMPAIRED PHYSICIANS; TREATMENT.

Levy Merrick, Elizabeth S., Joanna Volpe-Vartanian, Constance M. Horgan, and Bernard McCann. "Revisiting Employee Assistance Programs and Substance Use Problems in the Workplace: Key Issues and a Research Agenda." *Psychiatric Services* 58, no. 10 (October 2007): 1,262–1,264.

Roman, Paul M., and Terry C. Blum. "The Workplace and Alcohol Problem Prevention." *Alcohol Research & Health* 26, no. 1 (2002): 49–57.

enablers　A term for women or men who may prevent individuals with alcohol dependence from seeking treatment because they help the alcoholic avoid the consequences of his or her actions. For example, if a person does not get up and go to work because he or she is too hungover from an alcoholic binge, the enabler may call up the boss and say that the person is "too sick" to go to work. The person who does *not* enable the alcoholic, on the other hand, does nothing when the person fails to go to work, and instead allows him or her to suffer the consequences of the absence, such as docked pay or even termination from employment. It is often very difficult for many people to understand that their partners or adult children will usually not change their behavior unless they suffer from the consequences of that behavior, including a loss of employment, lack of money, an eviction, sickness, or imprisonment.

Individuals who are enablers are usually spouses, partners, parents, or others who love (or say that they love) the alcoholic person, and they may believe that only they can truly understand the problems of the alcoholic. They often deny that there *is* any problem with ALCOHOLISM, despite an environment replete with evidence (such as empty whiskey bottles or numerous discarded beer cans, vomit from the evening before, and so forth).

In addition, the behavior of the alcoholic may be ignored and explained away by the enabler as caused by "stress" or "depression"—yet this stress or depression is not treated by a psychiatrist or other physician. This behavior is somewhat similar to the behavior of the woman who is beaten by her husband or partner and tells others it is "really nothing" or "he didn't mean it and he's really sorry now." In fact, the alcoholic may be guilty of domestic abuse as well.

Sometimes the alcoholic is also a child abuser or neglects a child, and the child maltreatment is explained away or even ignored by the enabling parent, which can lead to lifelong psychological scarring in the child's adulthood. In fact, when told by social services that because of the abuse or neglect of the child by the alcoholic person, they must leave him or her in order to have custody of their children, some enablers will choose the alcoholic and let the children go into foster care.

The enabler gains some psychological benefit from the enabling behavior, such as a feeling of power and/or selflessness, otherwise the behavior would not continue. In some cases, the enabler is financially and/or emotionally dependent on the alcoholic, and the potential removal of this person from their life is perceived as catastrophic. If the alcoholic does seek treatment, the enabler may thwart the individual's continued recovery. This behavior may or may not be consciously executed as a plan or strategy.

Adjuncts to ALCOHOLISM MUTUAL AID SOCIETIES, such as Al-Anon and Alateen, provide support for spouses and others and teach them to stop their enabling behavior so that the alcoholic is more likely to seek treatment and remain in recovery. Ending enabling may still not stop the alcoholic from his or her drinking, but it will usually make it more difficult or uncomfortable and may eventually convince the alcoholic that he or she needs to seek treatment. It will also force the enabler to make difficult choices, such as seeking a job to attain financial independence, possibly ending the relationship with the alcoholic to attain emotional independence, and so forth.

In a study of enabling behavior in a sample of 42 alcoholic clients and their partners, reported by Rotunda, West, and O'Farrell in the *Journal of Substance Abuse Treatment* in 2004, the researchers found that most of the partners of the alcoholic person took over duties and chores at various points, and they also used drugs or drank along with the client and made excuses to others to cover for the client's failings due to alcoholism.

Some examples of enabling behaviors that were reportedly exhibited included cleaning up vomit or urine after the alcoholic person was ill, having sex with the alcoholic when the enabler really did not wish to but the alcoholic had been drinking and wanted sex, and borrowing money to pay for bills incurred in some way by the alcoholic person's drinking. Enabling behaviors were also significantly related to beliefs held by the enabler; for example, some beliefs included the following:

- thinking that their alcoholic partner could not get along without them
- believing that they should do their best to protect the alcoholic person from his or her own behavior
- blaming themselves as one of the reasons for the substance abuse problem
- believing it was important to do whatever it took to hold the relationship together, no matter what

According to the researchers, the most common enabling behavior, exhibited by the broad majority of enablers, was to lie or make excuses to others in order to attempt to hide the alcoholic's drinking.

Identifying enabling behaviors and beliefs is important for counselors who wish to help families with alcoholic clients because, according to Rotunda and colleagues, it may "(1) help those that engage in enabling to decrease or eliminate these behaviors; (2) teach and foster the use of positive coping responses in what are usually very difficult situations; (3) help family members provide a socially supportive environment for recovery without becoming overly responsible for the impaired individual; and (4) help mitigate psychological and physical strain that may result from frustration and long-term interaction with those struggling with alcohol or drug dependence."

See also CODEPENDENCY; DENIAL; EXCESSIVE DRINKING AND NEGATIVE SOCIAL CONSEQUENCES; FAMILIES AND ALCOHOL; STAGES OF CHANGE; TREATMENT.

Rotunda, Rob J., Laura West, and Timothy J. O'Farrell. "Enabling Behavior in a Clinical Sample of Alcohol-dependent Clients and Their Partners." *Journal of Substance Abuse Treatment* 26, no. 4 (2004): 269–276.

ethanol   See ACETALDEHYDE.

excessive drinking and health consequences Alcohol abuse and dependence as well as bouts of BINGE DRINKING or heavy drinking increase the risk for many very serious health problems, including CANCER, cardiovascular disease (including cardiac disorders and hypertension), gastrointestinal disorders, alcoholic lung disease, and other health problems. For example, kidney and liver diseases are more common among those who abuse or are dependent on alcohol, as are sleep disorders, pancreatic disorders, and musculoskeletal disorders. Psychiatric disorders are also more common among those who drink to excess. Falls and other types of accidents cause injuries more frequently among heavy drinkers. In addition, the stroke risk is higher for individuals who engage in binge drinking, based on recent research. Excessive drinking can also lead to blood disorders, such as anemia, and an estimated 90 percent of all alcoholics have alcohol-induced macrocytosis, or enlarged red blood cells, the treatment for which is ABSTINENCE.

It is also true that individuals who are dependent on or abuse alcohol are significantly less likely to take medications that they need to control other common chronic disorders, such as diabetes or hypertension, thus increasing their risk for needing medical care including EMERGENCY TREATMENT. The children of pregnant women with ALCOHOLISM are at risk for suffering from FETAL ALCOHOL SYNDROME/FETAL ALCOHOL SPECTRUM DISORDERS. However, a pregnant woman need not be an alcoholic for her child to have a problem—any amount of alcohol is considered potentially toxic to the developing fetus.

Alcoholic individuals are also more likely to suffer from vitamin and mineral deficiencies and poor nutrition than others. Some alcoholics obtain all or nearly all their nutrition from alcohol alone, and thus they become severely deficient in many vitamins and minerals.

Individuals who are alcohol-dependent are also more likely to suffer from falls and many other types of accidents that are directly alcohol-related and which require emergency treatment. For example, about 17,000 Americans die from alcohol-related car crashes every year, and about 258,000 are injured. Interestingly, according to Nicole T. Flowers et al. in their 2008 article on alcohol-impaired driving in the United States for *Alcoholism: Clinical and Experimental Research,* in at least half of the cases of impaired drivers, they are not heavy drinkers or alcoholics. Instead, they are more likely to have engaged in binge drinking; 84 percent of alcohol-impaired drivers were binge drinkers based on data from 2006.

Formerly alcoholic individuals who receive organ transplants may subsequently relapse, and some researchers have developed a means to predict possible relapse. However, some alcoholics may be denied organ transplants by major medical centers (particularly in the case of liver transplants, because the liver is the most susceptible to harm from heavy alcohol consumption). This is particularly true if the individual has liver damage that was caused by alcohol consumption combined with a viral form of HEPATITIS, especially hepatitis C.

It is also true that some individuals combine the use of ALCOHOL AND OTHER DRUGS, further increasing their risk for health problems.

According to the Centers for Disease Control and Prevention (CDC), an estimated 79,646 individuals of all ages who consumed a medium to high level of alcohol each day died of alcohol-related deaths in 2005, based on data from the Alcohol-Related Disease Impact (ARDI) software for 2001–05. Males were more likely to die from alcohol-related deaths (57,429 male deaths compared to 22,217 female deaths). Medium consumption was defined as equal to or greater than 3.1 drinks per day for men and equal to or greater than 1.6 drinks for women. High consumption was defined as equal to or greater than 4.5 drinks per day for males and equal to or greater than 3.0 drinks per day for females.

See Table 1 for a breakdown of the chronic and acute causes of death by disease; for example, of chronic death causes, alcoholic liver disease caused the single greatest number, or 12,219 deaths, followed by 7,055 deaths from liver cirrhosis. The data also shows that 2,382 people died from alcohol abuse, and 3,857 died from alcohol dependence. Thus, although their misuse of alcohol contributed to their deaths, most people who abused or were dependent on alcohol and who died from alcohol-related causes died from other causes.

Among those who died from acute causes, the largest number (13,819) of deaths was from motor vehicle traffic crashes, followed by homicide (7,787), and then suicide (7,235 deaths). A small number (204) died of aspiration; i.e., they choked to death on their own vomit.

TABLE 1
ALCOHOL-ATTRIBUTABLE DEATHS, ALL AGES, MEDIUM AND HIGH AVERAGE DAILY CONSUMPTION, UNITED STATES, 2001–2005, BY CAUSE AND GENDER. AVERAGE DEATHS PER YEAR.

	Male	Female	Total
Total for All Causes	**57,429**	**22,217**	**79,646**
Acute pancreatitis	366	320	695
Alcohol abuse	1,868	514	2,382
Alcohol cardiomyopathy	389	59	448
Alcohol dependence syndrome	3,037	820	3,857
Alcohol polyneuropathy	1	0	1
Alcohol-induced chronic pancreatitis	248	63	311
Alcoholic gastritis	17	4	21
Alcoholic liver disease	8,938	3,281	12,219
Alcoholic myopathy	1	0	1
Alcoholic psychosis	568	183	751
Breast cancer (females only)	0	355	355
Chronic hepatitis	2	2	4
Chronic pancreatitis	118	112	229
Degeneration of nervous system due to alcohol	77	14	91
Epilepsy	102	88	191
Esophageal cancer	426	52	478
Esophageal varices	53	20	74
Fetal alcohol syndrome	2	1	3
Fetus and newborn affected by maternal use of alcohol	0	1	1
Gastroesophageal hemorrhage	16	13	29
Hypertension	753	610	1,363
Ischemic heart disease	609	277	886
Laryngeal cancer	207	30	237
Liver cancer	598	187	786
Liver cirrhosis, unspecified	4,134	2,921	7,055
Low birth weight, premature, IUGRL death	108	52	160
Oropharyngeal cancer	320	56	376
Portal hypertension	26	14	40
Prostate cancer (males only)	232	0	232
Psoriasis	Less than 1	Less than 1	Less than 1
Spontaneous abortion (females only)	0	Less than 1	Less than 1
Stroke, hemorrhagic	1,472	303	1,775
Stroke, ischemic	495	181	676
Superventricular cardiac dysrhythmia	85	102	187
Subtotal	**25,269**	**10,646**	**35,915**
Acute Causes			
Air-space transport	104	21	125
Alcohol poisoning	292	78	370
Aspiration	109	95	204
Child maltreatment	96	72	168
Drowning	716	152	868
Fall injuries	2,888	2,644	5,532
Fire injuries	692	466	1,158
Homicide	108	15	123
Hypothermia	182	87	269
Motor-vehicle nontraffic crashes	147	36	183
Motor-vehicle traffic crashes	10,802	3,016	13,819
Occupational and machine injuries	130	7	137
Other road vehicle crashes	165	45	210
Poisoning (not alcohol)	3,669	1,747	5,416
Suicide	5,778	1,457	7,235
Suicide by and exposure to alcohol	22	9	31
Water transport	87	11	98
Subtotal	**32,159**	**11,572**	**43,731**

Adapted from computer-generated report from the Alcohol-Related Disease Impact (ARDI) software. Available online. URL: https://apps.need.cdcgov/ardi. Accessed May 12, 2009.

Alcoholic Liver Disease

Alcoholic liver disease refers to the progression of disease from fatty liver disease to alcoholic hepatitis to CIRRHOSIS. Fatty liver disease is a common problem among those who severely abuse alcohol, and 90 percent or more of heavy drinkers have a fatty liver, which is characterized by an enlarged liver (hepatomegaly). If the individual continues to drink, fatty liver disease progresses to alcoholic hepatitis. If the patient still does not stop drinking, the disease progresses further to cirrhosis, which is generally unrecoverable.

Symptoms and signs of alcoholic hepatitis are fever, appetite loss, jaundice, and right upper-quadrant abdominal pain. Enlarged liver is also common. The patient may also experience abnormal blood clotting and bleeding from esophageal varices (veins).

Some factors increase the risk for the development of alcoholic liver disease; for example, female alcoholics are significantly more likely to develop alcoholic liver disease than male alcoholics, and the disease also progresses more rapidly in women. Obesity and the presence of diabetes mellitus are additional risk factors leading to the development of fatty liver disease in alcoholics.

It should also be noted that the ingestion of acetaminophen, even at normal therapeutic dosages, can be harmful to the liver, because of the combination of alcohol and acetaminophen, which can cause hepatotoxicity.

Treatment for alcoholic liver disease includes an enforced abstinence from alcohol consumption, sometimes with the use of DISULFIRAM, a drug that causes nausea and copious vomiting among patients who drink alcohol after taking the drug. Other drugs such as acamprosate and NALTREXONE are used to treat alcohol dependence. (See TREATMENT.) Nutritional evaluation and therapy is often needed because the alcoholic may be malnourished, and malnourishment hastens the progression of liver disease.

An estimated 10 percent of alcoholics have cirrhosis. About 60 percent of patients with both alcoholic hepatitis and cirrhosis die within about four years.

Many patients with cirrhosis are also infected with hepatitis C, which makes the decision whether to transplant a needed liver a difficult one, since the new liver would become infected with the disease. If the patient is anticipated to continue to drink, then a liver transplant would usually be denied. According to Eugene R. Schiff, M.D., and Nuri Ozden, M.D., in their article on hepatitis C and alcohol for *Alcohol Research & Health* in 2003, patients who are alcoholics and infected with hepatitis C also have an increased risk for the development of liver cancer. Even moderate drinking is dangerous to the patient with hepatitis C. Individuals with hepatitis C

have an impaired response to interferon, which is an important drug for those who receive a liver transplant.

Alcoholic Lung Disease

According to the National Institute on Alcohol Abuse and Alcoholism (NIAAA), it is known that excessive alcohol consumption contributes to oxidative stress on the lung and that it can compromise lung function. Alcoholics are also at risk for infection with bacterial pneumonia, and in some cases, this disorder may be fatal. According to authors Corey D. Kershaw, M.D., and David M. Guidot, M.D., in their article on alcoholic lung disease for *Alcohol Research & Health* in 2008, not only are alcoholics at risk for pneumonia but they also have a three to four times greater risk for developing acute respiratory distress syndrome (ARDS), a severe form of lung injury which kills up to 50 percent of the people who develop it. ARDS causes a marked oxygen deficiency in the bloodstream.

Kershaw and Guidot also state that it has been known for over a century that alcohol abuse is a serious risk factor for pulmonary disease among alcoholics. Say the authors, "For example, alcoholic patients are at increased risk for infection with tissue-damaging gram-negative pathogens, such as *Klebsiella pneumoniae,* or for the spread of bacteria in the blood (i.e. bacteremia) and shock from typical pathogens, most notably *Streptococcus pneumoniae.* Importantly, alcoholics also are at increased risk for infections with *Mycobacterium tuberculosis.*"

The authors explain how and why alcoholics are at increased risk for such infections. "The mechanisms by which alcohol abuse increases the risk of pneumonia likely are multiple and include increased risk of aspiration of gastric acid and/or microbes from the upper part of the throat (i.e. oropharyngeal florida), decreased mucous-facilitated clearance of bacterial pathogens from the upper airway, and impaired pulmonary host defenses."

It should also be noted that many drinkers are also smokers; consequently, damage to the lungs can be caused by both alcohol and nicotine, as well as the two drugs in combination.

Cancer

Chronic alcoholism is a major risk factor for several forms of CANCER, including esophageal cancer, cancer of the pharynx and of the larynx, and oral cancer, according to the National Institute of Alcohol Abuse and Alcoholism (NIAAA). In addition, alcoholism is also strongly linked to liver cancer and colorectal cancer. Experts suspect that alcoholism may also be linked to pancreatic cancer and lung cancer. For women, particularly menopausal females, alcoholism is linked to the development of breast cancer.

It is unknown how heavy chronic consumption of alcohol causes or contributes to the development of cancer, but is believed that the formation of ACETALDEHYDE that is generated as alcohol is metabolized may be a factor in causing cancer. Alcoholism may also suppress the immune function. Many people who are alcoholics (up to 80 percent) also smoke, and the combination of smoking and drinking increases the risk for cancer, because alcohol increases the bioavailability of carcinogens. Alcohol may also increase estrogen rates in menopausal women, increasing the risk for breast cancer.

Cardiovascular Disease

Heavy alcohol users are at an increased risk for heart disease and stroke. Heavy drinking can lead to cardiomyopathy, which causes arrhythmias and left-ventricular dysfunction of the heart. Some experts believe that alcoholic cardiomyopathy may be more common than was previously believed because of an underdiagnosis of alcohol dependence. Note that drinking in moderation can enhance the health of the heart. (See MODERATE DRINKING AND HEALTH BENEFITS.)

Atrial fibrillation is a common heart disorder whose existence is exacerbated by excessive drinking. It is more common among long-term drinkers who consume more than 36 grams per day of alcohol. There are about 14 grams of alcohol in a 1.5-ounce jigger of brandy or a mixed drink or 8 ounces of malt liquor. Thus, it would take only about two and a half shots of brandy/mixed drink or about 24 ounces of malt liquor consumed on a regular basis to risk atrial fibrillation.

Binge drinkers are particularly at risk for stroke, based on a study by Laura Sundell, M.D., and colleagues, published in *Stroke* in 2008. In this study of subjects drawn from 15,965 Finnish men and women ages 25 to 64 years, the researchers defined binge drinking as consuming six or more drinks of the same alcoholic beverage in men and four or more drinks in women. (This is an amount that is greater than the standard binge drinking definition in the United States.) The study group, which included 1,053 women and 2,505 men with binge drinking patterns compared to 12,407 non-bingers, was followed up for both fatal and nonfatal strokes. In the Finnish study, binge drinking was independently correlated to an increased risk for total strokes and ischemic strokes, with a higher risk for ischemic strokes.

Falls and Accidents

Studies have shown that excessive alcohol consumption is linked to an increased risk for falling down; for example, in a study in New Zealand by B. Kool and colleagues, reported in *Alcohol,* the researchers studied 335 individuals ages 25–60 years who either were admitted to the hospital or had died as a result of an injury from a fall at home. They found a direct correlation between alcohol consumption and a risk for falling down within six hours after drinking. The researchers reported that the subjects who consumed two drinks were 3.7 times more likely to have experienced an injury from a fall than those who did not drink. In addition, those who consumed three or more drinks were 12.9 times more likely to be injured in a fall than those who did not drink.

The researchers concluded that 20 percent of all fall injuries in the population that was studied were alcohol-related.

Fetal Alcohol Syndrome/ Fetal Alcohol Spectrum Disorders

Women who abuse or are dependent on alcohol during their pregnancies may harm the developing fetus and cause the surviving child to suffer lifelong development delays and disorders, as well as a panoply of medical problems that depend on the severity of the drinking and when it occurred during fetal development.

If physicians are suspicious that a pregnant woman may be drinking, they may run tests on biological samples. Table 2 shows the type of sample that is used and describes both the advantages and disadvantages of such use; for example, it is easy to obtain a large sample of urine, but the disadvantage is that urine is readily tampered with; for example, the mother could switch out her urine with another woman's urine. Breast milk may also be tested for alcohol in the new mother, but there may be a narrow window of opportunity for collection if the doctor wishes to test the first milk produced by the mother. With a fetus, the blood can be tested, but this is an extremely invasive procedure and most obstetricians would resist this test for fear of endangering the fetus.

Gastrointestinal Disorders

Individuals who misuse alcohol have an increased risk for PANCREATITIS (inflammation of the pancreas), as well as for the development of gastro-esophageal reflux disease (GERD, also known as chronic heartburn), peptic ulcers, and esophagitis (inflammation of the esophagus, or food tube). Excessive drinking is the primary cause of chronic pancreatitis and represents the cause of about 70 percent of the cases of chronic pancreatitis.

Severe vomiting caused by alcoholic gastritis can cause tears in the gastroesophageal junction. Both long-term and short-term alcohol consumption can cause both gastric and duodenal (small intestine) irritation and even hemorrhage. Heavy drinking can also destroy the islet cells in the pancreas that produce insulin, thus causing the patient to develop diabetes mellitus. As a result, these patients will need to take insulin.

The alcoholic may experience poor absorption of vitamins, particularly thiamine and B12 and also of minerals such as calcium and magnesium. When the alcoholic relies mostly or solely on alcohol for nutrition, he or she may become malnourished. Alcoholics may also become deficient in key vitamins such as A, C, D, E, and K, as well as B vitamins. Because these vitamins maintain cells and wound healing, deficiencies may lead to serious problems; for example, a deficiency of Vitamin K, the vitamin that causes blood clotting, can result in excessive bleeding from a minor injury. A vitamin D deficiency is associated with decreased bone density. Diseases such as WERNICKE-KORSAKOFF

SYNDROME may develop as a result of insufficient thiamine.

Hematological Disorders

In addition to macrocytosis, alcoholic individuals may have decreased red blood cell function, often caused by an iron deficiency that is linked to gastrointestinal bleeding or a nutritional folate deficiency.

Some alcoholics have an impaired immune system, and as a result, they have recurrent infections. These may be due to leukopenia, or a significant drop in the neutrophil count and function. It may also be caused by liver cirrhosis and an enlarged spleen, both of which can lower the white blood cell count.

Some studies show that up to 80 percent of alcoholics who are hospitalized for any reason have mild thrombocytopenia, which is a blood platelet count of less than 150,000. This may be caused or related to an enlarged spleen caused by alcoholic cirrhosis, but the alcohol itself has a direct effect on the platelets.

Infectious Diseases

Alcoholics have an increased risk for developing infectious diseases and some studies have shown that up to half of the patients admitted to hospitals for pneumonia are alcoholics. Tuberculosis is another disease that is more commonly found among those who are alcohol-dependent. Alcoholics may also have bacterial meningitis and other serious and less-serious infections.

Injuries and Deaths from Car Crashes

Deaths from injuries sustained in car crashes are common and also the leading cause of death in the United States among individuals ages 1–34 years old, according to data from the 2006 Behavior Risk Factor Surveillance System (BRFSS), produced by the Centers for Disease Control and Prevention (CDC). The National Highway Traffic Safety Administration says that about 40 percent of all traffic-related deaths involved alcohol.

According to researchers Nicole T. Flowers and colleagues in *Alcoholism: Clinical and Experimental Research* in 2008, about 5 percent of current drinkers reported at least one episode of alcohol-impaired driving in the past 30 days, and the highest percentage of alcohol-impaired drinking occurred among binge/heavy drinkers, or 22.2 percent. The binge drinkers were less likely to be wearing their seat belts than the non-binge drinkers.

Among the heavy drinkers/binge drinkers, the highest rates of alcohol-impaired driving occurred in males older than age 40, and factors of income, race, education, and ethnicity were not relevant. Some binge drinkers were college graduates with annual incomes exceeding $75,000 per year.

Said Flowers et al., "Although BRFSS does not collect information about alcohol dependence, most AI [alcohol-impaired] drivers drank during fewer than half the days in the preceding month, and binge drank less than once per week on average. Other studies that have accessed alcohol dependence among AI drivers demonstrate that only 10–15% of binge drinkers are alcohol dependent. As such, our findings are consistent with the notion that most AI drivers are not alcohol dependent, and therefore should be responsive to broad-based environmental alcohol control policies (e.g., increased alcohol excise taxes) and from brief counseling interventions by health care providers."

The researchers also added their recommendations: "Examples of effective interventions to reduce AI driving include lowering legal BACs [blood alcohol concentrations], promptly suspending the licenses of people arrested for driving while impaired, sobriety checkpoints, alcohol ignition interlock programs for convicted AI driving offenders, and sustained public education and enforcement. In conclusion, efforts to reduce AI driving should focus on preventing excessive drinking behaviors—particularly binge drinking—that are so strongly associated with AI driving."

Musculoskeletal Disorders

Chronic heavy alcoholism leads to an increased risk of low bone mass, decreased bone formation, and an increased risk for bone fractures, according to the NIAAA. Interestingly, one drink per day *reduces* the risk for a hip fracture, while two or more drinks per day *increase* the risk for fracture. Thus, there is a mild benefit to one drink per day, which is eradicated if the individual doubles his or her alcohol consumption.

Heavy alcohol use also increases the risk for osteoporosis, or deficiency in bone mass. This problem is more likely to occur in females who abuse or are dependent on alcohol. (See ALCOHOL AND WOMEN.)

Psychiatric Disorders

Those who misuse, abuse, or are dependent on alcohol also have an increased risk for suffering from a variety of PSYCHIATRIC COMORBIDITIES, such as ANXIETY DISORDERS, ATTENTION-DEFICIT/HYPERACTIVITY DISORDER, DEPRESSION, ANTISOCIAL PERSONALITY DISORDER, BIPOLAR DISORDER, CONDUCT DISORDER, SCHIZOPHRENIA, and many other possible coexisting psychiatric disorders. Many individuals who misuse alcohol have more than one type of psychiatric disorder. Sometimes it is difficult or impossible to determine whether the psychiatric disorder preceded or followed the alcohol abuse or dependence, as with depression.

Sleep Disorders

Chronic sleep disorders are common among those who abuse or are dependent on alcohol. Some studies indicate that alcohol affects and impedes the body's natural circadian rhythm. Many individuals who are alcohol-dependent do not fall asleep naturally but rather "pass out" from their intoxication. This can lead to chronic insomnia and daytime sleepiness.

Alcoholics who are under treatment may experience severe insomnia, and alcoholics with this problem have a greater risk for relapse than others.

Vitamin and Mineral Deficiencies

Those who are heavy alcohol users often have a high risk for deficiencies in vitamin A, vitamin B complex, vitamin C, carnitine, folic acid, magnesium, selenium, and zinc. This is particularly likely if the individual also suffers from malnourishment, and some alcoholics obtain some or all of their caloric intake from alcohol alone. Some studies have demonstrated that alcohol dependence is the leading cause of malnutrition among adults in the United States. Malnutrition impedes the absorption, digestion, and metabolism of key vitamins.

TABLE 2
BIOLOGICAL SAMPLES FOR DETECTING DRINKING DURING PREGNANCY

Sample	Advantages	Disadvantages
Maternal samples		
Urine	Large sample size	Tampering possible
Hair	May indicate timing of exposure	May not be desirable, requires special analytical techniques
Blood	Battery of biomarkers may be used	Invasive, painful
Breath	Easy to obtain large quantities	Requires special equipment, technology is limited
Saliva	Easy to obtain	Sample size limited
Gases acquired through skin patch	Easy to obtain	Requires special equipment, technology is limited
Breast milk	Large sample, noninvasive (or "first milk") is required	Narrow window of opportunity to collect if colostrum
Fetal samples		
Blood	Measures proximal exposure	Sample size limited, extremely invasive
Chorionic villus	Measures very early exposure	Sample size limited, extremely invasive
Amniotic fluid	Can be sampled from 18 weeks on	Sample size limited, extremely invasive
Newborn		
Cord blood	Large volume available, discarded sample, battery of biomarkers may be used	Narrow window of opportunity to collect, single time point for measurement
Placenta	Large sample size, discarded sample	Narrow window of opportunity to collect
Umbilical cord	Large sample size, discarded sample	Narrow window of opportunity to collect
Amniotic fluid	Large sample size, discarded sample	Difficult to collect, narrow window of opportunity to collect
Urine	Concentrates metabolites, discarded sample	Difficult to collect
Hair	May indicate timing of exposure	May not be available, may not be acceptable to parent
Breath	Easy to obtain	Requires special equipment, technology is limited
Saliva	Easy to obtain	Small sample
Vernix	Discarded sample	Narrow window of opportunity to collect, not present on all babies, little background information available
Gases acquired through skin patch	Easy to obtain	Requires special equipment, technology is limited
Meconium	Easy to obtain, discarded sample, may indicate timing of exposure	Does not measure exposure prior to second trimester

Source: Bearer, Cynthia F., MD., et al. "Biomarkers of Alcohol Use in Pregnancy." National Institute on Alcohol Abuse and Alcoholism. Available online. URL: http://pubs.niaaa.nih.gov/publications/arh28-1/38-43.htm. Accessed April 8, 2009.

Failure to Comply with Treatment for Chronic Medical Problems

Those who misuse alcohol are much more likely to fail to comply with their normal medication regimens. This is particularly problematic in chronic and severe diseases such as hypertension but is also important in many other chronic medical diseases and disorders as well, as in chronic severe infections such as hepatitis C or the human immunodeficiency virus (HIV).

Chris L. Bryson, M.D., and colleagues analyzed alcohol screening scores and medication non-adherence for patients treated for diabetes, hypertension, and hyperlipidemia, publishing their results in the *Annals of Internal Medicine* in 2008. The researchers analyzed the results for 5,473 patients who were taking a statin medication (for hyperlipidemia), 3,468 patients taking oral hypoglycemic agents for type 2 diabetes, and 13,279 patients taking antihypertensive agents for hypertension.

The patients were given the Alcohol Use Disorder Identification Test-Consumption (AUDIT-C questionnaire) and from these results were divided into nondrinkers, those with low-level alcohol use, and those with mild, moderate, and severe alcohol misuse. The researchers found that about 20 percent of all the subjects had AUDIT-C scores of 4 or more, indicating alcohol misuse. Medication compliance was defined as filling their prescriptions (based on pharmacy records) for at least 80 percent of the time.

The researchers found that non-adherence with taking their medication was associated with higher AUDIT-C scores among the patients treated for hypertension and hyperlipidemia but not for those who were treated for diabetes. (This may be because there was a higher proportion of nondrinkers among the diabetic subjects.) The researchers also found that subjects with an AUDIT score of 8 or more (of 40 possible points) were 2.6 times more likely to miss doses or to take them off-schedule.

The researchers concluded, "This study demonstrated that alcohol misuse is a possible risk factor for lower medication adherence among patients taking common medications. Moreover, the measure of alcohol misuse is a practical 3-item alcohol screening questionnaire that is increasingly used for routine screening in large health care systems. Because research has shown that brief counseling interventions decrease drinking, intervention studies are needed to assess whether brief counseling that leads to decreased drinking will also improve medication adherence. In the meantime, this study adds to the already strong evidence for the potential medical relevance of routine screening in medical settings." (See INTERVENTION, BRIEF.)

Relapse after Organ Transplants

Some formerly alcoholic patients who receive organ transplants may relapse. In a study of 387 patients who had a liver transplant because of alcoholic cirrhosis in Switzerland and France from 1989–2005, Andrea De Gottardt, M.D., and colleagues evaluated the risk of relapse to drinking, publishing their findings in *Archives of Internal Medicine* in 2007. They developed factors likely to indicate a relapse, such as:

- abstinence from alcohol for a period less than six months when placed on the transplant waiting list
- the presence of psychiatric comorbidities
- a score of higher than 3 on the High-Risk Alcoholism Scale

If more than one of these factors was present, according to the researchers, then the risk of relapse was increased. According to the researchers, "In conclusion, the results of the present study warrant further consideration, not only because 3 parameters (short abstinence, presence of psychiatric comorbidity, and higher HRAR score) were associated with alcohol relapse but also because the combination thereof assumed a particular importance. In fact, while 1 factor alone was associated with a risk of recidivism [relapse] below 20%, the combination of 2 or 3 factors resulted in a risk of recidivism exceeding 60%. Based on these findings, we suggest that the evaluation before LT [liver transplant] for ALD [alcoholic liver disease] should include these 3 parameters and that a patient presenting with 2 or 3 of them should be considered at very high risk of recidivism."

See also AGE AND ALCOHOL; ALCOHOL AND MEN; ALCOHOL POISONING; CHILD ABUSE AND NEGLECT; DELIRIUM TREMENS; DRIVING UNDER THE INFLUENCE/DRIVING WHILE INTOXICATED; EXCESSIVE DRINKING AND NEGATIVE SOCIAL CONSEQUENCES; HOSPITAL PATIENTS AND ALCOHOL-RELATED ADMISSIONS; LIVER DISEASE, ALCOHOLIC.

Bearer, Cynthia F., M.D., et al. "Biomarkers of Alcohol Use in Pregnancy." National Institute on Alcohol Abuse and Alcoholism. Available online. URL: http://pubs.niaaa.nih.gov/publications/arh28-1/38-43.htm. Accessed April 8, 2009.

Bryson, Chris L., M.D. "Alcohol Screening Scores and Medication Nonadherence." *Annals of Internal Medicine* 149, no. 11 (2008): 795–803.

De Gottardi, Andrea, M.D., et al. "A Simple Score for Predicting Alcohol Relapse After Live Transplantation: Results from 387 Patients Over 15 Years." *Archives of Internal Medicine* 167 (June 11, 2007): 1,183–1,188.

Epstein, Murray, M.D. "Alcohol's Impact on Kidney Function." *Alcohol Health & Research World* 21, no. 1 (1997): 84–93.

Flowers, Nicole T., et al. "Patterns of Alcohol Consumption and Alcohol-Impaired Driving in the United States." *Alcoholism: Clinical and Experimental Research* 32, no. 4 (2008): 639–644.

Kershaw, Corey D., M.D., and David M. Guidot, M.D. "Alcoholic Lung Disease." *Alcohol Research & Health* 31, no. 1 (2008): 66–75.

Kool, B., et al. "The Contribution of Alcohol to Falls at Home Among Working-Aged Adults." *Alcohol* 42, no. 5 (2008): 383–388.

Lieber, Charles S., M.D. "Relationships between Nutrition, Alcohol Use, and Liver Disease." *Alcohol Research & Health* 27, no. 3 (2003): 220–231.

Maraldi, Cinzia, M.D., et al. "Impact of Inflammation on the Relationship among Alcohol Consumption, Mortality, and Cardiac Events: The Health, Aging, and Body Composition Study." *Archives of Internal Medicine* 166, no. 14 (July 24, 2006): 1,490–1,497.

Mukamal, Kenneth J., M.D., et al. "Alcohol and Risk for Ischemic Stroke in Men: The Role of Drinking Patterns and Usual Beverage." *Annals of Internal Medicine* 142, no. 1 (2005): 11–19.

Mukamal, Kenneth J., M.D., Stephanie E. Chiuve, and Eric B. Rimm. "Alcohol Consumption and Risk for Coronary Heart Disease in Men with Healthy Lifestyles." *Archives of Internal Medicine* 166, no. 19 (October 23, 2006): 2,145–2,150.

Schiff, Eugene R., M.D., and Nuri Ozden, M.D. "Hepatitis C and Alcohol." *Alcohol Research & Health* 27, no. 3 (2003): 232–239.

Sundell, Laura, et al. "Increased Stroke Risk Is Related to a Binge Drinking Habit." *Stroke* 39, no. 12 (2008): 3,179–3,184.

Tolstrup, Janne, et al. "Prospective Study of Alcohol Drinking Patterns and Coronary Heart Disease in Women and Men." *British Medical Journal* 332, no. 7752 (2006): 1,244–1,248.

Vonlaufen, Alain, M.D., et al. "Role of Alcohol Metabolism in Chronic Pancreatitis." *Alcohol Research & Health* 30, no. 1 (2007): 48–54.

Wilson, Jennifer F. "Alcohol Use." *Annals of Internal Medicine* Supp. (2009): ITC3-1–ITC3-16.

Wright, Clinton B., et al. "Alcohol Intake, Carotid Plaque, and Cognition: The Northern Manhattan Study." *Stroke* 37, no. 5 (2006): 1,160–1,164.

excessive drinking and negative social consequences Heavy and/or chronic drinking can cause considerable distress to the individual himself or herself as well as to an individual's family, friends, and coworkers. It is clear that excessive drinking is harmful to the individual, but it is not always clear what the negative consequences are to others in the person's life. Research has demonstrated that those who begin their drinking early (before age 14) are more likely to develop alcohol dependence as adults. In addition, individuals who drink are more likely to engage in risky behavior, such as having sex without using contraception. As a result of such behavior, they are more likely to have unplanned pregnancies. They are also more likely to become infected with sexually transmitted diseases. (See AGE AND ALCOHOL.) In addition, alcohol fuels violence in many people in the United States.

The consequences of excessive drinking are not limited to individuals in the United States. According to a 2005 report on interpersonal violence and alcohol published by the World Health Organization, alcohol increases the risk for violence in people in many countries worldwide.

Self-Harm or Harm to Others Linked to Alcohol

In the case of people who die violent deaths from suicide, homicide, or other causes, research has demonstrated that many individuals who suicide as well as many of the victims of violent deaths were intoxicated. For example, in a study of vio-

TABLE 1
NUMBER* AND PERCENTAGE OF VICTIMS TESTED FOR ALCOHOL AND DRUGS WHOSE RESULTS WERE POSITIVE,
BY TOXICOLOGY VARIABLE—NATIONAL VIOLENT DEATH REPORTING SYSTEM, 16 STATES, 2005[1]

	Tested		Positive	
Toxicology variable	Number	Percentage	Number	Percentage
Blood alcohol concentration (BAC)	12,340	78.2	3,849	31.2
BAC ≤0.08 mg/DL			1,470	38.2
BAC >0.08 mg/DL			2,273	59.1
Alcohol-positive, level unknown			106	2.8
Amphetamine	7,729	47.7	428	5.5
Antidepressant	7,142	44.1	1,442	20.2
Cocaine	9,181	56.7	1,409	15.4
Marijuana	5,828	36.0	709	12.2
Opiate	8,882	54.9	2,115	23.8
Other drug	7,685	47.5	3,256	42.4

* N = 15,962
[1] Alaska, Colorado, Georgia, Kentucky, Maryland, Massachusetts, North Carolina, New Jersey, New Mexico, Oklahoma, Oregon, Rhode Island,
South Carolina, Utah, Virginia, and Wisconsin.
Source: Centers for Disease Control and Prevention. "Surveillance for Violent Deaths—National Violent Death Reporting System, 16 States, 2005."
Morbidity and Mortality Weekly Report 57, no. SS-3, April 11, 2008, page 20.

lent deaths in 16 states in 2005, published by the Centers for Disease Control and Prevention (CDC), the researchers found that when the blood alcohol levels of the victims were tested, in 59.1 percent of the cases, the blood alcohol level exceeded 0.08 mg/DL, or the legal limit for drinking and driving. See Table 1 for more details on the presence of alcohol and other drugs in the victims of violent deaths. Intoxicated victims are less likely to be able to flee from intoxicated aggressors, and they are more likely to stand their ground when it would be far more advisable for them to leave the scene.

Alcohol is often involved in SUICIDE. According to the CDC, when the BLOOD ALCOHOL CONCENTRATION (BAC) of the suicide victims was measured in nearly 9,000 suicide deaths, alcohol was present at or about 0.08 in nearly two-thirds of the cases. (See Table 2.) In addition, an alcohol abuse problem was present in 19.3 percent of the males and 13.7 percent of females who suicided. (See Table 3.)

Violent Behavior among Those Who Drink

Many studies have shown that alcohol increases the rate of the commission of aggressive acts. This may be due to a disruption of brain chemicals, particularly serotonin. It may also be that alco-

hol weakens the normal restraining areas of the brain, allowing impulsive, aggressive behaviors to dominate. Alcohol may also trigger an underlying predisposition to violence in some individuals. Whatever the causes that make aggression increase when some individuals are under the influence of alcohol, they are clearly very powerful influences.

According to the Substance Abuse and Mental Health Services Administration (SAMHSA), young adult males are more likely than any other demographic group to be involved in alcohol-related assaults and homicides. In addition, SAMHSA reports that more than any other substance, alcohol has been the drug most clearly demonstrated to increase aggressive behavior.

Some violent perpetrators use only alcohol, while others use alcohol in combination with illicit drugs or misused prescription drugs. According to Lawrence A. Greenfield's 1998 report, *Alcohol and Crime*, in cases of spousal violence, alcohol alone was involved in 65 percent of the cases, while both alcohol and drugs were involved in 11 percent of the cases. The combined use of both drugs and alcohol was present in 18 percent of alcohol-involved rapes and sexual assaults, 36 percent of alcohol-involved robberies, 24 percent

TABLE 2
NUMBER* AND PERCENTAGE OF SUICIDE VICTIMS TESTED FOR ALCOHOL AND DRUGS WHOSE RESULTS WERE
POSITIVE, BY TOXICOLOGY VARIABLE—NATIONAL VIOLENT DEATH REPORTING SYSTEM, 16 STATES, [1] 2005

Toxicology variable	Tested		Positive	
	Number	Percentage	Number	Percentage
Blood alcohol concentration (BAC)	6,455	72.1	2,063	32.0
Blood alcohol ≤0.08 mg/DL			722	35.0
Blood alcohol >.08 mg/DL			1,282	62.1
Alcohol-positive, level unknown			59	2.9
Amphetamine	3,719	41.6	178	4.8
Antidepressant	3,586	40.1	902	25.2
Cocaine	4,335	48.4	406	9.4
Marijuana	3,214	35.9	243	7.6
Opiate	4,266	47.7	790	18.5
Other drug	3,802	42.5	1,871	49.2

* N = 8,949
[1] Alaska, Colorado, Georgia, Kentucky, Maryland, Massachusetts, North Carolina, New Jersey, New Mexico, Oklahoma, Oregon, Rhode Island, South Carolina, Utah, Virginia, and Wisconsin.
Source: Centers for Disease Control and Prevention. "Surveillance for Violent Deaths—National Violent Death Reporting System, 16 States, 2005." *Morbidity and Mortality Weekly Report* 57, no. SS-3, April 11, 2008, page 23.

of aggravated assaults in which the offender was drinking, and 15 percent of simple assaults when the offender was drinking.

According to research reported by Greenfield and Maureen A. Henneberg in *Alcohol Research & Health* in 2001, in about half the cases of violent crimes in which the victims survive, the victims report that the perpetrator had been drinking. In about 20 percent of the cases, the violence occurred within the home of the victim. In about a third of the cases, however, the violence occurred in a public place, such as on the street or in a bar. The time of the assault was also significant. In about half the cases of violent victimizations, the alcohol use of the perpetrator occurred between 6 P.M. and midnight. The fewest number of incidents occurred between 6 A.M. and noon.

Individuals who are on probation for crimes sometimes commit violent offenses, and according to Greenfield and Henneberg, male probationers

TABLE 3
NUMBER AND PERCENTAGE OF SUICIDES, BY SEX AND ASSOCIATED CIRCUMSTANCES—
NATIONAL VIOLENT DEATH REPORTING SYSTEM, 16 STATES, 2005

Associated circumstances, mental health/substance abuse	Male		Female		Total	
	Number	Percentage	Number	Percentage	Number	Percentage
Current depressed mood	2,744	44.6	836	49.7	3,580	45.7
Current mental health problem	2,274	36.9	1,023	60.8	3,297	42.1
Current mental health treatment	1,723	28.0	861	51.2	2,584	33.0
Alcohol abuse problem	1,185	19.3	230	13.7	1,415	18.1
Other substance abuse problem	928	15.1	292	17.3	1,220	15.6

Source: Centers for Disease Control and Prevention. "Surveillance for Violent Deaths—National Violent Death Reporting System, 16 States, 2005." *Morbidity and Mortality Weekly Report* 57, no. SS-3, April 11, 2008, page 23.

were more likely to report using alcohol at the time of their offense (41 percent) than female probationers (25 percent).

Research on Acts of Violence in Bars In the Bar Violence Study in Buffalo, New York, the researchers found that the more alcohol consumed by participants in barroom acts of violence, the more likely there was for a severe injury to occur. Researchers Brian M. Quigley and Kenneth E. Leonard provided further details on the study results in their article for *Alcohol Research & Health* in the 2004/2005 issue.

According to the researchers, "Not everyone who drinks at a bar experiences violence, and those who do become involved in violence often have unique personality characteristics and alcohol usage patterns. For example, men who had committed or been the target of a violent act in a bar scored higher on measures of anger-proneness and impulsiveness than did men who had not experienced bar violence (although they might have observed it). Men who had experienced violence also scored lower on measures of personality agreeableness. Men who had been involved in bar violence reported drinking more than men who had not been involved (i.e., nonviolent men); they also reported having more alcohol problems than nonviolent men."

Among women who had experienced bar violence, the researchers found that these women had consumed more alcohol in general than did women who did not experience barroom violence. Quigley and Leonard said, "This study also found that women who experienced severe violence in a bar had consumed more alcohol at the bar and were more likely to go to the bar alone or leave alone or with a stranger."

Alcohol Abuse in Youth Is Predictive for Later Violence Alcohol abuse at a young age is predictive of later violence, according to Kenneth Leonard in his chapter in *Alcohol and Violence: Exploring Patterns and Responses*, published in 2008.

According to Leonard, research reveals that the hazardous use of alcohol at age 16 is predictive for the commission of both violent and property offences at ages 18 and 21 years each. Leonard also discusses research that indicates that violent encounters are 2.5 times more likely to involve

alcohol than are nonviolent encounters, whether the violent encounter is a spousal assault or sexual assault. Leonard says that violent homicides are more likely to involve alcohol than less violent homicides. With spousal or intimate partner violence, an injury is more likely to occur if the man (it is usually the male who is violent) has been drinking.

Psychiatric Diagnoses and Violent and Criminal Behavior

Individuals with some psychiatric diagnoses are more likely to commit crimes than others; for example, those with ANTISOCIAL PERSONALITY DISORDER (ASPD) have an inherently high rate of criminal behavior. ASPD is a disorder in which the individual does not follow the laws or guidelines of society, although he or she is aware of these laws and basic rules. In addition, some studies show that when people with ASPD drink, their aggressive levels are significantly higher than among others who drink. Researchers have also found that those who are severely mentally ill with SCHIZOPHRENIA, BIPOLAR DISORDER, and other psychotic disorders and who consume alcohol also have an increased risk for exhibiting violent behavior. The violence is most often directed at those close to them. The risk is much less present among severely mentally ill people who do not drink.

Several studies have found that mentally ill people are more prone than others to acts of violence only if there is a substance abuse or dependence that is present as well as other stressors. Eric B. Elbogen and Sally C. Johnson, M.D., reported on the issue in their 2009 article for *Archives of General Psychiatry,* based on their research on almost 35,000 subjects with severe mental illnesses such as schizophrenia, bipolar disorder, and major DEPRESSION.

According to the researchers, "The current study aimed to clarify the link between mental disorder and violence, and the results provide empirical evidence that (1) severe mental illness is not a robust predictor of future violence; (2) people with co-occurring severe mental illness and substance abuse/dependence have a higher incidence of violence than people with substance abuse/dependence alone; (3) people with severe mental illness report histories and environmental stressors associated with elevated violence risk; and (4) severe mental illness alone is not an independent contributor to explaining variance in multivariate analyses of different types of violence."

They concluded, "As severe mental illness itself was not shown to sequentially precede later violent acts, the findings challenge perceptions that severe mental illness is a foremost cause of violence in society at large. The data shows it is simplistic as well as inaccurate to say the cause of violence among mentally ill individuals is the mental illness itself; instead, the current study finds that mental illness is clearly relevant to violence risk but that its causal roles are complex, indirect, and embedded in a web of other (and arguably more) important individual and situation cofactors to consider."

In another study by Mulvey and colleagues published in 2006 in the *Journal of Consulting and Clinical Psychology*, the researchers found that among mentally ill people who were at high risk of violence, drinking on one day was predictive for the commission of violence on the following day; however, violence itself was not predictive for subsequent drinking. That is, the violent person drank alcohol and then became violent the next day, but after committing violence, may or may not have consumed alcohol. Other researchers such as Fals-Stewart and colleagues have found that among men who are presumably not mentally ill, drinking on one day increased the probability that violence would occur on the same day, particularly if the man had antisocial personality disorder.

Antisocial Personality Disorder Combined with Alcohol: A Recipe for Aggression

Research has shown that individuals with antisocial personality disorder have a greater risk for alcohol dependence than others and that they are also significantly more aggressive than other individuals after consuming alcohol. An estimated 3 percent of men and 1 percent of women in the population have ASPD, and many (although not all) have had numerous encounters with the criminal justice system. The disorder is characterized by a disregard for the needs or safety of others as well as by impulsivity, irresponsibility, the repeated commission of criminal acts, and a lack of remorse.

There are still many unresolved questions about ASPD and alcohol.

Authors F. Gerard Moeller, M.D., and Donald M. Dougherty, in their 2001 article on the combination of alcohol and antisocial personality disorder for *Alcohol Research & Health*, wrote, "Human laboratory studies have led to significant advances in understanding the relationship between personality and alcohol-related aggression. Several questions remain, however, regarding the role of ASPD in this relationship. For example it is still unclear whether the association of alcohol-related aggression with ASPD results from some key feature of ASPD itself or from the difficulties that many people with ASPD have in controlling aggressive or impulsive behaviors."

They continued, "Similarly, researchers have not determined the neurological and biochemical factors underlying alcohol-related aggression. Once scientists have further elucidated these issues, researchers may be able to develop successful treatment approaches aimed at decreasing alcohol-related aggression. Because alcohol-related violence continues to be a significant public health problem, further research on the relationship between ASPD and alcohol-related aggression clearly is warranted."

Sexual Assaults

The risk of violent sexual assaults is increased when both the perpetrator and the victim use alcohol. For example, in a study by Jenna McCauley and colleagues, published in *Addictive Behaviors* in 2009, the researchers did a telephone interview of 1,980 college women ages 18–34 years old. (The average age was 19.89 years.) The researchers found a lifetime prevalence of any type of rape of 11.3 percent. However the prevalence of sexual assaults was higher (15.8 percent) for women who engaged in BINGE DRINKING. In addition, the rate was 19.8 percent if the women were substance abusers. The researchers found that the most common substance of abuse was alcohol, used by 99.7 percent of substance abusers. The next most common substance of abuse was marijuana, used by less than half (45.5 percent) of substance abusers. According to the researchers, "The present study also lends support to findings that alcohol/drug use

excessive drinking and negative social consequences

at the time of assault may not only have been a risk factor for the rape itself, but also an indicator of women's risk for current/future substance abuse."

According to Antonia Abbey and colleagues in their article on alcohol and sexual assault for *Alcohol Research & Health* in 2001, most sexual assaults that are reported to the police occur between strangers; however, at least 80 percent of all actual sexual assaults occur between people who know each other. In the case of alcohol-related assaults, however, the researchers report that in most cases the individuals do not know each other very well, as in the situation of casual dates.

Abbey et al. also noted that heavy drinkers often use their own intoxication as an excuse or justification to commit socially unacceptable acts, including sexual assaults. Some personality characteristics, such as impulsivity or antisocial behavior, also increase the risk for both heavy drinking and the commission of sexual assaults.

See Table 4 for a comparison of general ("distal") and situational factors among both perpetrators and victims of sexual assaults, based on the research from Abbey. For example, often both the perpetrator and the victim have been drinking heavily. In addition, the perpetrator may have expectancies that alcohol will cause him to become more aggressive and disinhibited, thus creating a self-fulfilling prophecy.

Abbey and colleagues report that there are two distinct points at which alcohol increases the likelihood that a sexual assault will occur. According to the researchers, "The first point is during the early stages of the interaction, when the man is evaluating the likelihood that his companion wants to have sex with him." At this point, say the researchers, the man may misinterpret the woman's behavior and believe that she is much more encouraging than she is because his cognitive function is impaired by alcohol. They also say that the woman who drinks also has a cognitive impairment. "Thus, if she feels that she has made it clear that she is not interested in sex at this point, alcohol consumption will make her less likely to process the man's cues indicating that he has misread her intentions."

The second point when alcohol affects the man's behavior is when he forces sex on the woman. According to Abbey and colleagues, when a man is intoxicated, he is focused on his own immediate sexual gratification, sense of entitlement, and his anger, instead of considering what is appropriate behavior or the possibility that he might be punished in the future for his actions.

TABLE 4
SUMMARY OF EXPLANATIONS FOR ALCOHOL-RELATED SEXUAL ASSAULT, INCLUDING DISTAL FACTORS, WHICH ARE TEMPORARILY REMOVED FROM THE ASSAULT, AND PERSONAL FACTORS, WHICH ARE TEMPORARILY CLOSE TO THE ASSAULT

	Perpetrators	Victims
Distal Factors	General, heavy alcohol consumption	General, heavy alcohol consumption
	Alcohol expectancies about sex, aggression, and disinhibition	Childhood sexual abuse
	Stereotypes about drinking women being sexually available and appropriate targets	
Situational Factors	Heavy drinkers spend time in bars and at parties	Heavy drinkers spend time in bars and at parties
	Drinking is used as an excuse for socially unacceptable behavior	Alcohol's cognitive impairments reduce ability to evaluate risk
	Alcohol's cognitive impairments enhance misperception of the woman's friendly cues as sexual	Alcohol's motor impairments reduce ability to resist effectively
	Alcohol's cognitive impairments facilitate an aggressive response if the man feels he has been "led on"	

Adapted from Abbey, Antonia, et al. "Alcohol and Sexual Assault." *Alcohol Research & Health* 25, no. 1 (2001): page 46.

Worldwide Interpersonal Violence and Alcohol

According to the World Health Organization (WHO) report on interpersonal violence and alcohol in 2005, alcohol-fueled violence is a serious problem in many countries throughout the globe. For example, Europe has the highest per capita consumption of alcohol worldwide, which is also tied to 73,000 deaths per year or about 1 percent of all the deaths in Europe. In addition, for every European person who dies from interpersonal violence, another 20–40 victims are believed to need hospital treatment, while still more victims of violent acts go untreated and unrecorded.

Some statistics are particularly disturbing; for example, according to the WHO report, 80 percent of the violent crimes that are committed by juveniles in Estonia are alcohol-related. In Switzerland, 33 percent of perpetrators and 9.5 percent of victims of intimate partner violence were intoxicated when the assault occurred. In Spain, nearly half (46 percent) of rapists had consumed alcohol before the rape occurred.

According to the WHO report, nearly 75 percent of individuals arrested for homicide in 1995 had consumed alcohol. In national survey data from 2003–04 in England and Wales, research revealed that violent perpetrators had been drinking in 50 percent of all violent incidents, or more than 1.3 million alcohol-related incidents of violence.

Child Maltreatment

Child maltreatment is another social issue among some who abuse or are dependent on alcohol. Children whose parents abuse or are dependent on alcohol have an increased risk for being abused or neglected. In addition, their own risk for alcohol abuse or dependence in adolescence and adulthood is elevated. (See CHILD ABUSE AND NEGLECT.)

Alcohol and drug abuse are key risk factors for the maltreatment of children, including all forms of abuse as well as neglect, and alcohol and/or other drugs are involved in at least half of all cases of child abuse and neglect. In addition, nearly four in 10 child victimizers admit they were drinking at the time of the crime, and about half of them said they had been drinking for six or more hours before abusing the child.

Parents impaired by alcohol and/or drugs cannot pay proper attention to their children and their needs. Intoxicated parents are also much less patient than are sober parents, and thus they are more likely to cause physical harm to a child, including a crying baby or toddler. They are also more likely to neglect the needs of a baby, and neglected babies may become very ill and could die.

According to *Understanding Substance Abuse and Facilitating Recovery: A Guide for Child Welfare Workers*, some indicators of alcohol or drug abuse in parents include the following factors:

- a report of substance use is included in the child protective services call or report
- paraphernalia is found in the home (a large number of liquor bottles or beer bottles, a syringe kit, pipes, charred spoon, or foils)
- the home or the parent may smell of alcohol, marijuana, or drugs
- a child reports alcohol and/or other drug use by parents or other adults in the home
- a parent appears actively under the influence of alcohol or drugs (slurred speech, inability to mentally focus, physical balance is affected, extremely lethargic or hyperactive, etc.)
- a parent shows signs of addiction (needle tracks, skin abscesses, burns on inside of lips, etc.)
- a parent admits to substance use
- a parent shows or reports experiencing physical effects of addiction or being under the influence, including withdrawal (nausea, euphoria, slowed thinking, hallucinations, or other symptoms)

Another report by J. D. Fluke and colleagues on child maltreatment, *Rereporting and Recurrence of Child Maltreatment*, published in 2005, which reported on children who were revictimized, reported that research has shown that children whose parents abused had a high likelihood of being re-reported for abuse or neglect to the child protective services system in their state.

Frequent drinking by teenagers is associated with poor school performance, truancy, and delinquency, and all of these behaviors increase the risk for suffering from physical abuse by the adolescent's caregivers.

In another study by S. H. Shin and colleagues, reported in the *American Journal of Addictions* in 2009, the researchers drew subjects from the National Study of Adolescent Health and found that all forms of abuse or combined forms of abuse (with the exception of physical abuse alone) were strongly predictive for adolescent alcohol use. As a result, in a vicious circle, the child was abused, turned to alcohol in adolescence, and was likely reabused.

According to the World Health Organization, alcohol is a problem in child maltreatment worldwide; for example, in Canada, alcohol or drug use was involved in 34 percent of all child welfare investigations. In the United Kingdom, parental substance abuse was a concern in more than half (52 percent) of families on the child protection register, and alcohol was the primary substance that was used.

Failure to Be Sexually Responsible

Human immunodeficiency virus (HIV) is another social issue among some people with alcohol dependence. According to the NIAAA, people who drink are less likely than others to be tested for HIV; however, if these individuals *are* tested and found positive for HIV, they are less likely than nondrinkers to comply with treatment regimens. In addition, they are more likely than others to continue risk-taking behaviors, such as engaging in unsafe sex (for example, failing to use condoms) and thus putting others at risk for HIV infection. The NIAAA also reports that up to 60 percent of HIV-infected individuals are alcohol abusers or dependent on alcohol.

Other sexually transmitted diseases (STDs) are affected by drinking behavior; for example, a study by Robert L. Cook and colleagues that screened young adults in a sexually transmitted disease clinic for alcohol use (average age 20.6 years) found that a third met the criteria for an alcohol use disorder, including 24 percent with alcohol abuse and 9 percent with alcohol dependence. In another study by Heidi E. Hutton et al. of clinic patients with sexually transmitted diseases, reported in *Alcoholism: Clinical and Experimental Research* in 2008, the researchers found that female binge drinkers had

five times the risk of contracting gonorrhea (10.6 percent) compared to abstainers from alcohol (2.2 percent). (Rates of risky sexual behaviors and STDs were high among men but were not affected by their use of alcohol.)

HIV and Alcohol

According to the NIAAA, chronic alcohol consumption actually facilitates contracting an infection of HIV in those who are exposed, and it also accelerates the disease progression to acquired immune deficiency syndrome (AIDS). There is also some evidence that alcohol consumption may interfere with antiretroviral treatment as well. It is also true that individuals with HIV may fail to seek treatment or may fail to show up for their treatment appointments due to homelessness, alcohol abuse, and other issues. The NIAAA also reports that HIV infection is an increasing problem among African-American males ages 25 to 44 years and that it is about seven times more prevalent among African Americans than whites. Hispanics also have a problem with HIV infection, which is about three times more common among Hispanics than whites.

HIV/AIDS is also a global problem. Many studies have shown that in sub-Saharan Africa, excessive drinking leads to greater sexual risks and higher rates of sexually transmitted diseases, including HIV/AIDS.

If individuals who consume alcohol are also intravenous drug users, their risk of contracting HIV is further increased. Other groups at risk for HIV are gay men and homeless individuals.

Unplanned Sex and Pregnancy

Not every pregnancy is planned, and an unplanned pregnancy is not necessarily a disaster; however, if the mother is an alcohol abuser or dependent on alcohol and cannot or will not stop drinking during pregnancy, then the fetus is at risk for mild to severe developmental delays. (See FETAL ALCOHOL SYNDROME/FETAL ALCOHOL SPECTRUM DISORDERS.) Even if the mother does not drink during pregnancy, as mentioned, children are at risk of abuse and neglect at the hands of their parents who drink.

Based on research by Hingson et al., COLLEGE STUDENTS who began drinking early (before age 14) were twice as likely to have unplanned sex than those who delayed drinking until after age 19 or older. The early drinkers were also 2.2 times more likely than were the other students to have experienced unprotected sex. As a result, they were at risk for unplanned pregnancies as well as for contracting sexually transmitted diseases.

See also ALCOHOL AND MEN; FAMILIES AND ALCOHOL; TREATMENT.

Abbey, Antonia, et al. "Alcohol and Sexual Assault." *Alcohol Research & Health* 25, no. 1 (2001): 43–51.

Centers for Disease Control and Prevention. "Surveillance for Violent Deaths—National Violent Death Reporting System, 16 States, 2005." *Morbidity and Mortality Weekly Report* 57, no. SS-3, April 11, 2008.

Cook, Robert L., et al. "Alcohol Screening in Young Persons Attending a Sexually Transmitted Disease Clinic." *Journal of General Internal Medicine* 20, no. 1 (2005): 1–6.

Fals-Stewart, W., K. E. Leonard, and G. R. Birchler. "The Occurrence of Male-to-Female Intimate Partner Violence on Days of Men's Drinking: The Moderating Effects of Antisocial Personality Disorder." *Journal of Consulting and Clinical Psychology* 73, no. 2 (2005): 239–248.

Fluke, J. D., et al. *Rereporting and Recurrence of Child Maltreatment: Findings from NCANDS.* Washington, D.C.: U.S. Department of Health and Human Services, Office of the Assistant Secretary for Planning and Evaluation, 2005.

Greenfield, Lawrence A. *Alcohol and Crime: An Analysis of National Data on the Prevalence of Alcohol Involvement in Crime.* Washington, D.C.: Bureau of Justice Statistics, 1998.

Greenfield, Lawrence A., and Maureen A. Henneberg. "Victim and Offender Self-Reports of Alcohol Involvement in Crime." *Alcohol Research & Health* 25, no. 1 (2001): 20–31.

Hutton, Heidi E., et al. "The Relationship between Recent Alcohol Use and Sexual Behaviors: Gender Differences among Sexually Transmitted Disease Clinic Patients." *Alcoholism: Clinical and Experimental Research* 32, no. 11 (2008): 2,008–2,015.

Leonard, Kenneth E. "The Role of Drinking Patterns and Acute Intoxication in Violent Interpersonal Behaviors." In International Center for Alcohol Policies. *Alcohol and Violence: Exploring Patterns and Responses,* 29–55. Washington, D.C.: International Center for Alcohol Policies, 2008.

McCauley, Jenna, et al. "Forcible, Drug-facilitated, and Incapacitated Rape in Relation to Substance Abuse Problems: Results from a National Sample of College Women." *Addictive Behaviors* 34, no. 5 (2009): 458–462.

Moeller, F. Gerard, and Donald M. Dougherty. "Antisocial Personality Disorder, Alcohol, and Aggression." *Alcohol Research & Health* 25, no. 1 (2001): 5–11.

Mulvey, E. P., et al. "Substance Use and Community Violence: A Test of the Relation at the Daily Level." *Journal of Consulting and Clinical Psychology* 74, no. 4 (2006): 743–754.

National Center on Substance Abuse and Child Welfare. *Understanding Substance Abuse and Facilitating Recovery: A Guide for Child Welfare Workers.* Rockville, Md.: Substance Abuse and Mental Health Services Administration, 2005.

Office of Applied Studies. "Substance Use and Dependence Following Initiation of Alcohol or Illicit Drug Use." *The NSDUH Report.* Bethesda, Md.: Substance Abuse and Mental Health Services Administration, March 27, 2008.

Quigley, Brian M., and Kenneth E. Leonard. "Alcohol Use and Violence Among Young Adults." *Alcohol Research & Health* 28, no. 4 (2004/2005): 191–194.

Shin, S. H., et al. "Relationship Between Multiple Forms of Maltreatment by a Parent or Guardian and Adolescent Alcohol Use." *American Journal of Addictions* 18, no. 2 (2009): 226–234.

World Health Organization. *Alcohol and Interpersonal Violence: Policy Briefing.* Rome, Italy: 2005.

families and alcohol Experts agree that when at least one person in the family is dependent on alcohol (particularly a parent), then the entire family is profoundly affected by this dependence. For example, the excessive alcohol consumption of a parent significantly increases the risk for him or her performing acts of child maltreatment. It also significantly increases the risk that the child will be an adult problem drinker, as illustrated by studies of adverse childhood events and many other studies. In addition, the greater the number of members of the household who abuse or depend on alcohol, the more likely that children in the family will be abused or neglected. (See CHILD ABUSE AND NEGLECT.)

Behavioral/Psychiatric Problems of Children of Substance-abusing Parents

According to the National Center on Addiction and Substance Abuse at Columbia University in their 2005 report *Family Matters: Substance Abuse and the American Family,* there are two broad types of psychiatric disorders that are common to children whose parents abuse drugs and/or alcohol. The authors say that these include "behavioral problems that are directed toward others such as attention deficit hyperactivity disorder, conduct disorder and oppositional defiant disorder; or, problems that are directed inward such as depression or anxiety. Outwardly directed disorders are more commonly found in boys and inwardly directed disorders are more commonly found in girls. Both types of disorders have been linked to increased risk for substance use in children and teens."

Child Abuse and Alcoholism in Adulthood

Child maltreatment is predictive of alcohol abuse and dependence in adulthood. In a study reported by Elisha R. Galaif in the *Journal of Studies on Alcohol* in 2001 of 426 adults ages 32–34 who were originally studied in adolescence at age 16–18 years, the researchers found that childhood maltreatment and child sexual abuse were each predictive of adult alcohol abuse. In contrast, the researchers also found that close (and normal) family relations were protective factors against the development of alcohol misuse in adulthood.

Adult Children of Alcoholics

Children of alcoholics have an increased risk for alcohol abuse and dependence themselves in adulthood. In a study of adults and the effect of alcoholism and DEPRESSION, reported in the *Journal of Alcohol* by Theodore Jacob and M. Winkle, the researchers studied 128 adult children of alcoholics, 138 adult children of normal parents, and 127 adult children of depressed parents. They found that the children of alcoholics were significantly more likely to be alcoholics in adulthood (40.6 percent) than either the children of depressed parents (26.8 percent) or the children of "nondistressed" normal parents (also 26.8 percent).

According to the researchers, "Family history of alcoholism is clearly a significant risk for both male and female COAs [children of alcoholics], seen in families of alcoholics without psychiatric comorbidity in the alcoholic parent or major psychopathology in the nonalcoholic parent." In addition, the authors said, "COAs' academic achievements were found to lag behind those of both comparison groups as did their overall socioeconomic status and rate of employment; this finding parallels and exceeds findings from earlier studies." (For further information on the impact of childhood experiences, see AGE AND ALCOHOL.)

Suggestions for Adult Children of Alcoholics In an article for the Center for Substance Abuse Prevention (CSAP) of the Substance Abuse and Mental Health Services Administration, Kathy Asper offers suggestions for the adult children of alcoholics, including the following:

1. Become involved in Al-Anon and/or Adult Children of Alcoholics (ACoA) meetings, and in individual therapy. By doing this, you will learn: you are not alone in your pain; and you can learn to move beyond the harm you experienced as a child. (If you are concerned that you cannot afford individual counseling, check with local clergy, as many offer counseling services. There are also mental health or treatment providers who offer their services based on income levels.) Your mental health is priceless. You owe it to yourself to seek options for becoming healthy.

2. Develop support systems by making those close to you aware of your decision to seek counseling. (Al-Anon or ACoA groups and counselors will help to provide such a system of support.) Share your decision with friends and family members who will encourage you. Do not share your decision with people who will question you or belittle your decision.

3. Learn how to ask for help. (If you go to an Al-Anon or ACoA group, counselors and fellow ACoAs can help you learn this. In time, you will learn whom you can trust with your struggles.)

4. Recognize that you have the right to talk about these issues and you have the right to experience and express emotions.

5. If you have children, learn about child development. Seek out and participate in a parent education course to learn skills for relating to your children.

6. Check with your local public library for books on this topic to help you understand and overcome a chaotic childhood.

Parents Need to Talk to Children about Alcohol The impact of parents on their children is often far greater than they realize, which is why it is very important for parents to talk to their children about such topics as UNDERAGE DRINKING, alcohol abuse, and ALCOHOLISM/ALCOHOL DEPENDENCE. Many parents mistakenly think that they have little or no influence over their children, assuming that the child's peers are the only individuals whose views matter to the child, particularly in the case of adolescents. Yet studies have shown that parental attitudes toward alcohol as well as their own drinking behavior directly affect the child and adolescent's later use or abuse of alcohol.

Protective Factors against Alcohol Dependence There are some protective factors against the development of alcohol dependence in children. Family closeness and the lack of alcoholism are protective factors against the abuse of alcohol in adulthood. In contrast, however, the adolescent who was sexually abused as a child is twice as likely to become a binge drinker than is the teenager who was not sexually abused. In addition, children exposed to parental alcoholics are significantly more likely to experience problems with drinking in their own adulthoods compared to adult children whose parents were not alcoholics, thus perpetuating the problem and leaving their children at risk for drinking problems when they grow up.

See also AGGRESSIVE BEHAVIOR AND ALCOHOL; BINGE DRINKING; CODEPENDENCY; DENIAL; ENABLERS; EXCESSIVE DRINKING AND HEALTH CONSEQUENCES; EXCESSIVE DRINKING AND NEGATIVE SOCIAL CONSEQUENCES; VIOLENCE.

Asper, Kathy. *Characteristics of Adult Children of Alcoholics.* Center for Substance Abuse Prevention. Undated. Available online. URL: http://captus.samhsa.gov/central/documents/4AdultChildrenofAlcoholics.pdf. Accessed April 1, 2009.

Galaif, Elisha R., et al. "Gender Differences in the Prediction of Problem Alcohol Use in Adulthood: Exploring the Influence of Family Factors and Childhood Maltreatment." *Journal of Studies on Alcohol* 62, no. 4 (2001): 486–493.

Jacob, Theodore, and M. Winkle. "Young Adult Children of Alcoholic, Depressed and Nondistressed Parents." *Journal of Studies on Alcohol* 61, no. 6 (2000): 836–844.

National Center on Addiction and Substance Abuse at Columbia University. *Family Matters: Substance Abuse and the American Family.* New York: National Center on Addiction and Substance Abuse at Columbia University, March 2005.

fatty liver disease, alcoholic   See EXCESSIVE DRINKING AND HEALTH CONSEQUENCES; LIVER DISEASE, ALCOHOLIC.

fetal alcohol syndrome/fetal alcohol spectrum disorders   A set of characteristics that presents in a child or adult that was caused by the alcohol abuse or ALCOHOLISM/ALCOHOL DEPENDENCE of the mother during her pregnancy. Fetal alcohol syndrome (FAS) was first identified by Seattle physicians K. L. Jones and D. W. Smith in 1973, and as a result of their discovery, pregnant women in the 21st century are actively discouraged from drinking any alcohol. The terminology later changed to fetal alcohol spectrum disorders (FASDS), a diagnosis that encompasses a range of disabilities including alcohol-related neurodevelopment disorder (ARND), alcohol-related birth defects (ARBD), and FAS; however, the term fetal alcohol syndrome continues to be more commonly known in much of the lay public and even among many physicians, and FAS is often used to mean any of the three types of fetal disabilities.

All of these disorders are completely preventable with ABSTINENCE from alcohol during pregnancy. As a result, the United States places warning labels on all alcoholic beverages to warn pregnant women away from consuming any alcohol. Armstrong and Abel argue that these labels have failed to achieve the desired result of preventing women from drinking during pregnancy; however, they point out that only a small proportion of children are born with FAS or lesser manifestations of drinking during pregnancy.

According to the Centers for Disease Control and Prevention (CDC), more than half of all births in the United States are unplanned, and thus any woman who might become pregnant should stop drinking. The CDC reports that an estimated one in 12 pregnant women use alcohol and that about one in 30 of them engage in BINGE DRINKING (having five or more drinks at one time).

According to the Substance Abuse and Mental Health Services Administration (SAMHSA), the prevalence of FAS is estimated to be 0.5 to 2 per 100,000 births. In considering fetal alcohol spectrum disorder, it is estimated that infants with FAS represent about 1 percent of all births, or about 40,000 newborns per year. SAMHSA reports that studies show that of individuals ages six to 51 years with a fetal alcohol spectrum disorder, they experience the following proportion of problems:

- 94 percent had mental health problems
- 83 percent lived dependently with others
- 79 percent had employment problems
- 60 percent of those ages 12 and older had problems with law enforcement officials
- 45 percent engaged in inappropriate sexual behavior
- 43 percent had dropped out of school
- 35 percent of adults and adolescents had been in prison, convicted of a crime
- 24 percent had alcohol and drug problems themselves
- 23 percent had received inpatient care for mental illness

Studies have also shown that of the women who have given birth to an infant with FAS, several risk factors for drinking during pregnancy were present, including the following:

- 96 percent had at least one mental illness
- 95 percent had a history of physical or sexual abuse
- 77 percent had an unplanned pregnancy, including 81 percent who used no birth control
- 61 percent were not high school graduates
- 59 percent had an annual gross family income of less than $10,000

A report published in *Maternal and Child Health Journal* by Anderson et al. in 2006, using data from the 2002 and 2004 federal Behavioral Risk Factor Surveillance System (BRFSS), stated that 54.5 percent of preconception women (not yet pregnant) have one or more of three risk factors for an adverse pregnancy, including frequent drinking, current smoking, and the absence of a test for the human immunodeficiency virus (HIV). This rate dropped to about a third (32 percent) for pregnant women. The researchers also found that women without insurance had a significantly higher risk for preconception or pregnancy risk factors; for example, 52.7 percent of pregnant women without health insurance had one or more risk factors compared to 29.4 percent of pregnant women with health insurance.

According to the authors, "Although it appears that some women reduce their risk for adverse pregnancy outcomes after learning of their pregnancy, the data suggest that a substantial proportion of women do not. Furthermore, if such change occurs it is often too late to affect outcomes, such as birth defects resulting from alcohol consumption during the periconception period."

Another study of 1,162 human services professionals working in child welfare/child protective services, foster care, and Medicaid enrollment in counties in New York was reported in 2008 in the *Canadian Journal of Clinical Pharmacology*. The researchers found that most of the professionals were aware and knowledgeable about the prevention of FAS and FASDs. However, their knowledge about how to identify children with these defects and how to work with these children was lower, and 90 percent said that they did not care for any children with FAS. For example, recognition of the physical features of FAS is important, but only about a third (36.5 percent) realized that a thin upper lip was a feature of FAS, and nearly half (46.7 percent) said that they did not know or were not sure which facial features were indicative of FAS.

The researchers concluded, "Given the large percent of children with FASD in the foster care, adoption, juvenile justice and mental health systems, professionals in these systems need to have a high index of suspicion that a child with behavioral or mental health problems has secondary disabilities resulting from in utero alcohol exposure. While the likelihood of a uniform FASD screening technique is important, the likelihood that children with FASD will be identified and referred would be increased if institutions or organizations have one or more individuals with the knowledge of best resources for diagnosis and treatment in their community, who is responsible for systematically following up the child."

Symptoms and Diagnostic Path

Children with FASD are often premature infants, and they are also small in size compared to other children. They may be developmentally delayed in intelligence, speech, and language, and they often have learning disabilities. They may be hyperactive and suffer from seizures. They may also have sleep disturbances as infants. The child may have facial abnormalities, such as a smooth philtrum (the area on the face between the upper lip and the nose). The child may also have thin upper lips.

Individuals with an FASD often have problems with their attention span, memory, problem solving, speech, and hearing. As adolescents and adults, they are also at high risk for having alcohol or drug abuse, mental health disorders, and getting into trouble with law enforcement officials. They may also have poor impulse control, which is why they experience difficulty with law enforcement officials and other authority figures. However, there are some protective factors against the worst outcomes; for example, if a child is diagnosed early, he or she can receive social services, as can the family. The child may also receive special education targeted to his or her individual abilities. If the child with FASD lives with a nurturing and loving family, this is also a protective factor aiding a child to fulfill his or her best potential. In contrast, if a child with FASD lives in an abusive or disruptive home, the child is more likely to become involved in youth violence and have a poor outcome.

Treatment Options and Outlook

Fetal alcohol syndrome and other FASDs cannot be cured, and only the symptoms and the manifestations of the disorder can be treated, with special education and a nurturing and loving family. However, as mentioned, early diagnosis and treatment improves the prognosis.

Risk Factors and Preventive Measures

Children whose mothers consumed alcohol during pregnancy are at risk for fetal alcohol spectrum disorder. The best preventive measure is for pregnant women to avoid alcohol completely during their entire pregnancy. Once a child is born with fetal alcohol syndrome, all that can be done is to treat whatever disorders or medical problems have been caused in the child because of the mother's drinking during her pregnancy, to help the child as much as possible.

See also ALCOHOL AND WOMEN; CHILD ABUSE AND NEGLECT; EXCESSIVE DRINKING AND HEALTH CONSEQUENCES; EXCESSIVE DRINKING AND NEGATIVE SOCIAL CONSEQUENCES; PREGNANCY.

Anderson, John E., Shahul Ebrahim, Louise Floyd, and Hani Atrash. "Prevalence of Risk Factors for Adverse Pregnancy Outcomes during Pregnancy and the Preconception Period—United States, 2002–2004." *Maternal and Child Health Journal* 10, Supp. 1 (2006): S101–S106.

Armstrong, Elizabeth M., and Ernest L. Abel. "Fetal Alcohol Syndrome: The Origins of a Moral Panic." *Alcohol & Alcoholism* 35, no. 3 (2000): 276–282.

Caley, Linda, Charles Syms, Luther Robinson, et al. "What Human Service Professionals Know and Want to Know about Fetal Alcohol Syndrome." *Canadian Journal of Clinical Pharmacology* 15, no. 1 (2008): e117–e123.

Jones, K. L., and D. W. Smith. "Recognition of the Fetal Alcohol Syndrome in Early Infancy." *Lancet* 3, no. 2 (1973): 999–1,001.

G

gamblers/pathological gambling Gamblers participate in games of chance for the opportunity to win money or other prizes. Pathological gamblers feel compelled to gamble, and they generally cannot walk away from a game if they have any chance at all of participating. Many pathological gamblers abuse or are dependent on alcohol. In fact, the locations where gambling occurs may offer free or discounted drinks to gamblers in order to encourage them to drink, particularly in large resort areas where local revenues are heavily dependent on money received from gamblers and gambling establishments.

Pathological gambling is categorized by the American Psychiatric Association in the *Diagnostic and Statistical Manual IV-TR* as an IMPULSE CONTROL DISORDER. Other impulse disorders are kleptomania (a compulsion to steal items that are not needed), pyromania (a compulsion to set fires), TRICHOTILLOMANIA (a compulsion to pull hair out of head and/or other parts of the body), and INTERMITTENT EXPLOSIVE DISORDER (an anger problem that arises suddenly and with little or no provocation and that may lead to violence).

Pathological gamblers experience serious life consequences, such as the loss of their jobs and the loss of their families through divorce. Some pathological gamblers turn to crime to obtain the money that is needed to continue gambling. They also have a significantly increased risk for alcohol abuse and ALCOHOLISM/ALCOHOL DEPENDENCE. However, male gamblers are more likely to have a substance abuse disorder than female gamblers. For example, in a study of pathological gamblers published in 2003 by Ibanez and colleagues, about a third (32 percent) of the men had a problem with either alcohol abuse or alcoholism, compared to 4.5 per-

cent of the female gamblers. In another study by Tavares et al., 27 percent of the male gamblers had an alcohol use disorder, compared to 6 percent of the female gamblers.

Symptoms and Diagnostic Path

Individuals who are pathological gamblers constantly think about gambling. Often they have repeatedly tried and failed to stop their gambling. They are often irritable and restless when they try to cut back or end their gambling. The pathological gambler may gamble to improve a bad mood or to avoid thinking about problems. Another symptom is that when the pathological gamblers lose, they frequently feel compelled to gamble again, reasoning to themselves that they need to recoup their losses. Some gamblers commit crimes to obtain the money they need to gamble. Often important personal and family relationships are jeopardized or lost because of gambling.

The psychiatrist who diagnoses pathological gambling discusses the importance of gambling to the individual and seeks to determine whether there are other disorders that are present, such as DEPRESSION, an ANXIETY DISORDER, and/or an alcohol use disorder.

Treatment Options and Outlook

Pathological gamblers may benefit from joining a mutual aid self-help group, such as Gamblers Anonymous, which is patterned on the 12 steps of Alcoholics Anonymous. Various therapies are used with pathological gamblers, such as cognitive-behavioral therapy (CBT), in which the gambler is taught to identify and challenge irrational beliefs, such as the belief that he or she is "due" for a win or of a need to gamble to obtain money for the gambler's family. In fact, if the person does win, he or she will use that money to gamble again.

Some physicians treat pathological gamblers with antidepressants in the class of selective serotonin reuptake inhibitors (SSRIs). According to Pallanti and colleagues in their chapter on pathological gambling in the *Clinical Manual of Impulse-Control Disorders,* the dosages of SSRIs that are needed to treat pathological gambling are generally higher than used to treat major depressive disorder—whether the individual also has depression or not. Some researchers have treated pathological gamblers with NALTREXONE, a medication also used to treat alcohol dependence.

The outlook for the pathological gambler largely depends on the personal commitment of the individual to stop gambling, with the help of therapy, self-help, and medications.

Risk Factors and Preventive Measures

Males are more likely to become pathological gamblers than females. Individuals in gangs or inmates incarcerated in prison have a risk for developing pathological gambling. In addition, according to authors William G. McCown and William A. Howatt in *Treating Gambling Problems,* head trauma and epilepsy should be ruled out in the pathological gambler, because brain injury can precipitate pathological gambling. In addition, they report that individuals with developmental problems such as ATTENTION-DEFICIT/HYPERACTIVITY DISORDER as well as those with neurological problems may be at an increased risk for pathological gambling and need to be evaluated by a neurologist.

There are no known preventive measures against pathological gambling. If the disorder develops, it should be treated as early as possible, including in adolescence or young adulthood.

See also BIPOLAR DISORDER; EXCESSIVE DRINKING AND NEGATIVE SOCIAL CONSEQUENCES; PERSONALITY DISORDERS; PSYCHIATRIC COMORBIDITIES.

Durdle, Heather, and Kevin M. Gorey. "A Meta-Analysis Examining the Relations Among Pathological Gambling, Obsessive-Compulsive Disorder, and Obsessive-Compulsive Traits." *Psychological Reports* 103, no. 2 (2008): 485–498.

Grant, Jon E., M.D., Matt G. Kushner, and Suck Won Kim, M.D. "Pathological Gambling and Alcohol Use Disorder." *Alcohol Research & Health* 26, no. 2 (2002): 143–150.

Ibanez, Angela, et al. "Gender Differences in Pathological Gambling." *Journal of Clinical Psychiatry* 64, no. 3 (2003): 295–301.

McGown, William G., and William A. Howatt. *Treating Gambling Problems.* New York: John Wiley & Sons, 2007.

Pallanti, Stevano, M.D., Nicolo Baldini Rossi, M.D., and Eric Hollander, M.D. "Pathological Gambling." In *Clinical Manual of Impulse-Control Disorders,* edited by Eric Hollander, M.D., and Dan J. Stein, M.D., Arlington, Va.: American Psychiatric Publishing, 251–289.

Pietrzak, Robert H., et al. "Gambling Level and Psychiatric and Medical Disorders in Older Adults: Results from the National Epidemiologic Survey on Alcohol and Related Conditions." *American Journal of Geriatric Psychiatry* 15, no. 4 (2007): 301–313.

Tavares, Hermano, et al. "Factors at Play in Faster Progression for Female Pathological Gamblers: An Exploratory Analysis." *Journal of Clinical Psychiatry* 65, no. 4 (2003): 433–438.

generalized anxiety disorder   Generalized anxiety disorder (GAD) is a condition of constant and pathological worrying that causes overwhelming anxiousness in an individual. This condition lasts for six months or more. The excessive worrying that typifies this condition is often groundless, or the individual worries about situations that he or she has little or no control over. People with GAD often are aware that they worry too much, yet despite this insight, they still cannot stop worrying. They cannot relax and they may have trouble getting to sleep or staying asleep. The lifetime prevalence of GAD is about 5 to 6 percent in the United States, and it has a one-year prevalence of about 3 percent. Some research suggests that GAD is the anxiety disorder that is the most associated with the use of alcohol and/or drugs in an individual's attempt to self-medicate its symptoms.

GAD is commonly associated with other psychiatric disorders, particularly depression, as well as with other ANXIETY DISORDERS; specifically, SPECIFIC PHOBIA, SOCIAL PHOBIA, and PANIC DISORDER. Many patients with GAD suffer from physical symptoms with no medical basis, known as "somatic" symptoms, including such symptoms as insomnia, muscle tension, and fatigue.

Symptoms and Diagnostic Path

Some common symptoms of individuals with GAD include:

- headaches
- fatigue for no apparent reason
- muscle pain and aches
- lightheadedness
- the need to use the bathroom frequently
- feeling out of breath
- chest pain
- general irritability

The physician diagnoses a person with GAD based on symptoms. The two primary elements of GAD are an unrealistic yet uncontrollable worry about two or more subjects at the same time with physical symptoms. Many medical problems may occur along with GAD, such as fibromyalgia, hyperthyroidism, hypoglycemia, seizure disorders, and so forth. Individuals with GAD worry about a variety of different things, and sometimes they worry about their worrying, a condition that is known as metaworry.

If the primary care physician notes that no serious medical problems are present, he or she may refer the individual to a psychiatrist. The psychiatrist diagnoses GAD based on the patient's symptoms. The doctor may also use a psychiatric instrument to evaluate the patient, such as the Hamilton Anxiety Rating Scale or the Anxiety Disorders Interview Schedule for *DSM-IV-TR*. The Penn State Worry Questionnaire is another instrument that is sometimes used.

Treatment Options and Outlook

GAD is generally treated with BENZODIAZEPINES (antianxiety medications) such as diazepam (Valium), lorazepam (Ativan), or alprazolam (Xanax). It is also treated with ANTIDEPRESSANTS, such as medications in the class of selective serotonin reuptake inhibitors (SSRI), such as paroxetine (Paxil), or escitalopram (Lexapro), as well as with antidepressants in the serotonin norepinephrine reuptake inhibitor (SNRI) class, such as venlafaxine XR (Effexor XR) or duloxetine (Cymbalta). Some patients are treated with beta blockers. Sometimes the antihistamine hydroxyzine is used to treat GAD.

Psychotherapy may also help the patient with GAD, particularly cognitive-behavioral therapy (CBT), in which the therapist teaches the individual to identify and challenge irrational thoughts. Relaxation therapy may provide improvement to those with GAD. Treatment can provide a great deal of relief to many people suffering from GAD.

Risk Factors and Preventive Measures

GAD affects about twice as many women as men. According to Kate Collins and Sanjay Matthew, M.D., in their 2008 article for *Perspectives in Psychiatry: A Clinical Update* (a supplement to *Psychiatric Times*), GAD is also more common among those who are single, widowed, or divorced rather than those who are married, as well as in those with a lower socioeconomic status and in ethnic and racial minorities. A family history of anxiety disorders is also a risk factor for GAD. About 90 percent of people with GAD have another psychiatric disorder at some point in their lives, according to Collins and Matthew. Patients with GAD are more likely to see both their primary care and gastroenterology physicians than individuals without GAD.

Collins, Kate, and Sanjay Matthew, M.D. "A Review of Generalized Anxiety Disorder." *Perspectives in Clinical Psychiatry: A Clinical Update.* Supplement to *Psychiatric Times.* September 2008, Issue 2 of 4, 3–8.

Huppert, Jonathan D., and Moira Ryan. "Generalized Anxiety Disorder." In *Clinical Manual of Anxiety Disorders,* edited by Dan J. Stein, M.D., 147–171. Washington, D.C.: American Psychiatric Press, 2004.

genetics and alcohol Twin studies and adoption studies have shown that some individuals have clear genetic predispositions to diagnoses of alcohol abuse and dependence; for example, adopted children whose birthparents are alcoholic (particularly the birthfather) have an increased risk for alcoholism themselves in adulthood, even when the adoptive parents do not use alcohol at all. However, in the unusual case when the adoptive father *is* an alcoholic, if the biological father is not an alcoholic, then the risk for the child becoming an alcoholic is very low. Twin studies have also shown that monozygotic (identical) twins with a family history of alcohol dependence have twice the risk of dizygotic twins (nonidentical twins) of becoming alcoholics.

Genetics is the study of inherited traits, including traits linked to alcohol dependence. According to the Online Mendelian Inheritance in Man (OMIM), a project that is genotyping the entire human genetic sequence, genetic links to alcohol dependence have been specifically identified on chromosomes 13q14-q2, 4q22, and 4p13-p12. These traits may actually become evident in the individual's behavior, or they may not because genetic traits are enhanced or decreased by environmental factors. Studies have shown that as high as 40–60 percent of the risk for ALCOHOLISM is apparently associated with genetic factors. The risk appears to be greater in men than women, although some experts contend that some research indicates the risk is high among females as well. (See ALCOHOL AND WOMEN.)

People cannot change the genes that they were born with, but some researchers are seeking to identify the problem genes contributing to alcoholism, while others are looking for the means to counteract existing problematic genes. For example, some researchers have attempted to perform genotherapy by treating individuals possessing certain genotypes with medications that are antagonists to the brain receptor that is associated with the gene. At the same time, it is important to keep in mind that genes are not destiny. Genes express or produce proteins and cause other changes in cellular functions. Some genes are switched on by stress, while stress turns other genes off. Some are turned on and stay on when the individual is exposed to tobacco or cocaine while in utero or during early childhood. Genes are best regarded as risks or odds, and these risks can be significantly altered by trauma, diet, exercise, mental health, drug exposure/use, and other factors. Genes have been shown to be useful in understanding medications, their metabolism, and the response to medications.

In a study reported in *Science* in 2008, researchers David T. George and colleagues said that the neurotransmitter substance P and its associated neurokinin-1 receptor (NK1R) were linked with alcohol dependence. They hypothesized that a medication that was a neurokinin-1 receptor antagonist could be used as a possible therapy. They first tested an experimental medication on mice and then tested it on alcoholic men recently discharged from treatment.

The researchers found that the medication suppressed the cravings for alcohol and also improved the overall well-being of the men. In addition, brain scans using magnetic resonance imaging (MRI) confirmed that there was a beneficial effect to the medication use. The medication is not approved for use by the Food and Drug Administration (FDA) for the general public, and further research is needed to verify its efficacy; however, this research may ultimately lead to better treatment and perhaps to individualized genotherapy for people with alcohol dependence.

Research continues to evolve. For example, a study conducted by Victor Karpyak and reported in 2009 in *Alcohol: Clinical and Experimental Research* isolated a gene linked to the severity of acute alcohol withdrawal and seizures in mice: the MPDZ protein. More dramatically, the researchers also found 67 new and largely rare variants of the human MPDZ genes when they studied 59 subjects of European ancestry with a history of alcoholic withdrawal without seizures. They found a significant correlation between the MPDZ in those with alcoholism but not seizures, compared to nonalcoholic subjects.

Some of the clearest evidence of a genetic link to alcoholism is that research that shows a predisposition to *not* drinking, as with the ALDH2 genetic variant. As many as 40 percent of Asians possess this genetic variant, which causes an ALCOHOL FLUSHING RESPONSE if they consume any amount of alcohol. Despite this, some Asians who have inherited the ALDH2 genetic variant drink anyway, as in the case of some Korean adolescent adoptees, particularly when an older sibling consumes alcohol. In such cases, environment apparently trumps genetics (and not in a good way).

Some adoption researchers have found a high risk of alcoholism among a subset of adoptees.

C. Robert Cloninger, M.D., was the first to identify what he called Type 1 and Type 2 alcoholism in 1981, based on detailed research made possible because of open access to adoption records in the Stockholm Adoption Study. According to subsequent research by Soren Sigvaradsson, Michael Bohman, M.D., and Dr. Cloninger in 1996, and reported in the *Archives of General Psychiatry,* adopted men with a genetic background for alcoholism had a six times greater risk for Type 2 alcoholism (a severe form of early onset alcohol dependence) than other adoptees, regardless of their subsequent postnatal environment.

Despite the increased risk of the biological children of alcoholics to develop alcoholism, most children of alcoholics do *not* become alcoholics. Also, children who have no known alcoholic relatives sometimes develop alcohol dependence. As a result, environmental impacts or other issues lead to alcoholism in some individuals; for example, researchers have demonstrated that adverse events in childhood, such as childhood abuse or neglect, can increase the risk for alcoholism in adulthood, and the greater the number of adverse events, the greater this risk is. (See AGE AND ALCOHOL.)

Some experts, such as Marc Schuckit, reporting in his 2009 article in the *Journal of Substance Abuse Treatment,* have found several key factors linked to genetics; for example, a low intensity response to alcohol is linked to an increased risk for alcoholism in adulthood. In addition, in an earlier article in *Journal of Studies on Alcohol* in 2000, Schuckit and T. L. Smith said they found that the sons of alcoholic fathers rated themselves lower than the sons of nonalcoholic fathers on such measures as dizziness, sleepiness, and drug effect after consuming alcohol, which indicates that the sons of alcoholic fathers had a less intense reaction to alcohol than did the sons of nonalcoholic fathers.

Other researchers have sought genetic linkages in the actual structure of the brain; for example, Shirley Y. Hill and colleagues reported in *Biological Psychiatry* in 2009 on their findings that an increased risk for alcoholism may be linked to a decreased volume of the right and left orbitofrontal cortex (OFC), an area of the brain that controls emotions and impulsive behaviors.

It can often be difficult to tease out which specific factors are related to genetic factors and which are tied to environmental factors. For example, if a child of an alcoholic parent grows up to become an alcoholic himself or herself, is this due to heredity or environment? Researchers continue to debate this issue. Some researchers say that there are some common mechanisms that may exist within a family and that may increase an individual's risk for alcohol dependence. In their article in *Archives of General Psychiatry* in 2004, John I. Nurnberger, M.D., and colleagues said that the presence of some psychiatric disorders within a family, such as ANTISOCIAL PERSONALITY DISORDER, ANXIETY DISORDERS, drug dependence, and mood disorders, are mechanisms by which alcohol dependence may develop in some families.

Genetic Risk Factors for Alcohol Dependence
In his 2009 article on the genetic influences in alcoholism, Marc A. Schuckit listed four primary intermediate genetic characteristics that interact with the environment and that may increase or decrease the risk for alcoholism, including:

1. A flushing response to alcohol, which tends to decrease the risk for alcohol dependence
2. A low level of response to alcohol, which tends to increase the risk for alcoholism
3. Personality characteristics such as impulsivity, sensation-seeking, and externalizing behaviors, which increase the risk
4. Psychiatric symptoms, which increase the risk

Flushing Response to Alcohol As mentioned, about 40 percent of Asians, particularly Japanese, Chinese, and Koreans, inherit a flushing response to even a small amount of alcohol, and this is generally predictive of a lower probability of alcohol dependence, since this response is obvious to others and embarrassing to the individual. These individuals have a mutation in the ALDH2 gene that produces an enzyme that does not metabolize alcohol as well as those without the mutated gene.

About 10 percent of Asians have two copies of the deficient gene; when they drink alcohol, it is as if they had taken the aversive drug DISULFIRAM (Antabuse), and they experience severe nausea and vomiting. There is an extremely low risk of alcoholism among individuals with this inherent internal "stop" mechanism.

Despite this innate mechanism, researchers have found that some Korean adoptees who have inherited the genetic mutation that causes the flushing response will drink anyway when an older nonbiological sibling in the family drinks, thus an environmental impact actually overrides genetics in this case. (The subjects were not genetically related to their adoptive parents or their siblings.)

As reported by Daniel E. Irons and colleagues in *Development and Psychopathology* in 2007, researchers genotyped 180 Asian adolescent adoptees to determine if they possessed the ALDH2 genetic deficiency. The adoptees were adopted as infants, with an average adoption age of 5.1 months. The researchers found 52 of the subjects were ALDH2 deficient. In most cases, the genetic deficiency acted as a protective factor and was significantly associated with lower rates of drinking and of becoming intoxicated. They also identified siblings rather than parents as the major familial effect on the adolescent's decision to consume alcohol.

The majority of the subjects with the deficient genotype were female (69.2 percent), and the average age of the subjects was 18. The researchers studied whether alcohol was ever used, and found that 63.5 percent of the subjects with the deficient ALDH2 status had ever used alcohol, compared to 71.9 percent of those who were not deficient. (It is not surprising that adoptees with the deficiency took their first drink, since these adolescents had no way to know ahead of time if their biological parents had the genetic deficiency.)

As for ever using alcohol in the past year, the researchers found that 66.4 percent of those subjects without the deficiency had used alcohol in the past year, compared to 48.1 percent with the deficiency. Only sibling alcohol use was significantly associated with adolescent alcohol use, while parental alcohol use was irrelevant.

The researchers concluded that even "in the presence of this, the single strongest known genetic protective factor against drinking behavior, family environment mattered. Adopted ALDH deficient individuals were still capable of being influenced, for example, by the alcohol use of their siblings, in such a way that their own alcohol use was elevated compared to ALDH deficient individuals with lower levels of exposure to such environmental influences."

Lower Level of Response to Alcohol   Some individuals react slower than others to the effects of alcohol, which is sometimes referred to as a low intensity response and which also appears to be a genetic intermediate characteristic, also known as an endophenotype. It seems paradoxical, but often because such individuals have to drink *more* alcohol in order to achieve the euphoric and other disinhibiting effects of alcohol, they have a greater risk for the subsequent development of alcoholism. Some racial and ethnic groups have a low intensity response to alcohol, including Koreans and Native Americans.

Research published by Geoff Joslyn and colleagues in a 2008 issue of *Proceedings of the National Academy of Sciences* found that two genetic markers that showed a strong association with lung cancer and nicotine dependence were also associated with a low intensity of response to alcohol. These markers were found on chromosome 15q25.1, although it was not possible to isolate the specific gene out of six possibilities. Among 367 siblings, the researchers found that two markers from nicotine studies shows a linkage with several low intensity response phenotypes.

According to the researchers, "Level of response (LR) to alcohol is an intermediate phenotype for AUDs [alcohol use disorders], and individuals with a low LR are at increased risk. A high rate of concurrent alcohol and nicotine use and dependence suggests that these conditions may share biochemical and genetic mechanisms."

Impulsivity, Disinhibition, and Sensation-seeking   Individuals who are impulsive, sensation-seeking, and externalizing are more likely to get into trouble than others. Alcoholism is only one type of problem that they may experience. Externalizing behaviors are linked to a diagnosis of oppositional defiant disorder, a diagnosis of behavior that is defiant and blaming of others for self-generated problems in childhood, and antisocial personality disorder in adulthood. These diagnoses increase the risk for an early onset of alcohol abuse and alcohol dependence.

A study of mostly Korean adoptees (68 percent), drawn from the Minnesota Sibling Interaction and Behavior Study (SIBS), that compared them to nonadoptees was reported by Serena M. King and colleagues in *Addiction* in 2009. The sample size included 132 adopted and 113 nonadopted adolescents with at least one parent with a lifetime diagnosis of alcoholism. Of these children, 78 nonadopted and 71 adopted were exposed to at least one symptom of alcohol abuse or alcoholism within their lifetimes. The researchers found that higher levels of disinhibition were present only among the biological children of parents with alcohol dependence; however, they also found the adopted children were about four times more likely to consume alcohol when the adoptive parent was an alcoholic.

Among the adolescents who were *not* adopted, parental alcoholism was associated with an increased risk for antisocial attitudes, aggressive personality, delinquent behavior, impulsive personality, tobacco use, and alcohol use. Among the adoptees, however, the sole effect of the parental dependence was a *decreased* level of impulsivity, that is, they were less impulsive. Said the researchers, "These results imply that what is transmitted genetically is a general tendency toward behavioral disinhibition, one that extends across substance use, personality traits, attitudes, and behaviors."

Psychiatric Disorders that Increase the Risk for Alcohol Use Disorders Some psychiatric disorders with a high rate of heritability also increase the risk for alcoholism, particularly antisocial personality disorder, as well as SCHIZOPHRENIA, BIPOLAR DISORDER, and some anxiety disorders, such as PANIC DISORDER, POSTTRAUMATIC STRESS DISORDER, and SOCIAL PHOBIA. (See PSYCHIATRIC COMORBIDITIES.)

In their 2002 article on childhood antisocial behavior and adolescent alcohol use disorders in *Alcohol Research & Health,* authors Duncan B. Clark, M.D., Michael Vanyukov, and Jack Cornelius, M.D., reported that antisocial behaviors in childhood and adolescent alcohol use disorders may share both genetic and environmental influences. The child with antisocial behaviors may be diagnosed with oppositional defiant disorder (ODD) or a more severe diagnosis of CONDUCT DISORDER (CD). The child with CD is actively aggressive toward other people and animals, destroys property, lies, steals, starts fights, and exhibits other problem behaviors. The child with ODD argues with adults, easily loses his or her temper, purposely annoys others, blames others for his or her own behavior, and expresses anger or vindictiveness toward others.

Severe ODD or CD persists throughout childhood and adolescence. CD may develop into the adult diagnosis of antisocial personality disorder (ASPD), known in the past as sociopathic behavior. ASPD is defined by behavior such as stealing and causing harm to others, and many prisoners have ASPD. (Not everyone with ASPD goes to jail, however, such as high-functioning sociopaths who elude detection.)

Clark and colleagues note that the environment is also important, and say, "For example, for AUDs to develop, alcohol availability in the environment (e.g. from family or friends) is a necessary but not sufficient condition. An adolescent who chooses peers who use alcohol and other drugs may be more frequently exposed to alcohol than is an adolescent with a different peer group." The adolescent with CD, however, is more likely to be drawn to those adolescents who *do* drink and use drugs.

Other Adoption and Twin Studies

In a study that was reported by Richard J. Rose and Danielle M. Dick in *Alcohol Research & Health* in 2004/2005, the authors analyzed studies of alcohol and drinking patterns among adopted adolescents, and they reported that "these studies indicate that drinking initiation is determined primarily by environmental influences, whereas the establishment of drinking patterns is determined by genetic factors, which themselves are subject to moderation by the environment."

The authors also noted that there are apparent gene-environment correlations, whereby individuals actively seek those environments that specifically match their own genetic predispositions. For example, the acting-out adolescent will be more attracted to other acting-out adolescents. He or she is also more likely to be rejected by adolescents who are devoted to their studies. Thus, the acting-out adolescent is unlikely to be accepted by the honor students or the cheerleaders.

The authors also discussed a study of Finnish twins (known as the FinnTwin studies) which found that the role of the environment shared by the twins played the largest role in causing the twins to use alcohol by age 14 or be abstinent. The authors said, "These factors—which included the familial environment and the nonfamilial environments of peers, schools and neighborhoods—accounted for 76 percent of the variation in drinking initiation in both boys and girls."

The FinnTwin study also looked at the frequency of the diagnosis of conduct disorder and found a high rate; 44 percent had one or more symptoms of CD, and 12 percent met the full diagnostic criteria for CD. Most of the twins diagnosed with CD were boys: 65 percent. The researchers found that genetic factors had a substantial impact in the diagnosis of CD. Said the authors, "One inference from these results is that CD is an early manifestation of a genetic predisposition that later contributes to the development of alcohol-related problems and alcohol dependence." Thus, experts should focus on adolescents with symptoms of CD to work on preventive measures against alcoholism.

The Ability to Produce and Amass Acetaldehyde

Some researchers have found that higher levels of ACETALDEHYDE, the substance that metabolizes alcohol, are protective against alcohol dependence. In a study by Young-Gyu Chai and colleagues, published in the *American Journal of Psychiatry* in 2005, the researchers tested three groups of Korean men, including 38 nonalcoholic control subjects, 48 men with an onset of alcoholism after age 25 (sometimes known as type I alcoholism and which is also found in women), and 24 men with an early inherited onset of alcohol dependence (also known as type II alcoholism, which is found only in men).

They found distinct genetic differences in the men with type II alcoholism compared to the nonalcoholic men and those with type I alcoholism, who were about the same genetically. The researchers found a significantly higher frequency of low-active ADH2 (43 percent) and ADH3 (58 percent) in the men with type II alcoholism than in the men with type I alcoholism (23 percent of ADH2 and 24 percent of ADH3). The control group

had results that were about the same as the men with type I alcoholism.

The researchers said, "Subjects with type II alcoholism are genetically less likely to experience adverse physiological consequences of alcohol consumption than those with type I alcoholism." (As mentioned earlier, an ability to consume larger quantities of alcohol from when drinking started is a risk factor for alcohol dependence.) Said the authors, "We presume that the genetic characteristics of alcohol metabolism of type I alcoholism fall between nonalcoholism and type II alcoholism."

In a related study, Camila Guindalini and colleagues compared the genetic variants of alcohol dehydrogenase 4 in patients with and without alcoholism, reporting on their findings in the *American Journal of Psychiatry* in 2005. According to the researchers, the gene for ADH4 is mapped to 4q22. The researchers found that the 92 healthy subjects were much more likely to have two genetic alleles that were associated with active forms of the ADH4 than were the 92 patients with alcohol dependence. According to the researchers, "These preliminary results suggest that ADH4 may play a role in the etiology of alcohol dependence."

Brain Differences

In their research on the orbitofrontal cortex among the offspring of families with parental alcohol dependence, Shirley Y. Hill and colleagues found a genetic susceptibility for alcoholism in some subjects, evidenced by a disruption of their orbitofrontal cortex laterality. This means the subjects had a decreased volume in the right hemisphere of the orbitofrontal cortex, which is a factor that is also significantly linked to variations in such genes as the 5-HTT and BDNF genes.

The researchers studied 107 subjects with an average age of 17.6 years. Sixty-three of the subjects were considered high-risk because of their family history of alcohol dependence, and each high-risk subject had an average of four first and second degree relatives who were alcoholics. The 44 low-risk offspring had no first or second degree relatives with either alcohol or drug dependence. Prior to the brain scan, the high-risk subjects had a much greater rate of DEPRESSION (20.7 percent) compared to the low-risk group (3.6 percent). In addition, 24.1 percent of the high risk group had ATTENTION-DEFICIT/HYPERACTIVITY DISORDER (ADHD) compared to zero with ADHD in the low risk group. The presence of oppositional defiant disorder was much higher in the high-risk group, or 17.2 percent compared to 7.1 percent in the low-risk group. More of the individuals in the high-risk group had already been diagnosed with alcohol or drug abuse (6.9 percent) compared to those in the low-risk group (3.6 percent).

The brain scan revealed that the high-risk (HR) group had significant brain differences compared to the low-risk (LR) group. The researchers said, "Our results suggest that the reduced volume of right OFC seen in HR offspring has implications for behavioral disinhibition and development of SUDs [substance use disorders, such as alcohol abuse/alcoholism or drug abuse/drug addiction]. Development changes in disinhibition appear to be most profound during adolescence and young adulthood."

The researchers noted it was not the total volume of the OFC that was different between the HR and LR groups, but instead, the right side of the OFC had a greater volume than the left side in the high-risk group. They noted that some animals react more rapidly when a predator appears on their left side, and there are benefits and risks associated with lateralization. At some time long past, speculated the researchers, a reduced volume of the OFC in the right hemisphere might have conferred an advantage; for example, risk-takers are faster to move on to new environments under adverse circumstances. According to the researchers, "However, risk-taking during adolescence can have lethal consequences. Identification of genetic variations associated with an OFC reduction and increased impulsivity may provide important clues for medication development for those at highest risk."

Differences in Neurotransmitters

Some researchers seeking to find differences in the genetic susceptibility to alcoholism (and sometimes to alcohol abuse) concentrate on neurotransmitters, specifically with regard to brain chemicals associated with the metabolism of alcohol, such as dopamine, gamma amino butyric acid (GABA), glutamate, and other biochemicals.

In a study by Gunter Schumann, M.D., and colleagues, reported in *Archives of General Psychiatry* in 2008, the researchers analyzed genetic variations in neurotransmission genes for the glutamate neurotransmitter, based on a study of 1,337 patients and 1,555 controls in several different studies. They found that genetic variations in NR2A had the greatest linkage to a diagnosis of alcohol dependence. These genes were also associated with an early onset of alcoholism, a family history of alcohol dependence, and risky drinking patterns among adolescents.

Other neurotransmitters that may increase susceptibility to alcohol dependence are those that affect the release of dopamine, which activates the brain's reward system. Low levels of serotonin, another neurotransmitter, are linked with increased rates of social withdrawal, impulsivity, aggression, and increased drinking. N-methyl-D-asparte (NMDA) has been implicated with alcoholism. Alcohol decreases the impact of NMDA, which may cause the depressant effects of alcohol. Gamma aminobutyric acid (GABA) is another neurotransmitter implicated in alcoholism, and alcohol increases the actions of GABA.

Endogenous opioids (not to be confused with misused drugs stemming from opiates, which are also referred to as opioids) are natural neurotransmitters, and alcohol causes their release and also alters opioid receptors. Research may show that natural opioids are implicated in alcohol dependence.

See also ADOPTION AND TWIN STUDIES AND ALCOHOL.

Chai, Y. G., et al. "Alcohol and Aldehyde Dehydrogenase Polymorphisms in Men with Type I and Type II Alcoholism." *American Journal of Psychiatry* 162, no. 5 (2005): 1,003–1,005.

Clark, Duncan B., M.D. "Childhood Antisocial Behavior and Adolescent Alcohol Use Disorders." *Alcohol Research & Health* 26, no. 2 (2002): 109–115.

Dick, Danielle M., and Arpane Agrawal. "The Genetics of Alcohol and Other Drug Dependence." *Alcohol Research & Health* 31, no. 2 (2008): 111–167.

Edenberg, Howard J. "The Genetics of Alcohol Metabolism: Role of Alcohol Dehydrogenase and Aldehyde Dehydrogenase Variants." *Alcohol Research & Health* 30, no. 1 (2007): 5–13.

George, David T., et al. "Neurokinin 1 Receptor Antagonism as a Possible Therapy for Alcoholism." *Science* 319 (2008): 1,536–1,539.

Guindalini, C., et al. "Association of Genetic Variants of Alcohol Dehydrogenase 4 with Alcohol Dependence in Brazilian Patients." *American Journal of Psychiatry* 162, no. 5 (2005): 1,005–1,007.

Hampton, Tracy. "Interplay of Genes and Environment Found in Adolescents' Alcohol Abuse." *Journal of the American Medical Association* 295, no. 15 (2006): 1,760–1,762.

Hill, Shirley Y., et al. "Disruption of Orbitofrontal Cortex Laterality in Offspring from Multiplex Alcohol Dependence Families." *Biological Psychiatry* 65, no. 2 (2009): 129–136.

Irons, Daniel E., et al. "Mendelian Randomization: A Novel Test for the Gateway Hypothesis and Models of Gene-Environment Interplay." *Development and Psychopathology* 19, no. 4 (2007): 1,181–1,195.

Joslyn, Geoff. "Chromosome 15q25.1 Genetic Markers Associated with Level of Response to Alcohol in Humans." *Proceedings of the National Academy of Sciences* 105, no. 51 (2008): 20,368–20,373.

Karpyak, Victor M., et al. "Sequences Variations of the Human MPDZ Gene and Association with Alcoholism in Subjects with European Ancestry." *Alcohol: Clinical and Experimental Research* 33, no. 4 (2009): 712–721.

King, Serena M., et al. "Parental Alcohol Dependence and the Transmission of Adolescent Behavioral Disinhibition: A Study of Adoptive and Non-Adoptive Families." *Addiction* 104, no. 4 (2009): 578–586.

Köhnke, Michael D. "Approach to the Genetics of Alcoholism: A Review Based on Pathophysiology." *Biochemical Pharmacology* 75, no. 1 (2008): 160–177.

Liu, I-Chao, M.D. "Genetic and Environmental Contributions to the Development of Alcohol Dependence in Male Twins." *Archives of General Psychiatry* 61 (2004): 897–903.

Nurnberger, John I., Jr., M.D., et al. "A Family Study of Alcohol Dependence: Coaggregation of Multiple Disorders in Relatives of Alcohol-Dependent Probands." *Archives of General Psychiatry* 61, no. 9 (2004): 1,246–1,256.

Rose, Richard J., and Danielle M. Dick. "Gene-Environment Interplay in Adolescent Drinking Behavior." *Alcohol Research & Health* 28, no. 4 (2004/2005): 222–229.

Schuckit, Marc A., M.D. "An Overview of Genetic Influences in Alcoholism." *Journal of Substance Abuse Treatment* 36, Suppl. 1 (2009): S5–S14.

Schuckit, M. A., and T. L. Smith. "The Relationships of a Family History of Alcohol Dependence, a Low Level of Response to Alcohol and Six Domains of Life Functioning to the Development of Alcohol Use Disorders." *Journal of Studies on Alcohol* 61, no. 6 (2000): 827–835.

Schumann, Gunter, M.D., et al. "Systematic Analysis of Glutamatergic Neurotransmission Genes in Alcohol Dependence and Adolescent Risky Drinking Behavior." *Archives of General Psychiatry* 65, no. 7 (2008): 826–838.

Sigardsson, Sören, Michael Bohman, M.D., and C. Robert Cloninger, M.D. "Replication of the Stockholm Adoption Study of Alcoholism: Confirmatory Cross-Fostering Analysis." *Archives of General Psychiatry* 53, no. 8 (1996): 681–687.

health issues and alcoholism See EXCESSIVE
DRINKING AND HEALTH CONSEQUENCES.

hepatitis Inflammation of the liver that is caused
either by infection with one of three primary hepatitis viruses (hepatitis A, B, C) or by chronic and
excessive drinking. It is also possible for a person
who is a very heavy drinker with an inflamed liver
and an impaired immune system to contract a viral
form of hepatitis and thus suffer from *both* forms
of the disease.

If the hepatitis is caused by drinking, this is
called alcoholic hepatitis. Alcoholic hepatitis is the
second stage of alcoholic liver disease (ALD). The
first major stage is fatty liver disease. The third
stage is CIRRHOSIS of the liver, an irreversible condition that eventually requires a liver transplant for
the individual to survive. In addition, a person with
cirrhosis has an increased risk for the development
of liver CANCER.

The prevalence of viral hepatitis has been declin-
ing in recent years. According to the National Center for Health Statistics in 2009, incidences of acute
hepatitis A have plummeted from a high of 28.9
cases per 100,000 population in 1971 to the 2006
level of 1.2 cases per 100,000 people. The high
for hepatitis B was 11.5 cases per 100,000 people
in 1985, down to 1.6 cases per 100,000 people in
2006. Acute hepatitis C was at its highest level of
2.4 cases per 100,000 people in 1993, and the rate
was 0.3 cases per 100,000 people in 2006 or less
than 1 person for every 100,000 people.

Symptoms and Diagnostic Path

Hepatitis A is a common infection that is transmitted through contaminated food or drink. It
generally causes no problems or even any symptoms, although symptoms may include nausea,
fatigue, abdominal pain, headache, and light-
colored stools. Hepatitis B is more problematic
and is transmitted through contact with the body
fluids of another person, such as blood or semen.
Men who have sex with other men are at risk for
hepatitis B, as are intravenous drug addicts who
share needles. Most people with the early stages
of hepatitis B have no symptoms, but if symptoms
are present, they are similar to the symptoms of
hepatitis A. Children in the United States today
are vaccinated against both hepatitis A and B in
early childhood.

Hepatitis C is a virus transmitted through body
fluids such as blood and dirty needles. The symptoms of hepatitis C are similar to those of hepatitis
A and B, or abdominal pain, fatigue, fever, diarrhea, and a lack of appetite. Hepatitis C is the
leading cause of scarring of the liver, according to
hepatitis expert Charles S. Lieber, M.D.

Treatment Options and Outlook

If an individual has only alcoholic hepatitis and
no viral forms of hepatitis, the treatment is to end
drinking. If the person stops drinking, the outlook
is generally favorable.

If an individual has a viral form of hepatitis,
the treatment depends on the virus. Hepatitis A
patients must avoid all alcohol to prevent further
damage to the liver. Individuals with hepatitis B are
also treated with interferon injections. Hepatitis C
is treated with interferon and ribavarin.

If the person with hepatitis C continues to
drink, he or she doubles the risk of developing
hepatocellular carcinoma, a form of liver cancer.
Continued drinking also markedly reduces the
ability of interferon to counteract the effects of the
disease.

Risk Factors and Preventive Measures

According to liver expert Charles Lieber, M.D., infection with hepatitis C is common in alcoholics, and the course of the disease can be hastened with alcohol consumption. According to Lieber, "Therefore, the reduction or complete cessation of alcohol consumption should be a primary focus of the treatment of HCV-infected patients. In addition, there is a persistent need for novel effective and safe treatments to arrest or reverse disease progression to the dismal end-stages. Various antioxidant and antifibrotic agents have shown promise in experimental animals, and some of these are being studied in HCV-infected humans."

According to Dr. Schiff and Dr. Ozden in their article on hepatitis C, nearly a third of alcoholics with clinical symptoms of liver disease are infected with hepatitis C.

See also EXCESSIVE DRINKING AND HEALTH CONSEQUENCES; LIVER DISEASES, ALCOHOLIC.

Lieber, Charles S., M.D. "Alcohol and Hepatitis C." *Alcohol Research & Health* 25, no. 4 (2001): 245–254.
Schiff, Eugene R., M.D., and Nuri Ozden, M.D. "Hepatitis C and Alcohol." *Alcohol Research & Health* 27, no. 3 (2003): 232–239.

histrionic personality disorder See PERSONALITY DISORDERS.

hospital patients and alcohol-related admissions Alcohol is the cause of, or at least a significant factor in, many traumatic injuries, accidents, and illnesses. In some cases, a patient may be dependent on alcohol, while in other cases, the intoxication is not linked to alcoholism. Ronald V. Maier, M.D., wrote in 2005 in the *Journal of Trauma,* "Alcohol intoxication is the leading risk factor for injury. It is a well-established fact that alcohol consumption contributes to unintentional and intentional injury and to mortality overall." Unintentional injuries may be caused by intoxicated individuals involved in car crashes or falls, while intentional injuries, according to Maier, may be caused by the antisocial and disruptive behaviors that alcohol can induce, with the most severe behaviors including homicide and SUICIDE. Alcohol is also a key link to hospital admissions related to DEPRESSION.

According to Maier, "For more than 20 years, alcohol has been consistently linked in 40% to 50% of deaths resulting from motor vehicle crashes; 20% to 70% of deaths caused by occupational and domestic incidents, fires, and drowning; and approximately 50% to 60% of deaths attributable to intentional injuries."

According to Ting-King Li, M.D., of the National Institute on Alcohol Abuse and Alcoholism (NIAAA) in a 2004 presentation, from 20–40 percent of hospital admissions are alcohol-related. Yet experts report that as many as half of those who have alcohol use disorders and are admitted to hospitals for health problems are not diagnosed as alcohol abusers by physicians. As a result, many experts believe that patients admitted to the hospital, particularly for an emergency or a trauma, should be briefly screened for their alcohol use.

According to Larry M. Gentilello, M.D., in his article for the *Journal of Trauma* in 2007, some trauma patients remain at high risk of reinjury or death for years after their discharge from the hospital. Gentilello says, "The characteristic that most readily identifies this high risk group is excessive alcohol use. After trauma center discharge, the unexpected death rate for patients with a positive blood alcohol test [for alcohol intoxication] is almost 200% greater than for patients who were not drinking at the time of injury, with most of these deaths occurring as a result of repeat injuries." In other words, those patients who had been drinking when they were severely injured were likely to drink again—and to be injured again.

In their article in the *Journal of the American College of Surgery* in 2008, Francine Terrell and colleagues reported that evidence supports the effectiveness of screening patients in acute-care medical and surgical settings, despite their initial diagnosis. In their study of trauma unit facilities nationwide, the researchers found that greater than 70 percent of the surveyed sites were using laboratory tests to screen trauma patients for alcohol, while others used questionnaires with the patients to perform their screening.

Dr. Gentilello said that studies have shown that patients randomized to either a brief intervention group or to standard trauma care in the hospital have shown distinctive differences, with a 47 percent reduced readmission rate for the brief intervention group.

For those who worry that it is too expensive to provide such services in the hospital, Gentilello says, "Feasibility studies have shown that the intervention needs of even the busiest trauma centers in the United States can be met by approximately one half-time employee, and that individuals without prior expertise in alcohol counseling can provide effective interventions after relatively little training."

According to a study in Australia by Anne M. Roche, Toby Freeman, and Natalie Skinner reported in *Drug and Alcohol Dependence* in 2006, an analysis of 65 studies and 100,980 patients revealed that blood alcohol levels taken from the patients were nearly twice as likely to yield a rate indicating intoxication compared to the self-reports of patients. In addition, males were two to four times more likely than females to screen positive for intoxication. In hospital emergency rooms, patients ages 20–40 years old were the most likely to be drunken, as were hospital inpatients ages 30–50 years old.

Roche and her colleagues strongly supported screening patients for alcohol and said, "Hospitals are particularly well suited to screening for problematic alcohol use. They often have large numbers of alcohol-related admissions from both acute (e.g. accidents and injuries, violence, deliberate self harm, acute alcohol poisoning) and chronic drinking (e.g. cardiac arrhythmias, pancreatitis)."

Some patients are discharged from short-stay community hospitals with an alcohol-related diagnosis. For example, according to Chiung M. Chen and Hsiao-Ye Yi in their report for the NIAAA in 2007, there were 441,000 discharge episodes for patients ages 15 and older with a first-listed alcohol-related diagnosis. There were also 1.6 million discharge episodes in which patients had any alcohol-related diagnosis.

The researchers noted that for the first time in 2005, ALCOHOLIC PSYCHOSIS diagnoses surpassed diagnoses for alcohol dependence; alcoholic psychosis represented 36 percent of principal diagnoses, followed by alcohol dependence (30 percent), then CIRRHOSIS of the liver (26 percent), and then nondependent alcohol abuse. Most patients with alcohol-related diagnoses were males ages 45 to 64 years.

See also ALCOHOL AND WOMEN; ALCOHOLISM/ ALCOHOL DEPENDENCE AND ALCOHOL ABUSE; EXCESSIVE DRINKING AND HEALTH CONSEQUENCES; EXCESSIVE DRINKING AND SOCIAL CONSEQUENCES; IMPAIRED PHYSICIANS; INTERVENTION, BRIEF.

Chen, Chiung M., and Hsiao-ye Yi. *Trends in Alcohol-Related Morbidity Among Short-Stay Community Hospital Discharges, United States, 1979–2005.* Washington, D.C.: National Institute of Alcohol Abuse and Alcoholism, August 2007.

Gentilello, Larry M., M.D. "Alcohol and Injury: American College of Surgeons Committee on Trauma Requirements for Trauma Center Intervention." *Journal of Trauma: Injury, Infection, and Critical Care* 62, Supp. (2007): S44–S45.

Li, Ting-Kai, M.D. *Alcohol Use Disorders and Co-occurring Conditions.* Bethesda, Md.: National Institute on Alcohol Abuse and Alcoholism, June 24, 2004.

Maier, Ronald V., M.D. "Controlling Alcohol Problems among Hospitalized Trauma Patients." *Journal of Trauma: Injury, Infection and Critical Care* 59, no. 3 (2005): S1–S2.

Terrell, Francine, et al. "Nationwide Survey of Alcohol Screening and Brief Intervention Practices at US Level 1 Trauma Centers." *Journal of the American College of Surgery* 207, no. 5 (2008): 630–638.

impaired physicians Doctors whose work performance is negatively affected by the excessive use of alcohol. In the case of physicians, formal agencies in most states in the United States provide state licensing boards that administer programs to doctors who have been identified as having an alcohol and/or drug problem that impedes their work. In general, the doctor may be referred to a rehabilitative program by colleagues or by regulatory agencies or others. An evaluation of the physician is made, and then he or she is given the opportunity to sign a contract agreeing to supervision until formal treatment and at least five years of regular urine testing reveals that the physician is no longer impaired.

In a study by McLellan et al. of 904 doctors enrolled in 16 formal treatment programs from 1995 to 2001, the researchers found that 19.3 percent of the physicians failed the program, most failing right away. This means that the majority of the physicians, 80.7 percent, succeeded with the program, an excellent success rate. Of the physicians who continued their practices under supervision, 19 percent were found to have an alcohol or drug misuse within the five-year period of supervision. At the point of their five-year follow-up, the researchers reported that 78.7 percent of the doctors were still licensed and practicing physicians, while 10.8 percent had had their medical licenses revoked, 3.5 percent had retired, 3.7 percent had died, and the status of 3.2 percent was unknown. This is a very positive success rate.

A similar success rate was described in a 21-year follow-up of 100 alcoholic doctors in England, reported in *Alcohol & Alcoholism* in 2002. According to author Gareth Lloyd, there was a 73 percent recovery rate among the doctors over the long-term, and there was a direct correlation between ABSTINENCE and recovery (although 3 percent of the formerly alcoholic doctors were reportedly able to drink normally rather than abstaining altogether from alcohol). In the first six months of the physicians' recovery from their alcohol dependence, there was also direct correlation between success and their attendance at mutual aid self-help groups; however, attendance eventually fell off, and after 20 years, only 14 doctors still attended regular meetings.

Some of the doctors relapsed to drinking, but of the 49 physicians who relapsed, 45 of them ultimately recovered. This is an astonishing 92 percent success rate among those who relapsed. It is testimony to the fact that a relapse does *not* mean that a person who relapses cannot recover. Instead, relapses are considered common among many people with alcohol dependence.

A total of 20 of the doctors in this study did *not* recover from their alcoholism, and they ultimately died of alcohol-related deaths, according to their relatives; for example, five of the doctors reportedly died of liver failure, five died of an overdose of alcohol and drugs, three physicians died of a gastrointestinal hemorrhage, two died from inhaling car exhaust fumes, two died from inhaling vomit, and the cause of death was not provided in three cases. In addition, as mentioned, five of the doctors recovered but then relapsed and died, including two who died of an overdose of alcohol and drugs, two who died of liver failure, and one who died of an inhalation of car exhaust fumes.

In another study of 100 physicians in a substance abuse program in Ontario, the Canadian doctors in the program were treated for alcohol or drug abuse. In this study, most of the participants were male (90 percent) and were married or living with a partner (66 percent). About half (51 percent) were alcohol abusers. The researchers also found that smokers were overrepresented in this program; 38 percent of the impaired doctors were smokers, compared to 5 percent of doctors in general in Canada. The doctors, who were enrolled in the Ontario Physician Health Program for substance dependence, had a high rate of success; 85 percent completed the program. Of the 85 percent, 71 percent had no known relapse, while 14 percent relapsed and then subsequently completed the program.

Finally, in a study reported by Erica Frank and colleagues on 2,316 medical students at 16 medical schools in the United States and their alcohol consumption, the researchers found that 78 percent of the students reported drinking in the past month and a third reported excessive (binge) drinking. The researchers concluded that BINGE DRINKING was common among medical students, although it was less common than among their same-age, nonmedical peers in the population (or about 40 percent among adults ages 25–34 years). Men were more likely to engage in binge drinking (43 percent) than women (24 percent).

The researchers recommended that medical schools screen their students for alcohol misuse and also work to discourage heavy drinking among medical students. They said, "Medical students' personal and clinical attitudes about alcohol have important implications for their current care of patients. Furthermore, drinking practices in young adulthood help to establish patterns for later drinking. If medical students are better educated about guidelines for low risk drinking and screening and counselling for alcohol misuse, they might be more likely to adhere to clinical guidelines and be better equipped to identify and reduce excessive drinking among their patients. Medical schools should also consider supporting the implementation of effective interventions to reduce excessive drinking among medical students and the general population."

See also EMPLOYEE ASSISTANCE PROGRAMS; EXCESSIVE DRINKING AND HEALTH CONSEQUENCES; OCCUPATIONS; STAGES OF CHANGE; TREATMENT.

Brewster, Joan M., et al. "Characteristics and Outcomes of Doctors in a Substance Dependence Monitoring Programme in Canada: Prospective Descriptive Study." *British Medical Journal* 337 (2008): a2,098.

Frank, Erica, et al. "Alcohol Consumption and Alcohol Counselling Behaviour among U.S. Medical Students: Cohort Study." *British Medical Journal* 337 (2008): a2,155.

Lloyd, Gareth. "One Hundred Alcoholic Doctors: A 21-Year Follow-Up." *Alcohol & Alcoholism* 37, no. 4 (2002): 370–374.

McLellan, A. Thomas, et al. "Five Year Outcomes in a Cohort Study of Physicians Treated for Substance Use Disorders in the United States." *British Medical Journal* 337 (2008): a2,038.

impulse control disorders   Disorders that are characterized by extreme impulsivity and compulsivity, and which cause serious distress and harm to the individual's life. Impulse control disorders, as defined by the American Psychiatric Association, include PATHOLOGICAL GAMBLING, PYROMANIA (compulsive fire setting), KLEPTOMANIA (compulsive stealing), TRICHOTILLOMANIA (compulsive pulling of the hair), and INTERMITTENT EXPLOSIVE DISORDER, or uncontrollable rage leading to property damage or physical harm to others (the most commonly known example is "road rage").

Some studies have found that individuals with Parkinson's disease have an increased risk for some impulse control disorders, such as intermittent explosive disorder and pathological gambling. According to Daniel Weintraub, M.D., risk factors for a Parkinson's patient developing an impulse control disorder include such factors as a family or personal history of substance abuse or BIPOLAR DISORDER, male gender, a younger age at the onset of Parkinson's disease, a previous history of impulsive disorder symptoms, and an impulsive personality. Treatment with dopamine agonists (medications used to treat Parkinson's disease), particularly at high dosages, may exacerbate the problem.

In each of these cases, the risk for alcohol abuse and ALCOHOLISM is elevated compared to individuals who do not have these disorders. For example, according to Robert H. Piertrzak et al., among older adults, the risk for an alcohol use disorder (alcohol abuse or alcohol dependence) is 12.8 percent among non-gamblers but rises to more than half (53.2 percent) among "disordered" (pathological) gamblers. In addition, "recreational gamblers" (or problem gamblers, a lower order of disorder than pathological gambling) had an alcohol use disorder rate of 30.1 percent.

Authors Eric Hollander et al. have written about the commonalities between all impulse control disorders in their chapter in *Clinical Manual of Impulse Control Disorders*, and they say that there are three areas that dominate each impulse control disorder. The first problem is the inability to delay gratification, which is present in every form of impulse control disorder. Next is a high level of distractibility, or an inability to remain focused on a task. The last feature of an impulse control disorder is disinhibition, or the inability to restrain their behavior to accepted social and cultural norms.

Some researchers have found a link between dopamine and the presence of impulse control disorders such as pathological gambling in individuals with Parkinson's disease. According to Daniel Weintraub in his article for *Annals of Neurology* in 2008, there is no evidence that psychiatric medications that may help individuals with impulse disorders but who do not have Parkinson's disease will have any efficacy at all in those with Parkinson's disease.

It is also true that prior to committing the impulsive act, the person with an impulse control disorder experiences an increasing tension or a sense of arousal. This feeling is replaced with one of gratification or pleasure as well as the relief of this tension when the act is committed, whether it is setting a fire, stealing an item, or another act associated with the disorder.

See also ADDICTIVE PERSONALITY; ANTISOCIAL PERSONALITY DISORDER/ANTISOCIAL BEHAVIOR; ANXIETY DISORDERS; ATTENTION-DEFICIT/HYPERACTIVITY DISORDER; BIPOLAR DISORDER; CONDUCT DISORDER; DEPRESSION; PERSONALITY DISORDERS; PSYCHIATRIC COMORBIDITIES; SCHIZOPHRENIA.

Adamec, Christine. *Impulse Control Disorders.* New York: Chelsea House, 2008.

Grant, Jon E. *Impulse Control Disorders: A Clinician's Guide to Understanding and Treating Behavioral Addictions.* New York: W.W. Norton, 2008.

Hollander, Eric, M.D., Bryann R. Baker, Jessica Kahn, and Dan J. Stein, M.D. "Conceptualizing and Assessing Impulse-Control Disorders." In *Clinical Manual of Impulse-Control Disorders,* edited by Eric Hollander, M.D. and Dan J. Stein, 1–18. Washington, D.C.: American Psychiatric Publishing, Inc., 2006.

LaSalle, V. Holland, et al. "Diagnostic Interview Assessed Neuropsychiatric Disorder Comorbidity in 334 Individuals with Obsessive-Compulsive Disorder." *Depression and Anxiety* 19, no. 3 (2004): 163–173.

Lejoyeux, Michel, et al. "Study of Impulse-Control Disorders among Alcohol-Dependent Patients." *Journal of Clinical Psychiatry* 60, no. 5 (1999): 302–305.

New, Antonia S., et al. "Low Prolactin Response to Fenfluramine in Impulsive Aggression." *Journal of Psychiatric Research* 38, no. 3 (2004): 223–230.

Weintraub, Daniel, M.D. "Dopamine and Impulse Control Disorders in Parkinson's Disease." *Annals of Neurology* 64, Supp. (2008): S93–S100.

initiation of drinking   See AGE AND ALCOHOL; EXCESSIVE DRINKING AND NEGATIVE SOCIAL CONSEQUENCES.

intermittent explosive disorder   *Intermittent explosive disorder* refers to recurrent extreme rages that are out of all proportion to whatever is going on around the individual. People with "road rage" may have intermittent explosive disorder (IED), as do others who suddenly fly into a state of extreme anger. Individuals with IED may be violent. They are also at risk for alcohol abuse; Kessler et al. found that 32.9 percent of those with IED abused alcohol, and 17 percent were alcoholics.

Symptoms and Diagnostic Path

Individuals with IED have exhibited past rages that have damaged property and sometimes harmed individuals. In these episodes, the rage usually is short-lived, and then the individual with IED may act like he or she wonders why others are very distressed. For the person with IED, their anger is completely over, like a fast-moving summer storm.

Treatment Options and Outlook

It is difficult to treat IED. The disorder may be treated with anger management therapy as well as with mood stabilizers, antidepressants, and beta blocker medications. In some cases, antipsychotic drugs such as risperidone (Risperdal) are prescribed as treatment for IED. If the patient has ATTENTION-DEFICIT/HYPERACTIVITY DISORDER in addition to IED, then drugs in the serotonin norepinephrine reuptake inhibitor class may be prescribed, such as duloxetine (Cymbalta) or venlafaxine (Effexor).

Risk Factors and Preventive Measures

Men are more likely than women to have IED, although some females have the disorder. According to Ronald Kessler, the lifetime prevalence of IED is 6.3 percent, and the average age of onset is 14 years. IED is linked to alcohol dependence; for example, in a study by Michel Lejoyeux et al. of 79 patients hospitalized for detoxification, 24 percent also met the criteria for IED. (In addition, 9 percent met the criteria for PATHOLOGICAL GAMBLING.)

See also IMPULSE CONTROL DISORDERS.

Kessler, Ronald C., et al. "The Prevalence and Correlates of DSM-IV Intermittent Explosive Disorder in the National Comorbidity Survey Replication." *Archives of General Psychiatry* 63, no. 6 (2006): 669–678.

intervention, brief An attempt by a physician (and sometimes by a psychologist or social worker) to identify problem drinking (alcohol abuse and sometimes BINGE DRINKING) and, if it is present, to assist the patient in determining what steps should be taken to resolve the problem. A brief intervention is *not* the same as when family and friends join together to try to compel an individual to enter a rehabilitative facility and to overcome his or her DENIAL that there is a problem with alcohol. Brief interventions usually are not effective in individuals with alcohol dependence, who require inpatient or intensive outpatient treatment as well as an ongoing association with a successful support group, such as Alcoholics Anonymous.

The National Institute on Alcohol Abuse and Alcoholism (NIAAA) recommends that all patients be interviewed each year regarding their alcohol use. A brief intervention may occur in a regularly scheduled patient visit. It may also occur in the course of EMERGENCY TREATMENT. Some studies have shown that about a third of emergency room patients and as many as half of severely injured trauma patients test positive for alcohol.

Yet experts report that many physicians are very hesitant to address possible problem drinking with their patients, perhaps for fear of upsetting or offending them or because they do not wish to take the time to perform the screening. They may also dislike treating patients with alcohol use problems.

According to Charles O'Brien in his article on the use of the CAGE questionnaire for the *Journal of the American Medical Association,* only about 30 percent of primary care physicians routinely perform brief interventions, and more than half (55 percent) use the CAGE questionnaire. Says O'Brien, "The tendency to omit substance abuse from diagnostic consideration often has a major effect on quality of care. Abuse of alcohol or other drugs is frequently the underlying cause of other diseases about which physicians find less discomforting to inquire."

O'Brien said that doctors are generally pessimistic about the success of treatment for alcohol dependence, and they often do not realize that individuals with alcohol issues can recover. He added of doctors, "They do not like working with patients who have these disorders and do not find treating these patients rewarding. Numerous studies analyzing the amount of time spent on substance abuse in medical school and residency curricula compared with the measures of clinical importance find that the subject is under-represented in the curricula of most medical schools." Yet O'Brien says that up to 40 percent of all hospital admissions and 20 percent of general outpatient visits are linked to alcohol abuse or dependence and/or drug dependence.

Brief interventions have proven effective in identifying outpatients with alcohol disorders, and many have subsequently sought treatment. A meta-analysis of 19 studies by Nicolas Bertholet, M.D., and colleagues found that brief alcohol intervention was effective in reducing alcohol consumption at the six- and 12-month point. Said the researchers, "The typical effective BAI [brief alcohol intervention] takes no more than 15 minutes, is accompanied by written material, and offers an opportunity for the patient to schedule a follow-up. Positive effects seem to be sustained beyond a year and can last for as long as 48 months."

If alcohol problems are identified during a brief intervention, the physician should recommend cutting back on the use of alcohol; for example, the NIAAA says that adults without contraindications to alcohol (who may drink alcohol safely, and who have no health or medication reasons to preclude such drinking) may safely drink as follows:

- women: seven or fewer drinks per week and three or fewer drinks on one occasion
- men: 14 or fewer drinks per week and no more than four drinks on one occasion
- elderly: no more than one drink per day for those ages 65 and older

The alcohol screening can begin by the physician asking the patient if he or she sometimes drinks alcoholic beverages. If the answer is "no," then no further screening is needed. If the answer is "yes," then the physician needs to ask the average number of drinks per week.

Goals for the Physician during the Brief Intervention

According to the NIAAA, a brief intervention to reduce alcohol consumption among patients who drink heavily (whether they are alcoholics or not) should include the following:

- feedback on the doctor's clinical assessment and discussion of the adverse effects of alcohol
- comparison to national drinking norms

- recommendation to cut back the patient's drinking to a specific level
- provide patient education material from the NIAAA
- provide a daily self-monitoring log from the NIAAA
- schedule repeated office sessions to check on the patient's drinking issues

Physicians also need to know that among patients who are alcoholics, recovery is possible and likely, if the patient wishes to recover and is well-motivated. Individuals who have the greatest risk for a relapse after one year are those with PSYCHIATRIC COMORBIDITIES, poor social support, and low motivation.

See also AGE AND ALCOHOL; ALCOHOL AND MEN; ALCOHOL AND WOMEN; STAGES OF CHANGE; TREATMENT.

Bertholet, Nicolas, M.D., et al. "Reduction of Alcohol Consumption by Brief Alcohol Intervention in Primary Care." *Archives of Internal Medicine* 165, no. 9 (May 9, 2005): 986–995.
O'Brien, Charles P., M.D. "The CAGE Questionnaire for Detection of Alcoholism: A Remarkably Useful but Simple Tool." *Journal of the American Medical Association* 300, no. 17 (2008): 2,054–2,056.

kleptomania Kleptomania is an impulse disorder characterized by the compulsion to steal items the individual does not need and that he or she could often simply purchase. The impulse lies in the sudden need to steal the item, and the individual is seeking more of the excitement of the moment rather than whatever item is stolen. Kleptomaniacs sometimes also suffer problems with alcohol use.

Symptoms and Diagnostic Path

The key symptom of kleptomania is impulsive theft. The individual with kleptomania actively seeks to hide his or her symptoms from others; if discovered (as when the individual is arrested), an active psychological probing will reveal there have been other instances of stealing.

Treatment Options and Outlook

Patients with kleptomania may be treated with psychotherapy. Some experts treat the patient with kleptomania with NALTREXONE, which is a drug also used to treat alcohol dependence. Antidepressants, lithium, and topiramate have also been used to treat kleptomania, as have BENZODIAZEPINES. As with many psychiatric disorders, the outlook depends on the commitment of the patient toward recovery.

Risk Factors and Preventive Measures

Females are more likely to be kleptomaniacs than males. There are no known preventive measures against kleptomania.

See also IMPULSE CONTROL DISORDERS.

liver disease, alcoholic A progression of severe liver diseases that individuals with alcoholism may develop; approximately 15 percent of all alcoholics in the United States develop alcoholic liver disease (ALD). However, alcoholics are not the only people who develop ALD. The liver is the organ that metabolizes alcohol; consequently, when alcohol consumption is excessive, the liver becomes overstressed and may become damaged. The first stage of alcoholic liver disease is fatty liver disease (steatosis), a disorder which is common among heavy drinkers who consume five to six drinks per day. The liver disease progresses further to alcoholic HEPATITIS in up to a third of heavy drinkers, and progresses further still to CIRRHOSIS in about 20 percent. About 7,000 people die each year from cirrhosis in the United States, and more than half of individuals with alcoholic hepatitis and cirrhosis die within four years. Individuals with cirrhosis are also at an elevated risk for the development of liver CANCER.

Women develop alcoholic liver disease at an accelerated rate compared to men. They are also more likely to die from cirrhosis than male alcoholics. African Americans are more susceptible to ALD than whites. Cirrhosis caused by alcoholic liver disease is the second most common reason in the United States for an individual needing a liver transplantation. (The most common reason is chronic hepatitis C.) If individuals have both alcoholic liver disease and hepatitis C, the prognosis is poorer than if they have either disease alone. The prognosis is so poor that the person may be denied a liver transplant.

Fatty liver disease may be reversible, but if the disease has progressed to cirrhosis, it is not reversible, even if the individual stops drinking completely. The only possible cure at that point is a liver transplantation. Whether the person is eligible for a liver transplantation is decided by a medical panel, which must determine whether or not the person is at a significant risk for resuming alcohol abuse after receiving a transplant and destroying a new liver.

Symptoms and Diagnostic Path

Fatty liver disease is marked by a buildup of fat within the liver cells. If drinking stops, the condition is reversible. Many of the symptoms and signs of alcoholic fatty liver disease are similar to those of nonalcoholic fatty liver disease (NAFLD), including the following:

- insulin resistance
- hyperglycemia
- hypertriglyceridemia
- hypertension
- abdominal body fat that is out of proportion to the overall body

If drinking continues, alcoholic hepatitis may develop. The symptoms of alcoholic hepatitis are nausea and vomiting, abdominal pain, fever, jaundice, and tenderness in the area of the liver. The individual may also show mental confusion as well. If patients with alcoholic hepatitis stop drinking at this point, the condition is still reversible. If drinking continues, however, then cirrhosis may develop, and this condition may not be reversible, depending on how advanced it is.

Physicians diagnose alcoholic liver disease based on medical history as well as laboratory tests, such as tests for liver enzymes, including gamma-glutamyltransferase (GGT), aspartate aminotransferase (AST), and alanine aminotransferase (ALT).

If the AST level is greater than twice the level of the ALT, then liver disease is likely.

Another disease that may accompany ALD is skeletal myopathy, or muscle damage. This problem occurs in about 42 percent of alcoholic males with ALD, according to Abhinandana Anantharaju, M.D., and David H. Van Thiel, M.D. Cardiomyopathy (damage to the heart muscles) is another problem among patients with ALD, although the percentage of patients with this disorder is unknown. Patients with ALD are often malnourished and deficient in vitamins and minerals, according to Charles S. Lieber, M.D. Patients suffering from ALD may also have osteopenia or osteoporosis, which is more severe, and require treatment with vitamin D and calcium supplements. Up to 30 percent of patients with ALD are infected with hepatitis C (HCV). The treatment for HCV is interferon, but this treatment is less effective among patients with ALD.

Treatment Options and Outlook

The person with alcoholic fatty liver disease must stop drinking completely. In many cases, the cessation of drinking provides the liver with an opportunity to self-heal. Patients should also stop smoking, because studies have shown that damage is more rapid among patients with ALD who also smoke cigarettes. If drinking does not stop, then the disease will progress to alcoholic hepatitis and then cirrhosis. If the liver is destroyed, then only a liver transplantation will enable the person to survive. Studies have shown that as long as patients are abstinent, there is a good survival rate for patients with ALD, and about 61 percent have survived at the five-year point.

Lieber says early treatment is essential: "Treatment of alcoholic liver disease must be started as early as possible in the disease process because patients are more likely to die as the disorder advances. For example, one study of patients with alcoholic liver disease found that 70 percent

of patients with fatty liver still were alive after 4 years, whereas less than 50 percent of patients with cirrhosis still were alive after the same amount of time. If the cirrhosis was associated with inflammation (i.e., alcoholic hepatitis), the outlook was even worse, with only about 33 percent of patients still alive after 4 years. Unfortunately, these high mortality rates, higher than those for many cancers, attract relatively little attention from the public or the medical professional because many people believe that no effective treatment of alcoholic liver disease is available. However, new insights into the mechanisms contributing to the disorder have resulted in prospects for improved treatments, including nutritional management approaches that can lead to better outcomes."

Risk Factors and Preventive Measures

Individuals who drink excessively and frequently over time are at risk for fatty liver disease as well as for the development of the other subsequent stages of alcoholic liver disease. Some studies have shown that individuals who drink and smoke have a more rapid scarring of the liver than those who drink and do not smoke.

See also ALCOHOLISM/ALCOHOL DEPENDENCE AND ALCOHOL ABUSE; DISULFIRAM; EXCESSIVE DRINKING AND HEALTH CONSEQUENCES; PANCREATITIS.

Anantharaju, Abhinandana, M.D., and David H. Van Thiel, M.D. "Liver Transplantation for Alcoholic Liver Disease." *Alcohol Research & Health* 27, no. 3 (2003): 257–268.

Lieber, Charles S., M.D. "Relationships Between Nutrition, Alcohol Use, and Liver Disease." *Alcohol Research & Health* 27, no. 3 (2003): 220–231.

Marsano, Luis S., M.D., et al. "Diagnosis and Treatment of Alcoholic Liver Disease and Its Complications." *Alcohol Research & Health* 27, no. 3 (2003): 247–256.

National Institute on Alcohol Abuse and Alcoholism. "Alcoholic Liver Disease." *Alcohol Alert* 64 (January 2005).

maintenance stage   See STAGES OF CHANGE.

medication interactions with alcohol   Refers to the combined effects of alcohol that is consumed with or at about the same time as taking over-the-counter or prescribed drugs. Depending on the medication, alcohol may increase the action of a drug, decrease its action, or change it in some other way. Even such commonly accepted and frequently used drugs as aspirin and acetaminophen (Tylenol) interact with alcohol, and the combination may cause, respectively, stomach bleeding and liver damage. In addition, some herbal remedies may also interact with alcohol. (See Table 1.) In some cases, the medication interaction with the alcohol is so strong that it can cause an accidental overdose, leading to brain damage or even to death.

Women have a greater risk for experiencing medication interactions with alcohol than men, because even when women and men drink the same amount of alcohol, the alcohol in the woman's bloodstream generally reaches a higher level. This is also true because women usually have less water in their bodies than men. (See ALCOHOL AND WOMEN.) Older people are also at a high risk

TABLE 1
COMMONLY USED MEDICATIONS (PRESCRIPTION AND OVER-THE-COUNTER) THAT INTERACT WITH ALCOHOL

Symptoms/Disorders	Medication Brand Name	Medication Generic Name	Some Possible Reactions with Alcohol
Allergies/Colds/Flu	• Alavert • Allegra, Allegra-D • Benadryl • Clarinex • Claritin, Claritin-D • Dimetapp Cold & Allergy • Sudafed Sinus & Allergy • Triaminic Cold & Allergy • Tylenol Allergy Sinus • Tylenol Cold & Flu • Zyrtec	Loratidine Fexofenadin Diphenhydramine Desloratidine Loratidine Brompheniramine Chlorpheniramine Chlorpheniramine Chlorpheniramine Chlorpheniramine Cetirizine	Drowsiness, dizziness; increased risk for overdose
Angina (chest pain), coronary heart disease	• Isordil	Isosorbide Nitroglycerin	Rapid heartbeat, sudden changes in blood pressure, dizziness, fainting

(continues)

(continued)

Symptoms/Disorders	Medication Brand Name	Medication Generic Name	Some Possible Reactions with Alcohol
Anxiety and epilepsy	• Ativan • Klonopin • Librium • Paxil • Valium • Xanax	Lorazepam Clonazepam Chlordiazepoxide Paroxetine Diazepam Alprazolam	Drowsiness, dizziness; increased risk for overdose; slowed or difficulty breathing; impaired motor control; unusual behavior; and memory problems
	• Herbal preparations (Kava Kava)		Liver damage, drowsiness
Arthritis	• Celebrex • Naprosyn • Voltaren	Celecoxib Naproxen Dicloffenac	Ulcers, stomach bleeding, liver problems
Blood clots	• Coumadin	Warfarin	Occasional drinking may lead to internal bleeding; heavier drinking also may cause bleeding or may have the opposite effect, resulting in possible blood clots, strokes, or heart attacks
Cough	• Delsym, Robitussin Cough • Robitussin A-C	Dextromethorphan Guaifenesin + codeine	Drowsiness, dizziness; increased risk for overdose
Depression	• Anafranil • Celexa • Desyrel • Effexor • Elavil • Lexapro • Luvox • Norpramin • Paxil • Prozac • Serzone • Wellbutrin • Zoloft • Herbal preparation (St. John's Wort)	Clomipramine Citalopram Trazodone Venlafaxine Amitriptyline Escitalopram Fluvoxamine Desipramine Paroxetine Fluoxetine Nefazodone Bupropion Sertraline	Drowsiness, dizziness; increased risk for overdose; increased feelings of depression or hopelessness in adolescents (suicide)
Diabetes	• Glucophage • Micronase • Orinase	Metformin Glyburide Tolbutamide	Abnormally low blood sugar levels, flushing reaction (nausea, vomiting, headache, rapid heartbeat, sudden changes in blood pressure)

Symptoms/Disorders	Medication Brand Name	Medication Generic Name	Some Possible Reactions with Alcohol
Enlarged prostate	• Cardura • Flomax • Hytrin • Minipress	Doxazosin Tamsulosin Terazosin Prazosin	Dizziness, light headedness, fainting
Heartburn, indigestion, sour stomach	• Axid • Reglan • Tagamet • Zantac	Nizatidine Metoclopramide Cimetidine Ranitidine	Rapid heartbeat, sudden changes in blood pressure (metoclopramide); increased alcohol effect
High blood pressure	• Accupril • Capozide • Cardura • Catapres • Xozaar • Hytrin • Loporessor HCT • Lotensin • Minipress • Vaseretic	Quinapril Hydrochlorothiazide Doxazosin Clonidine Losartan Terazosin Hydrochlorothiazide Benzapril Prazosin Enalapril	Dizziness, fainting, drowsiness; heart problems, such as changes in the heart's regular heartbeat (arrhythmia)
High cholesterol	• Advicor • Altocor • Crestor • Lipitor • Mevacor • Niaspan • Pravachol • Pravigard • Vytorin • Zocor	Lovastatin + Niacin Lovastatin Rosuvastatin Altovastatin Lovastatin Niacin Pravastatin Pravastatin + Aspirin Exetimibe +Simvastatin Simvastatiin	Liver damage (all medications); increased flushing and itching (niacin); increased stomach bleeding (pravastatin + aspirin)
Infections	• Acrodantin • Flagyl • Grisactin • Nizoral • Nydrazid • Seromycin • Tindamax	Nitrofurantoin Metronidazole Griseofulvin Ketokonazole Isoniazid Cycloserine Tiniadazole	Fast heartbeat, sudden changes in blood pressure; stomach pain, upset stomach, vomiting, headache, or flushing or redness of the face; liver damage (isoniazid, ketokonazole)
Muscle pain	• Flexeril • Soma	Cyclobenzaprine Carisoprodol	Drowsiness, dizziness; increased risk of seizures; increased risk for overdose; slowed or difficulty breathing; impaired motor control; unusual behavior; memory problems

(continues)

(continued)

Symptoms/Disorders	Medication Brand Name	Medication Generic Name	Some Possible Reactions with Alcohol
Nausea, motion sickness	• Chamomile • Echinacea • Valerian	Various preparations	Alcohol may accentuate the drowsiness that is associated with these herbal preparations.
Pain (such as headache, muscle ache, minor arthritis pain), fever, inflammation	• Advil • Aleve • Excedrin • Motrin • Tylenol	Ibuprofen Naproxen Aspirin, Acetaminophen Ibuprofen Acetaminophen	Stomach upset, bleeding and ulcers; liver damage (acetaminophen); rapid heartbeat
Seizures	• Dilantin • Klonopin	Phenytoin Clonazepam Phenobarbital	Drowsiness, dizziness; increased risk of seizures
Severe pain from injury, postsurgical care, oral surgery, migraines	• Darvocet-N • Demerol • Fiorinal with codeine • Percocet • Vicodin	Propoxyphene Meperidine Butalbital + codeine Oxycodone Hydrocodone	Drowsiness, dizziness; increased risk for overdose; slowed or difficulty breathing; impaired motor control; unusual behavior; memory problems
Sleep problems	• Ambien • Lunesta • Prosom • Restoril • Sominex • Unison	Zolpidem Eszopiclone Estazolam Temazepam Diphenhydramine Doxylamine	Drowsiness, sleepiness, dizziness; slowed or difficulty breathing; impaired motor control; unusual behavior; memory problems
	• Herbal preparations (chamomile, valerian, lavender)		Increased drowsiness

Source: National Institute on Alcohol Abuse and Alcoholism. *Harmful Interactions: Mixing Alcohol with Medicines.* Bethesda, Md.: National Institutes of Health, 2007. Available online. URL: http://pubs.niaaa.nih.gov/publications/Medicine/medicine.htm. Downloaded June 27, 2008.

for medication interactions, because aging often slows down the ability of the body to break down (metabolize) the alcohol. In addition, older people are much more likely than younger people to be taking one or more of the medications that interact with alcohol. (See AGE AND ALCOHOL; ELDERLY AND DRINKING ISSUES.)

See also EXCESSIVE DRINKING AND HEALTH CONSEQUENCES; TREATMENT.

men and alcohol   See ALCOHOL AND MEN.

military veterans/combat and active-duty military
Military veterans are individuals who have served in the military. If they are combat veterans, they have served in wars in other countries or regions, such as Vietnam, the Persian Gulf, and more recently, Iraq and Afghanistan. Combat veterans may continue to serve in the military, or they may have been discharged. Active-duty military people are those who are currently serving and who may or may not have served under combat conditions. Many individuals in the National Guard and Reserves are called to active duty during conflicts for about a year, such

as in the wars in Iraq and Afghanistan. Some major studies indicate that all active-duty personnel are at an increased risk for alcohol abuse or alcohol dependence, particularly those who become combat veterans and who may suffer from POSTTRAUMATIC STRESS DISORDER (PTSD).

Some experts believe that military culture encourages heavy drinking. According to Genevieve Ames and Carol Cunradi in their 2004/2005 article for *Alcohol Research & Health*, "The easy availability of alcohol, ritualized drinking opportunities, and inconsistent policies contribute to a work culture that facilitates heavy and binge drinking in this population." They added that "Navy underage recruits reported that they had easy access to alcohol in bars, in the barracks, or in hotel rooms near the base. On shore leave in foreign ports, alcohol was reportedly inexpensive, bars were located near the point of disembarkation, few ports had underage drinking laws, and most sailors who wanted to drink organized drinking groups before disembarking."

Ames and Cunradi recommended an increase in the price of alcohol and noted that the Department of Defense's Alcohol Abuse Prevention Strategic Plan states a policy that alcohol sold by the military at base or post outlets should be no more than 5–10 percent less than the price in local stores in most states. This policy has been inconsistently implemented, however. Ames and Cunradi also recommended that alcohol use be "deglamorized," by offering nonalcoholic beverages at functions where alcohol is also served and by stressing that alcohol use during or before work hours is not acceptable.

A major study of active-duty military personnel was reported by Robert M. Bray and colleagues in December 2006: the *2005 Department of Defense (DoD) Survey of Health Related Behaviors Among Active Duty Personnel*. In this survey, the researchers analyzed the anonymous responses of 16,146 military personnel, including 4,524 in the Air Force, 3,639 in the Army, 3,356 in the Marine Corps, and 4,627 in the Navy. (This study is performed every 3–4 years.) One of the behaviors considered was alcohol use.

The researchers divided respondents into five drinking levels, including

1. abstainers
2. infrequent/light drinkers

3. moderate drinkers
4. moderate/heavy drinkers
5. heavy drinkers

Heavy drinkers were defined as those who drank five or more drinks on one occasion at least once a week in the 30 days before the survey. The researchers also looked at BINGE DRINKING, which was defined as having five or more drinks on a single occasion at least once in the past 30 days. Thus, heavy drinkers were more problematic than binge drinkers, because heavy drinkers had multiple episodes of binge drinking. (Note that the definition of "heavy drinking" may vary with the research that is performed, and consequently, its definition should always be sought.)

The researchers also looked at the negative effects of alcohol use, including losing a promotion because of drinking, receiving a lower job performance rating because of drinking, losing a week or more from work because of an alcohol-related illness, punishment under the Uniform Code of Military Justice because of drinking, an arrest for drinking, and other consequences.

They found that the rate of heavy drinking was significantly higher overall among the military compared to their civilian counterparts—a heavy drinking rate of 16.1 percent for the military compared to 12.9 percent of civilians. The primary difference was accounted for by the age of the respondents, and military personnel ages 18 to 25 years had a heavy drinking rate of 24.8 percent compared to 17.4 percent among civilians. The drinking rates for those ages 26 to 55 who were on active duty were not significantly different for the military (9.7 percent) compared to the rate for same-age civilians (9.5 percent).

Interestingly, military personnel were much less likely to have used any illicit drug than the rate for civilians in the past 30 days, or 4.6 percent for military members compared to 12.8 percent for those not in the military. This was true across all age groups, services, and for males and females. Clearly, illicit drug use is actively discouraged in the military.

The researchers found that RELIGION was an important factor in decreasing drinking, and individuals who considered themselves highly religious or spiritual were much less likely to have drinking issues than those with low religiosity/spirituality. According to the researchers, 20 percent of the military personnel said they were highly religious, and 54 percent said they had a medium level of religiosity/spirituality.

There were significant differences between the heavy drinking rates of members of different services. The percentage of heavy drinkers in 2005 was 25.4 percent among the Marine Corps, followed by 24.5 percent among Army members, 17.0 percent among Navy members, and 10.3 percent among members of the Air Force.

Binge-drinking rates were problematic for some members, and more than half (53.2 percent) of Marines acknowledged at least one binge-drinking episode in the past month. The rates were lower (but still comparatively high) for other service members: 52.8 percent for Army members, 41.7 percent for Navy members, and 33.9 percent for Air Force personnel.

The researchers also found that almost a quarter of the heavy drinkers said that they had experienced one or more serious consequences as a result of their drinking. In addition, the researchers identified possible alcohol dependence in 11.6 percent of the heavy drinkers.

In looking at gender differences, the researchers found that more military men said that they used alcohol to cope with stress (29.9 percent) than did women in the military (21.8 percent).

The researchers also found higher risks for heavy drinking among the following groups: those with a high-school education versus college graduates; those who were either single or married but the spouse was absent; those in lower pay grades, such as E1–E3 (enlisted grades) and O1–O3 (officer grades).

Risks of being a heavy drinker were lower among African Americans, non-Hispanics, and those of "other" race categories compared to white non-Hispanics and those stationed within the continental United States (the 48 states excluding Alaska and Hawaii) compared with those stationed outside the continental United States.

Combat Veterans

Many studies have shown that combat veterans have an increased risk for both alcohol abuse and ALCOHOLISM. For example, a study reported in the *Journal of the American Medical Association* in 2008 revealed that National Guard and Reservists who had returned from deployment to Iraq had a high rate of binge drinking and alcohol dependence.

The researchers found that 9 percent of the "citizen-soldiers" exhibited heavy weekly drinking (for men, more than 14 drinks per week, and for women, more than 7 drinks per week), 53.6 percent exhibited binge drinking (five or more drinks per day or on one occasion), and 15.2 percent had alcohol-related problems. Their risk of drinking was about 60 percent higher than among Guard and Reserve troops who were not deployed to Iraq or Afghanistan, according to the Associated Press. At some points, the Guard and Reserve comprised more than half of the combat forces, which may have increased their stress levels.

The study also found among all deployed soldiers, those born after 1980 were at 6.7 times increased odds of new-onset binge drinking and 4.7 times increased odds of new-onset alcohol-related problems. Those with PTSD and depression were at increased odds of new-onset and continued alcohol-related problems at follow-up.

In contrast, among active-duty personnel who were deployed to Iraq, the rates of drinking problems among individuals in combat conditions were also high, but not as high as among Reserve and Guard personnel; the rate of heavy weekly drinking was 6.0 percent, the rate of binge drinking was 26.6 percent (about half the rate seen among Reserve and Guard personnel), and the rate of alcohol-related problems was 4.8 percent, versus the 15.2 percent among the Reserve and Guard personnel. These high percentages may be related to the presence of PTSD in some of the returned veterans.

See also AGE AND ALCOHOL; ALCOHOL AND MEN; ANXIETY DISORDERS; SUICIDE.

Ames, Genevieve, and Carol Cunradi. "Alcohol Use and Preventing Alcohol-Related Problems among Young Adults in the Military." *Alcohol Research & Health* 28, no. 4 (2004/2005): 252–257.

Bray, Robert M., et al. *2005 Department of Defense Survey of Health Related Behaviors Among Active Duty Personnel: A Component of the Defense Lifestyle Assessment Program.* December 2006.

Jacobson, Isabel J., et al. "Alcohol Use and Alcohol-Related Problems before and after Military Combat Deployment." *Journal of the American Medical Association* 200, no. 6 (August 13, 2008): 663–673.

moderate drinking and health benefits   Moderate drinking is generally defined as two drinks per day or less for men and one drink per day or less for women, although some researchers vary this definition or have one definition for both males and females. It is readily apparent and backed up by a great deal of evidence that excessive drinking or heavy episodic drinking (BINGE DRINKING) can cause a broad array of very serious health problems. Many people do not realize, however, that moderate drinking may confer some health benefits on some individuals, especially those in their middle years and older years. Benefits are primarily seen to the cardiovascular system, in terms of a decreased risk for a heart attack and stroke. It should also be noted that although some health benefits have proven to accrue with moderate drinking, these benefits disappear altogether should an individual revert to heavy drinking or binge drinking.

Moderate drinking may help some individuals with diabetes mellitus to maintain a favorable glycemic level. One study reported by Chris L. Bryson and colleagues in the *Journal of the American College of Cardiology* in 2001 studied patients over a period of 12 years. The researchers found that those diabetic patients who drank one or two drinks per day were 80 percent *less* likely to die of heart disease when they were compared to other diabetic individuals who did not drink.

In another study of 91 moderate drinkers with diabetes, published by I. Shai and colleagues and reported in *Diabetes Care* in 2007, the researchers found that the fasting blood glucose level significantly decreased among the subjects in the moderately drinking alcohol group, but it did not decrease in the control group subjects. Interestingly, individuals with a more severe form of diabetes were those who showed the most improvement from their moderate drinking.

Research has also shown that moderate drinkers have lower death rates than both abstainers and heavy drinkers, based on studies in the United States, China, Great Britain, Japan, and many other countries. For example, a study of 86,000 nurses, reported in the *New England Journal of Medicine* by Fuchs and colleagues in 1995, found that women consuming one to three drinks per week had a lower death rate than did abstainers from alcohol.

In some studies, the type of alcohol that is consumed is important; for example, a study published in a 2008 issue of *Hepatology* by W. Dunn and colleagues found that the moderate consumption of wine was associated with a decreased prevalence of nonalcoholic fatty liver disease (NFLD). The same protective benefits were not found among moderate consumers of either beer or distilled spirits. Other studies have shown that one glass of wine daily decreases the risk for Barrett's esophagus, a precancerous condition. However, in other studies, the type of the alcohol that is consumed moderately is irrelevant to the benefits from moderate drinking, and benefits are found with wine, beer, or distilled spirits.

Moderate alcohol consumption may also be protective against low bone density and also protective from the fractures that are caused by osteopenia and the more severe osteoporosis. In a meta-analysis of studies analyzed by K. M. Berg and colleagues, published in 2008 in the *American Journal of Medicine*, the researchers identified several studies that found that moderate alcohol use was associated with a decreased bone loss over time compared to the higher level of bone loss among individuals who were abstainers.

The risk for kidney dysfunction may be decreased among some individuals who are moderate consumers of alcohol. In the Physicians' Health study of 11,023 men, there was a reduced risk of kidney dysfunction among the moderate drinkers.

Some studies have shown that moderate alcohol consumption decreases the risk for the development of gallstones. In the Nurses' Health Study, those women who consumed two to three drinks minimum per week were less likely to develop gallstones than were the abstainers. Other studies have shown that this particular benefit of moderate drinking also extends to men, who also develop fewer gallstones.

Research has shown that the moderate consumption of alcohol may have many other benefits.

It may be linked to a decrease in the incidence of Barrett's esophagus, a precancerous condition linked to the often deadly esophageal cancer. There may be some cognitive benefits attributable to moderate drinking, particularly with regard to a decreased risk for vascular dementia (although this benefit has not been found with Alzheimer's disease). Moderate drinking may also decrease the risk for kidney failure.

Some physicians have expressed concern that moderate drinking should not commence among abstainers, should there be a risk for alcohol abuse or dependence. However, a study by D. E. King and colleagues, published in the *American Journal of Medicine* in 2008, revealed that moderate drinking was beneficial among former abstainers and that the risk for the development of an alcohol use disorder is low.

In this study of 7,697 patients of ages 45–64 years with no history of cardiovascular disease and who were not drinkers at the beginning of the study, 6 percent of the subjects began moderate drinking. The researchers found that after four years, the new moderate drinkers had decreased their risk for cardiovascular disease by 38 percent, compared to the nondrinkers. They also found that people who began consuming alcohol in middle age rarely consumed alcohol beyond the recommended amounts.

Some individuals, such as those who are pregnant or have a family or personal history of alcohol dependence, should not drink any amount of alcohol. In addition, individuals with any form of liver or pancreatic disease should avoid alcohol altogether. Those with an active case of gastritis or esophagitis should also avoid all alcohol, as should individuals with a family history of breast CANCER.

Alcohol and Healthy Hearts

In their study reported in a 2006 issue of the *Journal of the American College of Cardiology*, researchers Chris L. Bryson, M.D., and colleagues found that moderate drinking was associated with a lower risk for congestive heart failure (CHF) among older adults, including older adults who had already had a myocardial infarction (heart attack). This research was based on 5,595 subjects who were at risk for CHF, and the researchers compared the cardiac results for those who drank moderately to those who abstained from alcohol.

The National Health and Nutrition Examination Survey I and the Epidemiologic Follow-up Survey found that those individuals who consumed two to seven drinks per week had the lowest risk for coronary heart disease. The risk was lowered as well for men who were otherwise generally healthy, and were not obese, were nonsmokers, consumed a health diet, and those who engaged in regular exercise.

Researchers have found that moderate drinking increases high-density lipoprotein (HDL) cholesterol, or the "good" cholesterol. The levels of HDL cholesterol may increase by as much as 10 percent among those who consume two to three drinks of alcohol per day. Researchers believe that it is this increase in HDL cholesterol which may provide the cardiac benefit of moderate drinking.

Research has also shown that regular moderate drinkers have lower levels of C-reactive protein (CRP) compared to those who drink infrequently or not at all. Lower levels of CRP are linked to lower levels of health problems.

In a study published in 2009 by Satoyo Ikehara and colleagues in *Alcoholism: Clinical and Experimental Research,* the researchers studied data on 19,356 men ages 40–69 years who were participants in the Japan Public Health Center-Based Prospective Study. The researchers looked at alcohol consumption and the risk for stroke and coronary heart disease over 9.9 years. They found that light to moderate alcohol consumption was linked to a reduced risk for coronary heart disease and total cardiovascular disease, while heavy alcohol consumption increased the risk of stroke, especially hemorrhagic stroke. The researchers also found evidence that social support may have increased the benefits of light to moderate alcohol consumption with regard to cardiovascular disease risks.

According to the researchers, "We also found the reduced risks of total stroke, ischemic stroke, and total cardiovascular disease associated with light-to-moderate drinking were more pronounced in men with higher social support. These associations were unexplained by the difference of alcohol consumption because mean value of alcohol consumption did not differ in the light-to-moderate drinkers between the low and high social support groups." The researchers noted that other studies have found social support to be a protective risk factor against cardiovascular disease in healthy subjects.

In their article on alcohol and cardiovascular health in the *Journal of the American College on Cardiology* in 2007, James H. O'Keefe, M.D., and colleagues said that the possible cardiovascular benefits that are associated with light to moderate drinking appear to be the most important health benefits accruing to drinking in moderation.

The authors reported, "In the INTER-HEART study, involving 27,000 patients from 52 countries, regular alcohol consumption was associated with a reduced incidence of myocardial infarction (MI) in both genders, and in all adult age groups. Light to moderate drinking is associated with improved CV health in higher-risk individuals, such as those with known CHD [coronary heart disease] and/or diabetes, but it also may reduce CV risk even in lower-risk individuals. A subgroup study taken from the total cohort of 51,000 men in the Health Professionals Follow-Up Study focused on the effects of alcohol in the 8,867 men (mean age 57 years) who followed all 4 of the major healthy life-style behaviors (abstention from smoking, maintain a body mass index <25 kg/m^2, exercising at least 30 min daily, and eating a healthy diet). That study found that even in men who were already following a very healthy lifestyle, the consumption of 1 or 2 drinks per day was associated with 40% to 50% decreased risk of MI."

However, the authors stopped short of recommending that nondrinkers start drinking in moderation, because "sobering statistics warn that moderate daily drinking is a slippery slope that many individuals cannot safely navigate." They added, "Until we have more randomized outcome data, and tools for predicting susceptibility to problem drinking, it would seem prudent to encourage physicians and patients to focus on more innocuous interventions to prevent CHD [coronary heart disease]."

In a study published in 2009 in *Age and Ageing*, researchers Wanda M. Snow et al. found a cardiovascular benefit to moderate drinking but said that the benefit may not become evident until middle age or the older years. In this study, 1,154 subjects ages 18–64 years were evaluated on their alcohol consumption use. The researchers found a benefit of moderate drinking among middle-aged and older men, while the cardioprotection that moderate drinking afforded women was more apparent only in the youngest women. Of course, heavy episodic drinking (binge drinking) did *not* afford cardiac benefits.

The authors wrote, "The present findings do not suggest a decreased cardioprotective effect of usual alcohol as a function of age but rather a preservation of its beneficial effects, at least in men and at the generally modest levels of consumption seen in our sample. We found no indication of a 'safer' level of usual consumption for older adults as compared to younger groups. However, these results suggest that the harmful effects of HED [heavy episodic drinking] may become more pronounced with age, especially among men. These findings suggest that HED should be limited in older individuals and emphasise the importance of evaluating pattern in addition to level of consumption when making patient recommendations regarding alcohol use."

Moderate Drinking and Diabetes Improvements

Light to moderate drinking among men with type 2 diabetes has been associated with improved cognitive function, based on a study of 20 drinkers and 99 abstainers. In this study by Fan and colleagues and published in 2008, the researchers found that the drinkers performed significantly better in three of five cognitive tests. Moderate consumption also appears to improve insulin sensitivity.

Among older diabetics, moderate drinking may be protective against death from coronary heart disease; for example, in a study of 983 diabetics whose average age was 69 years, reported by A. A. Howard and colleagues in 2004 in the *Annals of Internal Medicine*, the risk for death from coronary heart disease was significantly lower among moderate drinkers compared to the risk of death for both abstainers and heavy drinkers.

Some researchers have found that moderate drinking decreases the risk for the development of type 2 diabetes, such as research by L. L. Koppes and colleagues and published in *Diabetes Care* in 2005.

Of course, alcohol is not always beneficial to patients with diabetes, and some studies have shown that even modest amounts of alcohol can increase the risk for hypoglycemia (low blood sugar) among individuals who are diabetics. Alcohol may also worsen the prognosis of diabetic neuropathy.

Moderate Drinking and Mortality

Many states in the United States and worldwide have shown that moderate drinkers have a lower mortality (death) rate compared to both abstainers and heavy drinkers. Even among patients with hypertension whose blood pressure could be affected by alcohol, individuals with moderate drinking still showed a lower mortality. As mentioned, moderate drinking is particularly protective against individuals at risk for heart problems; thus, in general, older individuals gain a greater benefit from moderate drinking than younger individuals, because older people have a significantly greater risk of heart disease and heart attack.

In a meta-analysis of 34 studies of drinking and mortality among men and women, published by Augusto Di Castelnuovo and colleagues in *Archives of Internal Medicine* in 2006, the researchers found that low levels of alcohol consumption (one to two drinks per day for women and two to four drinks per day for men) were associated with lower death rates. However, higher levels of alcohol consumption were tied to higher mortality risks.

The researchers said, "In conclusion, this meta-analysis confirms the hazards of excessive drinking but also indicates the existence of potential windows of alcohol intake that may confer a net beneficial effect of drinking, at least in terms of survival, both in men and in women. Heavy drinkers should be urged to cut their consumption, but people who already regularly consume low to moderate amounts of alcohol should be encouraged to continue."

Effect of Alcohol on Specific Diseases and Organs

Studies have demonstrated the impact of moderate drinking on several specific diseases and disorders as well as certain body systems and organs.

Improvements in Bones A variety of studies have shown that moderate alcohol use is linked to an increased bone mineral density, possibly because of higher estrogen levels. In a study on moderate alcohol consumption, published by N. Zhang and colleagues in *Medical Hypotheses* in 2008, the researchers found that moderate alcohol consumption may decrease the risk for intervertebral disc degeneration, a very painful medical condition.

Reduced Risk for the Development of Gallstones According to K. M. Maclure and colleagues in 1989, female subjects in the Nurses' Health Study who drank at least two to three drinks per week experienced a 40 percent lower risk of developing gallstones compared to the risk for abstainers. However, research has shown that if patients drink heavily, the protective benefit of alcohol against gallstones completely disappears; in fact, studies have also shown a high rate of gallstones among patients who were diagnosed with alcoholic CIRRHOSIS.

Decreased Risk for Barrett's Esophagus Drinking one glass of wine every day may reduce the risk for Barrett's esophagus, a precancerous esophageal condition, by 56 percent, according to data reported in 2009. Researchers found a trend for a lower risk for Barrett's esophagus with moderate wine consumption; they also found an increased risk for the condition with heavy consumption of alcohol. There was no similar decrease in Barrett's esophagus among those who drank other forms of alcohol moderately. The investigators hypothesized that the antioxidants in wine may have counteracted damage caused by gastroesophageal reflux disease (GERD). It may also be that the wine drinkers typically consumed their wine while they ate a meal, reducing the risk of damage to esophageal tissue.

Cognitive Abilities According to an analysis by the National Institute on Alcohol Abuse and Alcoholism on moderate drinking, reported by Lorraine Gunzerath and colleagues in 2004 in *Alcoholism: Clinical and Experimental Research,* some studies have indicated a decreased risk for vascular dementia among moderate drinkers. Similar results have not been found with Alzheimer's disease.

Moderate Drinking and the Kidneys Some studies have shown that moderate drinking may confer a protective benefit on the kidneys, decreasing the risk of kidney failure. For example, a study of 473 apparently healthy men followed for over 14 years, reported by Elke S. Schaeffner, M.D., and colleagues in *Archives of Internal Medicine* in 2005, found an apparent inverse relationship between moderate drinking and kidney dysfunction. According to the researchers, "Beneficial effects of moderate alcohol consumption on renal function are plausible; in recent years, traditional risk factors for CVD [cardiovascular disease] have been associated with an increased risk of developing renal dysfunction. Furthermore, autopsy data suggested potential beneficial effects of alcohol consumption on the hyalinization in renal arterioles."

See also ALCOHOL AND MEN; ALCOHOL AND WOMEN; EXCESSIVE DRINKING AND HEALTH CONSEQUENCES.

Barclay, Laurie, M.D., and Desiree Lie, M.D. "Drinking a Glass of Wine Daily Lowers the Risk for Barrett's Esophagus." Medscape Medical News. March 9, 2009. Available online to subscribers. URL: http://www.medsape.com/viewarticle/589244. Accessed April 3, 2009.

Berg, K. M., et al. "Association Between Alcohol Consumption and Both Osteoporotic Fracture and Bone Density." *American Journal of Medicine* 121, no. 5 (2008): 406–418.

Bryson, Chris L., M.D., et al. "The Association of Alcohol Consumption and Incident Heart Failure: The Cardiovascular Health Study." *Journal of the American College of Cardiology* 48, no. 2 (2006): 305–311.

Corder, R., et al. "Red Wine Procyanidins and Vascular Health." *Nature* 444 (2006): 566.

Di Castelnuovo, Augusto, et al. "Alcohol Dosing and Total Mortality in Men and Women: An Updated Meta-analysis of 34 Prospective Studies." *Archives of Internal Medicine* 166, no. 22 (2006): 2,437–2,445.

Dunn, W., et al. "Modest Wine Drinking and Decreased Prevalence of Suspected Nonalcoholic Fatty Liver Disease." *Hepatology* 47, no. 6 (2008): 1,947–1,954.

Fan, X., et al. "Light to Moderate Alcohol Drinking Is Associated with Higher Cognitive Function in Males with Type 2 Diabetes." *Experimental Aging Research* 34, no. 2 (2008): 126–137.

Fuchs, C. S., et al. "Alcohol Consumption and Mortality among Women." *New England Journal of Medicine* 332, no. 19 (1995): 1,245.

Goh, Siew Simg, et al. "The Red Wine Antioxidant Resveratrol Prevents Cardiomyocyte Injury Following Ischemia-Reperfusion via Multiple Sites and Mechanisms." *Antioxidants & Redox Signaling* 9, no. 1 (2007): 101–113.

Gunzerath, Lorraine, et al. "National Institute on Alcohol Abuse and Alcoholism Report on Moderate Drinking." *Alcoholism: Clinical and Experimental Research* 28, no. 6 (2004): 829–847.

Howard, A. A., H. H. Arnstein, and M. N. Gourevitch. "Effect of Alcohol Consumption on Diabetes Mellitus: A Systematic Review." *Annals of Internal Medicine* 140, no. 3 (2004): 211–219.

Ikehara, Satoyo, et al. "Alcohol Consumption, Social Support, and Risk of Stroke and Coronary Heart Disease Among Japanese Men: The JPHC Study." *Alcoholism: Clinical and Experimental Research* 33, no. 4 (2009): 1–8.

King, Dana E., M.D., Arch G. Mainous III, and Mark E. Geesey. "Adopting Moderate Alcohol Consumption in Middle Age: Subsequent Cardiovascular Events." *American Journal of Medicine* 121, no. 3 (March 2008): 201–206.

Koppes, L., et al. "Moderate Alcohol Consumption Lowers the Risk of Type 2 Diabetes: A Meta-Analysis of Prospective Observational Studies." *Diabetes Care* 28, no. 3 (2005): 719–725.

Maclure, K. M., et al. "Weight, Diet, and the Risk of Symptomatic Gallstones in Middle-Aged Women." *New England Journal of Medicine* 321, no. 9 (1989): 563–569.

Mukamal, Kenneth J., M.D., Stephanie E. Chiuve, and Eric B. Rimm. "Alcohol Consumption and Risk for Coronary Heart Disease in Men with Healthy Lifestyles." *Archives of Internal Medicine* 166, no. 19 (October 23, 2006): 2,145–2,150.

Mukhamal, Kenneth J., M.D., et al. "Alcohol and Risk for Ischemic Stroke in Men: The Role of Drinking Patterns and Usual Beverage." *Annals of Internal Medicine* 142, no. 1 (2005): 11–19.

O'Keefe, James H., M.D., Kevin A. Bybee, M.D., and Carl J. Lavie, M.D. "Alcohol and Cardiovascular Health: The Razor-Sharp Double-Edged Sword." *Journal of the American College of Cardiology* 50, no. 11 (2007): 1,009–1,014.

Schaeffner, Elke S., M.D., et al. "Alcohol Consumption and the Risk of Renal Dysfunction in Apparently Healthy Men." *Archives of Internal Medicine* 165, no. 9 (2005): 1,048–1,053.

Shai, I., et al. "Glycemic Effects of Moderate Alcohol Intake among Patients with Type 2 Diabetes: A Multi-Center, Randomized Clinical Intervention Trial." *Diabetes Care* 30, no. 12 (2007): 3,011–3,016.

Snow, Wanda M., et al. "Alcohol Use and Cardiovascular Health Outcomes: A Comparison Across Age and Gender in the Winnepeg Health and Drinking Survey Cohort." *Age and Ageing* 38, no. 2 (2009): 206–212.

Tanasescu, M., et al. "Alcohol Consumption and Risk of Coronary Heart Disease Among Men with Type 2 Diabetes." *Journal of the American College of Cardiology* 38, no. 7 (2001): 1,836–1,842.

Zhang, N., et al. "Moderate Alcohol Consumption May Decrease Risk of Intervertebral Disc Degeneration." *Medical Hypotheses* 71, no. 4 (2008): 501–504.

motor vehicle accidents See DRIVING UNDER THE INFLUENCE/DRIVING WHILE INTOXICATED.

naltrexone A medication prescribed to treat ALCO-HOLISM and chronic BINGE DRINKING. Naltrexone effectively reduces the craving for alcohol as well as the euphoria that it may induce among many people who are alcoholics, thus, essentially removing the main reasons for drinking. For some people being treated with naltrexone, alcohol tastes "bad," and consequently, they drink less of it. This drug seems most effective among patients with a family history of drinking as well as patients with strong cravings for alcohol.

Naltrexone was originally used to treat heroin addicts, and it has been found to decrease the craving for other illicit drugs, such as cocaine. Since some patients use both alcohol and illegal drugs, the drug may be helpful for treating both types of substance dependence.

Naltrexone has been approved by the Food and Drug Administration (FDA) to treat alcohol dependence since 1994. It was long-awaited; naltrexone was the first drug approved to treat alcoholism since the approval of DISULFIRAM (Antabuse) in 1951. Note that naltrexone has not been studied with adolescents, and it is generally considered too risky to use with this population. Anecdotal reports indicate some success has occurred in using it to treat alcoholic adolescents; however, the drug may affect growth and puberty and should be avoided by people younger than 17 or 18 years old.

Oral naltrexone is available as the brand names Depade or ReVia, and it is taken once per day. In 2006, the Food and Drug Administration (FDA) approved an intramuscular injection of naltrexone, known by its brand name as Vivitrol, and the drug became available to patients in the United States in 2008. Vivitrol is injected once per month, thus avoiding a common problem with medication compliance. Some patients respond better to one form of naltrexone than to another.

Naltrexone should be avoided by patients using narcotics as well as those with HEPATITIS or CIRRHOSIS of the liver. As with all drugs, naltrexone may cause some side effects, including lightheadedness, nausea, and fatigue, but these symptoms usually abate in most patients. Some patients have noted an increased interest in sex as well as a weight loss, two side effects that most people would appreciate.

Other medications that are used to treat alcohol dependence include acamprosate (Campral) and disulfiram. Sometimes combined medication therapy is used to treat alcoholism, such as an anti-alcohol drug that is combined with an antiseizure medication or a BENZODIAZEPINE or ANTIDEPRESSANT. Naltrexone is sometimes used to treat psychiatric disorders, particularly when they are comorbid (co-occurring) with alcoholism.

Naltrexone blocks the receptors (the opioid receptors) that trigger the rewarding effects of alcohol, and it also blocks the craving for alcohol. This is important, because often the craving remains even when a person has undergone TREATMENT and recovery and the physical addiction is gone.

In the Combined Pharmacotherapies and Behavioral Interventions (COMBINE) study of 1,383 subjects located at 11 sites in the United States, patients who received naltrexone for 16 weeks responded better than those who received the placebo drug; for example, the days of abstinence from alcohol for those on naltrexone increased by 80.6 percent compared to 75.1 percent of those on placebo.

According to Raymond Anton in his article on naltrexone for the *New England Journal of Medicine* in 2008, "A typical patient who presents for treatment of alcohol dependence is drinking, on average, more than five drinks per day on about 50 to 80% of days (a standard drink is 5 oz [0.15 liter] of wine, 12 oz [0.35 liter] of beer, or 1.5 oz [0.04 liter] of liquor). Health risks increase when drinking exceeds two to three drinks per day." Anton also describes the ideal patient for naltrexone as one who "drinks on more than 50% of days, consumed more than five drinks a day, and has alcohol-related problems. Such a person has probably failed in attempts to quit drinking but has a relatively high motivation to be abstinent or at least to try abstinence for a while. A good indication of this motivation is the ability to abstain from drinking for several days before starting naltrexone."

Anton says that naltrexone use should be combined with an initial visit with a health care professional, and patients should undergo weekly visits thereafter for two weeks, followed by visits every two weeks for 10 weeks, and a visit after another month.

See also ALCOHOL AND OTHER DRUGS; STAGES OF CHANGE.

Anton, Raymond F., M.D. "Combined Pharmacotherapies and Behavioral Interventions for Alcohol Dependence: The COMBINE Study: A Randomized Controlled Trial." *Journal of the American Medical Association* 295, no. 17 (May 3, 2006): 2,003–2,017.

Anton, Raymond F., M.D., et al. "Naltrexone for the Management of Alcohol Dependence." *New England Journal of Medicine* 359, no. 7 (August 14, 2008): 715–721.

Kuehn, Bridget M. "New Therapies for Alcohol Dependence Open Options for Office-Based Treatment." *Journal of the American Medical Association* 298, no. 21 (December 5, 2007): 2,467–2,468.

narcissistic personality disorder See PERSONALITY DISORDERS.

Native Americans Individuals belonging to tribes that were present in North America prior to the colonial period in the United States as well as subsequent to that period and to date. Alcohol was first introduced to the Native Americans in the 17th century by Europeans, and the drug has caused this group great hardship since that time. Native Americans have a high rate of alco-

hol abuse and dependence. According to author and researcher William White, the first ALCOHOLISM MUTUAL AID SOCIETIES that concentrated on ABSTINENCE were actually launched by Native Americans, who believed that their physical and cultural survival depended on conquering the alcohol abuse and ALCOHOLISM suffered by their tribal members.

It is difficult to generalize about individuals who are members of more than 500 tribes with many differences among them. However, some common points can be made. In the 21st century, Native Americans and Alaska Natives have a higher rate of alcohol abuse and alcohol dependence than all other races and ethnicities, when statistical data is provided. Experts argue over the reason for this. Many believe that it may be a heretofore undiscovered genetic risk that is the underlying cause. Others believe that tribal influences may play a role, especially among Native Americans who live isolated lives on tribal reservations. Some believe that alienation from their Native American culture is a key issue.

Some experts have hypothesized that perhaps Native Americans are more susceptible to the effects of alcohol than other races or ethnicities. This hypothesis was studied by C. Garcia-Andrade and colleagues through research conducted with Mission Indians and reported in 1997. The researchers tested 40 healthy and nonalcoholic men ages 18–25 who were evaluated both before and after ingesting alcohol. They found that subjects with at least 50 percent Native American heritage said that they experienced less intense effects of alcohol than those with less than 50 percent Native American heritage.

The researchers said, "These results contradicted the 'firewater myth'—the theory that Native Americans are more sensitive to the effects of alcohol. Rather, the data indicate that Mission Indian men generally may be less sensitive to alcohol's effects, a physiological characteristic that has been shown to be associated with a greater risk for alcoholism in Caucasian populations. In addition, individuals with a greater percentage of Native American heritage may be less sensitive to the subjective effects of alcohol than individuals with a smaller percentage of Native American heritage."

According to Cindy L. Ehlers and colleagues, alcohol-related deaths are two to eight times higher among Native American women than among women in general. Alcohol-related deaths among male Native Americans occur at an even worse rate. Some studies, such as by May and Moran, have found that 26.5 percent of all deaths among Native Americans were alcohol-related, and the rate was 13.2 percent among Native American women. In contrast, only about 3.5 percent of all deaths in the United States are alcohol-related.

Some studies have found that in some tribes, such as the Southern Cheyennes, alcoholism is extreme and has an early onset of age 25. Researchers have also found a high rate of alcoholism among Alaska Natives.

Native American adolescents also have a high rate of alcohol abuse; for example, in a study in 1996, 34 percent of the adolescents reported having been drunk in the month prior to the study. Researchers have found that those Native American adolescents who are at the greatest risk for drinking problems live on reservations, go to boarding schools, or drop out of school. Risk factors for drinking include a family history of alcohol use disorders, poverty or lower income, being male, and family use of alcohol.

Another factor leading to alcohol issues, according to Szlembo and colleagues, is the acculturation or the adaptation of mainstream values over the values of the individual's tribe. The authors write, "Tribal elders report that many of today's problems are a result of a loss of traditional Native American beliefs and culture. Indeed tribal beliefs and values are almost universal in that they prohibit drug or alcohol use as well as violence toward others. Researchers have found that higher levels of substance use occur among those individuals who most closely identify with non-Native American values; they also found that the lowest rates of use occurred among individuals who were bicultural, that is, they were equally comfortable with Native and non-Native American values."

In a study of 754 Native Americans and Alaska Natives, published by Jay Shore, M.D., and colleagues in *Psychiatric Services* in 2002, the authors found that 56 percent of the subjects were positive for lifetime alcohol abuse and 27 percent were cur-

rent alcohol abusers. This was a high rate, and the authors said, "The high rate of positive screenings in our study may be attributable to several factors. First, previous studies have suggested that among American Indians and Alaska Natives, urban populations have a higher rate of alcohol use than rural populations, which have been the primary focus of past efforts. Second, primary care patients may have a higher rate of alcohol abuse, because persons who abuse alcohol are more likely to have comorbid conditions for which they seek medical treatment."

There were four significant risk variables that were related to screening positive for alcohol abuse, including male gender, single marital status, having ever reported being assaulted, mugged or robbed, and feelings of sadness or depression for at least two weeks in the past year. The researchers also noted a low concordance (agreement) rate of only 16 percent between the clinician's diagnosis of alcohol abuse and the screening results. They could not explain the reason for this, but suggested that cultural differences between physicians and Native American patients could play a role.

In another study of Mission Indians by Ehlers and colleagues, published in the *American Journal of Psychiatry* in 2004, of 407 participants, 70 percent of the men and 50 percent of the women met lifetime criteria for alcohol dependence. The researchers found that the onset of alcoholism was younger (age 20) and more rapid than among other large studies of alcoholics. The study subjects also had a high rate of BINGE DRINKING, driving while intoxicated and alcohol-related health problems. On the positive side, after diagnosis, remission from alcohol symptoms was high (77 percent).

Native Americans who are treated for alcohol dependence have used adaptations of Alcoholics Anonymous programs. Some experts believe that Native Americans are not amenable to standard treatments for Caucasians.

See also EXCESSIVE DRINKING AND HEALTH CONSEQUENCES.

Caetano, Raul, M.D., et al. "Alcohol Consumption among Racial/Ethnic Minorities: Theory and Research." *Alcohol Research & Health* 22, no. 4 (1998): 233–242.

Ehlers, Cindy L., et al. "The Clinical Course of Alcoholism in 243 Mission Indians." *American Journal of Psychiatry* 161, no. 7 (2004): 1,204–1,210.

Garcia-Andrade, C., T. L. Wall, and C. L. Ehlers. "The Firewater Myth and Response to Alcohol in Mission Indians." *American Journal of Psychiatry* 154, no. 7 (1997): 983–988.

May, P. A., and J. R. Moran. "Prevention of Alcohol Misuse: A Review of Health Promotion among American Indians." *American Journal of Health Promotion* 9 (1995): 288–299.

Shore, Jay, M.D., Spero M. Manson, and Dedra Buchwald. "Screening for Alcohol Abuse among Urban Native Americans in a Primary Care Setting." *Psychiatric Services* 53, no. 6 (2002): 757–760.

Szlemko, William J., James W. Wood, and Pamela Jumper Thurman. "Native Americans and Alcohol: Past, Present, and Future." *Journal of General Psychology* 133, no. 4 (2006): 435–451.

obsessive-compulsive disorder (OCD) OCD is a chronic and debilitating condition in which the individual has persistent thoughts or repetitive behaviors that last for at least an hour each day. The most familiar obsessions are with contamination with dirt and germs and the compulsion to wash one's hands excessively. There are many others, such as hoarding, pathologic doubt, and so on. According to Jon E. Grant, M.D., in his 2008 article for *Perspectives in Clinical Psychiatry: A Clinical Update,* this disorder is often both underdiagnosed and undertreated. Grant says that individuals with OCD may develop a substance use disorder (SUD), and if so, often the SUD is diagnosed rather than the OCD.

Some studies have found that of those with primary SUD, 23.2 percent had a lifetime (at some point in their life) diagnosis of an alcohol use disorder (alcohol abuse or dependence) and 13.3 percent had a lifetime diagnosis of a drug use disorder. According to Grant, "One explanation for the rates of SUDs in patients with OCD may be the very high levels of distress reported by these individuals."

The person with OCD knows that his or her behavior is irrational, but despite this, the person cannot control his or her behavior unless treated with medications and/or therapy. OCD impairs the person's daily life. Some individuals with OCD use alcohol to try to control their symptoms. OCD affects about 2.2 percent of adults in the United States, and about a third of the adults with OCD had symptoms as children.

Symptoms and Diagnostic Path
Symptoms of OCD include the following:

- spending an hour or more each day on thoughts or rituals

- performing the same repeated rituals, such as locking and unlocking doors, repeating the same steps, and counting items

- having repeated thoughts that the individual cannot control

- receiving no pleasure from behaviors or rituals but obtaining brief relief from the anxiety caused by the thoughts

OCD is usually diagnosed and treated by a psychiatrist, although a psychologist or other mental health professional may provide therapy to help deal with the disorder.

Treatment Options and Outlook
OCD is treated with ANTIDEPRESSANTS, such as medications in the selective serotonin reuptake inhibitor (SSRI) class as well as with tricyclic antidepressants (TCAs). Sometimes medications in the serotonin norepinephrine reuptake inhibitor (SNRI) class are used. BENZODIAZEPINES and beta blocker medications are also used to treat OCD. Sometimes treatment is augmented with antipsychotic medications, according to Barwin Bandelow, M.D., in his article on the medical treatment of obsessive-compulsive disorder and anxiety for *CNS Spectrums* in 2008.

Psychotherapy may provide relief as well. For example, exposure therapy that includes either gradual exposure to the anxiety-providing object or "flooding," which is intense and immediate exposure, can help. Cognitive-behavioral therapy (CBT) has also been found helpful in treating OCD.

Risk Factors and Preventive Measures
OCD affects men and women equally. The disorder cannot be prevented, but once it has been identified, it should be treated.

See ANXIETY DISORDERS; PSYCHIATRIC COMORBIDITIES.

Bandelow, Barwin, M.D. "The Medical Treatment of Obsessive-Compulsive Disorder and Anxiety." *CNS Spectrums* 13, no. 9, Supp. 14 (2008): 37–46.

Grant, Jon E., M.D., and Brian L. Odlaug. "Challenges in Diagnosing and Treating Obsessive-Compulsive Disorder." *Perspectives in Clinical Psychiatry: A Clinical Update.* Supplement to *Psychiatric Times.* September 2008, Issue 2 of 4, 25–30.

obsessive-compulsive personality disorder See PERSONALITY DISORDERS.

occupations The careers in which individuals are employed. Some studies have found that individuals in some occupations have a significantly greater risk for alcohol abuse or alcohol dependence than people employed in other careers; for example, data in the United Kingdom for 2007 indicated that individuals who either owned or worked in bars had a greater risk for an alcohol use disorder leading to death. In addition, research on workers in North Dakota from 2004–05, a state with a high rate of binge drinkers, indicates that ranch workers have a high rate of BINGE DRINKING.

Alcohol-related Deaths and Occupations

Some individuals have speculated that the risk for death related to alcohol may also be related to an individual's occupation. One study by Romeri, Baker, and Griffiths looked at alcohol-related deaths by occupation among men and women in England and Wales over the period 2001–05, reporting on their findings in *Health Statistics Quarterly* in 2007.

The researchers found that there were nearly 23,000 alcohol-related deaths among individuals ages 20–64 years over the period 2001–2005, so the subject was of concern. Bar owners and bar staff had the highest rates of alcohol-related deaths, while the lowest indicators were found among men who were farmers (in contrast to the study by Jarman et al.) and drivers and women who were childcare workers.

Other occupations with high alcohol-related mortality for men were individuals classified as seafarers, including barge and boat operatives.

Among women, other occupations in addition to bar staff and bar owners with high rates of alcohol-related deaths were those in office occupations and actors and entertainers.

Interestingly, the United Kingdom researchers noted that earlier studies had indicated that physicians were among groups with high alcohol-related deaths in the 1960s, 1970s, and 1980s. This no longer appears to be true. The researchers said, "This may be similar to the situation with smoking where, once the hazards were recognized in Britain, doctors gave up smoking earlier than the general population. Suggested reasons for this include: doctors 'heard the message' more quickly; a contradiction developed between doctors' devotion to health and their smoking behavior; smoking may also have become stigmatized in medical circles before it became so in the rest of society." The researchers suggested that similar reasons may have led to changes in the alcohol consumption behavior of physicians.

The researchers also said that some occupations may draw people who are already problem drinkers, or they may create problem drinkers through work pressures. They discussed earlier research in Edinburgh, which indicated eight factors which had emerged as possible explanations for why some occupations had higher rates of alcohol-related problems. These included access of alcohol at work, social pressure to drink at work, separation from social or family relationships, freedom from supervision, either very high or very low income levels, collusion by colleagues with regard to drinking, stress, and the recruitment of individuals predisposed to be heavy alcohol consumers.

The researchers concluded, "Despite the limitations and challenges which have long been reported when examining deaths by occupation, reports on alcohol-related deaths over more than a century have consistently identified similar occupations as being most at risk."

Alcohol-related Hospital Utilization and Death by Occupations in Sweden

Researchers in Sweden reported in 2001 in the *Scandinavian Journal of Work and Environmental Health* that for the period 1991–95 they found differences in occupations between those who were hospitalized because of alcohol use as well as occupations of those who had died.

For example, in considering about 50 different occupations and the risk for an increased rate of alcoholism among the long-term employed, among male workers, the occupations with the highest rates of alcoholism overall were forest workers (8.8), followed by bakers or pastry cooks (3.9). The lowest rates of alcoholism were seen among drivers (1.0) and construction carpenters (also 1.0). Among women who were employed long-term, the highest rates of alcoholism were seen among woodworking machine operators (11.3), followed by horticultural workers (9.9). The lowest rates of alcoholism among women who were employed long-term were seen among those who were metal-processing workers (0.1), followed by social workers (0.5).

The researchers concluded, "In this study manual workers showed the highest relative risk of alcoholism. The increased relative risks of alcoholism diagnoses found for several mostly manual, occupations seemed partly to be an effect of the selection of heavy drinkers into the same occupations. This conclusion is based on the evidence that new recruits into high-risk occupations often had increased relative risks of at least the same magnitude as those stable in the occupation for several years."

Past Data

Older statistical data about occupations and alcohol-related problems continue to be helpful; for example, a 1988 study by Dimich-Ward, as reported in the *Canadian Journal of Public Health,* found that there was a high death rate among bartenders and waiters, and this finding continues to hold true in the 21st century. In addition, in a study on death by CIRRHOSIS of the liver and occupation in 1992, Harford and Brooks found that the highest cirrhosis rates were found among blue-collar workers and employees at sites where alcohol was readily plentiful, such as bars. This is similar to later findings.

See also ALCOHOLISM/ALCOHOL DEPENDENCE AND ALCOHOL ABUSE; BINGE DRINKING; EXCESSIVE DRINKING AND HEALTH CONSEQUENCES; IMPAIRED PHYSICIANS; TREATMENT.

Dimich-Ward, Helen, et al., "Occupational Mortality among Bartenders and Waiters." *Canadian Journal of Public Health* 79, no. 3 (May/June 1988): 194–197.

Harford, Thomas C., and Sharon D. Brooks. "Cirrhosis Mortality and Occupation." *Journal of Studies on Alcohol* 53, no. 5 (1992): 463–468.

Hemmingsson, Tomas, and Gunille Ringback Weitoft. "Alcohol-related Hospital Utilization and Mortality in Different Occupations in Sweden in 1991–1995." *Scandinavian Journal of Work & Environmental Health* 27, no. 6 (2001): 412–419.

Jarman, D. W., T. S. Naimi, S. P. Pickard, W. R. Daley, and A. K. De. "Binge Drinking and Occupation, North Dakota, 2004–2005. *Preventing Chronic Disease* 4, no. 4 (2007). Available online. URL: http://www.cdc.gov/pcd/issues/2007/oct/06_0152.htm. Downloaded July 3, 2008.

Mandell, Wallace, William W. Eaton, James C. Anthony, and Roberta Garrison. "Alcoholism and Occupations: A Review and Analysis of 104 Occupations." *Alcoholism: Clinical and Experimental Research* 16, no. 4 (July/August 1992): 734–746.

Moen, Bente E., M.D., Sverre Sandberg, and Trond Riise. "Drinking Habits and Laboratory Tests in Seamen with and without Chemical Exposure." *Journal of Studies on Alcohol* 53, no. 4 (1992): 364–368.

Romeri, Ester, Allan Baker, and Clare Griffiths. "Alcohol-related Deaths by Occupation, England and Wales, 2001–05." *Health Statistics Quarterly* 25 (Autumn 2007): 6–12.

pancreatitis Severe and dangerous inflammation of the pancreas, which acts as both a digestive organ and an endocrine gland. Chronic alcohol abuse and ALCOHOLISM may lead to pancreatitis, a very serious and potentially life-threatening disease. Gallbladder disease or gallstones may also cause pancreatitis, as may a traumatic injury that harms the pancreas, and some medications, such as corticosteroids or diuretics. An attack of pancreatitis may be acute and severe or it may become a chronic condition. Alcoholic pancreatitis may be caused by the effects of toxic metabolites in the bloodstream, such as ACETALDEHYDE and fatty acid ethyl esters (FAEEs).

According to Alice L. Yang, M.D., and colleagues in their article for *Archives of Internal Medicine* in 2008, alcoholic pancreatitis is the most common hospital discharge diagnosis in the cases of alcohol-related liver or pancreatic complications, although alcoholic HEPATITIS with CIRRHOSIS has the greater death rate. Alain Vonlaufen, M.D., and his colleagues also stated in their article for *Alcohol Research & Health* that alcohol abuse is the major cause of chronic pancreatitis. These authors say that the stellate cells of the pancreas become activated in response to both ethanol and to acetaldehyde, a toxic byproduct that is made during the metabolizing of alcohol. The stellate cells are the cells that cause the development of connective tissue fibers in the pancreas, and if they are overactivated, this action may trigger chronic pancreatitis. The exact mechanism and sequence of events causing pancreatitis, however, is still under study by researchers.

Some experts warn that the withdrawal from alcohol dependence may trigger alcoholic pancreatitis. In a study of 76 patients reported by I. Nordback and colleagues in *Gastroenterology* in 2005, most (91 percent) had stopped drinking before they experienced nausea and vomiting as well as abdominal pain (68 percent) from pancreatitis. Of 83 patients who had been assessed prior to their pancreatitis symptoms, only 29 percent had developed some symptoms before consuming their last drink, while 43 percent developed their first symptoms on the first day they stopped drinking, and the rest developed symptoms on the second or third day after drinking. This study does not prove that withdrawal from alcohol causes pancreatitis, but it is one medical concern that physicians treating alcoholics should take into account.

Symptoms and Diagnostic Path

With acute pancreatitis, the following symptoms and signs may be present:

- abdominal pain that is the most severe in the upper left quadrant or upper middle
- fever
- nausea and vomiting
- perspiration
- mild jaundice
- low blood pressure
- edema
- rapid heart rate

With acute pancreatitis, laboratory tests will show elevated blood levels of amylase and lipase and elevated levels of amylase in the urine. An abdominal computerized tomography (CT) or magnetic resonance imaging (MRI) scan of the abdomen will reveal an inflamed pancreas. In addition, a plain chest X-ray may show abnormalities in about one-third of patients with acute pancreatitis, according to Santhy Swaroop Vege, M.D., and Suresh T. Chari, M.D., in their article for UpToDate, a private subscriber service offering information about medical problems. According to these authors, acute pancreatitis is classified as one of five grades, from Grade A (the mildest form) to Grade E (the most severe).

It is very important to differentiate whether acute pancreatitis is caused by alcoholism or by gallstones, because the cause affects the treatment; for example, gallstones can be removed surgically, while with alcoholism, the person must stop drinking.

In the case of chronic pancreatitis, the individual will often have the following symptoms and signs:

- severe abdominal pain, primarily in the upper abdomen, which may increase with eating or drinking
- fatty stools
- nausea and vomiting
- clay-colored or pale stools
- unintentional weight loss

Tests for chronic pancreatitis include blood tests for elevated levels of amylase, lipase, and trypsinogen. A fecal fat test may be ordered as well. In addition, an abdominal ultrasound or CT scan may reveal pancreatic inflammation as well as calcium deposits in the pancreas.

Treatment Options and Outlook

With acute pancreatitis, the main treatment is to relieve the severe pain and replace fluids intravenously. The patient is not given food or fluids orally so as to avoid activating the digestive system and any further aggravation of the pancreas. Rarely, surgery is required to remove dead (necrotic) tissue from the pancreas. Most patients recover within about a week; however, if the pancreas hemorrhages or the heart, liver, or kidneys become involved, the death rate is high. If the patient does recover, it is imperative that the patient give up drinking under the supervision of his or her physician. Some studies have also found that coffee can decrease the risk of alcohol-induced pancreatitis, apparently by partly blocking some channels within the pancreatic cells, although the mechanism of action is not entirely clear.

Narcotic pain medications or a surgical nerve block may be administered. When the pain is persistent, long-acting narcotics such as fentanyl patches or MS Contin may be used, according to Steven D. Freedman in his article for UpToDate.

The patient with pancreatitis may be placed on a low-fat diet and advised to eat small meals. Acid-blocker medications are given to avoid the production of gastric acid enzymes. Patients may also need to take oral vitamin D. If diabetes develops, the patient may be placed on insulin. Supplemental pancreatic enzymes may relieve some pain, although they are less effective among patients whose pancreatitis was caused by alcohol dependence. In some cases, surgery is required.

Risk Factors and Preventive Measures

To avoid either chronic or acute alcoholic pancreatitis, the individual who drinks should avoid consuming alcohol, since alcohol is a major risk factor for this serious medical problem.

See also ALCOHOL AND WOMEN; EXCESSIVE DRINKING AND HEALTH CONSEQUENCES; LIVER DISEASE, ALCOHOLIC.

Freedman, Steven D., M.D., and Michele D. Bishop. "Etiology and Pathogenesis of Chronic Pancreatitis in Adults." Private subscriber service online. URL: http://wwwupto date.com/online/content/topic.do?topicKey=pancdis/5929&selectedTitle4~79&source=search_result. October 6, 2008. Accessed March 12, 2009.

Nordback, I., et al. "Is It Long-Term Continuous Drinking or the Post-Drinking Withdrawal Period that Triggers the First Acute Alcoholic Pancreatitis?" Scandinavian Journal of Gastroenterology 40, no. 10 (2005): 1,235–1,239.

Swaroop Vege, Santhi, M.D., and Suresh T. Chari, M.D. "Clinical Manifestations and Diagnosis of Acute Pancreatitis." Official reprint from UpToDate. Private subscriber service online. URL: http://www.uptodate.com/online/content/topic.do?topicKey=pancdis/7667&selectedTit le=3~150&source=search_result. 22 September 2008. Accessed March 12, 2009.

Vonlaufen, Alain, M.D., et al. "Role of Alcohol Metabolism in Chronic Pancreatitis." Alcohol Research & Health 30, no. 1 (2007): 48–54.

Yang, Alice L., et al. "Epidemiology of Alcohol-Related Liver and Pancreatic Disease in the United States." *Archives of Internal Medicine* 168, no. 6 (March 24, 2008): 649–656.

panic disorder Panic disorder is a form of anxiety disorder that is characterized by recurrent panic attacks, which are attacks of an overwhelming fear and dread, often accompanied by a racing heart, and that may feel like a heart attack to the individual who is experiencing it. Individuals with recurrent panic attacks may try to "anesthetize" their fear through alcohol use; however, this is not an effective way to treat the disorder. According to the National Institutes of Mental Health (NIMH), about 6 million adults in the United States have panic disorder. Individuals with panic disorder are often ashamed of their disorder and feel like they should be able to control it.

Up to 40 percent of patients with panic disorder also have agoraphobia, which is an anxiety, fear, and avoidance of places from where the individual feels escape would be difficult or impossible. Some people with agoraphobia will not leave their city or sometimes even their own home because they fear that if they do, something terrible will happen to them.

Symptoms and Diagnostic Path

Common symptoms of a panic attack include difficulty with breathing, heart palpitations, heavy sweating, dizziness, and lightheadedness. A feeling of imminent doom is also a common and very frightening experience. The person may feel like he or she is dying and often seeks out EMERGENCY TREATMENT. When the emergency department doctor rules out a serious medical problem, often the person is embarrassed or confused.

Treatment Options and Outlook

Panic disorder can be treated with therapy and medications and is considered highly treatable, according to the NIMH. BENZODIAZEPINES are often used to treat panic disorder, and sometimes ANTI-DEPRESSANTS are prescribed. When panic disorder is accompanied by ALCOHOLISM, the alcohol dependence is treated separately. Panic disorder is also treated with psychotherapy, such as cognitive-behavioral therapy.

Risk Factors and Preventive Measures

Women are about twice as likely to suffer from panic disorder as men. Many people with SPECIFIC PHOBIA disorders have panic attacks although they may not have panic disorder. The only preventive measure is for the person who knows that he or she suffers from panic attacks to take medication to keep the disorder under control.

See also ANXIETY DISORDERS.

paranoid personality disorder See PERSONALITY DISORDERS.

parental influence See CHILD ABUSE AND NEGLECT; FAMILIES AND ALCOHOL; PARENTIFICATION.

parentification An invented term that was first used in 1965 by Boszormenyi-Ngy and which refers to children or adults who assume a quasi-parental role toward their own parents. This occurs because these parents cannot or will not provide the normal guidance and control of a parent, nor do they provide adequate (or any) emotional support. The parents may be alcoholics or drug addicts, or they could have other issues that prevent them from playing a normal parental role. The parents may fail to prepare food for their minor children as well as provide appropriate clothing because they are too intoxicated to perform this responsibility successfully. They may also fail to take their minor children to the doctor when they are sick. These are all forms of child neglect. (See CHILD ABUSE AND NEGLECT.)

The parents may unreasonably expect their children to fulfill the adult's personal needs (such as providing love, preparing food, and so forth), rather than realizing that it is the job of the parent to provide for the needs of their children. The parentified child may also feel forced to assume the responsibility and care of younger siblings. Children as young as two or three years old have been ordered by their alcoholic parents to watch over their younger siblings, sometimes to a tragic outcome.

In a study of depression and parentification among 207 adult children of alcoholics and "workaholics" that compared the two groups, reported by Jane J. Carroll and Bryan E. Robinson in *Family Journal: Counseling and Therapy for Couples and Families* in 2000, the adult children of alcoholics scored significantly higher on measures of parentification than did the children of workaholic parents. Children whose parents were *both* alcoholics and workaholics had even higher scores of parentification.

See also FAMILIES AND ALCOHOL.

Carroll, Jane J., and Bryan E. Robinson. "Depression and Parentification among Adults as Related to Parental Workaholism and Alcoholism." *Family Journal: Counseling and Therapy for Couples and Families* 8, no. 4 (2000): 360–367.

pathological gambling The pathological gambler has an addictive need to play games of chance, and he or she will gamble away the money needed for the rent, for food for a child, or money targeted for any other purpose, because the individual with this disorder is irresistibly drawn to gambling, despite the consequences and even when he or she has multiple losses. Many pathological gamblers also have problems with alcohol use. An estimated 1–3 percent of the general population are pathological gamblers.

Although pathological gambling has been described and categorized as an IMPULSE CONTROL DISORDER, many authorities believe that it is in fact far more akin to an addictive disorder. For example, in their editorial on pathological gambling written for the *Journal of Addictive Medicine* in 2007, authors Edward Gottheil, M.D., and his colleagues compare the diagnostic criteria for pathological gambling in the *DSM-IV*, published by the American Psychiatric Association, to the symptoms for substance dependence.

For example, the pathological gambler is preoccupied with gambling; similarly, the individual with substance dependence spends a great deal of time obtaining, using, or recovering from the effects of the substance. In addition, another diagnostic criterion is that the pathological gambler needs to spend increasingly greater amounts of money to achieve the same level of euphoria, just as the individual who is dependent on substances develops a tolerance to it and needs greater amounts to achieve the same level of intoxication.

In another comparison, the pathological gambler has tried and failed to stop gambling on many different occasions, just as the person who is dependent on alcohol or other drugs has also tried and failed to stop using the addictive substance. Last, the pathological gambler becomes irritable or restless when he or she tries to cut back or stop gambling altogether, just as the alcoholic experiences emotional withdrawal symptoms when he or she stops using the addictive substance.

The authors also point out that a gambling problem may be easier to hide than a substance dependence problem, because the gambler does not have direct observable physiological effects from the use of alcohol or a drug, such as dilation of the pupils of the eyes (with drugs) or a staggered gait (with alcohol). At the same time, however, the gambler may generate even more anger from family members, because of the penury into which he may have propelled them due to his or her gambling.

The authors also add that pathological gamblers often have substance dependence problems as well, and they state, "Recent data from the National Epidemiologic Survey on Alcohol and Related Conditions suggests that 73% and 38% of current pathologic gamblers meet criteria for an alcohol or drug disorder respectively. Thus approximately half of individuals experiencing problems related to gambling also experience problems related to 1 or more substances."

In her 2001 article for *Drug and Alcohol Dependence*, Nancy Petry also questioned whether pathological gambling is a disorder of impulse control. Says Petry, "While some research finds high levels of impulsivity in pathological gambling, other data indicate that pathological gamblers score no higher than controls, and sometimes even lower, on scales assessing impulsivity and related traits." Petry speculates that since at least half of all pathological gamblers have a substance use disorder, any increased levels of impulsivity may be related more to their substance use than to gambling.

In Petry's study of 90 male substance abusers, she found that 30 percent were also pathological gamblers. Performing a variety of scientific tests, Petry found that the subjects with both substance abuse and pathological gambling were significantly more impulsive than other subjects. However, Petry herself noted that she did not study impulsivity in pathological gamblers who were not substance abusers.

Petry also noted that, "Although some data indicate impulsiveness may be related to specific disorders such as ASP [antisocial personality disorder], substance abuse or pathological gambling, impulsiveness may also be regarded as a behavioral adaptation to chaotic and unpredictable environments. These same environments may place individuals at increased risk for drug abuse and pathological gambling."

In another report on gambling that addressed the specific brain mechanisms that are involved in "chasing losses" (continuing to gamble after major losses of money), Daniel K. Campbell-Meiklejohn and colleagues noted that the behavior of chasing losses apparently correlated with increased activity in the cortical areas of the brain associated with incentive-motivation and reward expectation, based on functional magnetic resonance imaging (fMRI) studies of neural activity in the brain when their healthy subjects either chose to continue to gamble or to stop gambling. (The subjects were not diagnosed with pathological gambling.) Future research with pathological gamblers as subjects should provide even more enlightening data.

Symptoms and Diagnostic Path

The pathological gambler is constantly thinking about gambling, whether he or she is engaged in gambling at the moment or not. He or she is unable to walk away from virtually any type of betting. Pathological gambling is diagnosed based on the individual's recent past behavior as well as the toll it has taken on his or her life; for example, pathological gamblers have a high rate of divorce compared to non-gamblers. They are often deep in debt. Some commit crimes in order to obtain the money needed to gamble. They will also steal from their family members, friends, and others in order to pursue gambling. They may rationalize that they

will "pay back" the money when they win; however, if the pathological gambler wins, the money is quickly gambled away.

In addition, noted Gottheil and colleagues, pathologic gamblers have cognitive distortions about randomness and chance, accompanied by an irrational overconfidence in their skill at predicting events. Some skill may play a role in some gambling activities, such as horse racing, but have no effect on slot machines or other random games of chance.

Treatment Options and Outlook

Some patients with pathological gambling benefit from treatment with NALTREXONE, a drug that is also used to treat alcohol dependence, while some studies have shown improvement with treatment with ANTIDEPRESSANTS in the selective serotonin reuptake inhibitor (SSRI) class; however, there is no drug approved by the Food and Drug Administration (FDA) for the treatment of gambling. Patients may also benefit from joining mutual aid support groups, such as Gamblers Anonymous, modeled on the highly successful Alcoholics Anonymous.

Therapy is also used with gamblers; however, according to Kit Sang Leung and Linda B. Cottler in their article for *Current Opinions in Psychiatry* in 2008, cognitive-behavioral therapy (CBT) has proven ineffective compared to other more cost-effective methods, such as brief psychiatric interventions with subjects and/or participation in organizations such as Gamblers Anonymous.

Risk Factors and Preventive Measures

In general, males are more likely to be pathological gamblers than females, although some females are gamblers. In addition, male pathological gamblers also have a greater risk for ALCOHOLISM than females who are pathological gamblers. Individuals with a family history of pathologic gambling have an increased risk for gambling, as do those with mood disorders, particularly DEPRESSION and anxiety. Individuals who have high levels of sensation-seeking also have an increased risk for pathological gambling.

Pathological gambling cannot be prevented, but once it has been identified, it is important for the individual to seek treatment.

See also PSYCHIATRIC COMORBIDITIES.

Campbell-Meiklejohn, Daniel K., et al. "Knowing When to Stop: The Brain Mechanisms of Chasing Losses." *Biological Psychiatry* 63 (2008): 293–300.

Gottheil, Edward, M.D., et al. "Pathologic Gambling: A Nonsubstance, Substance-Related Disorder?" *Journal of Addictive Medicine* 1, no. 2 (2007): 53–61.

Petry, Nancy M. "Substance Abuse, Pathological Gambling, and Impulsiveness." *Drug and Alcohol Dependence* 63 (2001): 29–38.

Sang Leung, Kit, and Linda B. Cottler. "Treatment of Pathological Gambling." *Current Opinions in Psychiatry* 22 (2008): 69–74.

personality disorders Specific aberrant psychiatric conditions affecting an individual's general outlook toward life, which lead to chronic behaviors and also cause the individual problems with his or her relationships at home and at work. These problems may range from mild to severe. People with personality disorders are also much more likely to abuse or become dependent on alcohol. A study by Mark Lenzenwegar et al. and reported in *Biological Psychiatry* used data from the National Comorbidity Survey Replication to determine the prevalence of personality disorders.

The researchers found a prevalence of 9.1 percent for any personality disorder in the general population. In looking at particular personality disorders, they found a prevalence rate of 1.4 percent for borderline personality disorder and less than 1 percent (0.6 percent) for ANTISOCIAL PERSONALITY DISORDER. (Not all personality disorders were evaluated for their prevalence.) Other researchers have found a higher rate of personality disorders among those with alcohol abuse or alcohol dependence. (See PSYCHIATRIC COMORBIDITIES.)

According to an analysis by Bridget F. Grant and colleagues of the data from the National Epidemiologic Survey on Alcohol and Related Conditions (NESARC), among individuals identified with a current alcohol use disorder, 28.6 percent had at least one personality disorder. In addition, of those individuals who had at least one personality disorder, 16.4 percent had a current alcohol use disorder. In considering subjects with alcohol dependence, 39.5 percent had a personality disorder. The most commonly occurring personality disorder among those who were alcoholics was antisocial personality disorder (18.3 percent), followed by paranoid personality disorder (15.8 percent), and obsessive-compulsive personality disorder (15.2 percent).

The researchers found that male alcoholics with personality disorders were the most likely to have dependent personality disorder, followed by histrionic personality disorder, while women alcoholics with personality disorders were most likely to have histrionic personality disorder, followed by antisocial personality disorder.

There are three "clusters" of personality disorder, Clusters A, B, and C. Cluster A includes personality disorders that are considered eccentric or odd, such as paranoid personality disorder, schizoid personality disorder, and schizotypal personality disorder. Cluster B personality disorders are those which include dramatic, emotional, or erratic behaviors, such as narcissistic personality disorder, borderline personality disorder, and antisocial personality disorder. Cluster C disorders are those which include anxious and fearful behaviors, such as obsessive-compulsive personality disorder, avoidant personality disorder, and dependent personality disorder.

Mark Lenzenwegar and colleagues reported in *Biological Psychiatry* in 2007 that Clusters A and C were the most commonly appearing, with a prevalence of 5.7 percent for Cluster A and 6.0 percent for Cluster C. The prevalence was 1.5 percent for Cluster B personality disorders.

Personality disorders are often considered difficult to treat.

In a study comparing individuals who were alcohol-dependent to their diagnosis of personality disorders by Echeburúa and colleagues and reported in 2007 in *Alcohol & Alcoholism,* the researchers found that 44.3 percent of the 158 alcohol-dependent patients had a personality disorder. The most common personality disorders identified among the alcoholic subjects were obsessive-compulsive personality disorders (12 percent), followed by antisocial, paranoid, and dependent personality disorders (7 percent each). Most of the subjects had one personality disorder only.

There are 10 specific types of personality disorders according to the *Diagnostic and Statistical Manual IV-TR,* as follows:

- antisocial personality disorder
- avoidant personality disorder
- borderline personality disorder
- dependent personality disorder
- histrionic personality disorder
- narcissistic personality disorder
- obsessive-compulsive personality disorder
- paranoid personality disorder
- schizoid personality disorder
- schizotypal personality disorder

Antisocial Personality Disorder

The person with antisocial personality disorder (ASPD) has exhibited a pattern of lying, stealing, and generally disregarding the rights of others, including family members and friends. Some people with ASPD are able to hide their lack of empathy and their general contempt for most people from others, and they are successful in business and politics; however, many are incarcerated as a result of their crimes. Many have also experienced legal problems, and they have a high risk for alcohol and drug abuse and dependence. The person with ASPD may also "rewrite" past circumstances in his or her mind, so that they were never at fault for anything negative that has occurred to them. This new version of events may often directly contradict what others recall, yet the person with ASPD insists that he or she is right.

Individuals with ASPD are fully aware of what the normal rules of society are; they just do not feel that they must follow them, and thus they often do *not* follow them. Many individuals in the prison population have ASPD, including both males and females who are incarcerated (although in the general public, ASPD occurs much more commonly among males than females).

Avoidant Personality Disorder

Individuals with avoidant personality disorder have an active pattern of extreme shyness and underlying feelings of inadequacy, which can affect success at work and in the family environment. They are disturbed by their excessive shyness but do not know how to change their behavior. An estimated 1 percent of the population has avoidant personal-ity disorder. This condition is different from social anxiety disorder in that it does not involve the extreme physical symptoms of anxiety that are seen with social phobia, such as severe perspiration, rapid heartbeat, and so forth. Individuals with avoidant personality disorder are at risk for substance abuse as well as for mood disorders. Avoidant personality disorder can be treated with therapy and ANTIDEPRESSANTS.

Some common symptoms of avoidant personality disorder include the following behaviors:

- a reluctance to become involved with others
- an avoidance of activities that involve interacting with others
- becoming overly hurt by the criticism of others
- shyness in social situations for fear of doing something wrong

Borderline Personality Disorder

Borderline personality disorder is a disorder of the regulation of emotion and moods. It affects an estimated 2 percent of adults, primarily young women. Individuals with borderline personality disorder often perceive other people in the extreme as either "good" or "bad"; there are no shades of gray to them.

Many women with this disorder engage in self-cutting their bodies, although they are not seeking to commit SUICIDE. They may engage in this behavior primarily to receive attention from others. Individuals with borderline personality disorder account for 20 percent of all psychiatric hospitalizations, according to the National Institute of Mental Health (NIMH). The person with borderline personality disorder may exhibit extreme anger, depression, or anxiety, although these mood changes last for no longer than a day. The disorder is not as severe as BIPOLAR DISORDER or major DEPRESSION, although it can cause severe instability in the lives of those who have it.

Some symptoms of borderline personality disorder may include the following:

- impulsivity in spending, sexual relationships, and eating
- inability to be alone

- frequent temper tantrums
- self-mutilation behaviors such as cutting the wrist, overdosing on drugs, or making cuts on various parts of the body

Some risk factors for the development of borderline personality disorder include sexual abuse, abandonment in childhood, and a chaotic family life.

Treatment includes group therapy so that the individual can learn from others with regard to appropriate behaviors. Medications may help with depression or mood swings. However, the prognosis is generally poor, because individuals with borderline personality disorder are often noncompliant with treatment recommendations.

Dependent Personality Disorder

The person with dependent personality disorder is excessively dependent on others to meet their needs. The disorder may begin in childhood although its onset may occur later in life. It is equally prevalent among men and women. The person with dependent personality disorder cannot trust his or her own decisions and is also extremely distressed by separation from those he or she is dependent upon. As a result, they may go to extremes to cling to a relationship.

Some behaviors that may be exhibited by a person with dependent personality disorder include the following:

- an avoidance of being alone
- an inability to meet the normal demands that life presents
- an extreme passivity in relationships with others
- an avoidance of any personal responsibility
- difficulty making decisions without receiving positive feedback from others
- a preoccupation with the fear of abandonment
- excessive distress when confronted with any criticism from others

The person with dependent personality disorder is at risk for alcohol abuse. He or she is also at risk for being victimized by others, physically, emotionally, and sexually. One of the worst partners for this individual is someone with antisocial personality disorder. Treatment with psychotherapy may be helpful.

Histrionic Personality Disorder

This disorder is present in the person who exhibits constant highly emotional behavior. People with histrionic personality disorder are sometimes referred to as "drama queens." It occurs more commonly in women than men and usually has its onset in early adulthood. Some symptoms of histrionic personality disorder include the following:

- constant seeking of approval and reassurance from other people
- a low tolerance for frustration or delayed gratification
- an excessive interest in his or her own personal appearance
- an excessive sensitivity to criticism from others
- acting or appearing overtly sexual
- easily influenced by others
- the belief that personal relationships are more intimate than they actually are
- blaming one's own failure on others

Individuals with histrionic personality disorder can usually hold a job, although they are frequently disappointed in their personal relationships with others. Treatment with therapy can provide improvement. Substance abuse can become a problem among this population.

Narcissistic Personality Disorder

As with the myth of Narcissus, the mythical person who fell in love with his own reflection (and who fell in a pool and then drowned), the person with narcissistic personality disorder has an excessive sense of his or her own importance. This disorder is believed to be present in less than 1 percent of the adult population in the United States. Alcohol abuse is a common complication of this disorder, as are depression and eating disorders. It usually has its onset in early adulthood and it is characterized by the following symptoms:

- requiring constant admiration and attention from others
- preoccupied with fantasies of ideal love, success, beauty, power, or intelligence
- exaggerates his or her own achievements out of proportion to their merit
- uses others to attain his or her goals
- reacts to any criticism with humiliation, rage, or shame, out of proportion to the criticism
- has unreasonable expectations of receiving favorable treatment from others
- lacks empathy toward others

According to the Mayo Clinic, some risk factors for the development of narcissistic personality disorder may include the following:

- unpredictable caregiving from parents
- severe childhood emotional abuse
- modeling of manipulative behaviors exhibited by parents
- overindulgence by parents
- an oversensitive temperament in childhood
- having received extreme admiration from adults for appearance or talents

Individual and group psychotherapy may help the person with narcissistic personality disorder develop a more rational and realistic self-image. Treatment of alcohol abuse or ALCOHOLISM that is present is also important.

Obsessive-Compulsive Personality Disorder

Obsessive-compulsive personality disorder is not the same disorder as obsessive-compulsive disorder (OCD); OCD is an ANXIETY DISORDER. There are some similarities, however, between the anxiety disorder and the personality disorder. With obsessive-compulsive personality disorder, the individual is obsessed with rules and order and is perfectionistic. In contrast, the person with OCD often feels compelled to repeat meaningless rituals, count items, or wash his or her hands to an excessive level.

The person with obsessive-compulsive personality disorder may exhibit the following symptoms:

- an inability to throw items away, even when they have no value
- a preoccupation with rules, lists, and details
- a reluctance to let others manage things
- an excessive devotion to work
- a limited display of affection to others

Treatment may involve antidepressants, combined with psychotherapy. The prognosis is better than with other personality disorders, because the person with this disorder is unlikely to abuse substances, as is common with individuals with other personality disorders.

Paranoid Personality Disorder

Individuals with paranoid personality disorder are extremely distrustful and suspicious of others and their motives. However, they are not psychotic, as with individuals who have paranoid SCHIZOPHRENIA. The disorder seems to appear more frequently in families with a history of schizophrenia. Individuals with paranoid personality disorder are at risk for extreme isolation, and they have a potential for violent behavior.

Some symptoms of paranoid personality disorder include the following:

- a belief that they will be used or exploited by others
- an inability to work with other people
- a poor self-image
- hostile behavior

Psychotherapy can help individuals with paranoid personality disorder, if they are willing to trust the therapist. Substance abuse may be a problem with this population.

Schizotypal Personality Disorder

The individual with schizotypal personality disorder exhibits odd and eccentric behavior and frequently seeks to avoid social contacts, including interactions with family members. He or she has few or no friends. Individuals with this personality disorder have magical thinking and odd beliefs, and they also have an inappropriate or decreased mood response to situations. The individual is suspicious of others and exhibits paranoid ideas; however, he or she is not psychotic. Many people with schizotypal personality disorder also have borderline personality disorder. They may believe in witches or aliens from other planets who are present on the earth, and these beliefs prevent them from establishing or maintaining normal relationships with others. Sometimes antipsychotic medications are used to treat this disorder, even though the individual is not psychotic. The prognosis for treatment success is poor, because few people with schizotypal personality disorder seek treatment. Alcohol abuse may be a problem in this population.

Schizoid Personality Disorder

Individuals with schizoid personality disorder have considerable difficulty with their relationships with others, and they also have unusual thinking patterns and behavior; however, they do not have schizophrenia, nor are they psychotic. Those with this disorder are solitary in their behavior, and they are emotionally flat, failing to respond to either criticism or praise from others. The individual with schizoid personality disorder has no interest in sexual activities with others. Few things—and sometimes nothing—give this person any pleasure.

In contrast to the person with schizotypal personality disorder, the person with schizoid personality disorder does not have perceptual or cognitive distortions in thinking.

Substance abuse may be a problem as well.

See also ADDICTIVE PERSONALITY; ADOLESCENTS AND DRINKING; ATTENTION-DEFICIT/HYPERACTIVITY DISORDER; CONDUCT DISORDER; IMPULSE CONTROL DISORDERS; TREATMENT.

Echebúria, Enrique, Richard Bravo de Medina, and Javier Aizpiri. "Comorbidity of Alcohol Dependence and Personality Disorders." *Alcohol & Alcoholism* 42, no. 6 (2007): 618–622.

Grant, Bridget F., et al. "Co-Occurrence of 12-Month Alcohol and Drug Use Disorders and Personality Disorders in the United States: Results from the National Epidemiologic Survey on Alcohol and Related Conditions." *Alcohol Research & Health* 29, no. 2 (2006): 121–130.

Lenzenweger, Mark, et al. "DSM-IV Personality Disorders in the National Comorbidity Survey Replication." *Biological Psychiatry* 62, no. 6 (2007): 553–564.

"Narcissistic Personality Disorder." Mayo Clinic. Available online. URL: http://www.mayoclinic.com/print/narcissistic-personality-disorders.html. Accessed December 16, 2008.

phobias, specific See ANXIETY DISORDERS.

polysubstance abuse See ALCOHOL AND OTHER DRUGS.

posttraumatic stress disorder (PTSD) Posttraumatic stress disorder (PTSD) is a form of an ANXIETY DISORDER characterized by severe stress that is directly linked to a highly traumatic event that was suffered by an individual, such as combat experience in a war zone, a rape, a severe beating, childhood abuse, or even extreme weather, such as fearing for one's survival in the midst of a severe hurricane or tidal wave. In each case, the individual felt severely threatened and may have believed that his or her life and/or the lives of loved ones were at extreme risk. As a result, the person responded to the traumatic event with horror, helplessness, and fear. PTSD is often accompanied by alcohol abuse.

The individual with posttraumatic stress disorder is at risk for turning to alcohol in an attempt to blot out the unpleasant experience, as well as to block the general anxiety that continues to torment him or her. Alcohol appears to provide some temporary relief from a loss or a trauma, but it also makes the development of PTSD more likely and increases the risk for chronic mental disorders. Individuals with PTSD are at an increased risk for DEPRESSION and for other anxiety disorders.

According to the National Institute of Mental Health (NIMH), about 7.7 million American adults age 18 and older, or about 3.5 percent of people in this age group, in a given year have PTSD, and the median age of the onset of PTSD is 23 years. An estimated 19 percent of Vietnam veterans experienced PTSD at some point after the war. Some veterans of the war in Iraq and Afghanistan also have experienced PTSD once they return home. Some studies have shown that National Guard and Reservist "citizen soldiers" who have returned from the war in Afghanistan and Iraq have an increased risk for BINGE DRINKING, alcohol abuse, and alcohol dependence. (See MILITARY VETERANS/COMBAT AND ACTIVE-DUTY MILITARY.)

It is likely that many of these veterans have PTSD, although many do not seek diagnosis due to feelings of guilt or shame as well as the fear that applying for benefits related to PTSD would stigmatize the individual and make it hard or impossible to obtain a job, particularly one that requires a security clearance.

Individuals with PTSD may experience flashbacks, feeling like they are actually reliving the traumatic event. They may have recurring, frightening dreams of the event. They may also experience severe survivor guilt, thinking about their friends and associates who died during the event. They may become emotionally numbed and may feel detached from others. They may refuse to make any plans for the future, having lost faith that they *will* have a future life. They may also seek to actively avoid people or places that remind them of the traumatic event.

There are three basic types of PTSD, including acute PTSD, when the symptoms have lasted for less than three months; chronic PTSD, when symptoms have lasted three months or longer; and PTSD with delayed onset, when six months or more have transpired between the traumatic event and the symptom onset.

Symptoms and Diagnostic Path

The individual with PTSD may experience the following symptoms:

- recurring thoughts of the stressful event that led to the development of PTSD
- sleep disorders, such as having great difficulty getting to sleep or experiencing frequent awakenings
- having angry outbursts, hypervigilance, and an exaggerated startle response—such as with the soldier newly returned from combat who dives for cover when he or she hears a car backfire
- an emotional numbness or flatness

Treatment Options and Outlook

Supportive psychotherapy is usually the best treatment for PTSD. Often cognitive-behavioral therapy (CBT) is used, which helps individuals to challenge their destructive and distressing thoughts and learn to think more logically. Exposure therapy helps the individual use such tactics as writing about the event, mental imagery, or even revisiting the site of the trauma to gain control over stress. Another form of CBT is stress inoculation training, which teaches the person coping skills to reduce PTSD symptoms.

Medications may also be used to treat PTSD, such as ANTIDEPRESSANTS or BENZODIAZEPINES. In a study by Kathleen Brady and colleagues and reported in *Alcohol: Clinical and Experimental Research* in 2005, the researchers treated 94 subjects with both alcohol dependence and PTSD in a 12-week trial. They found that subjects with less severe alcoholism and an early onset of PTSD improved with sertraline (Zoloft) as compared to placebo.

Most individuals eventually recover from PTSD with treatment.

Risk Factors and Preventive Measures

Individuals who have experienced a severe ordeal, such as combat stress, physical or sexual assaults, childhood abuse or neglect, or other severe traumatic experiences, are at risk for the development of PTSD. Some individuals develop PTSD after a major natural disaster causing an extreme loss of life and property, such as Hurricane Katrina. In general, women are more likely to develop PTSD than men. There are no known preventive measures to protect against PTSD because most extreme circumstances cannot be predicted in advance.

See also PSYCHIATRIC COMORBIDITIES.

Brady, Kathleen, M.D., et al. "Sertraline in the Treatment of Co-Occurring Alcohol Dependence and Post-Traumatic Stress Disorder." *Alcohol Clinical and Experimental Research* 29, no. 2 (2005): 395–401.
National Institute of Mental Health. "NIMH Fact Sheet: Post-Traumatic Stress Disorder Research." Bethesda, Md. Undated.

pregnancy The carrying of a fetus. Research has documented that alcohol abuse and ALCOHOL-ISM/ALCOHOL DEPENDENCE can be very harmful to the developing fetus. In fact, physicians advise against the consumption of *any* alcoholic beverages during pregnancy. If the woman does drink during pregnancy, the fetus has an increased risk for developing FETAL ALCOHOL SYNDROME/FETAL ALCOHOL SPECTRUM DISORDERS. One study reported by the National Institute on Alcohol Abuse and Alcoholism (NIAAA) reported that children born to women who drank heavily (four drinks per day) had nerve damage to their arms and legs that was still present a year later.

Unfortunately, up to half of women of childbearing age in the United States drink alcohol before they realize that they are pregnant. Among women who are moderate to heavy drinkers during pregnancy (consuming one to two ounces of alcohol per day) and those who are chronic alcoholics, the rate of fetal alcohol syndrome is as high as 50 percent.

According to Kartik Shankar and colleagues in their article for *Alcohol Research & Health* in 2007, "Although the harmful effects of alcohol (i.e. ethanol) on the growing fetus have been recognized for nearly three decades, alcohol continues to be the most common malformation-causing chemical (i.e., teratogen) ingested during pregnancy." Alcohol interferes with the nutritional supply to the fetus and negatively affects the fetus in many other ways, even if the child does not develop fetal alcohol syndrome. In addition, many pregnant women who drink also smoke cigarettes, further increasing the risk for harm to the fetus.

Some women mistakenly believe that if they have been drinking in early pregnancy, it is already too late to stop and there would be no benefit to ending their alcohol consumption; however, experts report that ending drinking even in late pregnancy can be beneficial to children born to women who have abused alcohol.

Assessing Heavy Drinking during Pregnancy

Because there are no laboratory tests to ascertain drinking over time (although tests can determine recent alcohol consumption), physicians generally rely on screening pregnant women for drinking by asking them questions, including using some screening instruments that have been developed by researchers.

According to Grace Chang, M.D., in her article on alcohol intake and pregnancy for UpToDate (a private subscriber online service), one screening instrument for alcohol that is sometimes used with pregnant women is TWEAK, developed by Marcia Russell. With this particular instrument T stands for tolerance for alcohol, W for worry or concern by family and friends about drinking behavior, E for eye opener, or the need to have a drink in the morning, A for amnesia or ALCOHOLIC BLACKOUTS that occur during drinking, and K for the individual's own belief that she needs to cut down on the use of alcohol. (The last should technically be a C but the creators of the instrument used a K.)

The scores for TWEAK range from 0 to 7. "Yes" answers to the tolerance and worry questions are given two points each, and "yeses" to the other three questions are given one point each. A score of 2 or more on the TWEAK indicates heavy drinking.

Another screening instrument for alcohol that is used with pregnant women is T-ACE, in which T is for tolerance, as in "How many drinks does it take to make you feel high?" The A is for "Annoyed," as in "Have people Annoyed you by criticizing your drinking?" The C is for cut down, as in "Have you ever felt you ought to Cut down on your drinking?" The E is for "Eye opener," as in, "Have you ever had a drink first thing in the morning to steady your nerves or get rid of a hangover?" According to Chang in her article for *Alcohol Research & Health* in 2001, a response of "more than two drinks" to question T receives two points and "yes" answers to the other questions receive one point each. A total score of 2 or more indicates risky drinking is occurring during pregnancy.

Medications and Pregnancy Categories

The medications that are used to treat alcohol dependence are all Pregnancy C category (with the exception of DISULFIRAM). This is a category that denotes a medication may be dangerous to a fetus based on criteria set in 1979 by the FDA, but that the benefit may outweigh the risks. There are five pregnancy categories.

With Category A drugs, animal and human studies have failed to demonstrate a risk to the fetus in the first trimester, and there is no evidence of any risk in later trimesters. Almost no drugs fall in this category. Category B includes drugs in which animal studies have demonstrated no risk to the fetus and there are no adequate studies in pregnant women. Many drugs, including acetaminophen (Tylenol) and prenatal vitamins fall in this category. Category C includes drugs in which animal studies have shown an adverse effect on the fetus, but there are no adequate studies on humans; however, the potential benefits of the drug may warrant the risk of use in pregnant women. Many drugs fall into the Category C classification. With Category D, there is evidence of human fetal risk, but the potential benefits may warrant use of the drug in pregnant women despite the risks. With Category X, both animal and human studies indicate fetal risk and the risks involved in the use of the drug with pregnant women clearly outweigh potential benefits. (The FDA has requested a change in the pregnancy labeling of drugs and wishes to include data on dangers during pregnancy and lactation. However, the older pregnancy categories are still used as of this writing.)

Risks with Caffeine

In addition to avoiding alcohol and cigarettes, pregnant women should avoid caffeine, including caffeine that is often present in so-called decaffeinated drinks. For example, one study found that decaffeinated espresso from popular takeout places had a range of from 3 to 15.8 mg present in the espresso. Caffeine is also present in products that contain chocolate, as well as in some over-the-counter (OTC) drugs, such as Excedrin pain reliever. It is also true that many people consume products that are known to include caffeine, such as soft drinks as well as high-energy drinks, which may include up to 77 mg of caffeine. Although the extent of the risk of caffeine in inducing miscarriage is debatable, it is best for pregnant women to avoid caffeine as well as alcohol.

See also ALCOHOL AND WOMEN; CHILD ABUSE AND NEGLECT; TREATMENT.

Chang, Grace, M.D. "Alcohol Intake and Pregnancy." UpToDate. Available online to subscribers only. Updated October 8, 2008.

———. "Alcohol-Screening Instruments for Pregnant Women." *Alcohol Research & Health* 25, no. 3 (2001): 204–209.

Graham, Noni A., Christopher J. Hammond III, and Mark S. Gold, M.D. "Caffeine in Miscarriages: It's Not Just in the Coffee." *American Journal of Obstetrics & Gynecology* 199, no. 5 (November 2008): e15.

National Institute on Alcohol Abuse and Alcoholism. "NICHD News Release: New Study Finds Babies Born to Mothers Who Drink Alcohol Heavily May Suffer Permanent Nerve Damage." Available online. URL: http://www.niaaa.hih.gov/NewsEvents/News-Releases/mothers_alcohol.htm. Accessed March 16, 2009.

Shankar, Kartik, Martin J. J. Ronis, and Thomas M. Badger. "Effects of Pregnancy and Nutritional Status on Alcohol Metabolism." *Alcohol Research & Health* 30, no. 1 (2007): 55–59.

psychiatric comorbidities Serious psychiatric or emotional diagnoses that are present along with (otherwise known as "comorbid") alcohol abuse or alcohol dependence, including such diagnoses as ANTISOCIAL PERSONALITY DISORDER, ANXIETY DISORDERS, ATTENTION-DEFICIT/HYPERACTIVITY DISORDER, BIPOLAR DISORDER, DEPRESSION, and SCHIZOPHRENIA, as well as some IMPULSE CONTROL DISORDERS, such as PATHOLOGICAL GAMBLING. Most psychiatrists rely upon the criteria and guidelines provided in the *Diagnostic and Statistical Manual (DSM) IV*, published by the American Psychiatric Association, to help them make psychiatric diagnoses. A psychiatric comorbidity that is present along with an alcohol use disorder is sometimes referred to as a dual diagnosis.

The most common comorbidity among individuals with alcohol use disorders (alcohol abuse and ALCOHOLISM) is SMOKING, and nicotine dependence as well as nicotine withdrawal are problems described in the *Diagnostic and Statistical Manual*. An estimated 80 percent of all alcoholics are smokers, compared to a rate of about 25 percent in the general public. The next most common comorbidities among individuals with alcohol use disorders are depression and anxiety disorders. This is significant in relation to smokers, because, according to Jill M. Williams and Douglas Ziedonis in their 2004 article in *Addictive Behaviors*, the metabolism of tobacco can drastically affect the blood levels of psychiatric medications by inducing P450 liver cytochrome (CYOP1A2) enzymes produced by the liver. As a result, smoking can slash the blood levels of some medications by up to 40 percent, particularly antipsychotic medications, but also some ANTIDE-PRESSANTS and other prescribed medications, as well as some over-the-counter (OTC) medications. Thus, the standard dosage of these medications will not work as well in smokers as they will in nonsmokers.

According to Williams and Ziedonis, "Rates of cigarette smoking appear to be highest among patients with psychotic and substance-use disorders but remain high also for depression, anxiety, and personality disorders. Nicotine may act as a conditioned cue for alcohol and illicit substance use."

Individuals who use ALCOHOL AND OTHER DRUGS, including those who misuse both prescribed and illicit drugs, have an increased risk for becoming dependent on alcohol. In addition, individuals who abuse alcohol have an increased risk for abusing or becoming dependent on other drugs, ranging from the nicotine in cigarettes to marijuana and other illicit drugs to prescription medications.

People with psychotic disorders have an elevated risk for both alcohol abuse and alcoholism. People who are psychotic are out of touch with reality and may experience delusions (false beliefs, such as that other people are plotting against them or that the television is sending them special encoded messages) and/or hallucinations (false sensory experiences, such as hearing voices that are not there or seeing visions that are not real). Schizophrenia is always a psychotic disorder, although it can sometimes be treated effectively with antipsychotic medications. Bipolar disorder may be a psychotic disorder, while depression is infrequently accompanied by psychosis.

It is not always clear which came first, the psychiatric disorder or the alcohol abuse or dependence. Experts have spent years debating and studying this issue, particularly with regard to such comorbidities as depression. Some research indicates that depression may precede alcoholism, while other research indicates that alcohol dependence causes depression. Some research has indicated that depression precedes alcohol dependence in women, while alcohol dependence may trigger depression in men.

According to Monica L. Zilberman and colleagues, women with alcohol use disorders as well as other drug use disorders have higher rates of psychiatric comorbidities than men with alcohol or drug use disorders, particularly in the case of mood and anxiety disorders. According to the authors, "Because psychiatric disorders, particularly depression and PTSD [posttraumatic stress disorder], are associated in women with increased risk for developing substance use disorders, careful psychiatric assessment and treatment of these conditions may prevent the occurrence of substance use disorders." (See ALCOHOL AND WOMEN.)

Psychiatrists try to determine which disorder is the most serious for the individual and which may be driving other psychiatric problems, so that the key disorder can be treated first. When at least two disorders are very problematic for the individual, however, psychiatrists often must treat both. For example, severe depression and alcoholism are risk factors for SUICIDE; thus, they both require treatment. In most cases, the doctor cannot wait for the depression (or alcoholism) to improve so that the next disorder can be treated.

Considering Overall Risks for Psychiatric Comorbidities

Research has shown that the risk for mood and anxiety disorders is significantly increased among those with alcohol dependence. For example, according to the National Institute on Alcohol Abuse and Alcoholism (NIAAA), the risk for major depression is increased by 3.7 times when a person is an alcoholic. See Table 1 for other risks; for example, the risk for manic disorder (a form of bipolar disorder) is increased by 5.7 times with alcohol dependence, and the risk for GENERALIZED ANXIETY DISORDER (GAD) is increased by 3.1 times when an individual is dependent on alcohol. Of course, sometimes the psychiatric disorder presents itself before the alcoholism. It should not be assumed that alcohol dependence necessarily caused the psychiatric problem.

It is also instructive to look at the percentage of those with alcohol use disorders who received treatment in the past 12 months and who have particular comorbidities. This information was provided by Bridget F. Grant and colleagues based on National Epidemiologic Survey on Alcohol and Related Conditions (NESARC) data and published in *Alcohol Research & Health* in 2006.

**TABLE 1
CO-OCCURRENCE RISK OF CURRENT (12-MONTH)
ALCOHOL DEPENDENCE AND MOOD
AND ANXIETY DISORDERS**

Disorder	With Alcohol Dependence
Major depression	3.7 X
Dysthymia	2.8 X
Manic disorder	5.7 X
Hypomania	5.2 X
Panic (with agoraphobia)	3.6 X
Panic (without agoraphobia)	3.4 X
Social phobia	2.5 X
Specific phobia	2.2 X
Generalized anxiety disorder	3.1 X

Source: Adapted from Li, Ting-Kai, M.D., Director, National Institute on Alcohol Abuse and Alcoholism. "Alcohol Use Disorders and Co-Occurring Conditions." Presentation on June 24, 2004 at the Complexities of Co-Occurring Conditions Conference, sponsored by the Substance Abuse and Mental Health Services Administration, the National Institute on Drug Abuse, the National Institute on Alcohol Abuse and Alcoholism, and the Agency for Healthcare Research and Quality. Washington, D.C.

Table 2 shows that of those mood and anxiety comorbidities that were considered, major depression was the most common one, occurring in 32.75 percent of the subjects with alcohol use disorders. SPECIFIC PHOBIA was also very common (17.24 percent), as was mania and generalized anxiety disorder. About a third of those with any alcohol use disorder have a drug use disorder.

Adolescents and Young Adults and Psychiatric Comorbidities

As with individuals of other ages, adolescents and young adults who are alcohol abusers or alcoholics often suffer from depression as well. Experts and policy makers are especially concerned about UNDERAGE DRINKING, because many studies show that those who start drinking early have an increased risk for alcohol dependence in adulthood.

In a study published in 2008 in the *American Journal of Drug and Alcohol Abuse* on 41 adolescents seeking treatment for their alcohol-related problems, Thiago Marques Fidalgo and colleagues found that 77 percent of the adolescents met the criteria for depression, and about half of the

teenagers who drank on a daily basis were at risk for or had anxiety disorders. The researchers also found that heavy users of alcohol were more likely to have anxious, depressive, and even psychotic symptoms.

The researchers said, "Co-morbid conditions are extremely common among [alcohol] dependent patients. Only by treating both the addiction as well as the associated psychiatric conditions will we approach the patient more comprehensively and as a consequence, will be able to offer the best fitting treatment."

According to Deborah Deas, M.D., and Suzanne Thomas in their article on the comorbid psychiatric factors contributing to adolescent alcohol and drug use, published in *Alcohol Research & Health* in 2002, studies have shown that some psychiatric comorbidities, particularly depression and anxiety disorders, predate substance abuse. Other risk factors for the adolescent abuse of alcohol or drugs are the behaviors of their peers and environmental factors, such as a low socioeconomic status or living

**TABLE 2
TWELVE-MONTH PREVALENCE OF MOOD AND
ANXIETY DISORDERS AMONG RESPONDENTS WITH
ANY ALCOHOL USE DISORDER WHO SOUGHT
TREATMENT IN THE PAST 12 MONTHS**

Disorder	Percent with Disorder, Percent
Any mood disorder	40.69
Major depression	32.75
Dysthymia	11.01
Mania	12.56
Hypomania	3.07
Any anxiety disorder	33.38
Panic Disorder	
With agoraphobia	4.10
Without agoraphobia	9.10
Social phobia	8.49
Specific phobia	17.24
Generalized anxiety disorder	12.35
Any drug use disorder	33.05

Grant, Bridget F., et al. "Prevalence and Co-Occurrence of Substance Use Disorders and Independent Mood and Anxiety Disorders: Results from the National Epidemiologic Survey on Alcohol and Related Conditions." *Alcohol Research & Health* 29, no. 2 (2006): page 117.

in an urban environment. Family factors, such as the use of alcohol and/or drugs by parents and/or siblings, and genetic factors are also relevant. A larger family size has also been found predictive for the abuse of alcohol and drugs, as is being born to parents under age 21.

The authors reported, "Adolescence is a dynamic period characterized by changes in many realms (e.g., physical, emotional, hormonal, and psychological), including AOD [alcohol and other drugs] use experience. Therefore, it is important that this period be viewed not as a single 'snapshot' of development, but rather as a period when risk factors for AOD use can and will change in their relative impact over time. For example, the literature suggests that peer influences and environmental influences are especially important in early adolescence and in the initiation of AOD use."

Abuse or Dependence on Other Drugs

Not all alcoholics use illegal drugs or misuse prescription drugs, but conversely, most people who abuse drugs also consume alcohol to excess. Individuals who abuse alcohol and other drugs may abuse marijuana, cocaine, and a wide array of other drugs, including prescription drugs, such as opioid prescription painkillers. When individuals abuse both cocaine and alcohol, the body forms a substance known as cocaethylene, which is more toxic than either substance alone.

Abuse of alcohol in concert with prescription drugs is often a cause of accidental death.

Sometimes it is difficult for experts to determine whether the death was a suicide or an accidental death. The difference is often important to the deceased's family and friends, and it can affect the position of insurance companies, which may exclude payments for suicide.

Anxiety Disorders

Many people who abuse or are dependent on alcohol suffer from anxiety disorders, and many people with an anxiety disorder have two or more such disorders. Sometimes they apparently "self-medicate" with alcohol, particularly among those with SOCIAL PHOBIA, generalized anxiety disorder, or PANIC DISORDER. Alcohol does not truly alleviate anxiety, although it may briefly mask symptoms for the individual.

The key anxiety disorders include generalized anxiety disorder, social phobia, panic disorder, POSTTRAUMATIC STRESS DISORDER (PTSD), specific phobia, and OBSESSIVE-COMPULSIVE DISORDER. Agoraphobia may occur with panic disorder; it is a fear of being in a situation where escape would be difficult or impossible, according to the individual's own assessment. Some people with agoraphobia will not leave their city or, in extreme cases, their homes, lest something terrible happen to them. Less than 1 percent of individuals ages 18 and older in the United States suffer from agoraphobia, although those with alcohol use disorders have an elevated risk for this disorder, as with all anxiety disorders.

Generalized Anxiety Disorder (GAD)   Generalized anxiety disorder (GAD) is present in an estimated 6.8 million Americans ages 18 and older, and its onset can occur at any time, although it generally develops in adulthood. GAD is characterized by an extreme generalized fear that impedes the individual's life, and this anxiety disorder is elevated among those with alcohol dependence. According to Kate Collins and Sanjay Matthew in their overview of GAD for *Perspectives in Psychiatry*, 90 percent of individuals with GAD have another psychiatric diagnosis at some point, and more than a third of them have alcohol abuse, social anxiety disorder (also known as social phobia), and specific phobia.

According to Ronald M. Doctor and colleagues in *The Encyclopedia of Phobias, Fears and Anxieties*, "Individuals with GAD are constantly tense and worried, even though most know their worries are irrational and unwarranted. Such individuals may worry constantly about their own health or the health of others or they may worry about money (when financial issues are not a problem), work, or other issues. Individuals with GAD often have problems with insomnia and may have physical symptoms such as fatigue, muscle pain, nausea, irritability, a frequent need to go to the bathroom, breathlessness, etc."

GAD is treated with therapy and antidepressants as well as antianxiety medications.

Obsessive-compulsive Disorder (OCD) A fairly rare disorder; only 1.2 percent of Americans meet the 12-month prevalence of a diagnosis of OCD, and about 2.3 percent meet the lifetime diagnosis of OCD, based on the National Comorbidity Survey Replication, according to A. M. Ruscio and colleagues in their 2008 article in *Molecular Psychiatry.*

An obsession is a repeated thought or impulse, while a compulsion is a repeated behavior or mental act that the person feels compelled to do, although in most cases, individuals with OCD know that both the obsession and compulsion are irrational, and they fervently wish to stop both the thoughts and the behaviors. (But they cannot stop them without professional intervention.) Some individuals with OCD are obsessed with contamination, and they feel compelled to constantly wash their hands, while others are obsessed with checking or counting things.

According to Ruscio et al., more than a third (38.6 percent) of adults with OCD have substance use disorders, and many of them also have other anxiety disorders (76.8 percent) as well as mood disorders (63.3 percent). Of those with substance use disorders, an estimated 23.7 percent of adults with OCD have alcohol dependence. According to the researchers, often it is only the severe cases of OCD that come to the attention of mental health professionals, and it is likely that many people with less severe cases attempt to cope with the illness on their own.

A 40-year follow-up of patients with OCD alone by Gunnar Skoog and Ingmar Skoog, published in the *Archives of General Psychiatry* in 1999, found that 83 percent of the 144 psychiatric patients had improved and 20 percent had completely recovered. An early age of onset and low social functioning as well as the presence of magical obsessions and compulsive rituals were linked with a worse prognosis. (An example of a magical obsession for an adult is to believe that if you step on a crack, you really will break your mother's back. Thus, the person with this obsession compulsively avoids all cracks in the sidewalk.) The researchers did not consider substance abuse issues, but their discovery of complete remission in some patients is important to consider.

The researchers also noted that the subjects' obsessions and compulsions seemed to change over time; for example, one patient who was followed from puberty to his 50s had guilt obsessions as a young man. In his late 20s, his obsession changed to one of doubt that was accompanied by severe checking behavior and agoraphobia. By the time the man was in his 50s, he had improved greatly but still had some vague avoidance symptoms, according to the researchers.

Panic Disorder Among the general public, about 2.7 percent of adults have panic disorder. Some people have one panic attack and never have another one, and they would not be diagnosed with panic disorder, which involves repeated panic attacks. The person with a panic attack often presents to the emergency room of the nearest hospital, convinced that he or she is dying because of a racing heart and a feeling of imminent doom. The doctor screens the person for obvious cardiovascular issues, and if none are present, may make the diagnosis of panic attack. About a third of those with panic disorder develop agoraphobia. Individuals with alcoholism have a three times greater risk of having panic disorder than nonalcoholics.

PTSD Posttraumatic stress disorder (PTSD) is a long-term reaction to extreme stress, such as witnessing or participating in combat or seeing or suffering from violence in noncombatant situations. About 3.5 percent of adults ages 18 and older have PTSD in any given year, according to the National Institute of Mental Health (NIMH), and most people develop PTSD as adults, although the disorder can occur in children and adolescents. Individuals with PTSD suffer from flashbacks, or a reliving of the traumatic incident as if it were actually happening all over again. To block such retraumatization, some individuals turn to alcohol for escape; however, alcohol can provide only a brief respite at best.

Social Phobia An estimated 6.8 percent of adults ages 18 and older have social phobia (also known as social anxiety disorder or SAD). This is a fear of interacting with others in public, and those with alcohol dependence have an increased risk for social phobia. Many people are fearful of public speaking, but the person with social phobia may be frozen with fear when compelled to communicate with others or even be in their presence. In general, the onset of social phobia occurs at around age 13 and in most cases, it precedes alcohol abuse and dependence. Theoretically, if social phobia were treated in the early stages, then the risk for alcohol dependence might be averted or at least decreased.

According to Lakshmi N. Ravindran, M.D., in his article on social anxiety disorder and comorbidities, the prevalence of alcohol use disorder among those with SAD ranges from 15 to 24 percent. Also, once an alcohol use disorder develops, it may work to maintain or worsen the social phobia.

Ravindran said, "Identifying SAD in individuals with AUDs [alcohol use disorders] poses a particular diagnostic challenge. Socially anxious individuals may be unaware of their disorder and attribute anxious symptoms (i.e., sweating, nausea) to alcohol withdrawal. In addition, the group treatment environment commonly used in AUD is likely to be a deterrent for patients with SAD. Finally, obtaining SAD treatment for this population may be complicated by the requirement of research trials and clinics to have substance use treated prior to addressing anxiety."

Specific Phobia Specific phobia refers to an extreme fear that an individual has among a wide array of possible feared objects, ranging from common fears, such as a fear of tunnels or insects, to bizarre phobias, such as autodysomophobia, the fear that one has a disgusting and repellant smell, or icthyophobia, the fear of fish. Specific phobia usually has its onset in childhood, particularly at age seven, according to the NIMH. About 8.7 percent of adults ages 18 and older have specific phobias, while those with alcohol use disorders have an elevated risk for specific phobias. The reason for this higher rate of specific phobias is unknown, but perhaps the "self-medication" theory of the cause for some alcohol abuse may apply in this case.

In his article on dual diagnosis in *Biological Psychiatry* in 2004, Ronald Kessler suggested that phobias nearly always precede substance abuse by as much as 10 years or more, and the substance abuse that subsequently follows phobias is especially common in adult female alcoholics. He concludes that interventions treating these phobias ahead of time might be extremely helpful at preventing substance abuse or at least teaching phobic individuals how to handle their fears.

Kessler says, "Based on this thinking, interventions might be aimed either at curing the phobia before secondary substance abuse begins or at teaching treatment-resistant phobics alternative strategies for managing their fears. There is good reason to believe that these strategies could be quite effective. If so, they would reduce a substantial percent of lifetime substance use disorders and an even greater percent of current disorders. This is because alcoholics and substance abusers with primary phobias are more chronic than primary alcoholics and substance abusers, presumably because continued fears precipitate further drinking."

Attention-deficit/Hyperactivity Disorder

Individuals with attention deficit hyperactivity disorder (ADHD) all have an increased risk for the development of alcohol use disorders. About 4.1 percent of adults have ADHD in the United States, according to the NIMH. According to data on ADHD from the National Comorbidity Survey Replication and reported by Ronald C. Kessler and colleagues in the *American Journal of Psychiatry* in 2006, 5.9 percent of adult respondents with ADHD had a diagnosis of alcohol abuse, compared to 2.4 percent among respondents without ADHD. In addition, the adults with ADHD had double the rate of alcohol dependence, or 5.8 percent compared to 2.9 percent of the non-ADHD subjects.

According to Timothy E. Wilens in his article on the nature of ADHD and substance use in the *Journal of Clinical Psychiatry* in 2007, about 20 percent of adults with a substance use disorder (SUD) have ADHD, and adults with an SUD and ADHD have a more complex and severe course of their SUD. (A substance abuse disorder is either alcohol abuse or alcoholism or drug abuse or drug addiction.) Treatment of ADHD in childhood may decrease the risk for both smoking and SUD in adulthood, according to Wilens.

In their analysis of adults with ADHD plus substance use disorders and their psychiatric comorbidities, published in the *American Journal on Addictions* in 2005, Wilens et al. studied four groups, including

1. individuals with ADHD but no substance use disorders

2. individuals with substance disorders but no ADHD
3. individuals with both ADHD and substance use disorders
4. a control group with neither ADHD nor substance use disorders

The highest rate of comorbidities was found among individuals with both ADHD and a substance use disorder; for example, only 5 percent of the control group with no disorders had major depression, but 15 percent of the ADHD group had depression, and 17 percent of the SUD-only group were depressed. Among those with both ADHD and an SUD, the rate of depression was 32 percent.

In the case of individuals with social phobia, none of the control group had this disorder, but 20 percent of the adults with ADHD only were socially phobic, as were 13 percent of those with only substance use disorders. However, when ADHD was combined with an SUD, then the rate of social phobia was 42 percent. Other disorders that were much higher when the individual had both ADHD and an SUD were bipolar disorder, antisocial personality disorder, panic disorder, and obsessive-compulsive disorder.

The researchers also found a much higher rate of smoking among those with both ADHD and an SUD, or 68 percent. In contrast, 32 percent of the control group smoked, as did 15 percent of the ADHD only group. (Other studies have found higher rates of smoking among ADHD, or up to two-thirds of adults with ADHD.) Those with a substance use disorder had a smoking rate of 52 percent. Clearly the combination of ADHD and substance use disorders in adults with ADHD is a harmful one.

ADHD is often treated with stimulants, but many physicians are concerned about prescribing stimulants to those who are abusing alcohol. Studies are mixed on whether treatment with stimulants is advisable in those who formerly abused substances.

Bipolar Disorder

Individuals with bipolar disorder have approximately a three-fold risk for the development of alcohol abuse or dependence. Some studies have shown that women with bipolar disorder have a 2.7 times greater risk for psychiatric comorbidities than men, while other studies state that the risk for a substance abuse is 7 times greater in a woman with bipolar disorder compared to a woman without bipolar disorder.

In an article on women with bipolar disorder who use alcohol and other drugs, authored by Diane Snow, Tonia Smith, and Susan Branham and published in the *Journal of Addictions Nursing* in 2008, the authors state that since women with bipolar disorder have an "extraordinarily high risk for alcoholism," mental health professionals who treat such women should also perform an assessment for the abuse of and dependence on alcohol and other substances.

According to Robert M. A. Hirschfeld and Lana A. Vornik in their 2005 article on bipolar disorder for the *American Journal of Managed Care*, alcohol is the most commonly abused substance among patients with bipolar disorder, and 33 percent of bipolar patients meet the criteria for alcohol abuse. (The next most commonly abused drug by those with bipolar disorder, according to the authors, is marijuana, which is abused by 16 percent of bipolar patients.)

According to Hirschfeld and Vornik, "Complications of substance abuse in bipolar disorder include higher rates of mixed and rapid cycling, prolonged recovery time, higher prevalence of medical disorders, including liver diseases, more suicide attempts, and suicide. Comorbidity with alcohol and drug abuse is often associated with poor adherence and poor treatment response compared with patients without comorbidity."

Depression

Many alcoholics (as many as 33 percent) have depression, in contrast to the general public, in which about 7 percent have depression in any given year, according to the National Institute of Mental Health. Up to 80 percent of men and women with alcohol dependence complain of depressive symptoms, but they do not all meet the criteria for depression. Treatment for alcoholism should cause remission in those who do not have a "true" depression.

Some research indicates that alcohol abuse or dependence may trigger depression. In a study by David M. Fergusson and colleagues, published in the *Archives of General Psychiatry* in 2009, the researchers analyzed data from 1,055 participants at different ages, including when the subjects were ages 17–18, 20–21 and 24–25 years. They found that it was more likely that alcohol led to an increased risk for major depression than the alternate theory that some people self-medicate their depression with alcohol.

Alcoholics with depression are often treated effectively with antidepressants such as medications in the class of selective serotonin reuptake inhibitors (SSRIs), such as fluoxetine (Prozac) and many other medications available in this class. Some individuals are treated with serotonin norepinephrine reuptake inhibitors (SNRs), such as venlafaxine (Effexor, Effexor XR) or duloxetine (Cymbalta). Bupropion (Wellbutrin, Wellbutrin XR) is an atypical antidepressant that is sometimes used to treat depression. Bupropion is also used to treat nicotine dependence; it is called Zyban when used for that application. Older medications known as tricyclic antidepressants may also be effective in treating depression.

According to the Office of Applied Studies in their report on major depressive episodes, released in May 2009, an estimated 16.5 million people ages 18 and older had one or more major depressive episodes in 2007, and about two-thirds of them received treatment. Of those who were treated, 68.8 percent saw a medical doctor and received a medication to treat their depression. The majority (61.9 percent) who saw a doctor for depression were treated by a family doctor or general practitioner, while 29.1 percent received treatment from a psychiatrist or psychotherapist, and 28.5 percent saw a psychologist.

Of those with depression in 2007, individuals who were age 50 or older had the lowest rate of depression (5.8 percent), but they also had the highest rate of receiving treatment (74.2 percent). Those who were in fair or poor health were the most likely to be depressed (14.2 percent) compared to those who were in excellent health (4.3 percent). See Table 3 for general demographic information on depression.

Impulse Control Disorders

Impulse control disorders are severely prob. behaviors that are beyond the control of the i.. vidual, such as pathological gambling, KLEPTOMANIA (compulsive stealing), TRICHOTILLOMANIA (compulsive hair pulling to the extent that some sufferers are bald), and INTERMITTENT EXPLOSIVE DISORDER, a rage control disorder. Several of these disorders are discussed here.

Pathological Gambling The majority of people who are addicted to gambling behavior are also alcohol abusers or alcoholics. Pathological gamblers gain a temporary euphoric high from gambling, but it is the rush from the gambling that they enjoy,

---

TABLE 3

ADULTS 18 AND OLDER WHO HAD AT LEAST ONE MAJOR DEPRESSIVE EPISODE (MDE) IN THE PAST YEAR, AND RECEIPT OF TREATMENT FOR DEPRESSION IN THE PAST YEAR AMONG ADULTS WITH MDE, BY DEMOGRAPHIC AND HEALTH CHARACTERISTICS: 2007.

Characteristic	Past Year MDE (%)	Received Treatment for Depression in the Past Year among Adults with Past Year MDE (%)
Total	7.5	64.5
Age Group in Years		
18 to 25	8.9	44.2
26 to 49	8.5	65.6
50 or older	5.8	74.2
Gender		
Male	5.3	57.9
Female	9.5	68.0
Marital Status		
Married	5.3	71.5
Widowed	7.9	Not available
Divorced/Separated	13.1	70.5
Never Married	9.2	52.1
Overall Health		
Excellent	4.3	54.6
Very good	5.9	59.0
Good	9.0	62.5
Fair or poor	14.2	78.4

Adapted from: Office of Applied Studies. "Major Depressive Episode and Treatment among Adults." *NSDUH Report.* Substance Abuse and Mental Health Services Administration: 1–4.

not the attainment of money, and thus they will immediately gamble any winnings away. In a study of pathological gamblers based on the National Comorbidity Survey Replication, published in *Psychological Medicine* in 2008, Ronald C. Kessler and colleagues reported that pathological gambling was associated with being male, young, and non-Hispanic black. Pathological gamblers reported an earlier age of gambling (average 16.7 years) than non-pathological gamblers, who started gambling at an average age of 23.9 years.

The researchers also found that the onset and continued persistence of pathological gambling was predictive by prior psychiatric comorbidities, including substance use disorders, anxiety disorders, mood disorders, and other impulse control disorders. Pathological gambling was also predictive for the subsequent onset of generalized anxiety disorder, PTSD, and substance dependence. The researchers found that among pathological gamblers, there was a 46.2 percent lifetime comorbidity for alcohol or drug abuse and a 31.8 percent lifetime comorbidity for alcohol or drug dependence. In addition, 63.0 percent of pathological gamblers were also smokers.

Intermittent Explosive Disorder Intermittent explosive disorder (IED) is a psychiatric diagnosis of sudden and often unprovoked extreme rages. Consumption of alcohol by someone suffering from IED is problematic because of the person's decreased inhibitions and the accelerated aggressive impulses that alcohol can trigger. According to research by Kessler and colleagues and reported in the *Archives of General Psychiatry* in 2006, 32.9–37.5 percent of individuals with IED have a diagnosis of alcohol abuse, and 17.0–18.6 percent are alcoholics. The only higher comorbidity found among those with IED is with major depressive disorder, which ranges from 37.3 to 37.9 percent of individuals with IED.

Nicotine Dependence

As mentioned, as many as 80 percent of individuals with alcohol dependence are smokers, and experts say that cigarettes may stimulate those who drink, while alcohol may act as a sedative to the stimulating effects of nicotine. Those who both smoke

and drink have serious health risks for CANCER and other illnesses. (See EXCESSIVE DRINKING AND HEALTH CONSEQUENCES.)

Many treatment facilities for alcohol dependence fail to provide patients with assistance in quitting smoking, often because the staff believes that alcoholism is so much "worse" than cigarette addiction. In fact, in some cases, staff members may even provide cigarettes and smoke breaks to patients as rewards for "good" behavior in the facility. However, increasing numbers of experts are encouraging treatment facilities as well as smokers who are alcoholic to seek to rid themselves of both addictions. Such experts view continued smoking as a gateway to relapse back to alcohol dependence.

Personality Disorders

PERSONALITY DISORDERS are aberrations of the personality that impede normal and healthy functioning in society, and the most commonly known personality disorder is antisocial personality disorder. This is a disorder in which the individual exhibits sociopathic behavior as well as little or no concern for others. Many individuals incarcerated in jail and prison have antisocial personality disorder.

Other personality disorders (PDs) include borderline PD, avoidant PD, dependent PD, obsessive-compulsive PD (not to be confused with obsessive-compulsive disorder), paranoid PD, schizoid PD, and histrionic PD. Individuals who are alcohol abusers or alcoholics have an increased risk for personality disorders.

In an analysis of individuals with a 12-month alcohol use disorder and their percentage of personality disorders (with the exclusion of borderline personality disorder), researchers Bridget F. Grant and colleagues reported that more than a third (39.5 percent) of subjects with any alcohol dependence have a personality disorder. The most common personality disorders among alcoholics are antisocial personality disorder (18.3 percent) and paranoid personality disorder (15.8 percent). The rates of other PDs are significantly lower among those who abuse alcohol, or 9.5 percent with obsessive-compulsive disorder followed by 7.4

TABLE 4
PREVALENCE OF PERSONALITY DISORDERS (PDS) AMONG RESPONDENTS WITH A 12-MONTH ALCOHOL USE DISORDER

Comorbid Disorder	Percent of Alcohol Abusers	Percent of Alcoholics
Any personality disorder	19.8	39.5
Avoidant PD	2.0	7.7
Dependent PD	0.3	2.5
Obsessive-compulsive PD	9.5	15.2
Paranoid PD	5.6	15.8
Schizoid PD	2.5	8.2
Histrionic PD	3.1	10.3
Antisocial PD	7.4	18.3

Adapted from Grant, Bridget F., et al. "Prevalence and Co-Occurrence of Substance Use Disorders and Independent Mood and Anxiety Disorders: Results from the National Epidemiologic Survey on Alcohol and Related Conditions." *Alcohol Research & Health* 29, no. 2 (2006): page 125.

percent with antisocial personality disorder. (See Table 4.)

In another study of alcohol dependence and personality disorders, researchers Enrique Echebúria and colleagues compared the prevalence of personality disorders among 158 alcoholics receiving treatment at a psychiatric outpatient clinic to the prevalence among 120 psychiatric patients without addictive disorders and also among 103 normal individuals in the community. They found that nearly half (44.3 percent) of the alcoholics had at least one personality disorder, compared to 21.7 percent of the clinical nonalcoholic patients and 6.8 percent of the normative group. The most common personality disorder among the alcoholics in this study was obsessive-compulsive personality disorder (12 percent), followed by antisocial personality disorder, paranoid personality disorder, and dependent personality disorder (7 percent each).

Schizophrenia

Only about 1–2 percent of the adult population has schizophrenia, a severe psychotic disorder. Studies indicate that individuals with schizophrenia often exhibit more violent behavior than others; however, many researchers have also found that schizo-phrenics with alcohol dependence are much more likely to be violent than those with schizophrenia who are not alcoholics. As with nonschizophrenics, alcohol lowers inhibitions and increases aggressive impulses in some schizophrenic individuals, thus also increasing their propensity to commit violent acts, based on their turbulent psychotic and often paranoid thoughts.

Suicide and Alcohol Dependence

Another risk factor among alcoholics is the high risk for suicide, and the lifetime suicide risk for those who are dependent on alcohol is about 10 percent, which is at least five times higher than the rate in the general population. Alcoholism that is combined with depression is the most common diagnosis among patients who commit suicide. Of those alcoholics who attempt suicide and then fail, an estimated 15 to 20 percent of them will reattempt suicide within five years of the first suicide attempt. Intoxication with alcohol increases the risk of impulsive acts, including suicide. It also increases the risk of violent and painful suicides.

See also AGE AND ALCOHOL; ALCOHOL AND MEN; ALCOHOLIC PSYCHOSIS; EXCESSIVE DRINKING AND NEGATIVE SOCIAL CONSEQUENCES; STAGES OF CHANGE; TREATMENT.

Collins, Kate, and Sanjay Mathew, M.D. "A Review of Generalized Anxiety Disorder." *Perspectives in Psychiatry: A Clinical Update.* Supplement to *Psychiatric Times* (2008): 3–8.

Deas, Deborah, M.D., and Suzanne Thomas. "Comorbid Psychiatric Factors Contributing to Adolescent Alcohol and Other Drug Use." *Alcohol Research & Health* 26, no. 2 (2002): 116–121.

Doctor, Ronald M., Ada P. Kahn, and Christine Adamec. *The Encyclopedia of Phobias, Fears, and Anxieties.* 3rd ed. New York: Facts On File, Inc., 2008.

Echebúria, Enrique, Ricardo Bravo De Medina, and Javier Aizpiri. "Comorbidity of Alcohol Dependence and Personality Disorders: A Comparative Study." *Alcohol & Alcoholism* 42, no. 6 (2007): 618–622.

Fergusson, David M., Joseph M. Boden, and L. John Horwood. "Tests of Causal Links Between Alcohol Abuse or Dependence and Major Depression." *Archives of General Psychiatry* 66, no. 3 (2009): 260–266.

Grant, Bridget E., et al. "Co-Occurrence of 12-Month Alcohol and Drug Use Disorders and Personality Disorders in the United States: Results from the National Epidemiologic Survey on Alcohol and Related Conditions." *Alcohol Research & Health* 29, no. 2 (2006): 121–130.

Grant, Bridget F., et al. "Prevalence and Co-Occurrence of Substance Use Disorders and Independent Mood and Anxiety Disorders: Results from the National Epidemiologic Survey on Alcohol and Related Conditions." *Alcohol Research & Health* 29, no. 2 (2006): 107–120.

Hirschfeld, Robert M. A., M.D., and Lana A. Vornik. "Bipolar Disorder—Costs and Comorbidity." *American Journal of Managed Care* 11, no. 3, Supp. (2005): S85–S90.

Kessler, Ronald C. "The Epidemiology of Dual Diagnosis." *Biological Psychiatry* 56, no. 10 (2004): 730–737.

———. "The Prevalence and Correlates of Adult ADHD in the United States: Results from the National Comorbidity Survey Replication." *American Journal of Psychiatry* 163, no. 4 (2006): 716–723.

Kessler, Ronald C., et al. "The Prevalence and Correlates of DSM-IV Intermittent Explosive Disorder in the National Comorbidity Survey Replication." *Archives of General Psychiatry* 63, no. 6 (2006): 669–678.

Kessler, Ronald C., et al. "The Prevalence and Correlates of DSM-IV Pathological Gambling in the National Comorbidity Survey Replication." *Psychological Medicine* 38, no. 9 (2008): 1,351–1,360.

Marques Fidalgo, Thiago, Evelyn Doering da Silveira, and Dartiu Xavier da Silveira. "Psychiatric Comorbidity Related to Alcohol Use Among Adolescents." *American Journal of Drug and Alcohol Abuse* 34, no. 1 (2008): 83–89.

National Institute of Mental Health. "The Numbers Count: Mental Disorders in America." Available online. URL: http://www.nimh.ni.gov/health/publications/the-numbers-count-mental-disorders-in-america/index.shtml. 2008. Accessed March 2, 2009.

Petrakis, Ismene L., M.D., et al. "Comorbidity of Alcoholism and Psychiatric Disorders." *Alcohol Research & Health* 26, no. 2 (2002): 81–89.

Ravindran, Lakshmi N., M.D. "Comorbidity and Social Anxiety Disorder: Prognostic Implications." *Perspectives in Psychiatry: A Clinical Update.* Supplement to *Psychiatric Times* (2008): 18–21.

Ruscio, A. M., et al. "The Epidemiology of Obsessive-Compulsive Disorder in the National Comorbidity Survey Replication." *Molecular Psychiatry* (2008). http://www.nature.com/mp/journal/vaop/ncurrent/abs/mp200894a.html. Accessed 11/27/09.

Skoog, Gunnar, M.D., and Ingmar Skoog, M.D. "A 40-Year Follow-up of Patients with Obsessive-Compulsive Disorder." *Archives of General Psychiatry* 56, no. 2 (1999): 121–127.

Snow, Diane, Tonia Smith, and Susan Branham. "Women with Bipolar Disorder Who Use Alcohol and Other Drugs." *Journal of Addictions Nursing* 19, no. 2 (2008): 55–60.

Wilens, Timothy E., M.D. "The Nature of the Relationship between Attention-Deficit/Hyperactivity Disorder and Substance Use." *Journal of Clinical Psychiatry* 68, Supp. 11 (2007): S4–S8.

Wilens, Timothy E., et al. "Characteristics of Adults with Attention Deficit Hyperactivity Disorder Plus Substance Use Disorder: The Role of Psychiatric Comorbidity." *American Journal on Addictions* 14, no. 4 (2005): 319–327.

Williams, Jill M., and Douglas Ziedonis. "Addressing Tobacco among Individuals with a Mental Illness or an Addiction." *Addictive Behaviors* 29, no. 6 (2004): 1,067–1,083.

Zilberman, Monica L., M.D., et al. "Substance Use Disorders: Sex Differences and Psychiatric Comorbidities." *Canadian Journal of Psychiatry* 48, no. 1 (2003): 5–15.

psychosis See ALCOHOLIC PSYCHOSIS.

psychotherapy See TREATMENT.

pyromania Pyromania is an irresistible impulse to start fires. It is not the same as arson-for-profit; instead, pyromania is an impulsive disorder in which the individual usually tries to avoid harming other people or animals. The fire-setting is a thrill for the person, as is the possibility of getting caught, although paradoxically, the pyromaniac does not apparently wish to be caught in the act.

Symptoms and Diagnostic Path
Fire-setting behavior is the key symptom of pyromania, but many pyromaniacs are never identified because they do not wish to be apprehended or punished. Because of their fascination with fire, pyromaniacs may also feel compelled to go to the scene of fires. Interestingly, in contrast to most other individuals with an impulse control disorder, research by Grant and Kim has shown that most

adolescent fire setters are not relieved after their impulsive act but are more distressed. They experience relief with the actual act of fire-setting, followed by elevated tension.

Treatment Options and Outlook

Pyromania is treated with therapy. Because pyromaniacs often have an alcohol dependence, this problem must be treated as well. Medications such as ANTIDEPRESSANTS are also used. Some researchers have reported success with treatment with topiramate, lithium, and clonidine.

Risk Factors and Preventive Measures

Males are more likely to be pyromaniacs than females. There are no known preventive measures to avoid the onset of pyromania.

See also IMPULSE CONTROL DISORDERS.

Grant, Jon E., and Suck Won Kim. "Clinical Characteristics and Psychiatric Comorbidity of Pyromania." *Journal of Clinical Psychiatry* 68, no. 11 (2007): 1,717–1,722.

R

recovery See STAGES OF CHANGE; TREATMENT.

relapses See ALCOHOLISM/ALCOHOL DEPENDENCE AND ALCOHOL ABUSE; STAGES OF CHANGE; TREATMENT.

religion Belief in a higher power, often called God but that is sometimes referred to by other names. Some mutual aid alcoholism societies such as Alcoholics Anonymous contend that it is essential for the alcoholic to acknowledge that there is a power greater than himself or herself in order to move toward recovery from alcoholism dependence. (This power need not necessarily be God or a god-like figure and can be the life force within the person or a related concept.) It should be noted that Muslims, members of the most rapidly growing faith group, forbid the use of alcohol. Many studies have also found that an individual's personal level of religiosity and spirituality is inversely related to his or her risk for alcohol abuse or dependence; that is, the more religious the person is, the less likely he or she is to have an alcohol abuse problem. Studies have also shown that women who are religious are less likely to drink alcohol. (See ALCOHOL AND WOMEN.) Yet other researchers contend that religious beliefs are not needed to recover from alcohol dependence.

In a study of 16,595 high-school seniors and the relationships between their religiosity and their use of alcohol, tobacco, and marijuana, J. M. Wallace Jr. and colleagues found that the higher the level of religiosity in the adolescents, the lower the probability of their having engaged in BINGE DRINKING, using tobacco, or using marijuana in the past year.

In a study of religiosity, alcohol expectancies and drinking motives by Luke W. Galen and W. M. Rogers, published in the *Journal of Studies on Alcohol* in 2004, the authors studied 265 undergraduates in college. They found that religiosity was inversely related to a positive expectancy of drinking, i.e., individuals who were more religious were significantly less likely to expect to drink. They were also less likely to actually drink, particularly among those who were members of conservative Protestant denominations.

The authors said, "For many individuals, it is likely that religiosity plays several roles in relationship to drinking, including directly reducing their willingness to consume through proscriptions [bans] and indirectly discouraging drinking through such mechanisms such as family and peer selection. Religion itself can mediate other influences, such as buffering the impact of life stress on substance use."

In a study by Laurence Michalak, Karen Trocki, and Jason Bond, the researchers analyzed results from telephone interviews from the 2000 National Alcohol Survey, reporting on their findings in *Drug and Alcohol Dependence* in 2007. The researchers found that religious preferences were significant in whether people were heavy drinkers or abstainers, as well as whether the individuals regarded themselves as religious or were proscriptive (condemning) of the use of alcohol. The importance of religion to the individual was also a factor; for example, about half (49.6 percent) of abstainers said that religion was very important, while 23.5 percent said religion was less important/not important.

In considering various religions or no religions, of those who drank, the highest percentage of heavy drinkers (50.2 percent) was among those with no

222

religion. This percentage was followed by Mormons who drank, or 50 percent. Of course, most Mormons do *not* drink, and the highest percentage of abstainers was found among Mormons, or 82.1 percent. The next highest percentage of abstainers were Church of God (79.1 percent). The lowest percentage of abstainers were Lutheran (19.9 percent), followed by those with no religion (25.1 percent) and Catholics (28.7 percent). (See Table 1.)

The researchers also noted that men were less likely to be religious than women as well as less likely to be proscriptive, affiliated with a religion, and abstainers, and they were more likely than women to be heavy drinkers. Married people were more likely to be religious and not heavy drinkers, but they were similar to unmarried people in terms of their attitudes toward proscription and abstention of alcohol. The researchers also found

TABLE 1
RELIGION AND DRINKING VARIABLES

		All respondents				Drinkers only	
	Number	Proscriptive (%)	Religiosity (%)	Affiliated (%)	Abstainers (%)	Number	Heavy Drinkers (%)
Importance of religion							
Less/not important	3,012	24.2	n/a	69.9	23.5	2,292	48.6
Very important	4,555	50.4	n/a	95.1	49.6	2,214	32.2
Preference							
No religion	1,123	n/a	18.9	n/a	25.1	832	50.2
Mormon	139	95.5	80.6	100.0	82.1	24	50.0
Assembly of God	25	92.9	93.1	100.0	71.4	7	12.5
Seventh Day Adventists	28	89.7	86.2	100.0	60.3	8	18.2
European Free Church	42	86.7	79.2	100.0	60.0	20	8.7
Church of God	81	80.2	93.0	100.0	79.1	16	50.0
Churches of Christ	45	77.4	77.4	100.0	60.4	18	31.8
Muslim	45	75.6	82.5	100.0	78.0	10	33.3
Pentecostal	127	74.6	90.9	100.0	68.6	36	47.4
Baptist	1,376	69.4	78.4	100.0	54.8	643	42.5
Protestant/miscellaneous denominations	118	61.5	72.3	100.0	61.2	47	32.7
United Church of Christ	89	58.8	63.7	100.0	47.5	49	14.8
Christian/no denomination	304	58.4	71.7	100.0	42.1	175	47.7
Protestant/no denomination	391	52.6	66.0	100.0	42.9	221	33.9
Methodist	527	50.2	56.9	100.0	39.7	312	33.2
Community Churches	64	48.4	77.0	100.0	29.7	47	33.3
Jehovah's Witness	89	33.3	94.2	100.0	34.8	56	37.0
Presbyterian	196	31.9	61.5	100.0	31.9	137	22.9
Catholic	1,916	26.4	57.4	100.0	28.7	1,350	44.5
Lutheran	365	25.3	55.6	100.0	19.9	287	33.4
Episcopal	160	17.6	59.2	100.0	35.1	116	30.2
Jewish	120	16.3	33.7	100.0	30.8	87	12.5

Source: Adapted from Michalak, Laurence, Karen Trocki, and Jason Bond. "Religion and Alcohol in the U.S. National Survey: How Important Is Religion for Abstention and Drinking?" *Drug and Alcohol Dependence* 87 (2007), page 271.

that African Americans were the most likely to be proscriptive, religious, and abstaining.

In his article on the anthropological aspects of alcohol in the *Annual Review of Anthropology* in 2006, Michael Dietler makes this observation about religion: "Because inebriation induces altered stages of consciousness, alcohol has frequently played a prominent role in rituals of both a religious and secular nature. Indeed, it is often treated as an indexical sign of a ritual event. But the relationship of alcohol to religion is complex. On the one hand, it is, and has been, an integral part of many religious practices around the world and throughout history, from the ritual consumption of wine in the Catholic mass to ancestor and spirit propitiation with beer in Africa. On the other hand, its consumption is proscribed by some religions (e.g., Islam and several Protestant Christian sects) to such an extent that abstention can become one of the most important defining symbols of piety and group membership."

See also CHILD ABUSE AND NEGLECT; FAMILIES AND ALCOHOL; MILITARY VETERANS/COMBAT AND ACTIVE-DUTY MILITARY.

Dieter, Michael. "Alcohol: Anthropological/Archaeological Perspectives." *Annual Review of Anthropology* 35 (2006): 229–249.

Galen, Luke W., and W. M. Rogers. "Religiosity, Alcohol Expectancies, Drinking Motives and Their Interaction in the Prediction of Drinking among College Students. *Journal of Studies on Alcohol* 65, no. 4 (2004): 469–476.

Michalak, Laurence, Karen Trocki, and Jason Bond. "Religion and Alcohol in the U.S. National Survey: How Important Is Religion for Abstention and Drinking?" *Drug and Alcohol Dependence* 87 (2007): 268–280.

Wallace, J. M., et al. "Religiosity and Adolescent Substance Abuse: The Role of Individual and Contextual Influences." *Social Problems* 54, no. 2 (2007): 308–327.

schizoid personality disorder See PERSONALITY DISORDERS.

schizophrenia A severe psychotic thought disorder that is characterized by delusions (false beliefs), such as the paranoid belief that others are plotting against a person, when there are no such plots, and hallucinations, such as hearing noises or voices that others do not hear, seeing items that others do not see, or even smelling odors that others do not smell. The individual may also believe that he or she receives secret coded messages that no one else can identify or interpret and which are transmitted through the television or the radio. This is a delusional thought. The exact cause of schizophrenia is not known. It may be an inherited disease, although it may also be triggered by the use of illicit drugs.

Individuals with schizophrenia may not make much or any sense to others when they are acutely psychotic and verbalizing their delusions or hallucinations. Some people with schizophrenia may be suspicious, reclusive individuals who do not say anything at all to others. It is difficult to impossible to convince a person with schizophrenia that his or her delusions or hallucinations are false, since these experiences are extremely vivid to them, and thus they seem very real. At best, some doubt may be interjected in the person's mind that the delusions and hallucinations *may* not be real.

Schizophrenia is a tragedy, not only for the person with the disease but also for their parents, siblings, and others; for example, parents often wonder what they did wrong to make their young adult child "crazy." Siblings may wonder if they will "get" the disease themselves, and they may fear that schizophrenia somehow lurks in the back of their minds, ready to pounce at some unknown future point. Psychiatrists in the mid-20th century, particularly those who considered themselves Freudian psychoanalysts, did believe that parents caused their children's schizophrenia by their actions or inactions; however, few psychiatrists today think that the disease is somehow induced by parental failings, unless the parents were egregiously abusive.

People with schizophrenia have an increased risk for both alcohol abuse and alcohol dependence as well as for the abuse of ALCOHOL AND OTHER DRUGS. People with schizophrenia may prefer abusing alcohol to taking their medications, particularly when they believe that there is nothing wrong with them, which is a lack of insight that is very common with schizophrenia. According to E. Fuller Torrey, M.D., author of *Surviving Schizophrenia*, people with schizophrenia abuse alcohol and drugs for many of the same reasons that nonschizophrenic people abuse substances: They like the effects. However, Torrey says that some people with schizophrenia may use alcohol and/or drugs to self-treat their symptoms of DEPRESSION and anxiety.

Alcohol and illegal drugs can decrease, increase, or otherwise change the effects of antipsychotic and other medications that the person takes and may also decrease the level of compliance with taking their medication—the individual either forgets to take or purposely chooses to not take the medication.

Most people with schizophrenia are not inherently violent individuals, but if they abuse alcohol and/or drugs, there *is* an elevated risk that they may become violent. According to Torrey, substance-abusing schizophrenics have more violent episodes than people with schizophrenia who are not substance abusers, and they also experience more symptoms than those who do not abuse substances. Such individuals are not readily treated by the mental health care system. According to Torrey, "The treatment of individuals with schizophrenia who also are severe substance abusers is quite unsatisfactory. Many are ping-ponged back and forth between the mental illness system and the substance abuse treatment system, rejected on both sides. They are the patients nobody wants."

Studies back Torrey up; for example, an analysis of individuals with schizophrenia in Sweden by Pirkko Rasanen et al., described in *Schizophrenia Bulletin* in 1998, revealed that men who were alcohol abusers and who were also diagnosed with schizophrenia were 25.2 times more likely to commit violent crimes than were mentally healthy men. In addition, patients with schizophrenia who did not abuse alcohol but who did commit a crime were rarely repeat offenders. In contrast, the risk for committing more crimes among those with schizophrenia who also abused alcohol was increased by 9.5 times. As a result, it is clear that it is important to treat individuals with schizophrenia for their comorbid alcohol abuse and dependence, not only for their own sakes but also for the sake of society itself.

People with schizophrenia also have an elevated risk for SUICIDE and any mention of suicide by the individual always should be followed up because a threat could become a plan and then an action.

Steven Batki and his colleagues studied 80 patients with schizophrenia or schizoaffective disorder who also had alcohol dependence and published their results in 2009 in *Schizophrenia Research*. They found that 83 percent of the subjects also had at least one other serious chronic disease, such as hypertension, high levels of cholesterol, and osteoarthritis. Batki and his colleagues found that compared to other patients in prior studies who had schizophrenia but no issues with alcohol, the subjects with both schizophrenia and alcohol dependence had 1.5 times the level of high cholesterol, twice the level of hypertension, and four times the level of osteoarthritis.

Other diseases, such as asthma and infection with the human immunodeficiency virus (HIV), were significantly more common among schizophrenics with alcohol issues than in schizophrenics without alcohol problems. In addition, the risk for having other serious chronic diseases increased with the level of alcohol that was consumed. As a result, treating individuals who have both schizophrenia and alcohol dependence for their ALCOHOLISM is important for many different health reasons.

Schizophrenia may first appear in men in their late teens or early twenties or to women who are in their mid-20s to late 30s. Sometimes symptoms occur earlier or later. Rarely, however, does schizophrenia appear for the first time before puberty or after age 45. About 1–2 percent of the population in the United States has schizophrenia.

Symptoms and Diagnostic Path

There are three primary types of symptoms in schizophrenia, including positive symptoms, negative symptoms, and cognitive symptoms. The *positive symptoms* of schizophrenia do not refer to good symptoms; instead, they refer to active and apparent symptoms that are causing acting-out behaviors, such as hallucinations, delusions, and unusual thoughts on which the person acts. Positive symptoms are often apparent to others because the individual exhibits overt actions, such as talking to himself or herself or acting frightened when there is nothing present to fear.

In contrast, *negative symptoms* refer to the lack of expressed emotions or abilities, such as the inability to make plans or even to speak or express emotion. The person may exhibit little or no emotion, despite what is going on in the surrounding environment. Negative symptoms sometimes may be misinterpreted by others as depression or laziness.

A third category of the types of symptoms of schizophrenia is *cognitive symptoms,* which are problems with memory, attention, and the executive functions that allow a person to make a plan and carry it out.

Schizophrenia is diagnosed by a psychiatrist, usually one who is experienced in treating psychotic disorders. Many psychiatrists treat people with transient life problems, and they do not treat individuals with severe or psychotic mental illnesses such as BIPOLAR DISORDER or schizophrenia, so it is important for patients to see a psychiatrist with appropriate experience.

Treatment Options and Outlook

Treatment is usually comprised of medication. One or more hospitalizations in a psychiatric facility may become necessary if the individual becomes a threat to himself or herself or to others. Psychotherapy may be offered but is usually considered ineffective with people who have schizophrenia, particularly when they are in a psychotic state and cannot relate to what the therapist is saying or asking.

In the recent past (the late 20th century), there were few effective antipsychotic medications available to counteract the psychotic features of schizophrenia, and most medications served only to sedate the individual and decrease symptoms of agitation. However, today atypical antipsychotics have been proven effective for many people with schizophrenia. The only way to know if an antipsychotic drug works on an individual is to try it for a period of time. If the symptoms do not abate, another medication is usually tried.

Older antipsychotics are sometimes still used to treat schizophrenia, but they may cause muscle spasms, restlessness, and other side effects. They may also cause chronic and permanent tics and involuntary movements, also known as tardive dyskinesia. Some examples of older antipsychotics include haloperidol (Haldol) and chlorpromazine (Thorazine). The newer antipsychotics do not cause tardive dyskinesia. Another side effect risk with older antipsychotics is akinesia, which causes a decrease in the spontaneous movements of the patient. Parkinsonian syndrome is also a risk with older antipsychotics. Patients with Parkinsonian syndrome may drool, have a loss of facial expression and exhibit a shuffling gait. There are drugs to reverse this syndrome, such as Cogentin.

Clozapine (Clozaril) is another antipsychotic drug used to treat schizophrenia. Because it has the risk of a life-threatening side effect known as agranulocytosis, patients taking clozapine must have regular blood tests (complete blood counts) to ensure that their blood levels are within the normal range.

Many antipsychotics, both old and new, cause significant weight gain, and they may also increase the risk for the development of type 2 diabetes as well as lead to high blood cholesterol levels. Atypical antipsychotics include such drugs as risperidone (Risperdal), olanzapine (Zyprexa), quetiapine (Seroquel), ziprasidone (Geodon), aripiprazole (Abilify), and paliperidone (Invega). Each of these drugs has side effects; for example, quetiapine may cause sedation and weight gain, as may olanzapine.

Medication compliance with antipsychotics is poor among those with schizophrenia, whether the drug is one of the older or the newer medications, based on a study reported by Marcia Valenstein and colleagues in a 2004 issue of the *Schizophrenia Bulletin*. In this study, researchers analyzed adherence among patients receiving one or two antipsychotics over the course of a year. There were 49,003 patients receiving one drug and 14,211 receiving two antipsychotics.

The researchers found that patients on atypical agents were more likely to be noncompliant (41.5 percent) than were patients on conventional older drugs (37.8 percent). They found that in one group of patients switching from a conventional to an atypical drug, the noncompliant percentage decreased from 46 percent to 40 percent, still not a good rate. African Americans and younger patients were the least likely to be compliant with their drug regimen. Some have speculated that patients on high dosages are more likely to be noncompliant, but the researchers found that the most poorly adherent patients were least likely to be prescribed high dosages.

Some studies indicate that either NALTREXONE or DISULFIRAM are effective medications to treat alcoholism when someone with schizophrenia also has alcohol dependence. For example, in a study by Ismene L. Petrakis, Charla Nich, and Elizabeth Ralevski, reported in 2006 in *Schizophrenia Bulletin*, the researchers found that over a 12-week course of treatment, either disulfiram or naltrexone was superior to placebo among the psychotic subjects. They also found very high medication compliance rates of 80 percent.

The subjects were 66 individuals enrolled in the Mental Illness Research Education Clinical Center Naltrexone Disulfiram Treatment Trial, including 11 diagnosed with schizophrenia, 7 diagnosed with schizoaffective disorder (often considered a disorder with features of both schizophrenia and either depression or bipolar disorder), and 48 with bipolar disorder. Other subjects in the study did not have a psychotic disorder but had major depressive disorder, POSTTRAUMATIC STRESS DISORDER (TSD), PANIC DISORDER, and GENERALIZED ANXIETY DISORDER (GAD). There were a total of 185 psychotic and nonpsychotic subjects, and many had more than one diagnosis. There were no significant differences in the drinking behavior of the psychotic versus the nonpsychotic subjects.

According to the researchers, "Results from this study suggest that individuals with psychotic spectrum disorders are particularly suited for treatment with medications for alcohol dependence. This may be because the medication is more effective in this group of patients or may be in part because patients with a psychotic spectrum disorder may not be able to benefit as fully from the forms of treatments that have been developed for noncomorbid alcohol-dependent individuals, so medication effects may be more readily apparent."

Some substance-abusing schizophrenics may gain benefit from joining groups such as Alcoholics Anonymous; however, some such groups discourage the use of psychiatric medications, which is a serious drawback for the individual with schizophrenia.

Risk Factors and Preventive Measures

There is a hereditary risk to schizophrenia, and researchers have found that about 10 percent of individuals with a first-degree relative with the disorder (such as a parent or sibling) will also develop schizophrenia. The identical twin of a person with schizophrenia has the most risk for developing the disorder; about 40–65 percent, according to the National Institute of Mental Health (NIMH). Some individuals with relatives who have schizophrenia may develop PERSONALITY DISORDERS.

Other risk factors may trigger a preexisting inherited risk for the disorder, such as severe stress, viruses, or other factors, although it is still unknown which factors act to precipitate the disorder. Drug abuse may trigger a psychotic break that resembles schizophrenia.

Medication compliance is a problem among many patients with schizophrenia (as it is among many people who need to take psychiatric or even nonpsychiatric medications on a regular basis), but if they stop taking their medicines that control their symptoms, then the symptoms will return.

See also ANTISOCIAL PERSONALITY DISORDER/ANTISOCIAL BEHAVIOR; ANXIETY DISORDERS; PSYCHIATRIC COMORBIDITIES; TREATMENT.

Batki, Steven L., et al. "Medical Comorbidity in Patients with Schizophrenia and Alcohol Dependence." *Schizophrenia Research* 107, no. 2–3 (2009): 139–146.

Gorman, Jack M., M.D. *The Essential Guide to Psychiatric Drugs.* 4th ed. New York: St. Martin's Griffin, 2007.

Petrakis, Ismene L., Charla Nich, and Elizabeth Ralevski. "Psychotic Spectrum Disorders and Alcohol Abuse: A Review of Pharmacotherapeutic Strategies and a Report on the Effectiveness of Naltrexone and Disulfiram." *Schizophrenia Bulletin* 32, no. 4 (2006): 644–654.

Rasanen, Pirkko, et al. "Schizophrenia, Alcohol Abuse, and Violent Behavior: A 26-Year Followup Study of an Unselected Birth Cohort." *Schizophrenia Bulletin* 24, no. 3 (1998): 437–441.

Torrey, E. Fuller, M.D. *Surviving Schizophrenia: A Manual for Families, Consumers, and Providers.* New York: Quill, 2001.

Valenstein, Marcia, et al. "Poor Antipsychotic Adherence among Patients with Schizophrenia: Medication and Patient Factors." *Schizophrenia Bulletin* 30, no. 2 (2004): 255–264.

schizotypal personality disorder   See PERSONALITY DISORDERS.

self-help groups   See ALCOHOLISM MUTUAL AID SOCIETIES.

smoking and alcohol   Many people who abuse or are dependent on alcohol are also addicted to nicotine, and up to 80 percent of those who abuse or are addicted to alcohol are also smokers of cigarettes. Individuals who smoke may unconsciously use alcohol for its sedating effect. Adolescents with alcohol abuse and dependence also have a high rate of smoking, and smoking among teenagers is further associated with use of illicit drugs, such as marijuana, according to Mark G. Myers and John F. Kelly. (See ALCOHOL AND OTHER DRUGS.) The combination of alcohol abuse or dependence and nicotine dependence has been found to be very dangerous to an individual's health and potentiates an increased risk for diseases such as CANCER.

In their article in 2007 in *Archives of Internal Medicine,* Sherry A. McKee and colleagues found that both daily and occasional smokers were more likely to abuse or be dependent on alcohol than nonsmokers, based on an analysis of 42,374 adults from the National Epidemiological Survey on Alcohol and Related Conditions in 2001–02. They suggested that an individual's smoking status could be a reminder for physicians to perform basic alcohol screening of patients. The researchers said, "Some have suggested that screening for smoking behavior be elevated to the status of a vital sign." (A vital sign includes such measures as taking the pulse and blood pressure of a patient.)

They added, "The spectrum of problem drinking behaviors that are amenable to office-based treatment in primary care is expanding from nondependent hazardous drinking to alcohol dependence. Thus, improved screening approaches such as one that uses smoking behavior as a 'trigger' to identify alcohol misuse becomes even more vital in promoting optimal patient management and outcomes."

Common Genetic Factors Affecting both Drinking and Smoking

Researchers Richard A. Grucza and Laura J. Bierut, M.D., discuss possible common genetic factors surrounding both drinking and smoking in their article in *Alcohol Research & Health* in 2006. They cite the Collaborative Study on the Genetics of Alcoholism (COGA), an ongoing family and genetic study, as a source for information on genetic factors that are linked to both alcohol and nicotine dependence. For example, COGA data to date has found that chromosomes 2 and 3 are linked to both alcohol and nicotine dependence, although the specific genes have not yet been identified. In contrast, some genes have been identified for alcohol dependence, such as the GABRA2 gene on chromosome 4 and the CHRM2 gene on chromosome 7. A genetic link has also been found to smoking: the GABAB2 gene on chromosome 9.

In looking at risk factors for family members to smoke, the COGA researchers found that the

siblings of an alcoholic person were 1.7 times more likely to be habitual smokers than the siblings of individuals who were *not* dependent on alcohol.

Controversy Surrounding Concurrent Treatment

According to an analysis of studies on smoking cessation among alcoholics by Molly Kodl and her colleagues, published in *Alcohol Research & Health* in 2006, most of the individuals receiving treatment for their alcohol dependence are more interested in addressing their alcoholism first and dealing with their nicotine addiction later, once they have attained a period of sobriety. According to the researchers, "Evidence suggests that effective smoking cessation interventions can be delivered but that their success often is short-term and dependent on treatment format. Experimental evidence also suggests potential for detriment to long-term sobriety among alcohol-dependent smokers who receive simultaneous smoking cessation intervention and alcohol treatment."

These authors recommended that nicotine dependence treatment could be incorporated as an option for patients who are completing their substance abuse treatment program. This way smokers leaving treatment for alcohol dependence could subsequently receive behavioral and medication treatment to quit smoking.

In contrast, some researchers argue that concurrent tobacco dependence treatment with treatment for substance dependence is not only feasible but also advisable. According to Douglas M. Ziedonis, M.D., and colleagues in their 2006 article for *Alcohol Research & Health* on barriers and solutions to addressing tobacco dependence in addiction treatment programs, the main problems are not the patients themselves but rather staff attitudes, lack of staff training in tobacco cessation issues, and unfounded fears about smoking cessation among the staff and administration. For example, the authors report that up to 40 percent of the treatment staff are themselves dependent on tobacco, compared to from 60 to 95 percent of the patients. (In the general population, about 22 percent are dependent on tobacco.)

The authors said, "Staff members who smoke most likely are not going to try to help a patient quit smoking—sometimes as a result of their own guilt and shame about their own smoking." In addition, say the authors, staff members may say that smoking alongside their patients can promote a better "therapeutic alliance."

The authors vigorously dispute this belief, saying, "Although spending nontreatment time with patients can be positive (such as taking walks, sharing meals, etc.), engaging in addictive behaviors with a patient is inappropriate and unhelpful for recovery. Smoking with patients also normalizes tobacco addiction and even enhances its value as a therapeutic event." Instead, the authors recommend a policy to ban staff from smoking around patients. The authors report that some facilities are hiring only nonsmoking employees and are also helping current staff quit smoking.

Another issue is a lack of training, according to Ziedonis and colleagues, who state that staff receive little or no training on treating dependence on tobacco, but that they quickly can grasp key concepts because of their understanding of other forms of addiction.

"Clinical lore" is another issue, say Ziedonis et al.; for example, the staff may not regard tobacco as a "real drug." They may also believe that quitting smoking at the same time as giving up alcohol would be far too stressful for patients with alcohol dependence. The authors said, "In fact, evidence suggests that the opposite can occur—the tobacco use can harm, rather than enhance, recovery from other substance use by its ability to trigger other substance use."

Cancer Risk among Drinkers Who Smoke

As mentioned, many drinkers are also smokers, and smoking combined with excessive drinking increases the cancer risk in an individual by about 50 times, according to researchers Helmut K. Seitz and Peter Becker in their article for *Alcohol Research & Health* in 2007. Certain types of cancer are more common among those who both drink and smoke; for example, Claudio Pelucchi and colleagues reported that the combination of alcohol and tobacco increases the risk for such cancers as oral cancer, esophageal cancer, and liver cancer. In the cases of oral and esophageal cancer, the tobacco and alcohol together work to escalate the risk of cancer synergistically. In contrast, alcohol

and tobacco use are each independent risk factors for the development of liver cancer.

See also EXCESSIVE DRINKING AND HEALTH CONSEQUENCES; INTERVENTION, BRIEF; PSYCHIATRIC COMORBIDITIES; TREATMENT.

Grucza, Richard A., and Laura J. Bierut, M.D. "Co-occurring Risk Factors for Alcohol Dependence and Habitual Smoking: Update on Findings from the Collaborative Study on the Genetics of Alcoholism." *Alcohol Research & Health* 29, no. 3 (2006): 172–178.

Kodl, Molly, Steven S. Fu, M.D., and Anne M. Joseph, M.D. "Tobacco Cessation Treatment for Alcohol-Dependent Smokers: When Is the Best Time?" *Alcohol Research & Health* 29, no. 3 (2006): 203–227.

McKee, Sherry A., et al. "Smoking Status as a Clinical Indicator for Alcohol Misuse in US Adults." *Archives of Internal Medicine* 167, no. 7 (2007): 716–721.

Myers, Mark G., and John F. Kelly. "Cigarette Smoking Among Adolescents with Alcohol and Other Drug Use Problems." *Alcohol Research & Health* 29, no. 3 (2006): 221–227.

Pelucchi, Claudio, et al. "Cancer Risk Associated with Alcohol and Tobacco Use: Focus on Upper Aerodigestive Tract and Liver." *Alcohol Research & Health* 29, no. 3 (2006): 193–198.

Seitz, Helmut K., M.D., and Peter Becker, M.D. "Alcohol Metabolism and Cancer Risk." *Alcohol Research & Health* 30, no. 1 (2007): 38–47.

Ziedonis, Douglas, M.D., et al. "Barriers and Solutions to Addressing Tobacco Dependence in Addiction Treatment Programs." *Alcohol Research & Health* 29, no. 3 (2006): 228–235.

social phobia   A social phobia, also known as social anxiety disorder (SAD), is a fear of being criticized or embarrassed while in the presence of others. Many people are fearful of giving a speech, but the person with a social phobia may be fearful of going out to dinner or going to a party. They may use alcohol to try to blunt their fear, which may cause them to act in ways that ultimately cause embarrassment to themselves or others. About 15 million people have social phobia, according to the National Institute of Mental Health (NIMH), and the lifetime prevalence of social phobia is about 12 percent among the entire population of the United States.

The majority of individuals with SAD have other psychiatric disorders, such as other ANXIETY

DISORDERS, DEPRESSION, PERSONALITY DISORDERS, or substance use (alcohol and/or drug) disorders. According to Lakshmi N. Ravindran, M.D., in his 2008 article on the comorbidities of SAD for *Perspectives in Psychiatry,* the prevalence of alcohol dependence ranges between 15 and 24 percent of all patients with SAD. He also notes that SAD and alcohol use may be linked, both due to a shared genetic cause and as a means for self-medication.

According to Ravindran, "In the latter case [self-medication], alcohol is used to provide relief from the cognitive and physiologically arousing symptoms of anxiety. This behavior is reinforced over time so that alcohol use is the conditioned response when an anxiety-provoking social interaction is anticipated. In support of this alcoholics with SAD were found to be more likely to drink to enhance functioning and sociability than alcoholics without SAD. They were also found to have greater severity of dependence and to have experienced a history of major depression. Suicide risk has also been shown to be elevated in males of this population."

According to Sarah W. Book, M.D., and Carrie L. Randall in their 2002 article for *Alcohol Research & Health,* about 20 percent of patients with social anxiety disorder are either alcohol abusers or alcoholics. As a result, patients requesting treatment for social anxiety disorder should also be evaluated to determine whether they have issues with alcohol as well. In addition, an estimated 15 percent of those receiving treatment for alcohol dependence have social anxiety disorder.

Individuals with social anxiety disorder may use alcohol as a coping mechanism to reduce their extreme tension in social situations, and up to 16 percent of those with SAD may abuse or depend on alcohol. Others may use marijuana.

Studies have shown that alcohol is not effective as a "social lubricant," and some studies have shown that it worsens anxiety. However, many people do not believe the researchers. Book and Randall write, "Regardless of whether researchers can demonstrate in the laboratory that alcohol reduces social fears, many people with social anxiety report that they expect alcohol to have that effect and that they use it to cope with their social anxiety. Because of their alcohol consumption, some of these individuals will eventually develop alcohol use problems in addition to their preexisting social anxiety."

Symptoms and Diagnostic Path

Social phobia is usually accompanied by physical symptoms when in the feared situation, such as excessive sweating, nausea, blushing, and trouble with talking. Social phobics usually try to avoid people or situations that they consider fearsome, such as going to parties, weddings, or other social events. It may be difficult to diagnose SAD, because subjects with this anxiety disorder generally try to avoid people and usually seek treatment only for another condition. If the individual also has alcohol dependence, he or she may express great resistance to receiving group therapy or to attending meetings with Alcoholics Anonymous, directly because of his or her phobia in social situations.

Treatment Options and Outlook

Social phobia is treated with therapy and also with medications such as ANTIDEPRESSANTS and BENZODIAZEPINES. Some people with social anxiety disorder are treated with beta blocker medications. Psychotherapy is also important in treating social anxiety disorder, and therapists may use cognitive-behavioral therapy (CBT) or exposure therapy in which the patient faces the feared situation in a gradual manner. With CBT, the therapist teaches the patient how to challenge irrational and self-defeating thoughts in his or her own mind. With exposure therapy, the patient is taught how to handle social situations and then is placed in such situations and told to use those new skills. Some patients also benefit from relaxation training, in which they are trained to relax muscles throughout the body.

When a person with social anxiety disorder has an alcohol use disorder (AUD) as well (alcohol abuse or dependence), then benzodiazepines are usually avoided, because such drugs can be very dangerous in concert with alcohol. Antidepressants, particularly selective serotonin reuptake inhibitors (SSRIs), appear to be safe and they may be especially effective with alcoholism that has had a late onset—after age 25.

Serotonin norepinephrine reuptake inhibitors (SNRIs) are also effective at treating social anxiety disorder, according to Franklin R. Schneier, M.D., in his 2006 article on social anxiety disorder for the *New England Journal of Medicine.* Other drugs such as beta blockers may be used, particularly before the individual must engage in public speaking or other performance-related tasks. In such a case, the drug is taken about 30 minutes beforehand, and the effects will last for up to several hours.

Risk Factors and Preventive Measures

Most people with SAD develop the disorder between the ages of 11 and 19 years, although it may occur later or even in elderly adults. Researchers believe that there is a genetic link with social phobia, although no specific gene has been identified as of this writing. Women are more likely to suffer from social phobia than men. There is no way to prevent the onset of social phobia; however, once it has been diagnosed, it can be treated.

Book, Sarah W., M.D., and Carrie L. Randall. "Social Anxiety Disorder and Alcohol Use." *Alcohol Research & Health* 26, no. 2 (2002): 130–135.

Ravindran, Lakshmi N., M.D. "Comorbidity and Social Anxiety Disorder: Prognostic Implications." *Perspectives in Clinical Psychiatry: A Clinical Update.* Supplement to *Psychiatric Times,* Issue 2 of 4 (September 2008): 18–21.

Schneier, Franklin R., M.D. "Social Anxiety Disorder." *New England Journal of Medicine* 355, no. 10 (2006): 1,029–1,036.

specific phobia A phobia is an extreme fear of certain things, such as spiders, people wearing black hats, or nearly anything that can be imagined; for example, some people are afraid of bridges, tunnels, or a broad array of other objects. The fear is out of all proportion to the actual threat presented by the feared item. The individual with a specific phobia will go to extreme lengths to avoid the feared item. It may be triggered by a traumatic event or by seeing others undergo a traumatic event.

Researchers have found that individuals who fear items in the natural environment (such as water, storms, and so forth) generally have an onset of their phobia when they are from age five to nine years old. Fears of blood or injections also may develop during this time. Individuals who have situational phobias (such as a fear of elevators, tunnels, flying, and so forth) generally experience onset of the phobia when they are in their mid-20s.

In a study of college students and their noncollege peers, there was about the same level of specific phobias, or 8.1 percent of the college students with a specific phobia, compared to 8.8 percent of their noncollege peers. Phobic individuals may turn to alcohol in an attempt to "calm their nerves." According to the National Institute of Mental Health (NIMH), about 19.2 million Americans suffer from a specific phobia.

Symptoms and Diagnostic Path

The person with a specific phobia usually has a physical reaction, with racing heart, excessive perspiration, and trembling hands. The feared item is identified by the patient himself or herself or by the mental health professional. Even thinking about the feared item can cause a physical response.

Treatment Options and Outlook

Phobias are usually treated with psychotherapy, and the individual learns how to manage and quell his or her fears around the dreaded item. Desensitization therapy is one form of therapy which may be used, in which case the individual is slowly exposed to the feared object, but from a distance, later moving closer and closer to the object. Some therapists use a technique known as flooding, in which the patient is told to directly confront the object that is feared and to remain there. The therapist may or may not accompany the patient, depending on the situation.

Risk Factors and Preventive Measures

Women are about twice as likely as men to suffer from specific phobias. There is no known way to prevent the development of specific phobia.

See also ANXIETY DISORDERS.

stages of change The stages that the person with ALCOHOLISM (as well as individuals making other major changes, such as recovery from drug addiction) needs to go through in order to achieve a state of recovery. These stages include the following:

- precontemplation
- contemplation
- preparation
- action
- maintenance
- relapse

Precontemplation

In this stage, the alcoholic individual is not considering making any changes with regard to alcohol consumption. According to Carlo DiClemente, codeveloper of the stages of change of the transtheoretical model in his book *Addiction and Change,* "Precontemplation represents a status quo. An individual in the Precontemplation stage is satisfied with or at least unwilling to disrupt, a current behavior pattern. Precontemplators are not considering change in the foreseeable future most often defined as a period of 6 months to a year. This applies whether change means adopting, modifying, or stopping a behavior. Change is seen as irrelevant, unwanted, not needed, or impossible to achieve."

At this point, helping professionals who possess the skills needed to provide assistance to the alcohol-dependent person will explain to him or her the physical and psychological risks of continuing the behavior and also tell individuals that the decision to make a change (such as by stopping drinking or attending a meeting of Alcoholic Anonymous) is entirely theirs. When individuals are in this stage, they are not encouraged by experts to take action, because they are not perceived to be ready. Instead, they are urged to consider their current behavior and its consequences on themselves and others.

Contemplation

Within the contemplation stage, the individual *is* considering making a change with regard to his or her drinking problem but is also ambivalent about whether change is possible or is needed. It is clear that no changes are anticipated to be made by the individual within the next month or so.

Helping professionals assisting individuals in this stage should continue to tell alcoholic individuals that the choice to change is theirs. They also help him or her to consider the benefits and the risks of making changes. In addition, they reinforce positive expectations of making a change in their drinking habits.

Preparation

Within this stage, individuals are actively considering making changes to their excessive chronic drinking, and they *do* plan to act on this decision within the next month or so. The helping professional assists the person by discussing obstacles to making needed change and discussing how they can be removed. They also help the person find others who will support him or her socially during the process of change. This does not include his or her old drinking buddies, who would not want the person to change and who would actively discourage refraining from alcohol or no longer meeting at bars. The professional ascertains whether the individual has the ability to make the needed changes and if so, gently moves the person toward making "baby steps" toward improving their behavior.

Action

This is the stage in which the new behavior actually occurs. All the previous stages were necessary to lead up to this stage. DiClemente writes, "The old pattern retains its attraction and returning to it is often easier than sustaining a new pattern. It takes a long time to establish a new pattern of behavior. Three to six months is usually the time frame we have given for duration of the Action stage."

In this stage of change, the helping professional assists the alcoholic person to deal with sad feelings and feelings of loss. For example, when not intoxicated, the individual will have to face the consequences of his or her former actions, such as a failed marriage, children who are angry with him or her, failed job opportunities, and so forth. The individual knows that intoxication could prevent thinking about such things.

Maintenance

In the maintenance stage of change, the individual makes a sustained and long-term commitment to remain abstinent from alcohol. Explains DiClemente, "During this stage the new behavior pattern becomes automatic, requiring little thought or effort to sustain it. It truly becomes an established, habitual pattern. However, during maintenance there is still an ever-present danger of reverting to the old pattern. In fact, the new behavior becomes fully attained only when there is little or no energy or effort needed to continue it and the individual can terminate the cycle of change. The new behavior then becomes the status quo, and once again, there is little or no desire or intention to change, whether that be going back to the former pattern or moving onto another new pattern."

Helping professionals provide follow-up support as needed to individuals with alcohol dependence, which is important during the maintenance stage, as is also discussing the possibility of relapse with the person and telling the individual that a relapse does not mean that the individual cannot ever give up alcohol dependence.

Relapse

A relapse is a return to drinking and drunkenness, and relapses are common. A helping professional assists the person to determine what may have triggered the relapse. There are many reasons for a relapse, such as the death of a loved one, being terminated from a job, and so forth. However, sometimes the cause for the relapse may be internal rather than external to the individual, such as DEPRESSION or anxiety. The professional assists the individual who has relapsed to shore up his or her coping strategies and move back on the path to maintenance, hoping he or she can stay there.

See also HOSPITAL PATIENTS AND ALCOHOL-RELATED ADMISSIONS; TREATMENT.

Connors, Gerard J., Dennis M. Donovan, and Carlo C. DiClemente. *Substance Abuse Treatment and the Stages of Change.* New York: Guilford Press, 2001.
DiClemente, Carlo C. *Addiction and Change: How Addictions Develop and Addicted People Recover.* New York: Guilford Press, 2003.

suicide The ending of an individual's life by his or her own means or sometimes with the assistance of others. Individuals who abuse alcohol or who are alcoholics have an increased risk for suicide compared to others. In addition, if the person with an alcohol use disorder (alcohol abuse or ALCOHOLISM) also has a psychiatric disorder such as DEPRESSION or BIPOLAR DISORDER, then the risk for suicide is further escalated. In general, female alcoholics and alcohol abusers have a greater risk for suicide than male alcoholics. (See ALCOHOL AND WOMEN; PSYCHIATRIC COMORBIDITIES.)

Suicide may be attempted or committed by people of any age and is not limited to adults. According to the Centers for Disease Control and Prevention (CDC), an estimated 10.2 percent of Hispanic high-school students in 16 states attempted suicide in 2005, followed by 7.7 percent of African Americans, and 5.6 percent of white students. In considering the student's grade from ninth to 12th grade, the risk for suicide was the highest in the 10th grade (8.0 percent), followed by the ninth grade (7.9 percent). The risk declined to 5.8 percent for those in the 11th grade and further declined to 5.4 percent for high-school seniors.

In most cases, psychiatric problems are involved in suicide. In other research, according to the CDC data that was provided by the National Violent Death Reporting System, nearly half of the adults who took their own lives were depressed (45.7 percent), followed by those with a current mental health problem (42.1 percent). In addition 18.1 percent had an alcohol abuse problem, while 15.6 percent had another substance abuse problem. (See Table 1 for more details.)

Risk Factors for Suicide among Alcoholics

In an analysis of suicide attempt risk predictors among 1,237 alcoholics, both at an initial evaluation and later at a five-year follow-up point, researchers Ulrich W. Preuss, M.D., and colleagues found that there were 56 individuals who attempted suicide. These individuals were more likely than the other subjects to have made previous attempts at suicide. The researchers found that other factors related to suicide attempts were being divorced or separated, being younger, being dependent on other drugs in addition to alcohol, having substance-induced psychiatric disorders,

TABLE 1
NUMBER AND PERCENTAGE OF SUICIDES BY SEX AND ASSOCIATED CIRCUMSTANCES,
NATIONAL VIOLENT DEATH REPORTING SYSTEM, 16 STATES*, 2005

N = 7,838 (6,155 males and 1,683 females)

Associated Circumstances	Male		Female		Total	
	Number	Percent	Number	Percent	Number	Percent
Mental health/Substance abuse						
Current depressed mood	2,744	44.6	836	49.7	3,580	45.7
Current mental health problem	2,274	36.9	1,023	60.8	3,297	42.1
Current mental health treatment	1,723	28.0	861	51.2	2,584	33.0
Alcohol abuse problem	1,185	19.3	230	13.7	1,415	18.1
Other substance abuse problem	928	15.1	292	17.3	1,220	15.6
Relationship						
Intimate partner problem	2,031	33.0	439	26.1	2,470	31.5
Other relationship problem (nonintimate)	591	9.6	197	11.7	788	10.1
Death of family member or friend during previous 5 years	414	6.7	126	7.5	540	6.9
Suicide of family member or friend during previous 5 years	98	1.6	35	2.1	133	1.7
Perpetrator of interpersonal violence during previous month	419	6.8	29	1.7	448	5.7
Victim of interpersonal violence during previous month	29	0.5	25	1.7	54	0.7
Life stressor						
Crisis during previous two weeks	1,970	32.0	392	23.3	2,362	30.1
Physical health problem	1,341	21.8	379	22.5	1,720	21.9
Job problem	757	12.3	115	6.8	872	11.1
Recent criminal legal problem	804	13.1	62	3.7	866	11.1
Financial problem	713	11.6	150	8.9	863	11.0
Noncriminal legal problem	281	4.6	53	3.1	334	4.3
School problem	81	1.3	23	1.4	104	1.3
Suicide event						
Left a suicide note	1,895	30.8	633	37.6	2,528	32.3
Disclosed intent to commit suicide	1,773	28.8	464	27.6	2,237	28.5
Had history of suicide attempts	1,004	16.3	566	33.6	1,570	20.0

* States were Alaska, Colorado, Georgia, Kentucky, Maryland, Massachusetts, North Carolina, New Jersey, New Mexico, Oklahoma, Oregon, Rhode Island, South Carolina, Utah, Virginia, and Wisconsin.
Source: Karch, Debra L., et al. "Surveillance for Violent Deaths—National Violent Death Reporting System, 16 States, 2005." *Morbidity and Mortality Weekly Report* 57, no. SS-3 (April 11, 2008), page 23.

and having indicators of a worse prognosis of their alcohol dependence. Gender was not predictive for future suicide attempts.

The average age of the suicide attempters at follow-up was 33.3 years. Only about 21 percent were married. About two-thirds had drug dependence at some point in their lifetime in addition to their alcohol dependence. The most common dependency was on marijuana (39.3 percent), followed by cocaine (32.1 percent) and opioids (16.1 percent). About substance-induced psychiatric disorders that were identified, 46.4 percent had substance-induced depression, followed by 7.1 percent with substance-induced mania. Other substance-induced disorders were PANIC DISORDER (5.4 percent) and phobia (1.8 percent).

The researcher also found that half of the subjects who attempted suicide took pills (50 percent), while about a quarter of them (23.2 percent) cut their wrists or stabbed themselves.

According to the researchers, "As hypothesized, a past history of suicide attempts was an excellent predictor of such behavior during follow-up. More than half of the alcoholics who attempted suicide during the follow-up had prior attempts, compared with only 14% of the subjects with no prior suicidal behavior. An individual with a prior attempt has a 15.2% risk for a new attempt during the follow-up, compared with a 2.6% risk for the subjects without a prior attempt."

See also AGE AND ALCOHOL; ALCOHOL AND OTHER DRUGS; ANTISOCIAL PERSONALITY DISORDER/ANTISOCIAL BEHAVIOR; ANXIETY DISORDERS; ATTENTION-DEFICIT/HYPERACTIVITY DISORDER; CONDUCT DISORDER; EXCESSIVE DRINKING AND HEALTH CONSEQUENCES; EXCESSIVE DRINKING AND NEGATIVE SOCIAL CONSEQUENCES; IMPULSE CONTROL DISORDERS; PERSONALITY DISORDERS; SCHIZOPHRENIA; TREATMENT; VIOLENCE.

Akechi, Tatsuo, et al. "Alcohol Consumption and Suicide among Middle-aged Men in Japan." *British Journal of Psychiatry* 188 (2006): 231–236.

Centers for Disease Control and Prevention. "Youth Risk Behavior Surveillance—United States, 2007." *Morbidity and Mortality Weekly Report* 57, no. SS-4 (June 6, 2008).

Karch, Debra L., et al. "Surveillance for Violent Deaths—National Violent Death Reporting System, 16 States, 2005." *Morbidity and Mortality Weekly Report* 57, no. SS-3 (April 11, 2008).

Kelly, Thomas M., Jack R. Cornelius, and Duncan B. Clark. "Psychiatric Disorders and Attempted Suicide among Adolescents with Substance Use Disorders." *Drug and Alcohol Dependence* 73, no. 1 (2004): 87–97.

Mason, Barbara J. "Rationale for Combining Acamprosate and Naltrexone for Treating Alcohol Dependence." *Journal of Studies of Alcohol,* Supplement no. 15 (2005): 148–156.

Preuss, Ulrich W., M.D., et al., "Predictors and Correlates of Suicide Attempts over 5 Years in 1,237 Alcohol-Dependent Men and Women," *American Journal of Psychiatry* 160, no. 1 (January 2003): 56–63.

support groups See ALCOHOLISM MUTUAL AID SOCIETIES.

tolerance See ALCOHOLISM/ALCOHOL DEPENDENCE AND ALCOHOL ABUSE.

trauma patients See EMERGENCY TREATMENT.

treatment Treatment refers to the provision of services to stabilize a person with alcohol dependence or alcohol abuse and assist the individual toward the goal of the individual's no longer using alcohol (or toward attaining recovery). It primarily includes active attendance and involvement with mutual aid self-help groups such as Alcoholics Anonymous, as well as treatment with various forms of individual and group psychotherapy and specific medications for treating alcohol dependence. Individuals who are alcohol abusers and who are in danger of becoming alcoholics may also benefit from brief intervention therapy, in which the medical risks of their continued or escalated behavior are pointed out to them by a physician, therapist, or other trusted person.

Recovery is a more amorphous concept than treatment, and many individuals believe that an alcoholic is never truly "recovered" or "cured" and thus, is always at risk for suffering from a relapse. By this view, at best, the individual maintains the process of recovering from alcohol by a continued ABSTINENCE from drinking. Probably the best definition of recovery was provided by the Betty Ford Institute Consensus Panel in their article on recovery in 2007 for the *Journal of Substance Abuse Treatment*. They defined recovery as "a voluntarily maintained lifestyle composed [and] characterized by sobriety, personal health, and citizenship."

It is important to keep in mind that relapses should not be regarded as abnormal or as proof that the person cannot attain a state of abstinence from alcohol. Relapses are particularly common within the first six to 12 months after abstinence has started. As a result, most individuals treated for alcoholism will need to take their medication for a minimum period of three months, and treatment may need to continue for a year or longer. It is best that the person who enters treatment should be abstinent from alcohol for at least a few days prior to receiving any medications and therapy for their alcohol dependence. A longer period of abstinence is preferable.

In most cases, treatment is received voluntarily, but sometimes treatment is coerced or court-ordered. Coerced treatment is a policy used with some professionals, such as physicians who must undergo treatment, or they will not be allowed to practice medicine. (See IMPAIRED PHYSICIANS.) Coerced treatment is often very effective. In contrast, court-ordered treatment is usually applied to an individual who has been involved in the criminal justice system (for assaults upon others, drunken driving that caused accidents, or other crimes). In such cases, a judge may believe that alcohol abuse or dependence (or sometimes BINGE DRINKING) played a role in the commission of the crimes. According to the National Partnership on Alcohol Misuse and Crime, nearly half (43 percent) of all referrals to alcohol dependence treatment centers are made by the criminal justice system.

Some key issues complicate the treatment for alcoholism. For example, individuals of any age, ranging from adolescents to the elderly, may need treatment for alcohol dependence, and physicians must take into account whether treatment drugs are suitable for younger or older patients. They must also take into account other age-appropriate issues; for example, unlike adults, adolescents in treatment may balk at having regular blood tests, and may have (or perceive themselves to have) a lower capacity for pain than adults. Adolescents may also respond better to some types of psychotherapy, such as a contingency management program that provides rewards for some behaviors. Adolescent programs generally are much more structured and more supportive than programs offered to adults. Another issue to consider, and one which some parents may fail to take into account, is that adolescents may have been using other drugs in addition to alcohol, particularly marijuana, but also cocaine, methamphetamine, and misused prescription drugs. (See AGE AND ALCOHOL; ALCOHOL AND OTHER DRUGS.)

Another problem area is that many treatment facilities fail to provide treatment for individuals with both psychiatric disorders and alcohol dependence, yet the majority of patients who are alcoholics do have other serious psychiatric problems, such as DEPRESSION or ANXIETY DISORDERS or even psychotic disorders such as SCHIZOPHRENIA. Some alcoholic individuals have ANTISOCIAL PERSONALITY DISORDER, which is commonly linked to alcohol abuse and dependence as well as to the commission of aggressive acts that cause the individual to become incarcerated. (See PSYCHIATRIC COMORBIDITIES.) Another issue of concern is that the majority of alcoholics (an estimated 80 percent) are addicted to nicotine, but few treatment facilities provide any treatment for SMOKING.

Unfortunately, most individuals with problems with alcohol abuse or dependence in the United States do *not* receive any treatment. According to the Substance Abuse and Mental Health Services Administration (SAMHSA), about 19.3 million people ages 12 and older, or 7.8 percent of the population in 2007, needed treatment for alcohol abuse or alcoholism in the past year. According to SAMHSA, respondents to their study were classified as needing treatment for an alcohol problem if they met at least one of three criteria during the past year:

1. dependent on alcohol
2. abuse of alcohol
3. received treatment for an alcohol problem at a specialty facility (i.e., drug and alcohol rehabili-

tation facilities [inpatient or outpatient], hospitals [inpatient only], and mental health centers)

Of those who needed alcohol treatment, only 8.1 percent received their treatment in a specialty substance abuse treatment facility. The broad majority did *not* receive treatment, including 87.4 percent who received no treatment and who also did not believe that they needed any treatment, and 4.5 percent who thought that they needed treatment but who did not receive it.

According to the SAMHSA research, the predominant reason for the failure to seek treatment in 2007 was that many individuals with alcohol issues said that they were not ready to stop using alcohol (42.0 percent) while about a third of them (34.5 percent) attributed their failure to insurance barriers or the cost of treatment. Other reasons that were given for not seeking treatment were the social stigma that they believed was associated with treatment (18.8 percent) or their belief that they could handle their problem without receiving any treatment (11.6 percent). Some people (3.1 percent) said that they did not think that treatment would help them. (Some people provided more than one reason for not seeking treatment.)

Some who refuse treatment are in DENIAL that they have a problem with alcohol, or they may be embarrassed or afraid of repercussions at work or in the social network should they admit that they have an alcohol abuse or dependence problem. They may be unaware that many corporations offer EMPLOYEE ASSISTANCE PROGRAMS for individuals with problems with alcohol and/or drug abuse and dependence.

Another important point to consider is that before individuals can succeed at treatment, several factors need to be in play; for example, they need the motivation to recover as well as access to treatment facilities, and they also need the ability to comply with treatment recommendations (in terms of normal intelligence and other basic capabilities). For example, if an alcoholic has access to a rehabilitative facility and the intellectual ability to comply with the recommendations, but he or she lacks the motivation to change, then treatment will almost invariably fail. Similarly, a person may be highly motivated and capable of complying with treatment recommendations, but if a treatment facility is unavailable, then they cannot receive treatment. Some individuals argue that motivation to change is the most pivotal tool needed for successful treatment and is also what is most likely to be lacking among those dependent on alcohol. This belief seems borne out by the SAMHSA research.

The location of where treatment is provided varies. Treatment may be offered in an inpatient setting for one week to up to about one month. Some rehabilitation facilities offer programs lasting for up to one year. Sometimes treatment is offered to individuals as outpatients. In general, the longer that the treatment lasts, the better it is for the person.

Patients who are experiencing symptoms from DELIRIUM TREMENS are in a state of a medical emergency that was caused by withdrawal from alcohol. They urgently need to be hospitalized for their own medical safety and survival. They are usually treated in a local hospital rather than an alcohol treatment center for their immediate health needs.

Often individuals who receive inpatient treatment eventually "graduate" to continuing their treatment as outpatients. As part of the treatment process, it is important for the alcoholic to identify the people and places that are most likely to cause a relapse in order to avoid those individuals whenever possible; for example, if the person's best friend is a lifelong alcoholic who refuses treatment for alcoholism, then this friendship must be sacrificed. This is more difficult to achieve when it involves family members, such as parents, spouses, or even adult children.

Among those who received outpatient treatment for substance abuse (including alcohol and drugs) in 2005, the treatment completion rate was highest (46 percent) among those dependent on alcohol, according to a 2009 report from the Substance Abuse and Mental Health Services Administration. The success rate for alcohol treatment was followed by those treated for cocaine abuse (25 percent) and then those treated for primary opiate abuse (23 percent). In addition, the most successful percentage of treatment completers for all substances of abuse were referred by an employee through an employee assistance program (49 percent), followed by those referred by the criminal justice system (43 percent).

Some researchers, such as Joseph LoCastro in his 2008 article in the *Journal of Studies on Alcohol and Drugs,* have found that individuals seeking treatment for alcohol dependence for the first time (or "treatment-naive" clients) are very different in many ways from those seeking treatment for the second or third time and so on. For example, the subjects in the treatment-naive group had fewer psychological symptoms than the group who had already received treatment one or more times. In addition, the group of individuals who had received treatment three or more times had the most psychological symptoms of the three groups. (This research is discussed further later in this entry.)

Researchers, such as Carlo C. DiClemente, developed the concept of STAGES OF CHANGE that an alcoholic must go through in order to seek treatment and take the needed actions to achieve recovery from alcohol dependence. These stages include precontemplation (before the person has begun thinking about giving up alcohol), contemplation (when the person starts thinking about change), preparation (the person starts taking steps needed to change), action (the person actively works to change), and maintenance (the changes become a daily part of life).

Some individuals do not meet the criteria for alcoholism, but they are alcohol abusers, and their drinking behavior may be of concern, especially when it is escalating and may develop into a case of alcohol dependence. In such cases, brief intervention therapy may be very helpful. Physicians using brief intervention techniques talk to their patients about their excessive drinking and also encourage them to make changes. Brief interventions may be as brief as one session with a doctor and may also include several follow-up phone calls from a nurse. (See INTERVENTION, BRIEF.)

Locating a treatment facility can be challenging, but resources are available in the community and on the Internet to help individuals seeking treatment to find a suitable facility.

Mutual Aid Self-help Groups

According to the Substance Abuse and Mental Health Services Administration, about 2.3 million people attended self-help groups such as Alcoholics Anonymous for their alcohol use in 2007.

Individuals who attend meetings of Alcoholics Anonymous (AA) quickly learn that others have suffered like them, and they also discover that others have given up drinking, giving them hope that they can also stop drinking. Further attendance enhances and reinforces this belief.

Participation in a twelve-step program is often preceded by recommendations from physicians and others, who can explain why such groups exist and what they can accomplish as well as encouraging patients to become active members. These programs are often integral to overcoming alcoholism and alcohol abuse. (The Twelve Steps are specific steps created by Alcoholics Anonymous that the alcoholic must work through.)

According to John N. Chappell, M.D., and Robert L. DuPont, M.D., in their article on the Twelve Steps of AA and mutual help programs for addictive disorders, published in *Psychiatric Clinics of North America* in 1999, AA is a flexible and democratic fellowship that requires no dues and has only one criterion for membership, which is the desire to stop drinking. According to the authors, "The AA program is remarkable in many ways, including its freedom from any financial motivation because the care is free and the leaders of the groups are unpaid. No governmental or health care financing exists for the AA program. It is not licensed or monitored by any governmental regulatory agency. No records of attendance or clinical records of any kind are kept at AA meetings."

There are other mutual-help programs that exist in addition to AA, although AA is the best known; for example, Women for Sobriety, a group started in 1976, helps women with the unique problems of females who are dependent on alcohol. Secular Organizations for Sobriety (also known as Save Our Selves) is another organization, launched in 1986 as an alternative to twelve-step programs. Most of its members are agnostic or atheistic and are uncomfortable with AA's requirement to surrender internally to a higher power.

Chappell and DuPont said, "Modern epidemiology and treatment outcomes research confirms the common clinical experience that active involvement in one or more 12-step programs is a significant part of the process of getting well for many otherwise hopelessly addicted people."

In an addiction medicine review course given in 2004 by John Chappell, M.D., and Garrett O'Connor, M.D., they discussed twelve-step programs. They noted that it was important for individuals to choose a home group for their AA meetings, which could act as both an extended family and a recovery support system. They also discussed the importance of an AA sponsor, who is an individual who has experienced alcoholism himself or herself and who helps an alcoholic work through the Twelve Steps of AA, and thus helps to reduce the risk for relapse. They noted that Step One of the Twelve Steps is for the individual to admit that he or she is powerless over alcohol and that life has become unmanageable. This step addresses the denial of many alcoholics that they are addicted to alcohol and promotes the principle of honesty. Step Two is the step in which the alcoholic acknowledges that a greater power can restore the individual to sanity, thus recognizing that the person needs help. Chappell says this step promotes the principle of hope. (Other principles of AA are discussed in ALCOHOLISM/ALCOHOL DEPENDENCE AND ALCOHOL ABUSE.)

Medications Used to Treat Alcohol Dependence

Medications that are used to treat alcohol dependence and are approved by the Food and Drug Administration (FDA) include NALTREXONE (Depade, ReVia, Vivitrol), acamprosate (Campral), or DISULFIRAM (Antabuse). Medications that are used indirectly to treat alcoholism are sometimes used to mitigate some of the symptoms of alcohol withdrawal, such as BENZODIAZEPINES. Some medications are used off-label (they are not approved by the FDA to treat alcoholism, but still lawful for doctors to prescribe). For example, topiramate (Topamax) is a medication that is FDA-approved to treat seizures; however, some studies have shown that it is also efficacious in treating alcohol dependence, and as a result, some physicians have used the medication in an off-label manner to treat individuals with alcohol dependence.

Disulfiram is used as an aversive drug because of its extreme side effects; the medication causes extreme nausea and vomiting if the person taking it consumes any alcohol. This includes even alcohol in minute amounts such as in cooked food or mouthwash. The reason for this is that disulfiram blocks the body from metabolizing any alcohol. However, these very same side effects also cause patients to fail to take the drug.

Sometimes combination therapy is used to treat alcohol dependence. In a study reported by Helen M. Pettinati and colleagues in *Addictive Behaviors* in 2008, the researchers randomized 208 patients who were addicted to both cocaine and alcohol to treatment with either disulfiram alone, naltrexone alone, or a combination of disulfiram and naltrexone. (Many patients who abuse or are dependent on alcohol also use other drugs, such as cocaine.) In addition, another group received a placebo (sugar pill) drug.

The researchers found that medication adherence was low for the use of the treatment drugs, either alone or together. They also found that patients taking disulfiram alone or in combination with naltrexone fared the best, and they were also the most likely to abstain from either alcohol or cocaine. A further analysis three weeks later found that those patients who actually were taking the disulfiram-naltrexone combination were the most likely to be abstinent from both alcohol and cocaine.

See Table 1 for how alcohol dependence drugs work, as well as for contraindications against their use. For example, those who are currently taking opioid medications or who have hepatitis should not take naltrexone, and those with severe kidney impairment should not take acamprosate. The table also includes precautions, such as warnings for people with moderate kidney impairment or those with LIVER DISEASE and so forth. There are many precautions for those taking disulfiram, such as for those with a past or current history of psychosis, as well as patients with diabetes mellitus, epilepsy, and hypothyroidism. Note that all the drugs listed in Table 1 are pregnancy category C. This rating, provided by the FDA, means that animal studies have shown these drugs have an adverse effect on the fetus in pregnant women, but there are no adequate and well-controlled studies in actual pregnant women.

Considering Naltrexone Oral naltrexone (ReVia, Depade) is a medication that blocks endorphin receptors (endorphin is a neurochemical that causes pleasure or decreases pain), and thus, naltrexone prevents the euphoric feelings that people experience from consuming alcohol. As a result of the decreased craving for alcohol, ending drinking should be easier for those who are dependent on alcohol when they take naltrexone. The oral form of naltrexone was approved by the FDA as a treatment for alcoholism in 1994. Naltrexone is also available as an injection (Vivitrol) that lasts for about 30 days. According to the National Institute on Alcohol Abuse and Alcoholism (NIAAA), naltrexone cuts the risk of a relapse in the first three months of treatment by more than a third (36 percent) and is especially useful in patients prone to or likely to relapse.

According to Raymond F. Anton, M.D., in his 2008 article on naltrexone for the *New England Journal of Medicine*, "The ideal patient for naltrexone therapy would be a person who has moderate-to-severe alcohol dependence—for example, a person who drinks on more than 50% of days, consumes more than five drinks a day, and has alcohol-related problems. Such a person has probably failed in attempts to quit drinking but has a relatively high motivation to be abstinent or at least to try abstinence for a while. A good indication of this motivation is the ability to abstain from drinking for several days before starting naltrexone."

Common side effects of the use of naltrexone are dizziness, diarrhea, lightheadedness, and nausea, although these side effects generally disappear for most patients who experience them. In general, naltrexone is considered safe and effective in treating alcohol dependence. However, it is not recommended for adolescents who have not yet attained full maturity because naltrexone affects hormones such as growth hormone, prolactin, and luteinizing hormone, and its effects on the maturing adolescent may be risky.

Naltrexone appears most effective in individuals with a family history of alcoholism and a very high craving for alcohol. Extended-release naltrexone (Vivitrol) appears to be most effective in males and those who have been abstinent from alcohol for at least a week.

The Use of Disulfiram Approved by the Food and Drug Administration (FDA) in 1951 to treat alcohol dependence, disulfiram (Antabuse) blocks aldehyde dehydrogenase, a substance that helps

TABLE 1
MEDICATIONS FOR TREATING ALCOHOL DEPENDENCE

	Naltrexone (Depade, ReVia)	Extended-release injectable Naltrexone (Vivitrol)	Acamprosate (Campral)	Disulfiram (Antabuse)	Topiramate (Topamax)
Action	Blocks opioid receptors, resulting in reduced craving and reduced reward in response to drinking	Same as oral naltrexone, 30-day duration	Affects glutamate and GABA neurotransmitter systems, but its alcohol-related action is unclear	Inhibits intermediate metabolism of alcohol, causing a buildup of acetaldehyde and a reaction of flushing, sweating, nausea, and tachycardia if a patient drinks alcohol	Thought to work by increasing inhibitory (GABA) neurotransmission and reducing stimulatory (glutamate) neurotransmission
Contraindications	Currently using opioids or in acute opioid withdrawal, anticipated need for opioid analgesics, acute hepatitis, or liver failure	Same as oral naltrexone, plus inadequate muscle mass for deep intramuscular injection; rash or infection at the injection site	Severe renal impairment; patients who need pain medications	Concomitant use of alcohol or alcohol-containing preparations or metronidazole; coronary artery disease; severe myocardial disease; hypersensitivity to rubber (thiuram) derivatives	Hypersensitivity to topiramate
Precautions	Other hepatic (liver) disease, renal (kidney) impairment, history of suicide attempts or depression. If opioid analgesia is needed, larger doses may be required and respiratory depression may be deeper and more prolonged. Pregnancy Category C. Advise patients to carry a wallet card to alert medical personnel in the event of an emergency.	Same as oral naltrexone, plus hemophilia or other bleeding problems. Pregnancy Category C.	Moderate renal impairment; depression or suicidal ideation and behavior. Pregnancy Category C.	Hepatic cirrhosis or insufficiency, cerebrovascular disease or cerebral damage, psychoses (current or history), diabetes mellitus, epilepsy, hypo-thyroidism, renal impairment. Advise patients to carry a wallet card to alert medical personnel in the event of an emergency. Pregnancy Category C.	Narrow-angle glaucoma, kidney stones, renal or hepatic impairment, severely underweight, use of central nervous system antidepressants. Pregnancy Category C.
Serious adverse reactions	Will precipitate severe withdrawal if the patient is dependent on opioids; hepatoxicity [liver toxicity] (although does not appear to be a hepatoxin at the recommended doses)	Same as oral naltrexone, plus infection at the injection site; depression; and rare events including allergic pneumonia and suicidal ideation and behavior	Rare events include suicidal ideation and behavior	Disulfiram-alcohol reaction, hepatoxicity, optic neuritis, peripheral neuropathy, psychotic reactions	Metabolic acidosis, acute myopia and secondary narrow-angle glaucoma, oligohydrosis and hyperthemia

	Naltrexone (Depade, ReVia)	Extended-release injectable Naltrexone (Vivitrol)	Acamprosate (Campral)	Disulfiram (Antabuse)	Topiramate (Topamax)
Common side effects	Nausea, vomiting, decreased appetite, headache, dizziness, fatigue, anxiety	Same as oral naltrexone plus a reaction at the injection site; joint pain; muscle aches or cramps	Diarrhea, somnolence	Metallic aftertaste, dermatitis, transient mild drowsiness	Paresthesias, taste perversion, anorexia (lack of appetite) and weight loss, somnolence, cognitive dysfunction
Examples of drug interactions	Opioid medications (blocks action)	Same as oral naltrexone	No clinically relevant interactions known	Anticoagulants such as warfarin; isoniazid; metronidazole; phenytoin; any nonprescription drug containing alcohol	Other anticonvulsants, other carbonia anhydrase inhibitors, hydrochlorothiazide, metformin, pioglitazone, lithium, amtitriptyline
Usual adult dosage	*Oral dose:* 50 mg daily *Before prescribing:* Patients must be opioid-free for a minimum of 7 to 10 days before starting. If you feel that there's a risk of precipitating an opioid withdrawal reaction, administer a naloxone challenge test. Evaluate liver function. *Laboratory followup:* Monitor liver function	*Intramuscular dose:* 380 mg given as a deep intramuscular gluteal injection, once monthly **Before prescribing:** Same as oral naltrexone, plus examine the injection site for adequate muscle mass and skin condition *Laboratory followup:* Monitor liver function	*Oral dose:* 666 mg (two 333-mg tablets) three times daily; or for patients with moderate renal impairment, reduce to 333 mg (one tablet) three times daily *Before prescribing:* Evaluate renal function. Establish abstinence.	*Oral dose:* 250 mg daily (range 125 mg to 500 mg) *Before prescribing:* Evaluate liver function. Warn the patient (1) not to take disulfiram for at least 12 hours after drinking and that a disulfiram-alcohol reaction can occur up to 2 weeks after the last dose and (2) to avoid alcohol in the diet (e.g., sauces and vinegars), over-the-counter medications (e.g. cough syrups) and toiletries (e.g., cologne, mouthwash). *Laboratory followup:* Monitor liver function	*Oral dose:* initial dose 25 mgs at bedtime, increasing the dose by 25–50 mg daily each week, divided into morning and evening doses. Faster titration is more likely to cause adverse reactions. Target dose is 200 mg per day total dose, but patients unable to tolerate that dose may respond to lower doses. *Before prescribing:* Evaluate renal function, obtain serum electrolytes and bicarbonate *Laboratory follow up:* Monitor renal function, serum electrolytes and bicarbonate

Note: This chart highlights some of the properties of each medication. It does not provide complete information and is not meant to be a substitute for the package inserts or other drug reference sources used by clinicians. Whether or not a medication should be prescribed and in what amount is a matter between individuals and their health-care providers. The prescribing information provided here is not a substitute for a provider's judgment in an individual circumstance, and the National Institute of Health (NIH) accepts no liability or responsibility for use of the information with regard to particular patients. Also note that while topiramate may be prescribed "off-label" by a physician, it has not been approved for the treatment of alcohol dependence by the Food and Drug Administration (FDA).
Source: Adapted from *Helping Patients Who Drink Too Much: A Clinician's Guide.* Bethesda, Md.: National Institute on Alcohol Abuse and Alcoholism, December 2007, pages 8–9.

to metabolize alcohol. As a result, if an individual consumes any alcohol, this will cause a reaction of nausea and vomiting and the individual may also have difficulty with breathing. This reaction is similar to the reaction of some Asians who have a genetic lack of ability to metabolize alcohol. (See ALCOHOL FLUSHING RESPONSE.)

Disulfiram is most effective when it is monitored by someone else, such as a spouse or a clinic, or it is administered by a pharmacist or other person. Some patients who administer the drug to themselves take their disulfiram only when they consider themselves to be in a high-risk situation, such as a social situation where alcohol is served. (This is not the recommended manner of treatment.)

Disulfiram is generally the last choice of clinicians when other medications have failed to work because of the poor compliance with taking disulfiram. Sometimes treatment with disulfiram is court-ordered, and if the individual fails to show up to take the medication, then he or she will go to jail.

Acamprosate and Alcohol Dependence   The FDA approved acamprosate (Campral) for the treatment of alcohol dependence in 2004, and the medication first became available in the United States in 2005. As with naltrexone, acamprosate reduces the risk for relapse by reducing the craving for alcohol. Side effects of acamprosate include anxiety, insomnia, nausea, dizziness, and weakness. Some research also has demonstrated that acamprosate may worsen depression, and thus, patients who are depressed should be monitored carefully while on this medication. Studies on the effectiveness of this drug are mixed; some studies have shown acamprosate to be effective, while other studies have shown it to be less effective than naltrexone and disulfiram.

According to the NIAAA, acamprosate is believed to reduce the symptoms that are related to withdrawal from alcohol, such as anxiety, insomnia, and restlessness. However, several large trials in the United States have failed to confirm its efficacy. One study reported by Barbara J. Mason and colleagues in 2006 in the *Journal of Psychiatric Research* found that motivated patients were the most likely to succeed with this drug. Mason tested three groups of subjects. In one group, 258 subjects took the standard dose of 2 g, and in another group,

83 subjects took an exploratory 3 g dose. The placebo group included 260 subjects. All patients also received eight counseling sessions.

The researchers found that the placebo group had an abstinence rate of 52.3 percent, while the group taking 2 g had an abstinence rate of 58.2 percent. The group taking the higher dose of 3 g had an abstinence rate of 62.7 percent. However, when the study controlled for patients motivated for abstinence as a separate group, there was a significant effect with acamprosate: a rate of 57.1 percent for the placebo group, 70.0 percent for the group on 2 g acamprosate, and 72.5 percent for the group on 3 g of acamprosate.

According to Mason et al., "This study provides perhaps the most definitive evidence to date that acamprosate is not an effective treatment for alcohol dependence in non-motivated and non-abstinent populations." They added, "However, when statistical adjustments were made in keeping with prevailing theory on factors related to alcoholism treatment outcome and how acamprosate works in the brain, and what this mediating process implies about the therapeutic value of acamprosate treatment for alcohol dependence, significant efficacy was found."

Off-Label Medications Used to Treat Alcoholism   Some research has indicated that topiramate (Topamax), an antiseizure medication, is effective in decreasing heavy drinking among those who are alcoholics. Some preliminary research has also shown that aripiprazole (Abilify) may be effective in treating alcohol dependence, because it increases the sedating effects of alcohol and decreases the euphoric effects. Aripiprazole is an antipsychotic medication that is FDA-approved to treat schizophrenia and BIPOLAR DISORDER.

Ondanestron (Zofran) is a medication used to treat cancer patients to help them deal with the nausea and vomiting caused by chemotherapy. However, the medication has also been found to decrease dopamine levels and thus also decrease the rewarding impact of alcohol. Some studies have found oral ondanestron to be well tolerated in adolescents ages 14–20. The drug may be more effective in individuals with early-onset alcoholism, which has a greater link to antisocial behaviors.

Some experts have found some success with treating alcoholics with baclofen (Lioresal, Kemstro), a medication that is FDA-approved to relax the skeletal muscles and is used with patients with multiple sclerosis. It has been used with some success in patients with CIRRHOSIS, according to a study by Giovanni Addolorato, M.D., and colleagues, published in *Lancet* in 2007. Others have noted that levetiracetam (Keppra) has helped some patients who are alcoholics, although the drug is not FDA-approved to treat alcohol dependence.

Medications to Treat Withdrawal and the Side Effects of Treatment Benzodiazepines are often used to treat the common side effects of the withdrawal from alcohol dependence. Benzodiazepines should never be combined with alcohol, however, because this combination is dangerous and can be fatal. These drugs are effective at treating the symptoms of withdrawal from alcohol and often prevent the seizures that are sometimes linked to withdrawal as well.

Medication Compliance As with patients with a wide range of many other disorders, individuals who are being treated for alcohol dependence are often noncompliant at taking their medication. They may take fewer doses than ordered by the physician or may not take any of their medicine at all. According to Andrew M. Peterson in a 2007 issue of the *American Journal of Health-System Pharmacists,* nonadherence may result from the adverse effects caused by the drug or could be caused by frequent dosing. Patients may simply forget to take their medication if they must take it many times per day. When the drug is known to cause side effects, then patients are more reluctant to take the drug, as with disulfiram.

According to Peterson, "In one study, only 18.2 percent of the patients receiving disulfiram who had not been court-ordered to take it adhered to treatment; in stark contrast, medication adherence was 61 percent when the patient was under court order." Peterson also noted that in a large Veterans Administration study, adherence to medication regimens was only about 23 percent.

Compliance with acamprosate varies considerably, according to Peterson, ranging from studies reporting an adherence rate of 84.2 percent to much lower rates of 30 percent. In some studies, the medication compliance rate was very high because the drugs were dispensed directly by a doctor, nurse, physician assistant, or pharmacist.

In the case of oral naltrexone, studies also show a wide variability of medication adherence. Patients who receive cognitive-behavioral therapy (CBT) appear to have a higher rate of medication compliance than those who do not receive this form of therapy.

Peterson concluded that of all drugs used for alcohol dependence, "In controlled clinical trials, adherence to pharmacotherapy for alcohol dependence is highly variable, ranging from as low as 20% to almost 90%. However, it is thought that adherence may be even lower in less-controlled settings, such as the clinic and private practice."

He added, "Some psychosocial therapies have shown a positive effect on medication adherence. In addition, there are a variety of pharmacy tools available that have successfully improved adherence for other chronic disease states: these include medication refill reminders, use of easy-dosing regimens, including extended-release formulations and adherence packs, and pharmacist-based patient education. These interventions, if implemented, may improve adherence among patients receiving treatment for alcohol dependence and improve patient outcomes."

Psychotherapy

Psychotherapy is counseling provided to an individual alone or to individuals in a group in order to help them change their behavior. Psychotherapy by itself is usually insufficient to allow a person who is an alcoholic to recover from addiction; however, psychotherapy combined with membership in an ALCOHOLISM MUTUAL AID SOCIETY, such as Alcoholics Anonymous, as well as the use of targeted medication (such as naltrexone or disulfiram or a combination of drugs) can often provide much-needed help to the alcoholic.

There are a variety of different types of individual therapies that are generally used with alcoholics. Cognitive-behavioral therapy (CBT) is often used to treat individuals with alcohol dependence, while some therapists use motivational therapy or other forms of therapy, such as family therapy or group therapy. Contingency management is another approach, in which "good" behavior is rewarded with privileges, money, or other positive reinforcers. This approach may be most effective with adolescents. If the individual is not yet alcohol-dependent but appears at risk for alcoholism because of escalating alcohol abuse, then he or she may be a candidate for brief intervention therapy. Those who are already alcoholics, however, usually cannot benefit from brief intervention.

Cognitive-behavioral Therapy CBT is a popular form of therapy that helps a person identify his or her internalized irrational thoughts and learn how to challenge them within his or her own mind. For example, the thought that "Others should understand me" is one that is worthy of challenge, as is "I can't get better; I'm hopeless." The therapist trains the client to directly confront such thoughts and replace them with other thoughts, such as "It would be nice if others could always understand me, but they won't or can't" or "I can get better, but it may take a lot of work." CBT also includes a skills-training component in which the therapist aids the patient in learning skills to unlearn bad habits as well as develop skills to cope with existing or future problems. CBT requires the skills of a talented therapist working with a cooperative patient who can understand what the therapist says and is willing to make an attempt to comply with the goals of therapy.

Motivational Therapies According to Carlo C. DiClemente, Lori E. Bellino, and Tara M. Neavins in their article on motivation for change and alcoholism treatment in *Alcohol Research & Health* in 1999, motivation interviewing (MI) is based on the stages of change model and works on increasing and facilitating the patient's motivation. This approach seeks to help patients overcome their ambivalence about change, so that they can make needed life changes.

According to Lisa J. Merlo and Mark S. Gold, M.D., in their article on addiction research and treatment for *Psychiatric Times* in 2008, "Motivational interviewing is a brief, patient-centered, directive approach that emphasizes personal choice and responsibility. It has demonstrated efficacy with addiction populations related to both quitting/cutting down on substance abuse and accepting formal treatment. Some studies have indicated

that patients with high levels of anger do better with MET [motivation enhancement therapy] than with CBT."

According to DiClemente and colleagues,

One technique is reflective listening, a form of paraphrasing that enables patients to more fully tell their stories and to feel that they are being heard by the empathetic MI therapist. A second technique involves exploring the pros and cons of change, which may help patients realistically evaluate their behavior, and current situation, and, ideally, determine whether the pros of change outweigh the cons. A third MI technique, which supports the patient's self-efficacy, or confidence that he or she can change, can help bridge the gap between a patient's desire to change and concrete behavioral change. A fourth technique uses interview and assessment data to provide patients with personalized feedback regarding the problem behavior (e.g. comparing the patient's level of alcohol use with national drinking norms) as a means of increasing self-awareness and of highlighting the discrepancy between the patient's current behavior and the target behavior. Yet another technique involves eliciting self-motivational statements from the patient, such as recognition of the problem and concern for one's own welfare.

Another form of motivation therapy, or motivation enhancement therapy (MET), starts with an extensive assessment of the patient, including diagnostic testing, and then is composed of four treatment sessions over 12 weeks, according to DiClemente and colleagues. In the first session, the therapist talks to the patient about his or her drinking and the risk of serious health consequences faced from this drinking. The patient receives written feedback comparing his or her behavior and the results of diagnostic testing with other adults. In session two, the therapist uses MI techniques to help the patient create a plan. With sessions three and four, the therapist reviews the patient's progress and works on renewing the commitment to change and overcoming any remaining ambivalence.

Contingency Management Some therapists believe that behavior, including alcohol-seeking behavior, can be shaped with reinforcing consequences for some behaviors exhibited by patients (such as abstinence) and punitive measures for others (such as alcohol-seeking behavior). Stephen T. Higgins and Nancy M. Petry describe contingency management (CM) in their article for *Alcohol Research & Health* in 1999. According to the authors, of rewards and punishments, "For example, positive consequences for abstinence may include receipt of vouchers that are exchangeable for retail goods, whereas negative consequences for drinking may include withholding of vouchers or an unfavorable report to a parole officer." The contingency management approach may use written contracts between the patient and the facility.

In one study of CM, reported by Higgins and Petry, alcohol-dependent patients in two groups submitted breath samples that were tested for alcohol use daily for the first four weeks of treatment and then weekly thereafter. In the CM group, the patients had a chance to win a prize for every negative breath sample, ranging from $1 to $100. The allure of possibly winning prizes kept the CM patients coming back, and 84 percent remained in treatment for the entire eight weeks, compared to only 22 percent of the standard treatment group. In addition, by the end of the treatment period, only 31 percent of the CM treatment group had relapsed, compared to the nearly double relapse rate of 61 percent of the standard treatment group.

Group Therapy Group therapy is often beneficial in that others in the group who have experienced alcohol dependence can help challenge the irrational beliefs of an individual. In addition, he or she may be more likely to listen to others who have experienced an alcohol dependence rather than to an authority figure such as a counselor or a physician. Group therapy is offered in most treatment centers, whether they are inpatient or outpatient facilities.

Family Therapy The family is nearly always impacted severely in many ways by an alcoholic family member. Family therapy may help to get such issues out in the open where they may be dealt with, with the assistance of a trained family therapist. For example, family members may be ashamed, embarrassed, and angry with the alcoholic person. The alcoholic person may believe that family members have not been supportive or understanding of problems that he or she has faced. Family therapy meetings can sometimes become very heated, and they require a skilled therapist to transform the session into a positive one that is therapeutic and helpful—or at least one that is neutral.

In the past, the goal of family therapy was to figure out whose "fault" the alcohol dependence was, particularly if the person with alcohol dependence or alcohol abuse was an adolescent. In contrast, the more modern approach today is to determine what risk factors are present and to try to increase any protective factors in the environment. A risk factor could be that others in the family drink and should also seek treatment, or they may have to be avoided by the patient subsequent to treatment. A protective factor could be the individual's religious values and encouraging him or her to attend religious services. Those who are religious are generally less likely to abuse or be dependent on alcohol. (See RELIGION.)

Brief Intervention Therapy for Alcohol Abuse

Although alcoholism cannot be treated with brief intervention therapy, individuals with alcohol abuse often respond to it. With brief intervention therapy, the individual is advised by a physician in a nonconfrontational manner that there is an apparent problem and also told about the health consequences (such as liver disease, cancer, and so forth) that could result if this problem continues or escalates. Such an approach can be successful in helping individuals come to an acknowledgment that they do have a problem and that they need to take action to resolve it.

If patients indicate that they are willing to change, then physicians (or other professionals) can help the individual create a goal and a plan. If the patient is not willing to change, he or she can be urged to think about what was said by the doctor and what barriers they perceive that prevent them from changing. For all patients, a follow-up to further discuss the alcohol issue should be arranged, and patients with alcohol use issues should be screened on an annual basis.

First-time Alcohol Treatment Seekers Compared to Repeaters

Joseph LoCastro's research found that there are significant differences among those individuals who seek treatment for alcohol dependence for the first time compared to individuals who have experienced treatment once or twice as well as those who experienced treatment three or more times. For example, LoCastro's "treatment-naive" group (composed of individuals who had never been treated before) was significantly less committed to the goal of abstinence. Less than half (42.5 percent) of the treatment-naive group said that they were committed to abstinence as a goal. In sharp contrast, 70.0 percent of those individuals who had received treatment once or twice said they were committed to the goal of abstinence, and 80.7 percent of the group that had been treated three or more times said they were committed to abstinence as a goal.

There were also demographic differences; for example, the subjects in the treatment-naive group were more likely to be married females with jobs. According to the researcher, "These findings suggest that it is quite possible that women enter treatment after fewer years of drinking."

The levels of drinks consumed per day varied among the three groups. Subjects who had received treatment three or more times had the highest levels of daily drinking, while those who had received treatment once or twice were in the middle range, and the treatment-naive clients had the fewest drinks per day. Interestingly, however, the group with three or more prior treatment experiences reported the greatest number of days abstinent. According to LoCastro, "Supporting this finding, other studies have found that treatment-experienced patients slow down their drinking before entering treatment and are more likely to become abstainers than nonproblem drinkers."

The research also showed that those with prior incidents of treatment reported greater problems than the treatment-naive groups with social and emotional relationships and also said that they had a lower quality of life. LoCastro concluded,

> Treatment-experienced clients report even greater need for treatment than the first-time seekers by describing themselves as more severe alcoholics with lower levels of psychosocial functioning and quality of life. It may be important for alcohol treatment providers to understand that alcoholics with multiple prior treatments are quantitatively

and qualitatively different from first-time help seekers. These multiple treatment seekers may require more continuous treatment episodes based on abstinence approaches that also focus on a multiplicity of psychosocial needs. In contrast, first-time treatment seekers who report less motivation and commitment to abstinence may benefit more from cognitive-behavioral approaches that enhance motivation and build relapse prevention skills.

Programs for Substance-abusing Doctors

Some alcohol-dependent individuals receive coerced treatment, i.e., if they refuse treatment, then they risk losing their ability to practice in their professions. Coerced treatment programs for doctors have been very effective, and according to Robert L. DuPont, M.D., and colleagues in their 2009 article on this subject for the *Journal of Substance Abuse Treatment*, 78 percent of the participants in a study had no positive alcohol or drug test over the five-year period of intensive monitoring. This is a dramatic and unheard-of success rate.

The researchers studied 904 physicians who were admitted to 16 state physicians' health programs (PHPs) due to their addiction. These programs required the doctors to abstain from all alcohol and drugs of abuse for five years. Random testing was provided for up to five years and quickly identified any substance use. In the study, the 904 doctors were mostly men (86 percent). Their average age was 44 years. Many different specialties were represented, including family medicine (20 percent), internal medicine (13 percent), anesthesiology (11 percent), and so on. The primary drug of abuse was alcohol, which was abused by half the doctors, followed by opiates (33 percent), stimulants (8 percent), and other drugs of abuse.

More than half the doctors (55 percent) were required to enter the PHP by a hospital, licensing board, or other organization, and the researchers believe that the remaining doctors were informally pressured to enter the PHP.

The PHPs provide active care management and are not addiction programs per se. Instead, they create formal and binding contracts with the doctors for what will happen if they do or do not comply with the contract. The PHPs work with state licensing boards and provide a "safe haven" for doctors, as long as they are compliant. The researchers wrote, "Importantly, the contracts typically stipulate intense and ongoing treatment accompanied by regular monitoring of their substance use and addiction-related behaviors through random drug testing as well as unscheduled work site visits or work site monitors for extended periods—typically 5 or more years." Those doctors who are fully compliant obtain support and even advocacy from the PHPs with their state licensing boards.

The researchers added, "On the other hand, physicians who refuse the terms of the contract and/or are found to continue substance use risk report to their boards, which may result in loss of their licenses."

After the doctor signs a PHP contract, he or she usually enters a formal addiction program. The doctor is responsible for the cost of treatment as well as for urine monitoring and other costs. In addition, most PHPs expect alcoholic doctors to operate under the principles of Alcoholics Anonymous and also to regularly attend AA meetings.

In the first phase, the doctor enters three months of residential treatment or intensive outpatient treatment in a specialty program. Doctors withdraw from their practices during this phase of treatment, in most cases. The second phase lasts three to 12 months and involves less intensive outpatient treatment. Doctors may resume their practice in this phase, but are closely supervised by the PHP. Random alcohol testing, monitoring, and support is integral to this phase.

The use of pharmacotherapy for treatment in this program was very low; for example, 5 percent of the doctors were given naltrexone as adjunctive treatment, and one doctor was given methadone for an opiate addiction. About a third of the doctors were treated with ANTIDEPRESSANTS for depression or anxiety disorders. In contrast, 92 percent of the doctors attended meetings of Alcoholics Anonymous or Narcotics Anonymous, and they also relied upon aftercare groups from their formal treatment programs and follow-up with their PHP monitors.

Based on follow-up, 91 percent of the doctors who completed the program were practicing medicine, versus 28 percent of the non-completers. About half of the non-completers were not prac-

ticing medicine because they had left medicine, retired, surrendered their licenses, or their medical licenses had been suspended or revoked.

The researchers said, "Whatever the differences from other populations experiencing SUDs [substance abuse disorders], it is likely that the successful treatment of physicians with SUDs has important implications for SUD treatment in general. For example, if physicians were found to have significantly better outcomes than other groups when treated for diabetes or coronary artery disease, this would be of great public health interest. Recognizing that AUDs [alcohol use disorders] are biological disorders with major behavioral components (just like diabetes and coronary artery disease), the relatively high level of success exhibited by physicians whose care is managed by PHP is important with respect to the potential for success in addiction treatment generally. Indeed, the observed rate of success among physicians directly contradicts the common misperception that relapse is both inevitable and common, if not universal, among patients recovering from SUDs."

Coerced and Court-mandated Treatment

Some individuals are ordered to receive treatment by a court, and if they fail to comply with the court order, then they are sent to jail, as when a person is found guilty of driving under the influence of alcohol and is ordered to treatment. Treatment may involve classes about the risks of alcohol dependence as well as individual counseling. In addition, often the driver's license is suspended for at least three months—whether he or she receives treatment or not. However, the later return of the driver's license may depend on the proven receipt of treatment.

Other means of treatment coercion or pressure are employee assistance programs, which offer a person an opportunity to keep his or her job if the person seeks and completes treatment. In addition, sometimes family members meet for an "intervention" with an alcoholic family member, and with the help of a counselor, seek to compel the individual to enter treatment immediately. This means appears to be the least effective of the three means of coercion (court-mandated, employee assistance programs, or family interventions).

The key point to keep in mind is that, in most cases, if alcoholics do not receive treatment *and* remain in treatment until its completion, then they are usually unlikely to recover from their alcohol dependence. According to author Nancy Darbo in her article on issues related to coercion in substance abuse treatment, "The research indicates that the presence of coercion in treatment entry is a powerful predictor of treatment retention and hence treatment effectiveness. Coercion can also be a positive influence on motivation for treatment and readiness for change as well as engagement in treatment."

Darbo concluded, "Those in treatment often benefit from some form of pressure to complete it (extrinsic motivation). Those who remain in treatment long enough can develop the desire and motivation to voluntarily complete treatment (intrinsic motivation)."

Eric Goplerud and Laura Jacobus-Kantor said in their 2009 article for the National Partnership on Alcohol Misuse and Crime, "The threat of incarceration can be an extremely powerful motivator to encourage criminal offenders to initiate treatment, and probationary periods can provide courts with the opportunity and means to ensure treatment compliance. There is some evidence that regular contact with probation officers or court-designated monitors who have training in addiction can help reduce recidivism."

Another form of court-mandated treatment is the Secure Continuous Remote Alcohol Monitor (SCRAM), which is composed of an ankle bracelet, a modem, and a Web application. The bracelet can be worn 24/7, and it periodically tests for alcohol transdermally using the individual's perspiration. Up to 48 tests per day can be made. The SCRAM periodically downloads information to the Web site. It is believed to be a more cost-effective system than sending a person to jail or prison.

Finding a Treatment Facility

It can be challenging to find a treatment facility that meets most of an alcoholic's needs; however, a board-certified addiction specialist should be knowledgeable about local facilities. Members of the national New York–based American Society of Addiction Medicine can help; their Web site can be accessed at http://www.asam.org.

The Center for Substance Abuse Treatment, a division of the federal Substance Abuse and Mental Health Services Administration, recommends that individuals consider visiting the facility and finding the answers to the following questions when they are considering entering a particular treatment program:

1. Does the program accept your insurance? If not, will they work with you on a payment plan or find other means of support for you?
2. Is the program run by state-accredited, licensed, and/or trained professionals?
3. Is the facility clean, organized, and well run?
4. Does the program encompass the full range of needs of the individual (medical, including infectious diseases; psychological, including co-occurring mental illness; social; vocational; legal; etc.)?
5. Does the treatment program also address sexual orientation and physical disabilities as well as provide age, gender, and culturally appropriate treatment services?
6. Are long-term aftercare support and/or guidance encouraged, provided, and maintained?
7. Is there ongoing assessment of an individual's treatment plan to ensure it meets changing needs?
8. Does the program employ strategies to engage and keep individuals in longer-term treatment, increasing the likelihood of success?
9. Does the program offer counseling (individual or group) and other behavioral therapies to enhance the individual's ability to function in the family/community?
10. Does the program offer medication as part of the treatment regimen, if appropriate?
11. Is there ongoing monitoring of possible relapse to help guide patients back to abstinence?
12. Are services of referrals offered to family members to ensure they understand addiction and the recovery process to help them support the recovering individual?

Future Genomic Approaches to Treatment

Some studies have shown that some alcoholic individuals are genetically more responsive than others to medications such as naltrexone, and future studies may help to indicate which individuals possess the "candidate genes" that make them more responsive to medication therapy. For example, in a summary of the genomic approach in the *Archives of General Psychiatry* in 2008, the authors noted that naltrexone decreased alcohol stimulation in individuals carrying the Asp40 allele. Future physicians may be able to genotype individuals with alcoholism to determine the most effective medication.

See also ALCOHOL AND MEN; ALCOHOL AND WOMEN.

Addolorato, Giovanni, M.D., et al. "Effectiveness and Safety of Baclofen for Maintenance of Alcohol Abstinence in Alcohol-Dependent Patients with Liver Cirrhosis: Randomised, Double-Blind Controlled Study." *Lancet* 370, no. 9,603 (2007): 1,915–1,922.

Anton, Raymond F., M.D. "Naltrexone for the Management of Alcohol Dependence." *New England Journal of Medicine* 359, no. 7 (2008): 715–721.

Betty Ford Institute Consensus Panel. "What Is Recovery? A Working Definition from the Betty Ford Institute." *Journal of Substance Abuse Treatment* 33, no. 3 (2007): 221–228.

Chappell, John N., M.D., and Robert L. DuPont, M.D. "Twelve-Step and Mutual Help Programs for Addictive Disorders." *Psychiatric Clinics of North America* 22, no. 2 (1999): 425–446.

Chappel, John, M.D., and Garrett O'Connor, M.D. 12-Step Programs. Addiction Medicine Review Course, Foundations of Addiction Medicine: Evidence & Art. October 6–9, 2004. Slide presentation. Available online. URL: file:///C:/Documents%20and%20Settings/John%20Adamec/Local%20Settings/Temporary%20Internet%20Files/Content.IE5/QS16LJ1S/12Step%5B1%5D.ppt#288,42,RESPECT THE TRADITIONS. Accessed July 31, 2009.

Darbo, Nancy. "Overview of Issues Related to Coercion in Substance Abuse Treatment: Part I." *Journal of Addictions Nursing* 20, no. 1 (2009): 16–23.

DiClemente, Carlo C., Lori El Bellino, and Tara M. Neavins. "Motivation for Change and Alcoholism Treatment." *Alcohol Research & Health* 23, no. 2 (1999): 86–92.

DuPont, Robert L., M.D., et al. "Setting the Standard for Recovery: Physicians' Health Programs." *Journal of Substance Abuse Treatment* 36, no. 2 (2009): 159–171.

Garbutt, James C., M.D. "The State of Pharmacotherapy for the Treatment of Alcohol Dependence." *Journal of Substance Abuse Treatment* 36, Suppl. 1 (2009): S15–S23.

Gold, Mark S., M.D., and Mark D. Aronson, M.D. "Treatment of Alcohol Abuse and Dependence." UptoDate. Available online to subscribers. URL: http://www.uptodate.com. Accessed March 13, 2009.

Goplerud, Eric, and Laura Jacobus-Kantor. *Improving Criminal Justice Interventions for People with Alcohol Problems.* Washington, D.C.: National Partnership on Alcohol Misuse and Crime, March 2009.

Heilig, Markus, and Mark Egli. "Pharmacological Treatment of Alcohol Dependence: Target Symptoms and Target Mechanisms." *Pharmacology & Therapeutics* 111, no. 3 (2006): 855–876.

Higgins, Stephen T., and Nancy M. Petry. "Contingency Management: Incentives for Sobriety." *Alcohol Research & Health* 23, no. 2 (1999): 122–127.

Johnson, Bankole A., Norman Rosenthal, Julie A. Capece, et al. "Topiramate for Treating Alcohol Dependence: A Randomized Controlled Trial." *Journal of the American Medical Association* 298, no. 14 (2007): 1,641–1,651.

LoCastro, Joseph S. "Characteristics of First-Time Alcohol Treatment Seekers: the COMBINE Study." *Journal of Studies on Alcohol and Drugs* 69, no. 6 (2008): 885–895.

Mason, Barbara J., et al. "Effect of Oral Acamprosate on Abstinence in Patients with Alcohol Dependence in a Double-Blind, Placebo-Controlled Trial: The Role of Patient Motivation." *Journal of Psychiatric Research* 40, no. 5 (2006): 382–392.

Merlo, Lisa J., and Mark S. Gold, M.D. "Special Report—Frontiers in Psychiatric Research: Addiction Research and Treatment." *Psychiatric Times* 25, no. 7 (2009): 52–57.

Office of Applied Studies. *Results from the 2007 National Survey on Drug Use and Health: National Findings.* Rockville, Md.: Substance Abuse and Mental Health Services Administration, 2008.

Peterson, Andrew M. "Improving Adherence in Patients with Alcohol Dependence: A New Role for Pharmacists." *American Journal of Health-System Pharmacists* 64, Suppl. 3 (2007): S1–S17.

Pettinati, Helen M., et al. "A Double Blind, Placebo-Controlled Trial that Combined Disulfiram and Naltrexone for Treating Co-Occurring Cocaine and Alcohol Dependence." *Addictive Behaviors* 33, no. 5 (2008): 651–667.

"Prospects for a Genomic Approach to the Treatment of Alcoholism." *Archives of General Psychiatry* 65, no. 2 (2008): 132–133.

Substance Abuse and Mental Health Services Administration. Office of Applied Studies. *The NSDUH Report—Alcohol Treatment: Need, Utilization, and Barriers.* Rockville, Md. April 9, 2009.

Substance Abuse and Mental Health Services Administration. *The TEDS Report: Treatment Outcomes among Clients*

Discharged from Outpatient Substance Abuse Treatment. Rockville, Md. April 23, 2009.

Volpicelli, Joseph R., M.D. "New Options for the Treatment of Alcohol Dependence." *Psychiatric Annals* 35, no. 6 (2005): 484–491.

Wilson, Jennifer F. "Alcohol Use." *Annals of Internal Medicine* Suppl. (2009): ITC3-1–ITC3-16.

treatment facilities　See TREATMENT.

trichotillomania　Trichotillomania is the compulsion to pull out body hair, particularly on the head, but individuals may pull out their hair on other parts of the body. People with trichotillomania may be bald or have bald patches on their head, and often others think that the person has cancer and is receiving chemotherapy. The individual with trichotillomania knows that the behavior is irrational and wishes to end it, but cannot stop without treatment. Individuals suffering from trichotillomania may also experience problems with alcohol use.

Symptoms and Diagnostic Path

The constant pulling out of hair is the primary symptom of trichotillomania. The hair may be pulled out on the head and/or on other parts of the body. Some people with trichotillomania wear wigs to hide their problem. They may also actively avoid physicians or others who may discover their problem. If they do see a physician, the doctor can diagnose the problem by viewing the body and questioning the individual.

Rarely, individuals swallow the hair that they eat. Hair is indigestible, and in some cases, individuals with trichotillomania have suffered from blockages to their gastrointestinal systems, similar to a hair clog in a drain. Such blockages can be removed only by a physician.

Treatment Options and Outlook

Trichotillomania is treated with behavioral therapy as well as medications such as ANTIDEPRESSANTS and other drugs, such as clomipramine (Anafranil) and topiramate (Topamax, Epitomax, Topamac, and Opimax). Interestingly, sometimes topiramate is also used to treat alcoholism, so the person with both trichotillomania and alcohol dependence may benefit from this drug to treat both disorders.

Risk Factors and Preventive Measures

Most patients with trichotillomania are female. The reason for this gender prevalence is unknown. There are no known preventive measures, but when it is diagnosed, the disorder should be treated.

See IMPULSE CONTROL DISORDERS.

Franklin, Martin E., et al. "The Child and Adolescent Trichotillomania Impact Project: Descriptive Psychopathology, Comorbidity, Functional Impairment, and Treatment Utilization." *Journal of Developmental & Behavioral Pediatrics* 29, no. 6 (2008): 493–500.

twelve-step groups　See ALCOHOLISM MUTUAL AID SOCIETIES; STAGES OF CHANGE; TREATMENT.

twin studies　See ADOPTION AND TWIN STUDIES AND ALCOHOL; GENETICS AND ALCOHOL.

underage drinking The consumption of alcoholic beverages in the United States by individuals younger than age 21. Congress passed the National Minimum Drinking Age Act in 1984, which required all states to prohibit drinking by individuals under age 21 or forfeit a percentage of their federal highway funds. The law was challenged, and it was upheld by the U.S. Supreme Court in 1987. All states changed their laws to make age 21 the minimum legal drinking age, in order to comply with the federal law. According to the National Institute on Alcohol Abuse and Alcoholism (NIAAA), the preponderance of research has shown that minimum legal drinking age laws have decreased traffic crashes and deaths as well as SUICIDES and have also decreased alcohol consumption among those under age 21.

Despite improvements, however, underage drinking continues to be a major problem in the United States, and there are an estimated 10.8 million underage drinkers in the United States, according to the NIAAA. Alcohol is also a major contributor to deaths from injuries, and about 5,000 individuals under age 21 die each year from alcohol-related injuries involving underage drinking.

Many COLLEGE STUDENTS are underage drinkers, although some students are 21 years old or older, which often makes it difficult for campus administrators to monitor who may and who may not drink. Many times older students buy alcohol for younger students or loan them their identification so that the younger person may purchase alcohol. According to the Surgeon General's 2007 report, about 80 percent of college students drink alcohol, and 40 percent engage in binge drinking.

The Centers for Disease Control and Prevention (CDC) reports that in 2007, 44.7 percent of high-school students were current drinkers, or they had had at least one drink of alcohol on at least one day during the 30 days before the Youth Risk Behavior survey. Males and females were about equally likely to be current drinkers, in contrast to most other age groups, in which males are much more likely to consume alcohol than females. Of concern is that some evidence shows that consuming alcohol can affect brain development in adolescents, and some studies have shown that the hippocampus, the area of the brain that controls learning and memory, is smaller in size among adolescents who begin drinking at a young age. This may be why regular adolescent consumers of alcohol generally receive grades of Ds and Fs. In addition, high-school students who consume alcohol or other drugs have a five-fold increased risk for dropping out of high school.

An estimated 1.47 million adolescents ages 12–17 years fulfill the criteria for alcohol abuse or dependence, according to the National Household Survey on Drug Abuse; yet only about 15 percent receive any treatment for their alcohol problems.

In 2007, Acting U.S. Surgeon General Kenneth P. Moritsugu issued his "Call to Action on Underage Drinking" plan, which was developed with the National Institute on Alcohol Abuse and Alcoholism (NIAAA) and the Substance Abuse and Mental Health Services Administration (SAMHSA) in an attempt to combat adolescent and young adult drinking. Although all states prohibit drinking by individuals younger than age 21, their laws and policies continue to vary widely. There are no federal minimum drinking age laws on reservations owned and managed by NATIVE AMERICANS. An estimated 200 Native American tribes have created their own laws regarding who may consume alcohol.

Some states have prohibitions against underage drinking parties, issuing a liability to the owner of the home where they are held, whether the owners are present during the drinking party or not. In some cases, if an underage drinker subsequently gets into a car accident after the drinking party where a minor was allowed to drink, the state may prosecute the adult who allowed the party to occur. In addition, an injured third party may also be able to sue the host of the underage drinking event.

Some personality traits and psychiatric problems have been linked to underage drinking, as have some environmental issues. In addition, the tendency of adolescents and other underage drinkers to engage in risky behavior while drinking is very problematic. It is also true that a person's expectations about drinking are important; for example, adolescents who are at the greatest risk for drinking have positive expectations about the use of alcohol and its effects.

BINGE DRINKING is a problem among many adolescents; for example, an estimated 29 percent of 12th graders have engaged in binge drinking (defined as consuming five or more drinks on one occasion), as have 22 percent of 10th graders and 11 percent of eighth graders. Adolescents are more likely to engage in binge drinking than adults who drink.

All states have ZERO TOLERANCE LAWS, in which if an underage person who is driving a vehicle tests positive for a very minimal level of alcohol use (rather than the .08 percent standard for adults ages 21 and older), then it is a crime, although punishments for violating zero tolerance laws vary from state to state.

Some specific populations of adolescents have a higher risk for alcohol abuse or dependence than others, such as children of alcoholics and also detainees in juvenile facilities. For example, a study of adolescents who were screened as having alcohol problems compared to adolescents who did not have a problem with alcohol abuse and dependence was reported by Christine McCauley Ohannessian and Victor M. Hesselbrock in the *Journal of Adolescent Health* in 2008. The researchers found that children of alcoholics had higher levels of hostility, which predicted risk-taking and also significantly predicted substance abuse.

Some students are flagrant with their alcohol abuse, and they drink alcohol on school property, an act which is usually grounds for suspension. According to the youth surveillance summaries from the CDC, 7.5 percent of Hispanics, 3.4 percent of blacks, and 3.2 percent of whites drank alcohol on school property in 2007.

Early drinking is also associated with an increased risk for alcohol dependence in adulthood. According to the surveillance studies, 29.0 percent of Hispanics, 26.7 percent of blacks, and 21.5 percent of white high-school students drank alcohol for the first time before the age of 13 years. The risk for drinking alcohol was higher among males than females; for example, 24.2 percent of Hispanic high-school females drank alcohol before age 13, compared to 33.6 percent of male Hispanics. The rate for black females was 22.7 percent, compared to 30.7 percent for male high-school students. The rates for whites were 17.8 percent of females compared to 25.0 percent of male high-school students.

SMOKING is also associated with drinking, and some experts believe that cigarettes and alcohol enhance the effects of each other and increase the risk for nicotine dependence as well as alcohol dependence. According to the surveillance summaries, whites have the highest risk for smoking daily, and 14.9 percent of white female and 15.8 percent of white male high-school students were smokers in 2007. The rates were significantly lower for Hispanics: 7.1 percent for Hispanic females and 8.9 percent for Hispanic males. The rates for black high-school students were 5.0 percent for females and 7.3 percent for males.

Some studies have shown that the risk for teenage suicide is increased with alcohol abuse. According to researcher Michael Windle, suicide is the third leading cause of death among individuals ages 10–19 years, and teenage suicide is often associated with depression, impulsivity, and the use of ALCOHOL AND OTHER DRUGS. In addition, teenagers with peers who drink as well as those with low levels of family support are more likely to participate in binge drinking than others.

Underage Drinking Is Widespread
Data from the Monitoring the Future survey, an annual survey of drinking among students in

high school, shows that alcohol use is widespread among adolescents in the United States, and more than half (55 percent) of high school seniors and almost a fifth (18 percent) of eighth-graders in 2007 said that they had been drunk at least once in their lives. Of concern is that less than half (46 percent) of these adolescents perceived binge drinking as behavior that was greatly risky. The easy availability of alcohol for many teenagers is another factor in adolescent drinking, and 92 percent of the high school seniors who were surveyed said that it would be fairly easy or very easy for them to obtain alcohol if they wanted to drink.

Alcohol is commonly used by high-school students. According to the Centers for Disease Control and Prevention (CDC) in their Youth Risk Behavior Surveillance report for 2007, 75 percent of students nationwide have had at least one drink in their lifetime. Males and females were about equally likely to be current drinkers, in contrast to most other age groups, in which males are much more likely to consume alcohol than females. The prevalence was the highest among high-school seniors, or the majority (54.9 percent) of this population—85.2 percent among females and 80.2 percent among males. (The higher percentage for females is surprising, yet it is accurate.)

Some students are heavier drinkers than others; for example, according to the CDC, close to half (44.7 percent) of the adolescent subjects had had at least one alcoholic drink on at least one day in the past 30 days before the survey. The prevalence of current alcohol use was significantly higher among Hispanics (47.6 percent) and whites (47.3 percent) than among black students (34.5 percent). (See Table 1.)

According to the CDC, in the 30 days before the annual Youth Risk Behavior Surveillance, 29.1 percent of students nationwide said that they rode in a car driven by someone who had been drinking alcohol. The prevalence was the highest among Hispanic students (35.5 percent) compared to white (27.9 percent) or black (27.4 percent) students. In addition, 10.5 percent of the students said that they drove a car when they had been drinking alcohol one or more times in the 30 days before the survey. (See Table 2.)

TABLE 1
PERCENTAGE OF HIGH-SCHOOL STUDENTS WITH CURRENT ALCOHOL USE BY SEX, GRADE, RACE, AND ETHNICITY

Category	Female	Male	Total
Race/Ethnicity			
White	47.1	47.4	47.3
Black	34.9	34.1	34.5
Hispanic	47.5	47.7	47.6
Grade			
9	37.2	34.3	35.7
10	42.3	41.4	41.8
11	46.5	51.5	49.0
12	54.2	55.6	54.9
Total	44.6	44.7	44.7

Adapted from: Centers for Disease Control and Prevention. Youth Risk Behavior Surveillance—United States, 2007. *Morbidity and Mortality Weekly Report* 57, no. SS-4 (June 6, 2008), page 71.

In considering the state-by-state rates of high school students who rode in a car or another vehicle with a driver who had been drinking alcohol, the percentage was the highest in Texas, where more than a third of adolescents had committed this highly risky act (35.6 percent), and it was the lowest in Utah (14.8 percent). In addition, when considering adolescents who reported driving when they had been drinking, of the states that provided data, the rate was the highest in North Dakota (18.7 percent) and the lowest in Utah (4.7 percent). See Table 3 for further information.

Other risks for underage drinkers and drinkers in college, according to the Surgeon General's report, are as follows:

- about 1,700 college students ages 18–24 die every year from alcohol-related unintentional injuries, including car crashes
- about 600,000 college students are unintentionally injured while they are under the influence of alcohol
- about 700,000 college students are assaulted each year by other students who have been drinking
- about 100,000 students are victimized each year by alcohol-related sexual assaults or date rapes

TABLE 2
PERCENTAGE OF HIGH-SCHOOL STUDENTS WHO RODE IN A CAR OR OTHER VEHICLE DRIVEN
BY SOMEONE WHO HAD BEEN DRINKING ALCOHOL OR WHO DROVE A CAR OR OTHER VEHICLE
WHEN THEY HAD BEEN DRINKING ALCOHOL, BY SEX, RACE/ETHNICITY, AND GRADE IN SCHOOL, 2007

Category	Rode with a Driver Who Had Been Drinking Alcohol			Drove When Drinking Alcohol		
	Female	Male	Total	Female	Male	Total
Race/ethnicity						
White	28.0	27.8	27.9	9.3	13.9	11.6
Black	26.9	28.1	27.4	3.9	7.5	5.7
Hispanic	35.1	36.0	35.5	7.7	13.0	10.3
Grade						
9	27.6	27.6	27.6	4.1	6.8	5.5
10	30.4	27.1	28.7	7.3	10.0	8.7
11	26.8	31.4	29.2	9.1	13.7	11.5
12	30.5	32.5	31.5	13.1	23.6	18.3
Total	28.8	29.5	29.1	8.1	12.8	10.5

Source: Adapted from Centers for Disease Control and Prevention, "Youth Risk Behavior Surveillance—United States, 2007." *Morbidity and Mortality Weekly Report* 57, no. SS-4, June 6, 2008, page 41.

Risk Factors for Drinking

Some risk factors for alcohol abuse and dependence have been identified, such as childhood abuse, personality traits of the adolescent, and also parental issues, such as whether the child's parents abuse alcohol themselves. The presence of psychiatric problems also increases the risk for drinking during adolescence. There are also external environmental issues, such as viewing advertisements for alcohol and associating with peers who drink.

Personality Traits and Risks for Drinking According to the National Institute on Alcohol Abuse and Alcoholism, teenagers with certain personality traits or past circumstances are more at risk for alcohol consumption than others, including adolescents who have a strong sensation-seeking drive, as well as those with a past history of behavior problems and those who are experiencing family conflict or family alcohol problems. In addition, the NIAAA says that because adolescents are less prone to experiencing the negative after-effects of drinking, such as alcoholic hangovers, loss of physical coordination, or excessive sleepiness, they may enjoy the euphoric effects of drinking more than most adults.

Impulsiveness, aggression, and novelty-seeking are all traits that are directly related to the development of alcohol use disorders in adulthood. Behav-ioral undercontrol and a high level of rebelliousness are also tied to a risk for underage drinking.

Psychiatric Problems Increase the Risk for Underage Drinking According to *Alcohol Research & Health,* depression and anxiety in an adolescent are predictive for alcohol problems. In addition, psychiatric disorders such as CONDUCT DISORDER, oppositional defiant disorder, ATTENTION-DEFICIT/HYPERACTIVITY DISORDER, and borderline personality disorder are all linked to an increased risk for underage drinking. Some experts argue that disorders such as DEPRESSION do not precede drinking but instead they are are caused by heavy drinking. (See PSYCHIATRIC COMORBIDITIES.)

In a study by Thomas M. Kelly on psychiatric disorders in 63 adolescents compared to a matching community sample, published in *the Journal of Studies on Alcohol* in 2003, the subjects were evaluated for psychiatric disorders and compared to a community sample of non-ER patients. Kelly found a rate of alcohol use disorders (alcohol abuse or dependence) that was four times greater than among the sample of adolescents drawn from the community. He also found that the ER patients with alcohol disorders were drinking more to achieve an effect than their community peers, indicating a tolerance to alcohol.

TABLE 3
**PERCENTAGE OF HIGH-SCHOOL STUDENTS WHO RODE IN A CAR OR OTHER VEHICLE DRIVEN
BY SOMEONE WHO HAD BEEN DRINKING ALCOHOL OR WHO DROVE A CAR OR OTHER VEHICLE
WHEN THEY HAD BEEN DRINKING, SELECTED U.S. SITES, 2007**

State Surveys	Rode with a Driver Who Had Been Drinking Alcohol			Drove When Drinking Alcohol		
	Female	Male	Total	Female	Male	Total
Alaska	25.4	21.5	23.5	7.8	11.3	9.7
Arizona	29.5	32.7	31.2	9.7	14.8	12.3
Arkansas	30.0	27.2	28.5	8.5	13.8	11.1
Connecticut	27.4	27.0	27.3	8.4	11.8	10.2
Delaware	28.6	27.6	28.4	9.2	11.5	10.4
Florida	30.1	26.4	28.2	8.8	11.2	10.0
Georgia	23.0	24.7	23.9	7.5	10.6	9.1
Hawaii	33.7	34.1	33.9	7.9	8.1	8.0
Idaho	32.1	27.8	30.0	12.1	15.2	13.8
Illinois	31.4	25.9	28.6	9.9	12.8	11.3
Indiana	24.2	27.8	26.4	8.6	15.0	11.9
Iowa	28.1	25.1	26.5	11.3	13.9	12.6
Kansas	32.7	28.7	30.7	13.7	16.9	15.3
Kentucky	19.7	20.5	20.3	6.4	10.0	8.4
Maine	21.6	21.9	21.8	6.5	11.1	8.8
Maryland	31.0	26.7	28.9	7.2	9.5	8.5
Massachusetts	26.1	25.4	25.8	9.4	11.7	10.6
Michigan	28.3	26.7	27.6	8.3	9.8	9.1
Mississippi	28.9	31.9	30.5	8.1	15.3	11.8
Missouri	29.7	25.5	27.8	12.1	13.3	12.8
Montana	34.5	31.5	32.9	14.9	17.0	16.0
Nevada	24.3	22.4	23.4	8.7	8.6	8.7
New Hampshire	26.1	24.7	25.4	10.0	13.7	11.9
New Mexico	33.0	28.9	31.2	11.5	13.4	12.5
North Carolina	23.6	25.8	24.7	7.2	11.1	9.2
North Dakota	34.1	29.9	31.5	18.4	18.9	18.7
Ohio	21.7	23.6	22.8	7.9	10.9	9.5
Oklahoma	26.0	27.5	26.8	10.0	16.5	13.3
Rhode Island	26.4	28.5	27.5	7.4	12.3	9.8
South Carolina	25.6	26.7	26.3	8.3	11.2	9.9
South Dakota	24.3	24.0	24.3	13.2	12.0	13.0
Tennessee	24.8	23.4	24.2	6.4	10.6	8.5
Texas	35.6	35.5	35.6	10.8	18.6	14.7
Utah	14.1	14.8	14.8	3.5	5.8	4.7
Vermont	22.5	24.6	23.6	6.5	11.6	9.2
West Virginia	22.0	25.3	23.8	6.8	12.8	10.0
Wisconsin	33.7	29.4	31.5	11.9	16.6	14.3
Wyoming	31.1	27.5	29.4	14.1	16.8	15.6
Median	27.7	26.7	27.4	8.6	12.3	10.4

Source: Adapted from Centers for Disease Control and Prevention, "Youth Risk Behavior Surveillance—United States, 2007." *Morbidity and Mortality Weekly Report* 57, no. SS-4, June 6, 2008, page 42.

In addition, Kelly found a markedly increased rate of major depression (90 percent) among the ER patients, in comparison to the much lower rate of 1.6 percent among the community sample. Dysthymia (a low level of depression) was present among 3.2 percent of the ER sample, compared to none of the community sample subjects. He also found that 7.9 percent of the ER adolescents reported making persistent efforts to cut down on drinking, compared to 1.6 percent of the community sample. In addition, the rate of drinking more or over longer periods than was intended was 38.1 percent among the ER adolescents compared to 14.3 percent of the community sample.

Kelly also found a greater rate for some combined disorders; for example, 17.5 percent of the ER adolescents had a mood disorder and an alcohol abuse disorder, compared to 3.2 percent of the subjects in the community sample.

Advertising for Alcohol Adolescents are also affected by factors within their environment, such as product advertising of alcoholic beverages. Many ads for beer are televised during weekend sporting events, which are popular among young people. In addition, when they use alcohol, beer is often the form of alcohol underage drinkers most favor. Besides ads on television, underage drinkers view advertising on billboards and on the Internet. According to the Center of Alcohol Marketing and Youth, young people view 49 percent more beer ads than adults and 20 percent more ads for distilled spirits.

According to *Alcohol Research & Health* in their 2004/2005 article on environmental and contextual considerations, "A study of third, sixth, and ninth graders showed that the third-grade children who found alcohol ads desirable also were more likely to see positive benefits from drinking and to desire products with alcohol logos. Older children in the study who found the ads and logo products appealing were more likely to already be engaged in drinking behaviors."

Family Issues Children who have been abused have an increased risk for alcohol abuse, and women who were abused as children are up to twice as likely to abuse alcohol as are adults who were not abused in childhood.

Parental drinking (or the lack of drinking) also affects the drinking habits of youths ages 12–20;

for example, according to SAMHSA, rates of binge drinking among underage individuals were 17.6 percent among those whose mother was a past-year drinker versus a much lower rate of 9.3 percent for those whose mother was not a past-year drinker. In addition, the rate of binge drinking was 16.5 percent among those whose father was a past-year drinker versus 10.2 percent for those whose father was not a past-year drinker. Rates of binge drinking among underage individuals was also higher among those who lived with parents who were themselves binge drinkers, or 21.3 percent of underage youths who lived with a binge-drinking mother and 19.5 percent who lived with a binge-drinking father.

Children of alcoholics have an increased risk for alcohol abuse and dependence as adults, and they are between four and 19 times more likely to become alcoholics in adulthood (or earlier). According to the authors of an article on the scope of the problem in *Alcohol Research & Health,* "Some of the elevated risk is attributable to exposure and socialization effects found in alcoholic households, some to genetically transmitted differences in response to alcohol that make the drinking more pleasurable and/or less aversive, and some is attributed to elevated transmission of risky temperamental and behavioral traits that lead COAs [children of alcoholics], more than other youth, into increased contact with earlier-drinking and heavier-drinking peers."

Protective Factors against Drinking

Although many parents do not realize it, their own attitudes and discipline against drinking have a profound effect on whether teenagers drink. In addition, the relationships that children have with positive peers and in school can also veer them away from drinking. Awareness is an important first step in preventing drinking among adolescents. Parents are often completely unaware that their children drink. According to the Surgeon General's 2007 report, parents and other adults often have no idea their teenagers are drinking. According to the report, "They [parents] underestimate how early drinking begins, the amount of alcohol adolescents consume, the many risks that alcohol consumption creates for adolescents, and the nature and extent of the consequences to both drinkers and nondrinkers. Too often, parents are inclined to believe, 'Not my child.'"

Teaching Kids to Say "No" to Alcohol Peer pressure is a major problem among many adolescents and young adults, as well as underage college students. As a result, the Substance Abuse and Mental Health Services Administration advises teaching adolescents "comebacks" to pressures to drink, such as "No thanks," followed by "I don't like it, do you have a soda?" Or "Alcohol's not my thing." More aggressive comebacks include "Why do you keep pressuring me when I said NO!" and "Back off!"

Risky Behavior and Adolescents

Teenagers have an increased risk for engaging in risky behaviors that are related to alcohol use, often because of their underlying "magical" belief (and mistaken notion) that nothing bad could ever happen to them. When adolescents become intoxicated, they incur many risks because alcohol lowers their inhibitions and they lack maturity. For example, they may act in ways that they would not normally act if they were sober, such as having sex without contraception, attacking others physically and sexually, vandalizing property, and driving recklessly. In addition, females who consume alcohol are more prone to being victimized by physical and sexual assaults than girls who do not drink. (See VIOLENCE.)

According to the Substance Abuse and Mental Health Services Administration, Office of Applied Studies, of the 5,000 people under age 21 who die each year as a result of underage drinking, 1,900 die from fatal car crashes. In addition, the early use of alcohol is linked to an increased risk of the development of alcohol use disorder as well as the risk for involvement in violent behaviors, suicide attempts, and other problems. For example, based on data from 2002 to 2006, there are 3.5 million individuals ages 12 to 20 who meet the diagnostic criteria for alcohol abuse or alcohol dependence, or nearly 10 percent (9.4 percent) of all individuals in that age group.

Individuals who engage in underage binge drinking are more likely than those who do not binge drink to exhibit risky sexual behavior (such as failing to use contraceptives) and to become assaulted physically and/or sexually. Underage binge drinkers are also more likely than others to have academic and legal problems.

Serious consequences to underage drinking include the following:

- increased risk for suicide and homicide
- death from alcohol poisoning
- academic problems
- social problems
- unwanted and unintended sexual behavior
- memory problems
- alterations in the development of the brain, which can have lifelong consequences

Juvenile Detainees and Substance Abuse

Detainees in juvenile facilities are one problematic population at high risk for alcohol and drug abuse. In a study by Linda A. Teplin and colleagues, reported in the *Archives of General Psychiatry,* the researchers analyzed psychiatric disorders among 1,829 juvenile detainees ages 10–18 years old. They found that an estimated half of both the males and females had a substance use disorder, and about 60 percent of the males and greater than two-thirds of the females met the criteria for one or more psychiatric disorders. About 26 percent of the males and 27 percent of the females met the criteria for an alcohol use disorder (alcohol abuse or dependence), and 45 percent of the males and 41 percent of the females met the criteria for a marijuana use disorder.

ANXIETY DISORDERS were also common in this group. About 21 percent of the males and 31 percent of the females reportedly had an anxiety disorder. Depression was also a common problem, particularly among females (about 22 percent) compared to 13 percent for males. Interestingly, attention-deficit/hyperactivity disorder was more commonly diagnosed among the female adolescents (21 percent) than the males (17 percent).

In considering race alone for males, about 63 percent of the non-Hispanic white detainees had an alcohol use disorder, followed by 55 percent of the Hispanic males and 49 percent of the

African-American males. The females followed a similar pattern (although their rates of abuse were lower), with 39 percent of non-Hispanic whites with an alcohol use disorder, 34 percent of the Hispanic adolescents with an alcohol disorder, and 21 percent of the African-American females diagnosed with this problem.

The researchers concluded that this population is generally ill-served, and said, "The juvenile justice system is not equipped to provide adequate mental health services for the large numbers of detainees with psychiatric disorders. Although the mental health needs of youth in the juvenile justice system have been given much attention recently, there are still few empirical studies of the effectiveness of treatment and outcomes. This omission is critical."

Underage Military Members

Underage drinking is also a problem among military members; according to a 2005 Department of Defense Survey of Related Health Behaviors among Military Personnel, about two-thirds (62.3 percent) of underage military members drink at least twice per year. In addition, 21 percent of active-duty military personnel ages 20 and younger are heavy alcohol abusers or binge drinkers. Some experts believe that drinking is part of the military culture, especially in the Marine Corps and the Army.

Having experienced combat conditions can affect whether an underage military member consumes alcohol. Some studies have shown that National Guard and Reservists who had returned from deployment to Iraq had a high rate of binge drinking and alcohol dependence. Heavy drinking may be related to the presence of POSTTRAUMATIC STRESS DISORDER (PTSD) in some returned veterans. (See MILITARY VETERANS/COMBAT AND ACTIVE-DUTY MILITARY.)

Early Drinking and Alcohol Dependence

Some studies have shown that the younger an individual was when he or she first started consuming alcohol (such as in the early teens or even before then), the more likely they are as adults to have a problem with alcohol abuse or dependence. In fact, the highest prevalence of alcoholism in the entire United States population is among those ages 18 to 20 years old, according to the report by the Surgeon General. According to this report, "Underage drinking is deeply embedded in the American culture, is often viewed as a rite of passage, is frequently facilitated by adults, and has proved stubbornly resistant to change."

Some studies have shown that 10 percent of children ages 9–10 years have already started drinking, and others have shown that a third of adolescents began drinking before their 13th birthday. The peak years of initiation to alcohol are in the seventh and eighth grades.

A study by Grant and Dawson showed that those individuals who began their drinking before age 14 were four times as likely to become dependent on alcohol in adulthood when compared to individuals who started drinking after age 20. Other researchers have found an even greater gap; according to Hingson and colleagues, of those who began drinking before the age of 14 years, 47 percent became dependent on alcohol at some point in their lives, compared to 9 percent of those who delayed drinking until they were 21 years old became dependent on alcohol. According to the CDC, nearly a quarter of all high-school students (23.8 percent) took their first drink of alcohol before they were just 13 years old.

A Call to Action on Underage Drinking

The Surgeon General's Call to Action on Underage Drinking included six primary goals, as follows:

1. promoting healthy adolescent development and preventing as well as reducing underage drinking
2. involving parents, schools, government, communities, and youth in a national effort to prevent and reduce underage drinking and its consequences
3. advancing the understanding of underage drinking in general as well as gender, ethnic, and cultural differences
4. performing research on underage drinking and its consequences
5. increasing public health monitoring of underage drinking and policies regarding underage drinking
6. promoting consistency in policy throughout all levels of federal, state, and local governments

More information on the Call to Action can be found at the Surgeon General's Web site: http://www.surgeongeneral.gov.

State Laws and Policies on Underage Drinking

States have taken different approaches to underage drinking. Some states punish underage drinkers directly by prohibiting the use of false identifications to purchase alcohol. Zero tolerance laws cause underage drinkers to lose their driving privileges for minute quantities of alcohol in the bloodstream, in contrast to a .08 BLOOD ALCOHOL CONCENTRATION used for adults in all states to define DRIVING UNDER THE INFLUENCE/DRIVING WHILE INTOXICATED.

Other laws target those who sell alcohol; for example, states may have minimum ages for those who sell alcohol in retail establishments as well as for servers and bartenders in restaurants and bars. Some states have criminal penalties for those who host underage drinking parties.

Some states allow family members to give alcohol to their children under age 21, and according to the Alcohol Policy Information System of the NIAAA, five states had such a policy in 2008, including Montana, Ohio, Texas, Washington, and Wisconsin. Other states do not address the issue, nor do they specifically ban family members from providing alcohol to children in their home. In some states, the location of the drinking, such as the home, is considered as an exception. In other states, there are no exceptions to the drinking laws for minors, including in Alabama, Arizona, the District of Columbia, Idaho, Indiana, Kansas, Michigan, North Carolina, North Dakota, Pennsylvania, South Carolina, South Dakota, Tennessee, Utah, Vermont, and West Virginia.

Expert Recommendations for Combating Underage Drinking

According to Bonnie and O'Connell, editors of *Reducing Underage Drinking: A Collective Responsibility,* several actions should be taken to combat underage drinking. First, they recommend a national media effort on underage drinking, financed by the federal government. Next, they recommend that any parts of the alcohol industry that profit from underage drinking should join with private and public partners to create a nonprofit organization with the goal of preventing and reducing underage drinking.

The editors also recommend that alcohol companies, advertisers, and the commercial media should cease to use any promotional activities that have specific appeal to underage drinkers and that they should also be careful to avoid the exposure of youth to alcohol ADVERTISING and promotion.

Other recommendations include the development of an alcohol rating for movies, much like the *G* or *PG* rating, except in relation to films that depict underage drinking favorably or that have unsuitable alcohol content for youths. They also recommend that the music industry should not market recordings that glamorize the use of alcohol among young people.

Treatment Recommendations for Underage Alcohol-dependent People

Experts report that alcohol dependence in adolescents is not usually as severe as among adults, and hence detoxification is a more rapid process. Some organizations such as the Betty Ford Center have five-day programs for underage drinkers and their families. Once the program is completed, they may participate in outpatient sessions for 13 weeks.

In the past, treatment centered around finding out what was wrong with parents and how they had "made" the child into an alcoholic. Although it is true that parents who are alcoholic are more prone to having children with alcohol dependence, this is not a reasoned choice on the part of the parents. Treatment centers have moved away from this approach and are more actively centered on the present and therapies that work, such as cognitive-behavioral therapy (CBT), in which the patient learns to challenge his or her irrational ideas. One problem with treating adolescents, however, is that adolescents are noted for leaving alcohol treatment against the advice of physicians.

See also AGE AND ALCOHOL; EXCESSIVE DRINKING AND HEALTH CONSEQUENCES; TREATMENT.

Alcohol Policy Information System. "Exceptions as to Minimum Age of 21 for Consumption of Alcohol as of January 1, 2008." National Institute of Alcohol Abuse and Alcoholism. Available online. URL: http://www.alcoholpolicy.niaaa.nih.gov/index.asp?Type=BAS_APIS&SEC={0D5C719E-FCE8-4E15-A367-4145C655505F}&DE={E6F19624-0ADC-437F-917D-5E7CBC9F58B9}. Accessed March 12, 2009.

Bonnie, Richard J., and Mary Ellen O'Connell, eds. *Reducing Underage Drinking: A Collective Responsibility.* Washington, D.C.: National Academy of Sciences, 2004.

Centers for Disease Control and Prevention. "Youth Risk Behavior Surveillance—United States, 2007." *Morbidity and Mortality Weekly Report* 57, no. SS-4 (June 6, 2008).

Clark, Duncan B., et al. "Physical and Sexual Abuse, Depression and Alcohol Use Disorders in Adolescents: Onsets and Outcomes." *Drug and Alcohol Dependence* 69, no. 1 (2003): 51–60.

Deas, Deborah, M.D., and Suzanne Thomas. "Comorbid Psychiatric Factors Contributing to Adolescent Alcohol and Other Drug Use." *Alcohol Research & Health* 26, no. 2 (2002): 116–121.

"Environmental and Contextual Considerations." *Alcohol Research & Health* 28, no. 3 (2004/2005): 155–162.

Garland, Ann, et al. "Diagnostic Profile Associated with Use of Mental Health and Substance Abuse Services Among High-Risk Youths." *Psychiatric Services* 54, no. 4 (April 2003): 562–564.

Grant, B. F., and D. A. Dawson. "Age at Onset of Alcohol Use and Its Association with DSM-IV Alcohol Abuse and Dependence: Results from the National Longitudinal Alcohol Epidemiologic Survey." *Journal of Substance Abuse* 9 (1997): 103–110.

Johnston, Lloyd D., Patrick M. O'Malley, Jerald G. Bachman, and John E. Schulenberg. *Monitoring the Future: National Results on Adolescent Drug Use. Overview of Key Findings, 2007.* Bethesda, Md.: National Institute on Drug Abuse, 2008.

Kelly, Thomas M. "Psychiatric Disorders among Older Adolescents Treated in Emergency Departments on Weekends: A Comparison with a Matched Community Sample." *Journal of Studies on Alcohol* 64, no. 5 (2003): 616–622.

Newes-Adeyi, Gabriella, Chiung M. Chen, Gerald D. Williams, and Vivian B. Faden. *Surveillance Report #74: Trends in Underage Drinking in the United States, 1991–2003.* Bethesda, Md.: National Institute on Alcohol Abuse and Alcoholism, October 2005.

Office of Applied Studies. "Quantity and Frequency of Alcohol Use among Underage Drinkers." NSDUH Report. Substance Abuse and Mental Health Services Administration, March 31, 2008.

Ohannessian, Christine McCauley, and Victor M. Hesselbrock. "Paternal Alcoholism and Youth Substance Abuse: The Indirect Effects of Negative Affect, Conduct Problems, and Risk Taking." *Journal of Adolescent Health* 42, no. 2 (2008): 198–200.

Pemberton, Michael R., James D. Colliver, Tania M. Robbins, and Joseph C. Gfroerer. *Underage Alcohol Use; Findings from the 2002–2006 National Surveys on Drug Use and Health.* Rockville, Md.: Substance Abuse and Mental Health Services Administration, Office of Applied Studies, June 2008.

"Psychosocial Processes and Mechanisms of Risk and Protection." *Alcohol Research & Health* 28, no. 2 (2004/2005): 143–154.

"The Scope of the Problem." *Alcohol Research & Health* 28, no. 2 (2004/2005): 111–120.

Teplin, Linda A., et al. "Psychiatric Disorders in Youth in Juvenile Detention." *Archives of General Psychiatry* 59, no. 12 (2002): 1,133–1,143.

U.S. Department of Health and Human Services. *The Surgeon General's Call to Action to Prevent and Reduce Underage Drinking.* U.S. Department of Health and Human Services, Office of the Surgeon General, 2007.

Windle, M. "Suicidal Behaviors and Alcohol Use Among Adolescents: A Developmental Psychopathology Perspective. *Alcohol Clinical and Experimental Research* 28, no. 5 Suppl. (2004): 29S–37S.

veterans, military See MILITARY VETERANS/COMBAT AND ACTIVE-DUTY MILITARY.

victims of assault See AGGRESSIVE BEHAVIOR AND ALCOHOL; ALCOHOL AND MEN; ALCOHOL AND WOMEN; EXCESSIVE DRINKING AND NEGATIVE SOCIAL CONSEQUENCES; VIOLENCE.

violence Behavior that is usually meant to and/or that does cause physical harm to others, ranging from causing injury up to and including homicide. The broad majority of violent acts are committed by males, although both males and females may be victimized by violent people. Individuals who are intoxicated with alcohol have an increased risk for exhibiting physical violence toward others, and intoxicated individuals are more likely to be perpetrators of domestic violence and CHILD ABUSE than those who are not intoxicated.

In addition, those who begin their drinking early in life are more likely than others to become violent in adolescence after drinking. A study by Ralph Hingson, Timothy Heeren, and Ronda Zakocs in *Pediatrics* in 2001 reported that individuals who started drinking before age 17 were signifi-

cantly more likely to become involved in physical fights after drinking than those who started drinking at age 21 or older. Early drinkers were three times more likely to have been in a fight in the past year. This risk for the commission of physical violence continued beyond adolescence and into adulthood.

A study by Raul Caetano, M.D., and colleagues on intimate partner violence and alcohol was published in *Alcohol Research & Health* in 2001. The researchers found that partner violence among men who had been drinking was the highest among black men (41 percent), followed by whites (29 percent) and Hispanics (also 29 percent). Alcohol abstainers had a much lower rate of partner violence, or 18 percent among black males, 17 percent among Hispanic males, and 6 percent among white males. However, when the men drank five or more drinks on occasion at least once per week, the rates were significantly higher, or 40 percent for black men, 24 percent for Hispanic men, and 19 percent for white men. (See Table 1.)

Drinkers Who Become Victims of Violence

Individuals who are intoxicated have an increased risk of becoming a victim of physical violence that is perpetrated by others. (See ALCOHOL AND

TABLE 1
PERCENT OF MALE TO FEMALE PERPETRATORS OF PARTNER VIOLENCE AMONG ABSTAINERS AND SELECTED DRINKERS BY ETHNICITY

Drinking Level of Partner-Violence Perpetrator	White (n = 555)	Black (n = 358)	Hispanic (n = 527)
Abstainer	6	18	17
Drinks five or more drinks on occasion at least once per week	19	40	24

Source: Adapted from Caetano, Raul, M.D., et al. "Alcohol-Related Intimate Partner Violence among White, Black, and Hispanic Couples in the United States." *Alcohol Research & Health* 25, no. 1 (2001), page 62.

MEN; ALCOHOL AND WOMEN.) In a study by Janice Du Mont et al., reported in 2009 in the *Canadian Medical Association Journal*, the researchers found that of 882 victims of drug-facilitated sexual assaults, nearly 90 percent had consumed alcohol immediately prior to the assault. Women who are intoxicated with alcohol are less likely to be able to resist the sexual advances of others, and an excessive amount of alcohol is the equivalent of a self-administered "date rape drug." Some of the assaulted women had also consumed other substances within the 72 hours before the assault, such as street drugs or prescription drugs.

National Studies on Violent Deaths Associated with Alcohol

The Centers for Disease Control and Prevention studied issues related to violent deaths in 16 states in 2005, reporting on their findings in 2008 in the *Morbidity and Mortality Weekly Report*. The data came from the National Violent Death Reporting System (NVDRS), and the states covered included Alaska, Colorado, Georgia, Kentucky, Maryland, Massachusetts, New Jersey, New Mexico, North Carolina, Oklahoma, Oregon, Rhode Island, South Carolina, Utah, Virginia, and Wisconsin.

A violent death was defined as a death resulting from the intentional use of physical force or power against oneself (thus, SUICIDE was considered as a violent death by this definition), another person or a group or community, or a death caused by the unintentional use of a firearm. Deaths caused unintentionally by a firearm included deaths in which the evidence indicated the shooting was not directed at the person who was killed, such as a person who died from a self-inflicted wound while handling a firearm or someone who died from celebratory firing not intended to harm anyone.

One of the factors that was considered was whether there was alcohol present in the person who died, and of those deceased people who were tested for alcohol and who tested positive, in the majority of cases (59.1 percent), the person who died had a BLOOD ALCOHOL CONCENTRATION (BAC) that exceeded 0.08 percent, the legal limit in all states for driving a vehicle. In the case of suicidal decedents whose BAC was tested, the BAC exceeded 0.08 percent in 62.1 percent of the cases.

Of those who were murdered, tests for alcohol were performed on 84.3 percent of these homicide victims, and the majority (55.6 percent) of those who tested positive for alcohol had a blood alcohol level exceeding 0.08. When the case was an intimate partner homicide, in which the person who was killed was the spouse and/or sexual partner of the perpetrator, when decedent's BAC was tested, 61 percent had a BAC of 0.08 percent or greater. In a small number of cases (seven), a homicide was committed, and then the perpetrator killed himself or herself. In these cases, nearly half (47.7 percent) had a BAC of 0.08 percent or greater.

The researchers also looked at the rates for suicides. In the cases of former or current military personnel who suicided, the researchers found that in nearly two-thirds of the cases (63.4 percent), the deceased person had a BAC of 0.08 percent or greater. In addition, 17.2 percent had been diagnosed with an alcohol abuse problem, while an additional 7.7 percent had been diagnosed with another substance abuse problem.

In another study of the link between violence and mental disorder, the researchers looked at 34,653 subjects from the National Epidemiologic Survey on Alcohol and Related Conditions (NESARC). They were comparing the link between severe mental illness (SCHIZOPHRENIA, BIPOLAR DISORDER, and major DEPRESSION) and repeated acts of violence and the predictability of repeat acts. They found that severe mental illness alone was predictive of acts of violence only when the individual also had substance abuse and/or dependence. Other factors that played a role were environmental stressors and a past history of violence.

The researchers concluded that "(1) severe mental illness is not a robust predictor for future violence; (2) people with co-occurring severe mental illness and substance abuse/dependence have a higher incidence of violence than people with substance abuse/dependence alone; (3) people with severe mental illness report histories and environment stressors associated with elevated violence risk; and (4) severe mental illness is not an independent contributor to explaining variance in multivariate analyses of different types of violence."

Clearly, alcohol plays a major role in a variety of violent deaths and suicides.

See also AGE AND ALCOHOL; AGGRESSIVE BEHAVIOR AND ALCOHOL; ALCOHOLIC PSYCHOSIS; ANTISOCIAL PERSONALITY DISORDER/ANTISOCIAL BEHAVIOR; CONDUCT DISORDER; EXCESSIVE DRINKING AND NEGATIVE SOCIAL CONSEQUENCES; IMPULSE CONTROL DISORDERS; PSYCHIATRIC COMORBIDITIES.

Caetano, Raul, M.D., et al. "Alcohol-Related Intimate Partner Violence among White, Black, and Hispanic Couples in the United States." *Alcohol Research & Health* 25, no. 1 (2001): 58–65.

Du Mont, Janice, et al. "Factors Associated with Suspected Drug-Facilitated Sexual Assault." *Canadian Medical Association Journal* 180, no. 5 (2009): 513–519.

Elbogen, Eric B., and Sally C. Johnson, M.D. "The Intricate Link Between Violence and Mental Disorder: Results from the National Epidemiologic Survey on Alcohol and Related Conditions." *Archives of General Psychiatry* 66, no. 2 (2009): 152–161.

Haggård-Grann, Ulrika, John Hallqvist, Niklas Långström, and Jette Möller. "The Role of Alcohol and Drugs in Triggering Criminal Violence: A Case-Crossover Study." *Addiction* 101, no. 1 (2006): 100–108.

Hingson, Ralph, Timothy Heeren, and Ronda Zakocs. "Age of Drinking Onset and Involvement in Physical Fights After Drinking." *Pediatrics* 108, no. 4 (2001): 872–877.

Karch, Debra L., et al. "Surveillance for Violent Deaths—National Violent Death Reporting System, 16 States, 2005." *Morbidity and Mortality Weekly Report* 57, no. SS-3 (April 11, 2008).

vitamin deficiencies See EXCESSIVE DRINKING AND HEALTH CONSEQUENCES; WERNICKE-KORSAKOFF SYNDROME.

Wernicke-Korsakoff syndrome A severe brain disorder that is found among individuals who have experienced years of chronic ALCOHOLISM, and which is caused by an extreme deficiency of thiamine. Wernicke's encephalopathy lasts for a short period, and if it is untreated (or treatment fails), it is then followed by Korsakoff's psychosis. The two conditions together are referred to as Wernicke-Korsakoff syndrome. Wernicke's encephalopathy was first discovered by German psychiatrist Karl Wernicke in 1881, who observed that three of his patients had similar symptoms, including eye movement disorders, mental confusion, and poor motor coordination. Two of the patients had severe alcoholism, and the third had swallowed sulfuric acid.

Russian psychiatrist S. Korsakoff noted the symptom of anteretrograde amnesia in some severely alcoholic patients and documented it in a series of articles published from 1887–91. Anteretrograde amnesia means that the person cannot remember things which have just happened, although he or she has a remembrance of past experiences. Korsakoff named this syndrome "psychosis polyneuritica." In 1897, Murawieff suggested that a single cause was responsible for both syndromes.

Today, Wernicke's encephalopathy is considered the "acute" stage of the disease and Korsakoff psychosis (also known as Korsakoff's amnesic syndrome) is the chronic condition. However, as mentioned, if treated in time, patients with Wernicke's encephalopathy will not progress to Korsakoff psychosis.

Some doctors have a problem with the linkage of the two disorders. In an article published in *Alcohol & Alcoholism* in 2006, Allan D. Thomson and E. Jane Marshall say that the failure to diagnose and treat Wernicke's encephalopathy causes death in 20 percent of patients and leaves 75 percent of them with permanent brain damage. They also noted that patients who develop Wernicke's encephalopathy from a cause other than alcoholism rarely develop Korsakoff's psychosis and stated, "This may be because non-alcoholic patients may present at an earlier stage of WE [Wernicke's encephalopathy], may have more obvious symptoms, and may engender a more active treatment response."

With Wernicke's encephalopathy, heavy drinking can damage the mucosal layer of the intestines, causing thiamine absorption to be reduced by up to 90 percent. Chronic diarrhea and frequent vomiting can also impair thiamine absorption, as can LIVER DISEASE. Individuals with Wernicke's encephalopathy can develop a deficiency of thiamine over months. It may also occur during withdrawal from alcohol or an occurrence of DELIRIUM TREMENS. There may also be a genetic predisposition among some individuals to develop Wernicke's encephalopathy, which is then triggered by alcoholism. In individuals who carry the gene but do not drink or drink in moderation, the condition is not triggered.

Other disorders may trigger Wernicke-Korsakoff syndrome, such as eating disorders, prolonged vomiting (as with hyperemesis gravidarum—constant severe vomiting during pregnancy), and congestive heart failure. Long-term dialysis may also trigger the disorder.

Patients most at risk for Wernicke-Korsakoff syndrome appear to be those who are homeless alcoholics, elderly alcoholics living in isolation, and inpatients in some psychiatric institutions where the residents have access to alcohol and nutrition is poor. The age of onset ranges from age 30 to age

70. (With older people, there is a risk that they may be misdiagnosed with a form of dementia.)

Symptoms and Diagnostic Path

The key symptoms of Wernicke's encephalopathy are difficulty with muscle coordination, a paralysis of the eye muscles that control eye movements, and mental confusion. Some patients do not experience all three symptoms; however, the syndrome may be present even if only one symptom is exhibited. Sometimes the diagnosis is never made, because the patient does not exhibit "classic" symptoms or signs.

Other symptoms and signs (which are also symptoms of thiamine deficiency) may include the following:

- appetite loss
- nausea and vomiting
- fatigue
- insomnia
- anxiety
- double vision
- eye movement abnormalities
- drooping eyelids
- hallucinations
- unintentional weight loss

Many foods in the United States are thiamine-enriched, such as breads and cereals, but alcoholics may be thiamine deficient because of their extremely poor diet, as well as their poor absorption of thiamine.

Symptoms of Korsakoff's psychosis are difficulty with coordination and walking, memory problems, and learning difficulties. Individuals with Korsakoff's psychosis have difficulty with retaining any new information (anteretrograde amnesia). For example, the patient may be told something and then an hour later, have no memory of anything said in the conversation.

The condition is diagnosed by the patient's signs and symptoms as well as by laboratory tests; for example, blood thiamine levels are low, while blood or urine alcohol levels are high and liver enzymes may be high. A magnetic resonance imaging (MRI) scan will rarely show the brain damage which has occurred. Thiamine administration may improve symptoms of confusion, muscle coordination, and problems with the eyes in patients with Wernicke's encephalopathy; however, if the patient has advanced to Korsakoff's psychosis, thiamine will not help the loss of memory and intelligence.

Treatment Options and Outlook

Hospitalization of the patient is necessary. According to Thomson and Marshall, very high doses of thiamine are needed to treat Wernicke's encephalopathy (which has not advanced to Korsakoff psychosis), up to 1 gram in 24 hours. If the patient is in the more advanced stages of the syndrome, then the family is usually offered support and advice. About 25 percent of patients who have advanced to Korsakoff psychosis will require the care that is provided in an institution, such as a nursing home.

Thomson and Marshall say that patients at risk for Wernicke's encephalopathy should be treated *before* the condition develops. According to the authors, "The clear message is that patients (or individuals) at risk must be treated before they become thiamine deficient, in order to prevent the occurrence of this pernicious neurotoxicity. This is another reason why heavy drinkers are at increased risk: they are 'primed' for injury to occur as soon as brain thiamine reaches a critically low level!" Thomson and Marshall also state that preliminary trials indicate that treatment with mematine has proven effective in patients with Wernicke's encephalopathy.

Note that if an alcoholic patient also needs insulin, it is important for the doctor to supplement patients with thiamine *first* before giving an infusion of insulin, because if insulin is given first, this may precipitate Wernicke's encephalopathy in some patients who do not already have the disorder.

Risk Factors and Preventive Measures

The primary risk factor for Wernicke-Korsakoff syndrome is heavy chronic drinking, and the primary preventive measure is to avoid heavy chronic drinking. If the patient continues to drink, the disorder will kill him or her (if the patient does not die first from the many other risks that alcoholism presents).

See also ALCOHOLIC PSYCHOSIS; EXCESSIVE DRINKING AND HEALTH CONSEQUENCES.

National Institute on Alcohol Abuse and Alcoholism. "Alcohol's Damaging Effects on the Brain." *Alcohol Alert* 63 (October 2004): 1–7.

Thomson, Allan D., and E. Jane Marshall. "The Natural History and Pathophysiology of Wernicke's Encephalopathy and Korsakoff's Psychosis." *Alcohol & Alcoholism* 41, no. 2 (2006): 151–158.

Xiong, Glen L., M.D., et al. "Wernicke-Korsakoff Syndrome." Updated May 29, 2008. eMedicine Psychiatry. Available to subscribers online. URL: http://emedicine. medscape.com/article/288379-overview. Accessed March 21, 2009.

women   See ALCOHOL AND WOMEN.

Z

zero tolerance laws State laws that penalize individuals who are younger than age 21 and who consume small amounts (usually 0.2 percent or greater) or even *any* amount of alcohol while driving. The federal National Highway Systems Designation Act of 1995 required all states to pass zero tolerance laws against minors who were drinking and driving or lose federal highway funds by 1999. Predictably, by 1999, all states had passed such laws. Penalties for violating these zero tolerance laws vary from state to state and may range from fines and/or community service to the loss of a driver's license.

A study by R. B. Voas and colleagues, published in *Accident Analysis and Prevention* in 2003, found that zero tolerance laws reduced the percentage of underage drivers who were killed in fatal car crashes by nearly 25 percent. More recent research by James C. Fell and colleagues, published in *Alcoholism: Clinical and Experimental Research* in 2009, has estimated that the zero tolerance law combined with laws against the purchase and possession of alcohol by those under age 21 have saved 732 lives nationwide per year.

In another more recent study, Lan Liang and Jidong Huang analyzed the effect of zero tolerance laws on college students drinking away from home and reported their findings in *Health Economics* in 2008. Their subjects were drawn from the College Alcohol Survey. The researchers found that the zero tolerance laws *did* effectively decrease drinking and driving among college students. They also found that zero tolerance laws had the effect of decreasing drinking away from home by about 7 percent.

In addition, Liang and Huang pointed out that frequent drinking away from home is often associated with the commission of aggressive acts and with VIOLENCE among younger people. Less driving means fewer opportunities for drinkers to get into trouble away from home. The authors said, "Although the primary objective of the zero tolerance laws is to deter drinking and driving, the social benefit of the policy may be even larger if it also reduces the prevalence and intensity of alcohol use and drinking in public places for these young adults."

Note that the problem of heavy drinking and BINGE DRINKING on college campuses continues to be a major issue on many campuses throughout the United States.

Some employers and private and public schools have zero tolerance alcohol policies on their premises; for example, companies may have a policy to terminate workers who have been found to drink alcohol during working hours, and schools may suspend or expel students who use any amount of alcohol on the grounds of the school.

See also DRIVING UNDER THE INFLUENCE/DRIVING WHILE INTOXICATED; UNDERAGE DRINKING.

Fell, James C., et al. "The Impact of Underage Drinking Laws on Alcohol-Related Fatal Crashes of Young Drivers." *Alcoholism: Clinical and Experimental Research* 33, no. 7 (2009): 1–12.

Liang, Lan, and Jidong Huang. "Go Out or Stay In? The Effects of Zero Tolerance Laws on Alcohol Use and Drinking and Driving Patterns Among College Students." *Health Economics* 17, no. 11 (2008): 1,261–1,275.

Voas, R. B., A. S. Tippetts, and J. C. Fell. "Assessing the Effectiveness of Minimum Legal Drinking Age and Zero Tolerance Laws in the United States." *Accident Analysis and Prevention* 35, no. 4 (2003): 579–587.

APPENDIXES

APPENDIX I
IMPORTANT NATIONAL ORGANIZATIONS

Addiction Technology Transfer Center Network
ATTC National Office
University of Missouri—Kansas City
5100 Rockhill Road
Kansas City, MO 64110
(816) 482-1200

Adult Children of Alcoholics World Service Organization
P.O. Box 3216
Torrance, CA 90510
(310) 534-1815
http://www.adultchildren.org

AIDSinfo
P.O. Box 6303
Rockville, MD 20849-6303
(800) HIV-0440
http://www.aidsinfo.nih.gov

Al-Anon Family Groups, Inc.
Public Outreach Director
1600 Corporate Landing Parkway
Virginia Beach, VA 23454-5617
(888) 425-2666
http://www.al-anon.alateen.org

Alcoholics Anonymous World Services, Inc.
Grand Central Station
P.O. Box 459
New York, NY 10163
(212) 870-3400
http://www.alcoholics-anonymous.org

A Matter of Degree
Office of Alcohol and Other Drug Abuse
American Medical Association
515 North State Street
Chicago, IL 60610
(312) 464-5687

American Academy of Addiction Psychiatry
1010 Vermont Avenue, NW
Suite 710
Washington, DC 20005
(202) 393-4484
http://www.aaap.org

American Academy of Family Physicians
P.O. Box 11210
Shawnee Mission, KS 66207
(800) 274-2237
http://www.aafp.org

American Academy of Neurology
1080 Montreal Avenue
St. Paul, MN 55116
(800) 879-1960
http://www.aan.com

American Association for Cancer Education
9500 Euclid Avenue
Room 30
Cleveland, OH 44195
(216) 444-9827
www.aaceonline.com/index.asp

American Association for Marriage and Family Therapy
112 South Alfred Street
Alexandria, VA 22314
(703) 838-9808
http://www.aamft.org

American Association of Suicidology
5221 Wisconsin Avenue, NW
Washington, DC 20015
(202) 237-2280
http://www.suicidology.org

American Chronic Pain Association
P.O. Box 850

Rocklin, CA 95677-0850
(800) 533-3231
http://www.theacpa.org

American College of Health Care Administrators
300 North Lee Street
Alexandria, VA 22314
(703) 739-7900
http://www.achca.org

American College of Physicians
190 North Independence Mall West
Philadelphia, PA 19106
(800) 523-1546
http://www.acponline.org

American Council on Alcoholism
P.O. Box 25126
Arlington, VA 22202
(703) 248-9005
http://www.aca-usa.org

American Counseling Association
5999 Stevenson Avenue
Alexandria, VA 22304
(800) 347-6647
http://www.counseling.org

American Diabetes Association (ADA)
1701 North Beauregard Street
Alexandria, VA 22314
(800) 342-2383
http://www.diabetes.org

American Health Assistance Foundation
22512 Gateway Center Drive
Clarksburg, MD 20871
(800) 437-2423
http://www.ahaf.org

American Heart Association/American Stroke Association
7272 Greenville Avenue
Dallas, TX 75231-4596
(800) 242-8721 (Heart Association)
(888) 478-7653 (Stroke Association)
http://www.americanheart.org

American Hospital Association (AHA)
One North Franklin

Chicago, IL 60606
(312) 422-3000
http://www.aha.org

American Liver Foundation
75 Maiden Lane
Suite 603
New York, NY 10038
(800) 465-4837
http://www.liverfoundation.org

American Lung Association
61 Broadway
Sixth Floor
New York, NY 10006
(800) 586-4872
http://www.lungusa.org

American Medical Association
515 North State Street
Chicago, IL 60610
(312) 464-5000
http://www.ama-assn.org

American Nurses Association
8515 Georgia Avenue
Suite 400
Silver Spring, MD 20910
(800) 274-4262
http://www.nursingworld.org

American Osteopathic Association
142 East Ontario Street
Chicago, IL 60611
(800) 621-1773
http://www.osteopathic.org

American Pharmacists Association
1100 Fifteenth Street, NW
Suite 400
Washington, DC 20005
(800) 237-2742
http://www.pharmacist.com

American Psychiatric Association
1000 Wilson Boulevard
Suite 1825
Arlington, VA 22209
(703) 907-7300
http://www.psych.org

American Psychological Association
750 First Street, NE
Washington, DC 20002-4242
(800) 374-2721
http://www.apa.org

American Society of Addiction Medicine
4601 North Park Avenue
Upper Arcade
Suite 101
Chevy Chase, MD 20815
(301) 656-3920
http://www.asam.org

Anxiety Disorders Association of America
8730 Georgia Avenue
Suite 600
Silver Spring, MD 20910
(240) 485-1001
http://www.adaa.org

Arthritis Foundation
P.O. Box 7669
Atlanta, GA 30357
(800) 283-7800
http://www.arthritis.org

Association for Medical Education and Research in Substance Abuse
Center for Alcohol and Addiction Studies
Brown University
Box G-BH
Providence, RI 02912
(401) 785-8263
http://www.amersa.org/

Association of State and Territorial Health Officials
1275 K Street, NW
Suite 800
Washington, DC 20005
(202) 371-9090
http://www.astho.org

Better Hearing Institute
515 King Street
Suite 420
Alexandria, VA 22314
(800) 327-9355
http://www.betterhearing.org

Better Sleep Council
501 Wynthe Street
Alexandria, VA 22314
(703) 683-8371
http://www.bettersleep.org

Center for Substance Abuse Prevention (CSAP)
Substance Abuse and Mental Health Services Administration
1 Choke Cherry Road
Rockville, MD 20857
(240) 276-2000
http://prevention.samhsa.gov/

Center on Alcohol Marketing and Youth
Health Policy Institute
Georgetown University
Box 571444
3300 Whitehaven Street, NW
Suite 5000
Washington, DC 20057-1485
(202) 687-1019
http://www.camy.org

Centers for Disease Control and Prevention (CDC)
1600 Clifton Road, NE
Atlanta, GA 30333
(404) 371-5900
http://www.cdc.gov

Centers for Medicare and Medicaid Services (CMS)
7500 Security Boulevard
Baltimore, MD 21244
(800) 633-4227
http://www.cms.hhs.gov
http://www.medicare.gov

Child Welfare Information Gateway
Children's Bureau
Administration on Children, Youth, and Families
1250 Maryland Avenue, SW
Eighth Floor
Washington, DC 20024
(800) 394-3366
http://www.childwelfare.gov

Child Welfare League of America
440 First Street, NW

Third Floor
Washington, DC 20001
(202) 638-2952
http://www.cwla.org

Community Anti-Drug Coalitions of America
625 Slaters Lane
Suite 300
Alexandria, VA 22314
(800) 54-CADCA
http://cadca.org/

Depression and Bipolar Support Alliance
730 North Franklin
Suite 501
Chicago, IL 60610
(800) 826-3632
http://dbsalliance.org

**Depression and Related Affective Disorders
     Association**
8201 Greensboro Drive
Suite 300
McLean, VA 22102
(703) 610-9026
http://www.drada.org

Disabled American Veterans (DAV)
P.O. Box 14301
Cincinnati, OH 45250
(877) 426-2838
http://www.dav.org

Dual Recovery Anonymous
World Services Central Office
P.O. Box 8107
Prairie Village, KS 66208
(877) 883-2332 (toll-free)

Emergency Nurses Association
915 Lee Street
Des Plaines, IL 60016
(800) 900-9659 (toll-free)
http://www.ena.org

Employee Benefits Security Administration
Department of Labor
Frances Perkins Building
200 Constitution Avenue, NW
Washington, DC 20210
http://www.dol.gov/ebsa

Faces and Voices of Recovery
1010 Vermont Avenue, #708
Washington, DC 20005
(202) 737-0690
http://www.facesandvoicesofrecovery.org/

Families Anonymous
P.O. Box 3475
Culver City, CA 90231
(800) 736-9805
http://www.familiesanonymous.org

Family Caregiver Alliance
180 Montgomery Street
Suite 1100
San Francisco, CA 94104
(800) 445-8106
http://www.caregiver.org

**Fetal Alcohol And Drug Unit, University of
     Washington School of Medicine**
180 Nickerson Street
Suite 309
Seattle, WA 98109
(206) 543-7155
http://depts.washington.edu/fadu/

Food and Drug Administration (FDA)
5600 Fishers Lane
Rockville, MD 20857
(888) 463-6332 (toll-free)
http://www.fda.org

The Genetic Alliance
4301 Connecticut Avenue, NW
Suite 404
Washington, DC 20008
(202) 966-5557
http://www.geneticalliance.org

Governors Highway Safety Association
750 First Street, NE
Suite 720
Washington, DC 20002
(202) 789-0942
http://www.naghsr.org

Group for the Advancement of Psychiatry
P.O. Box 570218
Dallas, TX 75357

(972) 613-3044
http://www.groupadpsych.org

The Higher Education Center for Alcohol and Other Drug Prevention
Education Development Center, Inc.
55 Chapel Street
Newton, MA 02458
(800) 676-1730 (toll-free)
http://www.higheredcenter.org

Homelessness Resource Center
Substance Abuse and Mental Health Services
    Administration
c/o Institute on Homelessness and Trauma
189 Wells Avenue
Suite 200
Newton Centre, MA 02459
(617) 467-6014
http://www.homeless.samhsa.gov

Indian Health Service
The Reyes Building
Rockville, MD 20852
(301) 443-3593
http://www.ihs.gov

International Center for Alcohol Policies (ICAP)
1519 New Hampshire Avenue, NW
Washington, DC 20036
(202) 986-1159

International Commission for the Prevention of Alcoholism and Drug Dependency
12501 Old Columbia Pike
Silver Spring, MD 20904
(301) 680-6719
http://www.health20-20.org/icpa.htm

Join Together
715 Albany Street, 580
Third Floor
Boston, MA 02118
(617) 437-1500
http://www.jointogether.org/

Men For Sobriety
P.O. Box 618
Quakertown, PA 18951
(215) 536-8026

Mood and Anxiety Disorder Programs (MAP)
National Institute of Mental Health
9000 Rockville Pike
Bethesda, MD 20892
(866) 627-6464
http://intramural.nimh.nih.gov/mood

Mothers Against Drunk Driving (MADD)
511 East John Carpenter Freeway
Suite 700
Irving, TX 75062
(800) GET-MADD (toll-free)
http://www.madd.org

National Asian Pacific American Families Against Substance Abuse, Inc.
340 East Second Street
Suite 409
Los Angeles, CA 90012
(213) 625-5795
http://www.napafasa.org/

National Association for Children of Alcoholics
11426 Rockville Pike
Suite 301
Rockville, MD 20852
(888) 55-4COAS (toll-free)
(301) 468-0985
http://www.nacoa.net

National Association for Native American Children of Alcoholics
P.O. Box 2708
Seattle, WA 98111
(206) 903-6574

National Association of Addiction Treatment Providers
313 West Liberty Street
Suite 129
Lancaster, PA 17603
(717) 392-8480
http://www.naatp.org

National Association of Alcoholism and Drug Abuse Counselors
901 North Washington Street
Suite 600
Arlington, VA 22314-1535

(800) 548-0497
http://www.naadac.org/

National Association of Social Workers
750 First Street, NE
Suite 700
Washington, DC 20002
(800) 638-8799
http://www.naswdc.org

National Cancer Institute
Public Inquiries Office
6116 Executive Boulevard
Room 3036A, MSC 8322
Bethesda, MD 20892-8322
(800) 422-6237
http://www.cancer.gov

National Center for Complementary and Alternative Medicine Information Clearinghouse
P.O. Box 7923
Gaithersburg, MD 20898-7923
(888) 644-6226
http://nccam.nih.gov

National Center on Addiction and Substance Abuse at Columbia University
633 Third Avenue
New York, NY 10017
(212) 841-5200
http://www.casacolumbia.org

National Center on Birth Defects & Developmental Disabilities
Centers for Disease Control and Prevention (CDC)
Mail Stop E-86
1600 Clifton Road
Atlanta, GA 30333
(800) 232-4636
http://www.cdc.gov/ndbddd

National Center on Elder Abuse
c/o Center for Community Research and Services
University of Delaware
297 Graham Hall
Newark, DE 19716
(302) 831-3252
http://www.ncea.aoa.gov

National Center on Substance Abuse and Child Welfare
4940 Irvine Boulevard
Suite 202
Irvine, CA 92620
(714) 505-3525
http://www.ncsacw.samhsa.gov

National Clearinghouse for Alcohol and Drug Information (NCADI)
P.O. Box 2345
Rockville, MD 20847-2345
(800) 729-6686
http://ncadi.samhsa.gov

National Clearinghouse on Child Abuse and Neglect Information
330 C Street, SW
Washington, DC 20447
(703) 385-3206
http://nccanch.acf.hhs.gov

National Clearinghouse on Families & Youth
P.O. Box 13505
Silver Spring, MD 20911-3505
(301) 608-8098
http://ncfy.acf.hhs.gov

National Council on Alcoholism and Drug Dependence (NCADD)
22 Cortlandt Street
Suite 801
New York, NY 10007
(212) 269-7797
http://www.ncadd.org

National Criminal Justice Reference Service
P.O. Box 6000
Rockville, MD 20849-6000
(800) 851-3420
http://www.ncjrs.gov

National Diabetes Information Clearinghouse
One Information Way
Bethesda, MD 20892-3560
(800) 860-8747
http://diabetes.niddk.nih.gov

National Digestive Diseases Information Clearinghouse
Two Information Way
Bethesda, MD 20892-3570
(800) 891-5389
http://digestive.niddk.nih.gov

National Domestic Violence Hotline
P.O. Box 161810
Austin, TX 78716
http://www.ndvh.org

National Family Caregivers Association
10400 Connecticut Avenue
Suite 500
Kensington, MD 20895
(800) 896-3650
http://www.nfcacares.org

National Health Information Center
P.O. Box 1133
Washington, DC 20013-1133
(800) 336-4797
http://www.health.gov/nhic

National Heart, Lung, and Blood Institute Health Information Center
P.O. Box 30105
Bethesda, MD 20824-0105
(301) 592-8573
http://www.nhlbi.nih.gov

National Highway Traffic Safety Administration (NHTSA)
400 Seventh Street, SW
Washington, DC 20590
(888) 327-4236 (toll-free)
http://www.nhtsa.dot.gov

National Injury Information Clearinghouse
U.S. Consumer Product Safety Commission
4330 East-West Highway
Room 504
Bethesda, MD 20814
(301) 504-7921
http://www.cpsc.gov/about/clrnghse.html

National Institute of Mental Health
6001 Executive Boulevard
Room 8184, MSC 9663
Bethesda, MD 20892

(866) 615-6464
http://www.nimh.nih.gov

National Institute on Alcohol Abuse and Alcoholism
535 Fishers Lane
MSC 9304
Bethesda, MD 20892
(301) 443-0595
http://www.niaaa.nih.gov

National Kidney and Urologic Diseases Information Clearinghouse
Three Information Way
Bethesda, MD 20892
(800) 891-5390
http://www.kidney.niddk.nih.gov

National Kidney Foundation
30 East 33rd Street
New York, NY 10016
(800) 622-9010
http://www.kidney.org

National Liquor Law Enforcement Association
11720 Beltsville Drive
Suite 900
Calverton, MD 20705
(301) 755-2795
http://www.nllea.org

National Mental Health Association
2000 North Beauregard Street
Sixth Floor
Alexandria, VA 22311
(703) 684-7722
http://www.nmha.org

National Mental Health Consumers' Self-Help Clearinghouse
1211 Chestnut Street
Suite 1207
Philadelphia, PA 19107
(215) 751-1810
(800) 553-4539 (toll-free)
http://www.mhselfhelp.org

National Mental Health Information Center
P.O. Box 42557
Washington, DC 20015

(800) 789-2647
http://www.mentalhealth.samhsa.gov

National Organization for Victim Assistance
510 King Street
Suite 424
Alexandria, VA 23314
(703) 535-6682
http://www.try-nova.org

National Organization on Fetal Alcohol Syndrome (NOFAS)
900 17th Street, NW
Suite 910
Washington, DC 20006
(202) 785-4585
http://www.nofas.org

National Rehabilitation Information Center
200 Forbes Boulevard
Suite 202
Lanham, MD 20706
(800) 346-2742
http://www.naric.com

National Self-Help Clearinghouse
365 Fifth Avenue
Suite 3300
New York, NY 10016
(212) 817-1822
http://www.selfhelpweb.org

National Sheriffs' Association
1450 Duke Street
Alexandria, VA 22314
(703) 836-7827
http://www.sheriffs.org

National Student Assistance Association
1704 Charlotte Pike
Suite 200
Nashville, TN 37203
(800) 257-6310
http://www.nasap.org

National Women's Health Information Center
8270 Willow Oaks Corporation Drive
Fairfax, VA 22031
(800) 994-9662
http://www.womenshealth.gov

National Women's Health Network
514 10th Street, NW
Suite 400
Washington, DC 20004
(202) 347-1140
http://www.womenshealthnetwork.org

National Youth Violence Prevention Resource Center
P.O. Box 10809
Rockville, MD 20849-0809
(866) 723-3968
http://www.safeyouth.org

Office of Minority Health Resource Center
Office of Minority Health
P.O. Box 37337
Washington, DC 20013-7337
(800) 444-6472
http://www.omhrc.gov

Office on Smoking and Health
National Center for Chronic Disease Prevention and Health Promotion
Centers for Disease Control and Prevention
Mail Stop K-50, Publications
4770 Buford Highway, NE
Atlanta, GA 30341
(800) 232-4636
http://www.cdc.gov/tobacco

Pacific Institute for Research and Evaluation
11710 Beltsville Drive
Suite 125
Calverton, MD 20705
(866) 956-2253
http://www.pire.org

Secular Organizations for Sobriety/Save Our Selves
4773 Hollywood Boulevard
Hollywood, CA 90027
(323) 666-4295
http://www.cfiwest.org

Social Security Administration
Office of Public Inquiries
6401 Security Boulevard
Baltimore, MD 21235
(800) 772-1213
http://www.ssa.gov

Substance Abuse and Mental Health Services Administration (SAMSHA)
Department of Health and Human Services
One Choke Cherry Road
Rockville, MD 20850
(800) 729-6686
(800) 487-4889
http://www.samhsa.gov

Treatment Research Institute
600 Public Ledger Building
150 South Independence Mall West
Philadelphia, PA 19106
http://www.tresearch.org

Underage Drinking Enforcement Training Center
Pacific Institute for Research and Evaluation
11720 Beltsville Drive
Suite 900
Calverton, MD 20705-3102
(877) 335-1287 (toll-free)
(301) 755-2799 (fax)
http://www.udetc.org

Visiting Nurse Association of America
900 19th Street, NW
Suite 200
Washington, DC 20006
(202) 384-1420
http://www.vnaa.org

Women For Sobriety, Inc.
P.O. Box 618
Quakertown, PA 18951-0618
(215) 536-8026
http://www.womenforsobriety.org

APPENDIX II
U.S. STATE AND TERRITORIAL ORGANIZATIONS ON ALCOHOLISM AND SUBSTANCE ABUSE

Each state and most U.S. territories have an organization responsible for issues of substance abuse, including alcohol dependence and drug addiction. These agencies can help individuals to locate treatment facility centers. (Individuals may also call the 24-hour nationwide treatment referral service at (800) 662-HELP.)

States

ALABAMA

Substance Abuse Services Division
Alabama Department of Mental Health and
  Mental Retardation
P.O. Box 301410
100 North Union Street
Montgomery, AL 36130
(334) 242-3961
334-242-0759 (fax)
http://www.mh.alabama.gov/

ALASKA

Division of Behavioral Health
350 Main Street
Suite 214
P.O. Box 110620
Juneau, AK 99811
(907) 465-5808
(907) 465-2668 (fax)
http://www.hss.state.ak.us/dbh/

ARIZONA

Division of Behavioral Services
Arizona Department of Health Services

150 North 18th Avenue
Phoenix, AZ 85007
(602) 542-1000
(602) 364-4760 (fax)
http://www.azdhs.gov/

ARKANSAS

**Office of Alcohol and Drug Abuse
  Prevention**
Division of Behavioral Health Services
Department of Human Services
4800 West Seventh Street
Little Rock, AR 72205
(501) 686-9866
(501) 686-9035 (fax)
http://www.arkansas.gov/dhs/dmhs/alco_drug_
  abuse_prevention.htm

CALIFORNIA

Department of Alcohol and Drug Programs
1700 K Street
Fifth Floor
Sacramento, CA 95814
(800) 879-2772
(916) 323-1270 (fax)
http://www.adp.ca.gov/

COLORADO

Division of Behavioral Health
Colorado Department of Human Services
3824 West Princeton Circle
Denver, CO 80236
(303) 866-7480
(303) 866-7481 (fax)
http://www.cdhs.state.co.us/adad/

CONNECTICUT

Department of Mental Health and Addiction Services
P.O. Box 341431
410 Capitol Avenue
Fourth Floor
Hartford, CT 06134
(860) 418-6969
(860) 418-6690 (fax)
http://www.ct.gov/dmhas/site/default.asp

DELAWARE

Alcohol and Drug Services
Division of Substance Abuse and Mental Health
1901 North DuPont Highway
Room 180
New Castle, DE 19720
(302) 255-9399
(302) 255-4428 (fax)
http://www.dhss.delaware.gov/dsamh/index.html

DISTRICT OF COLUMBIA

Addiction, Prevention and Recovery Administration
1300 First Street, NE
Suite 300
Washington, DC 20002
(202) 727-8857
(202) 442-9433 (fax)

FLORIDA

Substance Abuse Program Office
Department of Children and Families
1317 Winewood Boulevard
Building 6, Room 334
Tallahassee, FL 32399
(850) 487-2920
(850) 487-2239 (fax)
http://www.dcf.state.fl.us/mentalhealth/sa/

GEORGIA

Addictive Diseases Program
Georgia Department of Human Resources
Two Peachtree Street, NW
22nd Floor, Suite 22-273
Atlanta, GA 30303
(404) 657-2331
(404) 657-2256 (fax)
http://mhddad.dhr.georgia.gov/portal/site/dhr-mhddad

HAWAII

Alcohol and Drug Abuse Division
Hawaii Department of Health
Kakuhihewa Building
601 Kamokila Boulevard
Room 360
Kapolei, HI 96707
(808) 692-7506
(808) 692-7521
http://hawaii.gov/health/substance-abuse

IDAHO

Division of Behavioral Health
Idaho Department of Health and Welfare
450 West State Street
Fifth Floor
Boise, ID 83720
(208) 334-5935
(208) 332-7305 (fax)
http://www.healthandwelfare.idaho.gov/site/3460/default.aspx

ILLINOIS

Division of Alcoholism and Substance Abuse
Department of Human Services
100 West Randolph Street
Suite 5-600
Chicago, IL 60601
(312) 814-3840
(312) 814-2419 (fax)
http://www.dhs.state.il.us/page.aspx?item=29725

INDIANA

Division of Mental Health and Addiction
Family and Social Services Administration
Indiana Government Building
402 West Washington Street
Room W353
Indianapolis, IN 46204
(317) 232-7895
(317) 233-3472 (fax)
http://www.in.gov/fssa/dmha/index.htm

IOWA

Division of Health Promotion, Prevention and Addictive Behaviors

Iowa Department of Public Health
Lucas State Office Building
321 East 12th Street
Fourth Floor
Des Moines, IA 50319
(515) 282-4417
(515) 281-4535 (fax)
http://www.idph.state.ia.us/bh/substance_abuse.
asp

KANSAS

Kansas Department of Social and Rehabilitation Services

Division of Health Care Policy, Addiction and
Prevention Services
Docking State Office Building
915 Southwest Harrison Street
10th Floor North
Topeka, KS 66612
(785) 291-3326
(785) 296-7275 (fax)
http://www.srskansas.org/services/alc-drug_assess.
htm

KENTUCKY

Division of Mental Health and Substance Abuse

Kansas Department for Mental Health
1000 Fair Oaks Lane
Suite 4E-D
Frankfort, KY 40621
(502) 564-2880
(502) 564-7152

LOUISIANA

Office for Addictive Disorders

Louisiana Department of Health and Hospitals
628 North Fourth Street
P.O. Box 2790
Baton Rouge, LA 70821
(225) 342-6717
(225) 342-3875 (fax)
http://www.dhh.louisiana.gov/offices/?ID=23

MAINE

Maine Office of Substance Abuse

41 Anthony Street
#11 State House Station
Augusta, ME 04333
(207) 287-2595
(207) 287-4334 (fax)
http://www.maine.gov/dhhs/osa/

MARYLAND

Alcohol and Drug Abuse Administration

Maryland Department of Health and Mental
Hygiene
55 Wade Avenue
Catonsville, MD 21228
(410) 402-8600
(410) 402-8601 (fax)

MASSACHUSETTS

Bureau of Substance Abuse Services

Massachusetts Department of Public Health
250 Washington Street
Third Floor
Boston, MA 02108
(617) 624-5111
(617) 624-5185 (fax)

MICHIGAN

Bureau of Substance Abuse and Addiction Services

Michigan Department of Community Health
Lewis Cass Building
320 South Walnut Street
Fifth Floor
Lansing, MI 48913
(888) 736-0253
(517) 335-2121 (fax)
http://www.michigan.gov/mdch/

MINNESOTA

Alcohol and Drug Abuse Division

Minnesota Department of Human Services
P.O. Box 64977
St. Paul, MN 55164
(651) 431-2460
(651) 431-7449 (fax)

MISSISSIPPI

Division of Alcohol and Drug Abuse
Mississippi Department of Mental Health
1101 Robert E. Lee Building
239 North Lamar Street
Jackson, MS 39201
(601) 359-1288
(601) 359-6295 (fax)
http://www.dmh.state.ms.us/substance_abuse.htm

MISSOURI

Division of Alcohol and Drug Abuse
Missouri Department of Mental Health
1706 East Elm Street
Jefferson City, MO 65102
(573) 751-4942
(573) 751-7814 (fax)
http://www.dmh.missouri.gov/ada/adaindex.htm

MONTANA

Addictive and Mental Disorders Division
555 Fuller Avenue
P.O. Box 202905
Helena, MT 59620
(406) 444-3964
(406) 444-9389 (fax)
http://www.dphhs.mt.gov/amdd/

NEBRASKA

Division of Behavioral Health
Nebraska Department of Health and Human
    Services Systems
P.O. Box 95026
Lincoln, NE 68509
(402) 471-7818
(402) 471-9449 (fax)
http://www.dhhs.ne.gov/sua/suaindex.htm

NEVADA

**Substance Abuse Prevention and Treatment
    Agency**
Mental Health and Developmental Services
4126 Technology Way
Second Floor
Carson City, NV 89706
(775) 684-4190
(775) 684-4185 (fax)
http://mhds.state.nv.us/

NEW HAMPSHIRE

Bureau of Drug and Alcohol Services
Department of Health and Human Services
109 Pleasant Street
Third Floor North
Concord, NH 03301
(603) 271-6110
(603) 271-6105 (fax)
http://www.dhhs.state.
    nh.us/dhhs/atod/a1-treatment

NEW JERSEY

Division of Addiction Services
Department of Human Services
120 South Stockton Street
Third Floor
P.O. Box 362
Trenton, NJ 08625
(609) 292-5760
(609) 292-3816 (fax)
http://www.state.nj.us/humanservices/das/index.
    htm

NEW MEXICO

Behavioral Health Services Division
Human Services Department
Harold Runnels Building
P.O. Box 2348
Santa Fe, NM 87504
(505) 476-9285
(505) 476-9277 (fax)

NEW YORK

**New York State Office of Alcoholism and
    Substance Abuse Services**
1450 Western Avenue
Albany, NY 12203
(518) 473-3460

NORTH CAROLINA

**Division of Mental Health, Developmental
    Disabilities and Substance Abuse Services**
North Carolina Department of Health and Human
    Services
3007 Mail Service Center
Raleigh, NC 27699
(919) 733-4670
(919) 733-4556 (fax)

NORTH DAKOTA

Substance Abuse Services
Division of Mental Health and Substance Abuse
  Services
North Dakota Department of Human Services
1237 West Divide Avenue
Suite 1C
Bismarck, ND 58501
(701) 328-8920
(701) 328-8969 (fax)

OHIO

Ohio Department of Alcohol and Drug Addiction Services
Two Nationwide Plaza
280 North High Street
12th Floor
Columbus, OH 43215
(614) 466-3445
(614) 752-8645 (fax)

OKLAHOMA

Substance Abuse Services
Oklahoma Department of Mental Health and
  Substance Abuse Services
1200 NE 13th Street
P.O. Box 53277
Oklahoma City, OK 73152
(405) 522-3619
(405) 522-0637 (fax)

OREGON

Department of Human Services
Health Services Building
Office of Mental Health and Addiction Services
500 Summer Street, NE
Salem, OR 97301
(503) 945-5763
(503) 378-8467 (fax)

PENNSYLVANIA

Bureau of Drug and Alcohol Programs
Pennsylvania Department of Health
62 Klein Plaza
Suite B
Harrisburg, PA 17104
(717) 783-8200
(717) 787-6285 (fax)

RHODE ISLAND

Behavioral Health Care Services
Department of Mental Health, Retardation and
  Hospitals
14 Harrington Road
Barry Hall
Cranston, RI 02920
(401) 462-1000
(401) 462-6078 (fax)

SOUTH CAROLINA

Division of Alcohol and Drug Abuse
South Dakota Department of Human Services
101 Executive Center Drive
Suite 215
Columbia, SC 29210
(803) 896-5555
(803) 896-5557 (fax)

SOUTH DAKOTA

Department of Human Services
East Highway 34
Hillsview Plaza
c/o 500 East Capitol
Pierre, SD 57501
(605) 773-3123
(605) 773-7076 (fax)

TENNESSEE

Bureau of Alcohol and Drug Abuse Services
Tennessee Department of Health
Cordell Hull Building
425 Fifth Avenue North
Third Floor
Nashville, TN 37247
(615) 741-1921
(615) 532-2419 (fax)

TEXAS

Mental Health and Substance Abuse Division
Department of State Health Department
P.O. Box 149347
Austin, TX 78714
(512) 206-5000
(512) 206-5718 (fax)

UTAH

Division of Substance Abuse and Mental Health
Utah Department of Human Services
120 North 200 West
Room 209
Salt Lake City, UT 84103
(801) 538-3939
(801) 538-9892 (fax)

VERMONT

Alcohol and Drug Abuse Programs
Vermont Department of Health
108 Cherry Street
Burlington, VT 05402
(802) 651-1550
(802) 651-1573 (fax)

VIRGINIA

Substance Abuse Services
Virginia Department of Mental Health, Mental Retardation and Substance Abuse
1220 Bank Street
Eighth Floor
Richmond, VA 23218
(804) 786-3906
(804) 786-4320 (fax)

WASHINGTON

Division of Alcohol and Substance Abuse
Washington Department of Social and Health Services
P.O. Box 45330
Olympia, WA 98504
(877) 301-4557
(360) 586-0341 (fax)

WEST VIRGINIA

Division of Alcoholism and Drug Abuse
Office of Behavioral Health Services
West Virginia Department of Health and Human Services
350 Capitol Street
Room 350
Charleston, WV 25301
(304) 558-2276
(304) 558-1008 (fax)

WISCONSIN

Bureau of Mental Health and Substance Abuse Services
One West Wilson Street
P.O. Box 7851
Madison, WI 53707
(608) 266-2717
(608) 266-1533 (fax)

WYOMING

Department of Health Substance Abuse Division
6101 Yellowstone Road
Suite 220
Cheyenne, WY 82002
(307) 777-3353
(307) 777-5849 (fax)

U.S. Territories

AMERICAN SAMOA

Department of Human and Social Services
P.O. Box 999534
Pago Pago, American Samoa 96799
(684) 633-2609
(684) 633-7449 (fax)

GUAM

Drug and Alcohol Treatment Services
Department of Mental Health and Substance Abuse
790 Governor Carlos G. Camacho Road
Tamuning, Guam 96913
(671) 647-5330
(671) 649-6948 (fax)

MICRONESIA

Department of Health, Education and Social Affairs
Federated States of Micronesia
P.O. Box PS 70
Palikir, Pohnpei Micronesia 96941
(691) 320-5520
(691) 320-5524 (fax)

PALAU

Ministry of Health
Behavioral Health Division

P.O. Box 6027
Koro, Republic of Palau 96940
(680) 488-1907
(680) 488-1211 (fax)

PUERTO RICO

**Puerto Rico Mental Health and Anti-
Addiction Services Administration**
P.O. Box 21414
San Juan, Puerto Rico 00928
(787) 274-3795, ext. 1229
(787) 765-5888 (fax)

VIRGIN ISLANDS

**Mental Health, Alcoholism & Drug
Dependency**
Virgin Islands Department of Health
Barbel Plaza South
Saint Croix, Virgin Islands 00820
(340) 774-4888
(340) 774-4701 (fax)

APPENDIX III
STATE MENTAL HEALTH AGENCIES

Individuals with problems with alcohol abuse and dependence often need mental health services. This appendix lists state agencies that offer assistance.

ALABAMA
Department of Mental Health
RSA Union Building
100 North Union Street
Montgomery, AL 36130
(334) 242-3454
http://www.mh.state.al.us

ALASKA
Division of Mental Health and Developmental Disabilities
P.O. Box 110620
Juneau, AK 99811
(907) 465-3370
http://www.hss.state.ak.us/dbh

ARIZONA
Department of Health Services
Division of Behavioral Health Services
150 North 18th Avenue
Suite 200
Phoenix, AZ 85007
(602) 364-4558
http://www.hss.state.az.us/bhs/index.htm

ARKANSAS
Division of Mental Health Services
Department of Human Services
4313 West Markham Street
Little Rock, AR 72205
(501) 686-9164
http://www.state.ar.us/dhs/dmhs

CALIFORNIA
Department of Mental Health
Health and Welfare Agency
1600 Ninth Street
Room 151
Sacramento, CA 95814
(916) 654-3565
http://www.dmh.cahwnet.gov

COLORADO
Colorado Mental Health Services
3824 West Princeton Circle
Denver, CO 80236
(303) 866-7400
http://www.cdhs.state.co.us/ohr/mhs

CONNECTICUT
Department of Mental Health and Addictions Services
410 Capitol Avenue
Hartford, CT 06106
(860) 418-6700
http://www.dmhas.state.ct.us

DELAWARE
Division of Substance Abuse and Mental Health
Department of Health and Social Services
Main Building
1901 North DuPont Highway
New Castle, DE 19720
(302) 255-9427
http://www.state.de.us/dhss/dsamh/dmhhome.htm

DISTRICT OF COLUMBIA
Department of Mental Health Services
77 P Street, NE

Fourth Floor
Washington, DC 20002
(202) 673-7440
http://dmh.dc/gov/dmh/site/default.asp

FLORIDA

Department of Children and Families
Building 1
1317 Winewood Boulevard
Room 202
Tallahassee, FL 32399
(850) 487-1111
http://www.state.fl.us/cf_web

GEORGIA

Division of Mental Health
Department of Human Resources
Two Peachtree Street, NW
Suite 22-224
Atlanta, GA 30303
(404) 657-2168
http://www.state.ga.us/departments/dhr/mhmrsa/
index.html

HAWAII

Behavioral Health Services Administration
Department of Health
P.O. Box 3378
Honolulu, HI 96801
(808) 586-4419
http://www.state.hi.us/doh/about/behavior.html

IDAHO

Department of Health and Welfare
450 West State Street
Boise, ID 83720
(208) 334-5500
http://www2.state.id.us/dhw/index.htm

ILLINOIS

Office of Mental Health
Department of Human Services
Centrum Building
319 East Madison Street
Third Floor
Springfield, IL 62701
(217) 785-6023
http://www.dhs.state.il.us

INDIANA

Division of Mental Health
Department of Family and Social Services
Administration
402 West Washington Street
Room W-353
Indianapolis, IN 46204
(317) 232-7844

IOWA

Division of Mental Health and Developmental Disabilities
Hoover State Office Building
1305 East Walnut Street
Des Moines, IA 50319
(515) 281-3573

KANSAS

Department of Social and Rehabilitation Services
Docking State Office Building
915 SW Harrison Street
Topeka, KS 66612
(785) 296-3959
http://www.srskansas.org

KENTUCKY

Department for Mental Health
Cabinet for Human Resources
100 Fair Oaks Lane
Frankfort, KY 40621
(502) 564-4527
http://mhmr.chs.ky.gov/Default.asp

LOUISIANA

Louisiana Office of Mental Health
Bienville Building
628 North Fourth Street
Baton Rouge, LA 70802
(225) 342-2540

MAINE

Adult Mental Health Services
Department of Behavioral and Developmental
Services
40 State House Station
Augusta, ME 04333
(207) 287-4200
http://www.state.me.us/dmhmrsa

MARYLAND

Department of Health and Mental Hygiene
201 West Preston Street
Baltimore, MD 21201
(410) 767-6860
http://www.dhmh.state.md.us

MASSACHUSETTS

Department of Mental Health
25 Staniford Street
Boston, MA 02114
(617) 626-8000

MICHIGAN

Department of Community Health
Lewis-Cass Building
320 South Walnut Street
Sixth Floor
Lansing, MI 48913
(517) 373-3500
http://www.michigan.gov/mdch

MINNESOTA

Department of Human Services
Mental Health Program Division
Human Services Building
444 Lafayette Road
Saint Paul, MN 55155
(651) 297-3510

MISSISSIPPI

Department of Mental Health
Robert E. Lee Building
239 North Lamar Street
Suite 1101
Jackson, MS 39201
(601) 359-1288
http://www.dmh.state.ms.us

MISSOURI

Department of Mental Health
P.O. Box 687
Jefferson City, MO 65102
(800) 364-9687
http://www.dmh.missouri.gov

MONTANA

Addictive and Mental Disorders Division
Department of Public Health and Human Services

555 Fuller
Helena, MT 59620
(406) 444-4928
http://www.dphhs.state.mt.us

NEBRASKA

**Office of Mental Health, Substance Abuse
and Addiction Services**
P.O. Box 98925
Lincoln, NE 68509
(402) 479-5166
http://www.hhs.state.ne.us/beh/mhsa.htm

NEVADA

**Mental Health & Developmental Services
Division**
Department of Human Resources
Kinkead Building
505 East King Street
Room 602
Carson City, NV 89701
(775) 684-5943
http://www.mhds.state.nv.us

NEW HAMPSHIRE

Division of Behavioral Health
Department of Health and Human Services
State Office Park South
105 Pleasant Street
Concord, NH 03301
(603) 271-8140
http://www.dhhs.state.nh.us

NEW JERSEY

Division of Mental Health Services
50 East State Street
Capitol Center, P.O. Box 727
Trenton, NJ 08625
(609) 777-0702
http://www.state.nj.us/humanservices/dmhs

NEW MEXICO

Behavioral Health Services Division
Harold Runnels Building
1190 Saint Francis Drive
Room North 3300
Santa Fe, NM 87505
(505) 827-2601
http://www.nmcares.org

NEW YORK

Office of Mental Health
44 Holland Avenue
Albany, NY 12229
(518) 474-4403
http://www.omh.state.ny.us

NORTH CAROLINA

Division of Mental Health, Developmental Disabilities and Substance Abuse Services
Department of Health and Human Resources
3001 Mail Service Center
Raleigh, NC 27699
(919) 733-7011
http://www.dhhs.state.nc.us/mhddsas

NORTH DAKOTA

Division of Mental Health and Substance Abuse Services
600 South Second Street
Suite 1D
Bismarck, ND 58504
(701) 328-8940

OHIO

Department of Mental Health
30 East Broad Street
Eighth Floor
Columbus, OH 43215
(614) 466-2337
http://www.mh.state.oh.us

OKLAHOMA

Department of Mental Health and Substance Abuse Services
P.O. Box 53277
Capitol Station
Oklahoma City, OK 73152
(405) 522-3908
http://www.odmhsas.org

OREGON

Oregon Department of Human Services
Mental Health and Addiction Services
500 Summer Street, NE
Number E6
Salem, OR 97301
(503) 945-5763
http://www.dhs.state.or.us/mentalhealth

PENNSYLVANIA

Office of Mental Health and Substance Abuse Services
P.O. Box 2675
Harrisburg, PA 17105
(717) 787-6443
http://www.dpw.state.pa.us/omhsas/dpwmh.asp

RHODE ISLAND

Department of Mental Health, Mental Retardation and Hospitals
14 Harrington Road
Cranston, RI 02920
(401) 462-3201
http://www.mhrh.state.ri.us

SOUTH CAROLINA

Department of Mental Health
2414 Bull Street
P.O. Box 485
Columbia, SC 29202
(803) 898-8581
http://www.state.sc.us/dmh

SOUTH DAKOTA

Division of Mental Health
Department of Human Services
Hillsview Plaza
East Highway 34
c/o 500 East Capitol
Pierre, SD 57501
(605) 773-5991
http://www.state.sd.us/dhs/dmh

TENNESSEE

Department of Mental Health and Developmental Disabilities
Cordell Hull Building
425 Fifth Avenue North
Third Floor
Nashville, TN 37243
(615) 532-6500
http://www.state.tn.us/mental/

TEXAS

Texas Department of Mental Health and Mental Retardation
Central Office
909 West 45th Street

Austin, TX 78751
(512) 454-3761
http://www.mhmr.state.tx.us

UTAH

Division of Mental Health
Department of Human Services
120 North 200 West
Fourth Floor
Suite 415
Salt Lake City, UT 84103
(801) 538-4270
http://www.hsmh.state.ut.us

VERMONT

**Department of Developmental and Mental
Health Services**
Weeks Building
103 South Main Street
Waterbury, VT 05671
(802) 241-2610
http://www.state.vt.us/dmh

VIRGINIA

**Department of Mental Health, Mental
Retardation and Substance Abuse
Services**
P.O. Box 1797
Richmond, VA 23218
(804) 786-3921
http://www.dmhmrsas.state.va.us/

WASHINGTON

Mental Health Division
Department of Social and Health Services

P.O. Box 45320
Olympia, WA 98504
(360) 902-0790
http://www.wa.gov/dshs/

WEST VIRGINIA

**Bureau of Behavioral Health and Health
Facilities**
Department of Health and Human Resources
350 Capitol Street
Room 350
Charleston, WV 25301
(304) 558-0627
http://www.wvdhhr.org/

WISCONSIN

Bureau of Community Mental Health
Department of Health and Family Services
One West Wilson Street
Room 433
P.O. Box 7851
Madison, WI 53702
(608) 267-7792
http://www.dhfs.state.wi.us/mentalhealth

WYOMING

Mental Health Division
Department of Health
6101 Yellowstone Road
Room 259-B
Cheyenne, WY 82002
(307) 777-7094
http://mhd.state.wy.us/

APPENDIX IV
STATE CHILD PROTECTIVE SERVICES AGENCIES

Children whose parents or primary caregivers are alcoholics or alcohol abusers are at risk for child maltreatment, including abuse and neglect. For this reason, this appendix is provided. At the end of this appendix are the state hotlines to report child abuse or neglect.

ALABAMA

Alabama Department of Human Resources
Family Services Division
50 North Ripley Street
Montgomery, AL 36130-1801
(334) 353-1045
(334) 242-0939 (fax)

ALASKA

Alaska Department of Health and Social Services
Office of Children's Services
751 Old Richardson Highway
Suite 300
Fairbanks, AK 99701
(907) 451-2650
(907) 451-2058 (fax)

AMERICAN SAMOA

American Samoa Department of Human and Social Services
Social Services Division
P.O. Box 997534
Pago Pago, AS 96799
(011) 684-633-2696, ext. 237
(011) 684-633-7852 (fax)

ARIZONA

Arizona Department of Economic Security
Administration for Children, Youth and Families
1789 West Jefferson Street
Third Floor
Site Code 940A
Phoenix, AZ 85007
(602) 542-2358
(602) 542-3330 (fax)

ARKANSAS

Arkansas Department of Human Services
Division of Children and Family Services
P.O. Box 1437
Slot S-569
Little Rock, AR 72203-1437
(501) 682-8008
(501) 682-6968 (fax)

CALIFORNIA

California Department of Social Services
Office of Child Abuse Prevention
744 P Street
MS 11-82
Sacramento, CA 95814
(916) 651-6960
(916) 651-6328 (fax)
Teresa.contreras@dss.ca.gov

COLORADO

Colorado Department of Human Services
Division of Child Welfare
1575 Sherman Street
Denver, CO 80203
(303) 866-5937
(303) 866-5563 (fax)

COMMONWEALTH OF THE NORTHERN MARIANA ISLANDS

Department of Community and Cultural Affairs
Division of Youth Services

P.O. Box 501000
Chalan Kanoa
Saipan, MP 96950
(670) 664-2550
(670) 664-2560 (fax)

CONNECTICUT

Connecticut Department of Children and Families
Child Welfare Services
505 Hudson Street
Hartford, CT 06106-7107
(860) 550-6542
(860) 566-7947 (fax)
karl.kemper@po.state.ct.us

DELAWARE

Delaware Department of Services for Children, Youth and Their Families
Office of Children Services/Division of Family Services
1825 Faulkland Road
Room 246
Wilmington, DE 19805
(302) 633-2663
(302) 633-2652 (fax)

DISTRICT OF COLUMBIA

District of Columbia Children and Family Services Administration
Office of Planning, Policy and Program Support
955 L'Enfant Plaza North
Suite P 101
Washington, DC 20024
(202) 724-7058
(202) 727-5619 (fax)

FLORIDA

Florida Department of Children and Families
Child Protective Investigations & Intervention Unit
1317 Winewood Boulevard
Tallahassee, FL 32399-0700
(850) 922-3862

GEORGIA

Georgia Department of Human Resources
Division of Family and Children Services
Two Peachtree Street

18th Floor, Room 101
Atlanta, GA 30303
(404) 657-3306
(404) 657-3406 (fax)

GUAM

Guam Department of Public Health and Social Services
Bureau of Social Services Administration
P.O. Box 2816
Agana, GU 96910
(671) 475-2640
(671) 472-6649 (fax)

HAWAII

Hawaii Department of Human Services
Social Services Division
810 Richards Street
Suite 400
Honolulu, HI 96813
(808) 586-5925
(808) 586-4806 (fax)

IDAHO

Idaho Department of Health and Welfare
Division of Family and Community Services
450 West State Street
Fifth Floor
P.O. Box 83720
Boise, ID 83720-0036
(208) 334-6618
(208) 334-6699 (fax)

ILLINOIS

Illinois Department of Children and Family Services
Division of Child Protection
10 West 35th Street
Chicago, IL 60616
(312) 328-2118
(217) 785-2513
(312) 328-2595 (fax)
(217) 328-2595 (fax)

INDIANA

Indiana Department of Child Services
402 West Washington Street
Room W-392
Indianapolis, IN 45204

(317) 234-1391
(317) 232-4490 (fax)

IOWA

Iowa Department of Human Services
Bureau of Protective Services
Hoover State Office Building
Fifth Floor
Des Moines, IA 50319
(515) 281-4625
(515) 242-6884 (fax)

KANSAS

**Kansas Department of Social and
  Rehabilitation Services**
Division of Children and Family Services
915 SW Harrison
Room 551-S
Topeka, KS 66612-1570
(785) 296-6030
(785) 368-8159 (fax)

KENTUCKY

**Kentucky Cabinet for Health and Family
  Services**
Department for Community-Based Services/
  Division for Protection and Permanency
275 East Main Street
3E-A
Frankfort, KY 40621
(502) 564-2136
(502) 564-3096 (fax)

LOUISIANA

Louisiana Department of Social Services
Office of Community Services
P.O. Box 3318
Baton Rouge, LA 70821
(225) 342-9928
(255) 342-9087 (fax)

MAINE

**Maine Department of Health and Human
  Services**
Office of Child and Family Services
211 State Street
Station 11

Augusta, ME 04333
(207) 287-2976
(207) 287-5282 (fax)

MARYLAND

Maryland Department of Human Resources
Social Services Administration
Fifth Floor
311 West Saratoga Street
Baltimore, MD 21201
(410) 767-7112
(410) 333-6556 (fax)

MASSACHUSETTS

**Massachusetts Department of Children and
  Families (DCF)**
24 Farnsworth Street
Boston, MA 02210
(617) 748-2350
(617) 261-6743 (fax)

MICHIGAN

Michigan Department of Human Services
Child Protective Services Program
235 South Grand Avenue
Suite 510
Lansing, MI 48909
(517) 335-3704
(517) 241-7047 (fax)

MINNESOTA

Minnesota Department of Human Services
Children and Family Services
444 Lafayette Road North
St. Paul, MN 55155-3830
(651) 296-2487
(651) 297-1949 (fax)

MISSISSIPPI

Mississippi Department of Human Services
Division of Family and Children
P.O. Box 352
Jackson, MS 39205
(601) 359-4479
(601) 359-4333 (fax)

MISSOURI

Missouri Department of Social Services
Children's Division

615 Howerton Court
Jefferson City, MO 65109
(573) 751-8927
(573) 526-3971 (fax)

MONTANA

Montana Department of Public Health and Human Services
Child and Family Services Division
P.O. Box 8005
Helena, MT 59604
(406) 444-1677
(406) 444-5956 (fax)

NEBRASKA

Nebraska Department of Health and Human Services
Office of Protection and Safety
P.O. Box 95044
Lincoln, NE 68509-5044
(402) 471-9733
(402) 471-9034 (fax)

NEVADA

Nevada Division of Child and Family Services
DCFS—Family Programs Office (FPO)
4126 Technology Way
Third Floor
Carson City, NV 89706
(775) 684-4483
(775) 684-4456 (fax)

NEW HAMPSHIRE

New Hampshire Department of Health and Human Services
Division for Children, Youth & Families/Bureau
of Quality Improvement
129 Pleasant Street, Brown Building
Fourth Floor
Concord, NH 03301
(603) 271-4684
(603) 271-4729 (fax)

NEW JERSEY

New Jersey Department of Children and Families
50 East State Street
Seventh Floor, CC#924
P.O. Box 717

Trenton, NJ 08625-0717
(609) 943-4181
(609) 633-8504 (fax)

NEW MEXICO

New Mexico Children, Youth & Families Department
Protective Services Division
Pera Building
Room 254, P.O. Drawer 5160
Santa Fe, NM 87502-5160
(505) 827-4490
(505) 827-7361 (fax)

NEW YORK

New York State Office of Children and Family Services
52 Washington Street
Room 331N
Rensselaer, NY 12144
(518) 474-9613
(518) 402-6824 (fax)

NORTH CAROLINA

North Carolina Department of Health and Human Services
Division of Social Services
325 North Salisbury Street
MSC 2408
Raleigh, NC 27699-2408
(919) 733-3360
(919) 715-6714 (fax)
http://www.dhhs.state.nc.us/dss

NORTH DAKOTA

North Dakota Department of Human Services
Children and Family Services Division
600 East Boulevard Avenue
Bismarck, ND 58505
(701) 328-3587
(701) 328-3538 (fax)

OHIO

Ohio Department of Job and Family Services
Protective Services
P.O. Box 182709
Columbus, OH 43218-2709

(614) 466-1213
(614) 466-0164 (fax)

OKLAHOMA

Oklahoma Department of Human Services
Division of Children and Youth Services
P.O. Box 25352
Oklahoma City, OK 73125
(405) 521-2283
(405) 521-4373 (fax)

OREGON

Oregon Department of Human Services
Child Protective Services
500 Summer Street, NE
E-68
Salem, OR 97301
(503) 945-6696
(503) 378-3800 (fax)

PENNSYLVANIA

Pennsylvania Department of Public Welfare
Office of Children, Youth, and Families
P.O. Box 2675
Harrisburg, PA 17105-2675
(717) 705-2912
(717) 705-0364 (fax)

PUERTO RICO

Puerto Rico Department of the Family
Aveue Seviloa #58
Plaza Seviloa
PO Box 194090
San Juan, PR 00910-4090
(787) 625-4900
(787) 977-2336 (fax)

RHODE ISLAND

Rhode Island Department for Children, Youth, and Families
Protective Services Division
101 Friendship Street
Providence, RI 02903
(401) 457-4943
(401) 528-3590 (fax)

SOUTH CAROLINA

South Carolina Department of Social Services
Division of Human Services

P.O. Box 1520
Columbia, SC 29202-1520
(803) 898-7514
(803) 898-7641 (fax)

SOUTH DAKOTA

South Dakota Department of Social Services
Child Protective Services
700 Governors Drive
Pierre, SD 57501
(605) 773-3227
(605) 773-6834 (fax)

TENNESSEE

Tennessee Department of Children's Services
Cordell Hull Building
436 Sixth Avenue, North
Eighth Floor
Nashville, TN 37243-1290
(615) 741-8278
(615) 253-0069 (fax)

TEXAS

Texas Department of Family and Protective Services
P.O. Box 149030
MC E-557
Austin, TX 78714-9030
(512) 438-3291
(512) 438-3782 (fax)

UTAH

Utah Department of Human Services
Division of Child and Family Services
120 North 200 West
Suite 225
Salt Lake City, UT 84103
(801) 538-4100
(801) 538-3993 (fax)

VERMONT

Vermont Department for Children and Families
Child Welfare and Youth Justice Division
103 South Main Street
Osgood Building
Waterbury, VT 05671-2401
(802) 241-2139
(802) 241-2407 (fax)

VIRGINIA

Virginia Department of Social Services
Child Protective Services Unit
Seven North Eighth Street
Richmond, VA 23219
(804) 726-7554
(804) 726-7895 (fax)

VIRGIN ISLANDS

Virgin Islands Department of Human Services
Division of Children, Youth and Families
3011 Golden Rock
Christiansted
St. Croix, VI 00820 1
(340) 773-2323, x 2004
(340) 773-4043 (fax)

WASHINGTON

Washington Department of Social and Health Services
Children's Administration
P.O. Box 45710
Olympia, WA 98504
(360) 902-0217
(360) 902-7903

WEST VIRGINIA

West Virginia Department of Health and Human Resources
Children and Adult Services
350 Capitol Street
Room 691
Charleston, WV 25301
(304) 558-2997
(304) 555-4563 (fax)

WISCONSIN

Wisconsin Department of Health and Family Services
Bureau of Programs and Policy
P.O. Box 8916
Madison, WI 53708-8916
(608) 266-1489
(608) 264-6750 (fax)

WYOMING

Wyoming Department of Family Services
Division of Social Services
2300 Capitol Avenue
Hathaway Building #376
Cheyenne, WY 82002
(307) 777-3570
(307) 777-7747 (fax)

APPENDIX V
STATE CHILD ABUSE REPORTING NUMBERS

These are the numbers to report in each state if child maltreatment is known or strongly suspected. Individuals may also obtain further information at each state's Web site. Most, but not all, are toll-free. Web sites are also provided for most states, which offer further information.

ALABAMA

(334) 242-9500
http://www.dhr.state.al.us/page.asp?pageid=304

ALASKA

(800) 478-4444 (toll-free)
http://www.hss.state.ak.us/ocs/default.htm

ARIZONA

(888) SOS-CHILD (888-767-2445) (toll-free)
https://www.azdes.gov/dcyf/cps/reporting.asp

ARKANSAS

(800) 482-5964 (toll-free)
http://www.state.ar.us/dhs/chilnfam/child_
    protective_services.htm

CALIFORNIA

http://www.dss.cahwnet.gov/cdssweb/PG20.htm
Click on the Web site above for information on reporting or call Childhelp® (800-422-4453) for assistance.

COLORADO

(303) 866-5932
http://www.cdhs.state.co.us/childwelfare/FAQ.htm

CONNECTICUT

(800) 624-5518 (TDD)
(800) 842-2288 (toll-free)
http://www.state.ct.us/dcf/HOTLINE.htm

DELAWARE

(800) 292-9582 (toll-free)
http://www.state.de.us/kids/

DISTRICT OF COLUMBIA

(202) 671-SAFE (202-671-7233)
http://cfsa.dc.gov/cfsa/cwp/view.asp?a=3&q=
    520663&cfsaNav =|31319|

FLORIDA

(800) 96-ABUSE (800-962-2873) (toll-free)
http://www.dcf.state.fl.us/abuse/

GEORGIA

http://dfcs.dhr.georgia.gov/portal/site
Access the Web site above for information on reporting or call Childhelp® (800-422-4453) for assistance.

HAWAII

(808) 832-5300
http://www.hawaii.gov/dhs/protection/social_
    services/child_welfare/

IDAHO

(800) 926-2588 (toll-free)
http://www.healthandwelfare.idaho.gov/
    site/3333/default.aspx

ILLINOIS

(217) 524-2606
(800) 252-2873 (toll-free)
http://www.state.il.us/dcfs/child/index.shtml

INDIANA

(800) 800-5556 (toll-free)
http://www.in.gov/dcs/protection/dfcchi.html

IOWA

(800) 362-2178 (toll-free)
http://www.dhs.state.ia.us/dhs2005/dhs_
    homepage/children_family/abuse_reporting/
    child_abuse.html

KANSAS

(800) 922-5330 (toll-free)
http://www.srskansas.org/services/child_
    protective_services.htm

KENTUCKY

(800) 752-6200 (toll-free)
http://chfs.ky.gov/dcbs/dpp/childsafety.htm

LOUISIANA

Call Childhelp® (800-422-4453) for assistance.

MAINE

(800) 963-9490 (TTY)
(800) 452-1999 (toll-free)
http://www.maine.gov/dhhs/bcfs/abusereporting.
    htm

MARYLAND

Call Childhelp® (800-422-4453) for assistance.

MASSACHUSETTS

(800) 792-5200 (toll-free)

MICHIGAN

Call Childhelp® (800-422-4453) for assistance.

MINNESOTA

Call Childhelp® (800-422-4453) for assistance.

MISSISSIPPI

(601) 359-4991
(800) 222-8000 (toll-free)
http://www.mdhs.state.ms.us/fcs_prot.html

MISSOURI

(573) 751-3448
(800) 392-3738 (toll-free)
http://www.dss.mo.gov/cd/rptcan.htm

MONTANA

(866) 820-5437 (toll-free)
http://www.dphhs.mt.gov/cfsd/index.shtml

NEBRASKA

(800) 652-1999 (toll-free)
http://www.hhs.state.ne.us/cha/chaindex.htm

NEVADA

(800) 992-5757 (toll-free)
http://dcfs.state.nv.us/DCFS_ReportSuspected
    ChildAbuse.htm

NEW HAMPSHIRE

(603) 271-6556
(800) 894-5533 (toll-free)
http://www.dhhs.state.nh.us/DHHS/BCP/default.
    htm

NEW JERSEY

(800) 835-5510 (TDD)
(800) 835-5510 (TTY)
(877) 652-2873 (toll-free)
http://www.state.nj.us/dcf/abuse/how/

NEW MEXICO

(505) 841-6100
(800) 797-3260 (toll-free)
http://www.cyfd.org/report.htm

NEW YORK

(518) 474-8740
(800) 369-2437 (TDD)
(800) 342-3720 (toll-free)
http://www.ocfs.state.ny.us/main/cps/

NORTH CAROLINA

Call Childhelp® (800-422-4453) for assistance.

NORTH DAKOTA

Call Childhelp® (800-422-4453) for assistance.

OHIO

Call Childhelp® (800-422-4453) for assistance.

OKLAHOMA

(800) 522-3511 (toll-free)
http://www.okdhs.org/programsandservices/cps/
    default.htm

OREGON

Call Childhelp® (800-422-4453) for assistance.

PENNSYLVANIA

(800) 932-0313 (toll-free)
http://www.dpw.state.pa.us/ServicesPrograms/
    ChildWelfare/003671030.htm

PUERTO RICO

(787) 749-1333
(800) 981-8333 (toll-free)
http://www.gobierno.pr/GPRPortal/StandAlone/
    AgencyInformation.aspx?Filter=177

RHODE ISLAND

(800) RI-CHILD (800-742-4453) (toll-free)
http://www.dcyf.ri.gov/child_welfare/index.php

SOUTH CAROLINA

(803) 898-7318
http://www.state.sc.us/dss/cps/index.html

SOUTH DAKOTA

Call Childhelp® (800-422-4453) for assistance.

TENNESSEE

(877) 237-0004 (toll-free)
http://state.tn.us/youth/childsafety.htm

TEXAS

(800) 252-5400 (toll-free)
https://www.dfps.state.tx.us/Child_Protection/
    About_Child_Protective_Services/report
    ChildAbuse.asp

UTAH

(800) 678-9399 (toll-free)
http://www.hsdcfs.utah.gov

VERMONT

(800) 649-5285
http://www.dcf.state.vt.us/fsd/reporting_child_abuse

VIRGINIA

(804) 786-8536
(800) 552-7096 (toll-free)
http://www.dss.virginia.gov/family/cps/index.html

WASHINGTON

(800) 624-6186 (TTY)
(866) END-HARM (866-363-4276) (toll-free)
(800) 562-5624 (after hours)
http://www1.dshs.wa.gov/ca/safety/abuseReport.
    asp?2

WEST VIRGINIA

(800) 352-6513 (toll-free)
http://www.wvdhhr.org/bcf/children_adult/cps/
    report.asp

WISCONSIN

http://dcf.wisconsin.gov/children/CPS/cpswimap.
    HTM

WYOMING

http://dfsweb.state.wy.us/menu.htm

APPENDIX VI

PAST YEAR AND MONTH ALCOHOL ABUSE AND DEPENDENCE AMONG UNDERAGE USERS, 2002–2006

As can be seen in the following table from the Substance Abuse and Mental Health Services Administration (SAMHSA), among individuals ages 12–20 years in the total United States, the majority (54.9 percent) have ever used alcohol in their lifetimes, and close to a half (46.5 percent) have used alcohol in the past year, based on data from 2002–2006.

An estimated 19.2 percent have binged on alcohol in the past month, and 6.2 percent were heavy users of alcohol in the past month. An estimated 9.4 percent abused or were dependent on alcohol in the past year. (Binge drinking is drinking five

or more drinks on the same occasion, at the same time or within a couple of hours of each other on at least one day in the past 30 days. Heavy drinking is defined as drinking five or more drinks on the same occasion in each of five or more days in the past 30 days. All heavy alcohol users are also binge alcohol users.

Some states have higher rates of alcohol abuse and dependence than others; for example, the highest rate was seen in Montana (17.8 percent) followed by North Dakota (17.7 percent). The lowest rates were seen in Mississippi (7.1 percent), followed by Georgia (7.3 percent).

TABLE 1
ALCOHOL USE IN THE LIFETIME, PAST YEAR, AND PAST MONTH: BINGE AND HEAVY ALCOHOL USE
IN THE PAST MONTH; AND ALCOHOL DEPENDENCE OR ABUSE IN THE PAST YEAR AMONG PERSONS
AGES 12 TO 20 YEARS, BY STATE: PERCENTAGES, ANNUAL AVERAGES BASED ON 2002–2006

State	Lifetime Use	Past Year Use	Past Month Use	Binge Use in Past Month	Heavy Use in Past Month	Dependence or Abuse in Past Year
Total United States	54.9	46.5	28.6	19.2	6.2	9.4
Alabama	52.5	42.4	25.7	17.0	5.4	7.9
Alaska	53.0	44.0	26.8	18.2	5.4	9.8
Arizona	54.9	44.8	28.5	19.4	6.1	9.7
Arkansas	55.6	44.6	27.0	19.8	7.1	10.4
California	51.5	42.5	25.3	16.2	4.2	8.6
Colorado	59.7	52.4	33.1	21.4	5.8	11.2
Connecticut	57.3	50.6	33.1	22.0	6.6	9.7
Delaware	57.2	47.9	29.5	19.2	5.7	8.2
District of Columbia	53.6	44.7	30.2	19.0	6.3	8.1
Florida	55.1	47.1	27.7	17.4	6.0	9.1
Georgia	50.5	40.7	23.5	15.0	4.1	7.3
Hawaii	53.7	43.9	26.7	18.9	5.2	9.9
Idaho	47.8	40.2	24.9	18.0	7.2	11.7

State	Lifetime Use	Past Year Use	Past Month Use	Binge Use in Past Month	Heavy Use in Past Month	Dependence or Abuse in Past Year
Illinois	54.9	47.4	29.7	20.5	6.6	10.2
Indiana	53.8	44.9	26.4	18.7	6.7	9.2
Iowa	58.0	51.8	33.4	24.8	9.9	13.2
Kansas	58.4	50.1	32.9	24.2	7.7	11.9
Kentucky	57.9	47.9	29.0	19.9	4.9	7.9
Louisiana	59.0	50.2	30.4	19.0	5.9	9.4
Maine	57.0	48.8	30.7	21.4	6.5	9.7
Maryland	53.8	46.1	27.6	16.3	5.9	8.1
Massachusetts	58.5	51.8	33.9	24.3	8.7	10.1
Michigan	55.6	48.1	30.0	20.5	6.7	9.6
Minnesota	56.1	49.5	31.7	22.6	7.3	10.9
Mississippi	51.9	40.4	24.1	15.9	5.6	7.1
Missouri	59.1	50.2	32.1	22.2	7.5	11.0
Montana	64.0	56.7	38.5	29.3	10.2	17.8
Nebraska	57.4	50.3	34.0	23.6	8.1	13.5
Nevada	56.0	45.8	27.1	17.4	5.5	9.3
New Hampshire	59.0	53.2	34.9	24.6	11.5	12.6
New Jersey	57.3	50.3	30.9	18.7	5.0	8.7
New Mexico	61.3	50.8	31.3	21.4	6.8	13.0
New York	57.3	50.2	32.0	21.2	7.1	9.4
North Carolina	51.5	42.3	25.1	16.8	4.6	7.7
North Dakota	66.2	59.1	41.2	31.7	12.9	17.7
Ohio	56.6	48.7	29.8	21.0	7.0	9.5
Oklahoma	55.3	46.3	26.9	18.9	5.9	10.2
Oregon	56.3	47.4	28.6	19.2	6.8	9.7
Pennsylvania	56.9	48.8	30.0	20.8	7.1	9.2
Rhode Island	61.0	54.8	37.8	26.2	9.9	12.2
South Carolina	52.0	40.6	24.2	16.0	5.3	7.7
South Dakota	63.6	56.8	37.2	27.9	8.9	15.9
Tennessee	50.1	41.3	22.7	14.4	5.0	7.7
Texas	54.0	44.7	26.8	17.2	5.5	8.2
Utah	37.1	30.0	9.3	14.1	4.6	8.0
Vermont	61.8	54.9	37.2	26.5	9.2	12.4
Virginia	52.8	45.0	28.6	19.5	6.4	9.4
Washington	56.4	47.6	30.3	20.3	7.1	10.4
West Virginia	57.1	48.0	29.0	21.6	6.7	10.6
Wisconsin	61.9	55.2	36.6	26.1	9.2	12.9
Wyoming	62.6	53.2	33.8	24.4	8.2	14.8

Source: Appendix C, Table 3.10B. Substance Abuse and Mental Health Services Administration, Available online at http://oas.samhsa.gov/underage2k8/AppC.htm. Accessed July 21, 2008.

APPENDIX VII

ALCOHOL USE IN THE UNITED STATES, LIFETIME, PAST YEAR, AND PAST MONTH AMONG PERSONS AGES 12 TO 20, BY GENDER, 2002–2007

This table shows that drinking among minors (under age 21) has declined since 2002, but it is still true that more than half of all individuals ages 12–20 have consumed alcohol and nearly half (45.1 percent) consumed alcohol in the past month in 2007. Males and females in this age group have about the same risk for alcohol consumption; for example, 28.4 percent of males consumed alcohol in the past month in 2007, compared to 27.3 percent of females. However, binge drinking was higher among males (21.1 percent in 2007) compared to 16.1 percent in females.

Gender/Alcohol Use	2002	2003	2004	2005	2006	2007
Total						
Lifetime	56.1	55.8	54.9	53.9	53.9	52.9
Past Year	47.0	46.8	46.6	46.3	46.1	45.1
Past Month	28.8	29.0	28.7	29.2	28.3	27.9
Binge alcohol use [1]	19.3	19.2	19.6	18.8	19.0	18.6
Heavy alcohol use [1]	6.2	6.1	6.3	6.0	6.2	6.0
Males						
Lifetime	56.5	55.0	54.9	53.7	54.0	53.0
Past Year	46.6	45.6	46.3	45.6	46.0	45.1
Past Month	29.6	29.9	29.6	28.9	29.2	28.4
Binge alcohol use [1]	21.8	21.7	22.1	21.3	21.3	21.1
Heavy alcohol use [1]	8.1	7.9	8.2	7.6	7.9	7.8
Female						
Lifetime	56.0	56.6	54.8	54.2	53.7	52.8
Past year	47.5	48.0	46.9	46.9	46.2	45.1
Past month	28.0	28.1	27.8	27.5	27.4	27.3
Binge alcohol use [1]	16.7	16.5	17.0	16.1	16.5	16.1
Heavy alcohol use [1]	4.2	4.2	4.3	4.2	4.3	4.2

[1]Binge alcohol use is defined as drinking five or more drinks on the same occasion (i.e., at the same time or within a couple of hours of each other) on at least one day in the past 30 days. Heavy alcohol use is defined as drinking five or more drinks on the same occasion on each of five or more days in the past 30 days; all heavy alcohol users are also binge alcohol users.
Source: Adapted from Substance Abuse and Mental Health Services Administration, Office of Applied Studies. *Results from the 2007 National Survey on Drug Use and Health: National Findings.* Rockville, Md., page 268 (2008).

APPENDIX VIII

ALCOHOL USE, BINGE ALCOHOL USE, AND HEAVY ALCOHOL USE IN THE PAST MONTH IN THE UNITED STATES AMONG PERSONS AGES 12 TO 20 BY DEMOGRAPHIC CHARACTERISTICS, PERCENTAGES, 2006 AND 2007

This table compares alcohol use to binge drinking and heavy alcohol use by gender and race; for example, as can be seen from the table, in 2007, the highest rate of any alcohol use among minors (those not legally allowed to drink) ages 12–20 years was found among whites (32.0 percent), followed by American Indians or Alaska Natives (28.3 percent), and the lowest rates were found among African Americans (18.3 percent). Whites also had the highest rate of heavy drinking in 2007, or 8.0 percent, while Asian youths had the lowest rates, or 1.9 percent.

In considering gender, males and females had almost the same rate of alcohol use, or 28.4 per-

cent of males and 27.3 percent of females in 2007. However, males were more likely to engage in binge drinking (21.1 percent) than females (16.1 percent) in 2007. Males were also more likely to engage in heavy alcohol use (7.8 percent) than females (4.2 percent).

Note that binge alcohol use is defined as drinking five or more drinks on the same occasion (at the same time or within a couple of hours of each other) on at least one day in the past 30 days. Heavy alcohol use is defined as drinking five or more drinks on the same occasion on each of five or more days in the past 30 days. (All heavy alcohol users are also binge alcohol users.)

| | Type of Alcohol Use | | | | | |
| | Alcohol use | | Binge Alcohol Use | | Heavy Alcohol Use | |
Demographic Characteristic	2006	2007	2006	2007	2006	2007
Total	28.3	27.9	19.0	18.6	6.2	6.0
Gender						
Male	29.2	28.4	21.3	21.1	7.9	7.8
Female	27.4	27.3	16.5	16.1	4.3	4.2
Hispanic Origin and Race						
Not Hispanic or Latino	29.0	28.6	19.5	19.1	6.5	6.4
White	32.3	32.0	22.7	22.4	8.2	8.0
Black or African American	18.6	18.3	8.6	8.4	1.3	1.5
American Indian or Alaska Native	31.3	28.3	23.6	Unknown	4.7	Unknown
Asian	19.7	24.7	16.5	16.7	4.8	4.1
Two or more races	27.5	26.2	20.7	16.4	6.3	5.0
Hispanic or Latino	25.3	24.7	16.5	16.7	4.8	4.1

(continues)

(continued)

Demographic Characteristic	Type of Alcohol Use					
	Alcohol use		Binge Alcohol Use		Heavy Alcohol Use	
	2006	2007	2006	2007	2006	2007
Gender/Race/Hispanic Origin						
Male, White, not Hispanic	33.2	32.7	25.2	25.1	10.3	10.2
Female, White, not Hispanic	31.4	31.2	20.0	19.5	5.9	5.6
Male, Black, not Hispanic	18.7	17.2	9.7	9.7	1.5	2.4
Female, Black, Not Hispanic	18.4	19.4	7.5	7.0	1.0	0.6
Male, Hispanic	26.7	25.8	19.4	19.2	6.6	5.6
Female, Hispanic	23.8	23.5	13.2	14.1	2.7	2.6

Source: Adapted from Table G.21, Substance Abuse and Mental Health Services Administration, Office of Applied Studies. *Results from the 2007 National Survey on Drug Use and Health: National Findings.* Rockville, Md., (2008) page 270.

APPENDIX IX

FEDERAL CITATIONS ON THE NATIONAL MINIMUM DRINKING AGE

This appendix provides citations on the federal law regarding the national drinking age and is current as of January 1, 2008. The information was provided by the Alcohol Policy Information System.

UNITED STATES CODE
Title 23-Highways
Chapter 1-Federal-Aid Highways
23 U.S.C.§ 158. National minimum drinking age.

(a) Withholding of Funds for Noncompliance.
(1) In general. The Secretary shall withhold 10 per centum of the amount required to be apportioned to any State under each of sections 104(b)(1), 104(b)(3), and 104(b)(4) of this title of the first day of each fiscal year after the second fiscal year beginning after September 20, 1985, in which the purchase or public possession in such State of any alcoholic beverage by a person who is less than twenty-one years of age is lawful.
(2) State grandfather law as complying. If, before the later of (A) October 1, 1986, or (B) the tenth day following the last day of the first session the legislature of a State convenes after the date of the enactment of this paragraph, such State has in effect a law which makes unlawful the purchase and public possession in such State of any alcoholic beverage by a person who is less than 21 years of age (other than any person who is 18 years of age or older on the day preceding the effective date of such law and at such time could lawfully purchase or publicly possess any alcoholic beverage in such State), such State shall be deemed to be

in compliance with paragraph (1) in each fiscal year in which such law is in effect.
(b) Effect of Withholding of Funds. No funds withheld under this section from apportionment to any State after September 30, 1988 shall be available for apportionment to that State.
(c) Alcoholic Beverage Defined. As used in this section, the term "alcoholic beverage" means:
(1) Beer as defined in section 5052(a) of the Internal Revenue Code of 1986,
(2) Wine of not less than one-half of 1 per centum of alcohol by volume, or
(3) Distilled spirits as defined in section 5002(a)(8) of such Code.

U.S. CODE OF FEDERAL REGULATIONS
Title 23 C.F.R. [Highways]
Chapter II: NATIONAL HIGHWAY TRAFFIC SAFETY ADMINISTRATION AND FEDERAL HIGHWAY ADMINISTRATION, DEPARTMENT OF TRANSPORTATION, SUBCHAPTER B—GUIDELINES.
Part 1208—NATIONAL MINIMUM DRINKING AGE

23 C.F.R. 1208.3. Definitions.

As used in this part:
Alcoholic beverages means beer, distilled spirits and wine containing one-half of one percent or more of alcohol by volume. Beer includes, but is not limited to, ale, lager, porter, stout, sake, and other similar fermented beverages brewed or produced from malt, wholly or in part or from any substitute therefore. Distilled spirits include alcohol, ethanol or spirits or wine in any form, including all dilutions and mixtures thereof from whatever process produced.

Public possession means the possession of any alcoholic beverage for any reason, including consumption on any street or highway or in any public place or in any place open to the public (including a club which is de facto open to the public). The term does not apply to the possession of alcohol for an established religious purpose; when accompanied by a parent, spouse or legal guardian age 21 or older; for medical purposes when prescribed or administered by a licensed physician, pharmacist, dentist, nurse, hospital or medical institution; in private clubs or establishments; or to the sale, handling, transport, or serve in dispensing of any alcoholic beverage pursuant to lawful employment of a person under the age of twenty-one years by a duly licensed manufacturer, wholesaler, or retailer of alcoholic beverages.

Purchase means to acquire by the payment of money or other consideration.

BIBLIOGRAPHY

Abbey, Antonia. "Alcohol-Related Sexual Assault: A Common Problem Among College Students." *Journal of Studies on Alcohol* Suppl. 14 (2002): 118–128.

Abbey, Antonia, et al. "Alcohol and Sexual Assault." *Alcohol Research & Health* 25, no. 1 (2001): 43–51.

Adamec, Christine. *Impulse Control Disorders.* New York: Chelsea House, 2008.

Ahlström, Salme K., and Esa L. Österberg. "International Perspectives on Adolescent and Young Adult Drinking." *Alcohol Research & Health* 28, no. 4 (2004/2005): 258–268.

Akechi, Tatsuo, et al. "Alcohol Consumption and Suicide among Middle-aged Men in Japan." *British Journal of Psychiatry* 188 (2006): 231–236.

Allen, Naomi, et al. "Moderate Alcohol Intake and Cancer Incidence in Women." *Journal of the National Cancer Institute* 101 (2009): 296–305.

Alling, C. "Revealing Alcohol Abuse: To Ask or to Test?" *Alcoholism: Clinical and Experimental Research* 29, no. 7 (2005): 1,257–1,263.

Ames, Genevieve, and Carol Cunradi. "Alcohol Use and Preventing Alcohol-Related Problems among Young Adults in the Military." *Alcohol Research & Health* 28, no. 4 (2004/2005): 252–257.

Ammerman, Robert T., Peggy J. Ott, and Ralph E. Tarter, Eds. *Prevention and Societal Impact of Drug and Alcohol Abuse.* Mahwah, N.J.: Lawrence Erlbaum Associates Publishers, 1999.

Anand, Preetha, et al. "Cancer is a Preventable Disease that Requires Major Lifestyle Changes." *Pharmaceutical Research* 29, no. 9 (2008): 2,097–2,116.

Anda, Robert, M.D. *The Health and Social Impact of Growing Up with Alcohol Abuse and Related Adverse Childhood Experiences: The Human and Economic Costs of the Status Quo.* Available online. URL: http://www.nacoa.net/pdfs/Anda%20NACoA%20Review_web.pdf. Accessed on April 1, 2009.

Anda, Robert F., M.D., et al. "Adverse Childhood Experiences, Alcoholic Parents, and Later Risk of Alcoholism and Depression." *Psychiatric Services* 53, no. 8 (August 2002): 1,001–1,009.

Anderson, John E., Shahul Ebrahim, Louise Floyd, and Hani Atrash. "Prevalence of Risk Factors for Adverse Pregnancy Outcomes during Pregnancy and the Pre-conception Period—United States, 2002–2004." *Maternal and Child Health Journal* 10 (2006): S101–S106.

Anton, Raymond F., M.D. "Combined Pharmacotherapies and Behavioral Interventions for Alcohol Dependence: The COMBINE Study: A Randomized Controlled Trial." *Journal of the American Medical Association* 295, no. 17 (May 3, 2006): 2,003–2,017.

Anton, Raymond F., M.D., et al. "Naltrexone for the Management of Alcohol Dependence." *New England Journal of Medicine* 359, no. 7 (August 14, 2008): 715–721.

Anton, Raymond F., M.D., et al. "Naltrexone Combined with Either Cognitive Behavior or Motivational Enhancement Therapy for Alcohol Dependence." *Journal of Clinical Psychopharmacology* 25, no. 4 (August 2005): 349–357.

Arias, Albert, M.D., and Henry R. Kranzler, M.D. "Treatment of Co-Occurring Alcohol and Other Drug Use Disorders." *Alcohol Research & Health* 31, no. 2 (2008): 155–167.

Armstrong, Elizabeth M., and Ernest L. Abel. "Fetal Alcohol Syndrome: The Origins of a Moral Panic." *Alcohol & Alcoholism* 35, no. 3 (2000): 276–282.

Arnaout, Bachaar, M.D., and Ismene L. Petrakis, M.D. "Diagnosing Co-Morbid Drug Use in Patients with Alcohol Use Disorders." *Alcohol Research & Health* 31, no. 2 (2008): 148–154.

Arnedt, J. Todd, et al. "Neurobehavioral Performance of Residents after Heavy Night Call vs. After Alcohol Ingestion." *Journal of the American Medical Association* 294, no. 9 (September 7, 2005): 1,025–1,033.

Ashton, Elizabeth. "Alcohol Abuse Makes Prescription Drug Abuse More Likely: Research Findings." NIDA Notes 21, 5 (March 2008). Available online. URL: http://www.drugabuse.gov/NIDA_notes/NNvol12N5/alcohol.html. Accessed on March 22, 2009.

Baan, Robert, et al. "Carcinogenicity of Alcoholic Beverages." *Lancet* 8 (2007): 292–293.

Babor, Thomas F., Jack H. Mendelson, Isaac Greenberg, and John Kuehnle. "Experimental Analysis of the 'Happy Hour': Effects of Purchase Price on Alcohol Consumption." *Psychopharmacology* 58 (1978): 35–41.

Back, Sudie E., and Kathleen T. Brady, M.D. "Anxiety Disorders with Comorbid Substance Use Disorders:

Diagnostic and Treatment Considerations." *Psychiatric Annals* 38, no. 11 (2008): 724–729.

Bagnardi, Vincenzo, et al. "Alcohol Consumption and the Risk of Cancer: A Meta-Analysis." *Alcohol Research & Health* 25, no. 4 (2001): 263–270.

Baltieri, Danilo Antonio, et al. "The Role of Alcoholic Beverage Preference in the Severity of Alcohol Dependence and Adherence to the Treatment." *Alcohol* 43 (2009): 185–195.

Barber, J. G., et al. "Intrapersonal versus Peer Group Predictors of Adolescent Drug Use." *Children and Youth Services Review* 21, no. 7 (1999): 565–579.

Barclay, Laurie, M.D., and Desiree Lie, M.D. "Drinking a Glass of Wine Daily Lowers the Risk for Barrett's Esophagus." *Medscape Medical News.* March 9, 2009. Available online to subscribers. URL: http://www.medsape.com/viewarticle/589244. Accessed on April 3, 2009.

Barlow, David H. "Anxiety Disorders, Comorbid Substance Abuse, and Benzodiazepine Discontinuation: Implications for Treatment." In *Treatment of Drug-Dependent Individuals with Comorbid Mental Disorders,* edited by Lisa Simon Onken, Jack D. Blaine, M.D., Sandra Genser, M.D., and Arthur MacNeill Horton, 33–51. Rockville, Md.: National Institute on Drug Abuse, 1997.

Batki, Steven L., et al. "Medical Comorbidity in Patients with Schizophrenia and Alcohol Dependence." *Schizophrenia Research* 107 (2009): 139–146.

Bearer, Cynthia F., M.D., et al. "Biomarkers of Alcohol Use in Pregnancy." National Institute on Alcohol Abuse and Alcoholism. Available online. URL: http://pubs.niaaa.nih.gov/publications/arh28-1/38-43.htm. Accessed on April 8, 2009.

Bedford, D., A. O'Farrell, and F. Howell. "Blood Alcohol Levels in Persons Who Died from Accidents and Suicide." *Irish Medical Journal* 99, no. 3 (2006): 80–83.

Beirness, Douglas J., and Erin E. Beasley. *Alcohol and Drug Use Among Drivers: British Columbia Roadside Survey, 2008.* Canadian Centre on Substance Abuse: Ottawa, Ontario, 2009.

Berg, K. M., et al. "Association Between Alcohol Consumption and Both Osteoporotic Fracture and Bone Density." *American Journal of Medicine* 121, no. 5 (2008): 406–418.

Berridge, Virginia, and Sarah Mars. "History of Addictions." *Journal of Epidemiology and Public Health* 58 (2003): 747–750.

Bertholet, Nicolas, M.D., et al. "Reduction of Alcohol Consumption by Brief Alcohol Intervention in Primary Care." *Archives of Internal Medicine* 165 (May 9, 2005): 986–995.

Betty Ford Institute Consensus Panel. "What Is Recovery? A Working Definition from the Betty Ford Institute." *Journal of Substance Abuse Treatment* 33 (2007): 221–228.

Biederman, Joseph, Michael C. Monuteaux, Thomas Spencer, et al. "Stimulant Therapy and Risk for Subsequent Substance Use Disorders in Male Adults with ADHD: A Naturalistic Controlled 10-year Follow-up Study." *American Journal of Psychiatry* 165, no. 5 (2008): 597–603.

Blanco, Carlos, M.D., et al. "Mental Health of College Students and Their Non-College-Attending Peers: Results from the National Epidemiologic Study on Alcohol and Related Conditions." *Archives of General Psychiatry* 65, no. 12 (2008): 1,429–1,437.

Blow, Frederic C., and Kristen Lawton Barry. *Use and Misuse of Alcohol among Older Women.* Bethesda, Md.: National Institute on Alcohol Abuse and Alcoholism, 2003. Available online. URL: http://pubs.niaaa.nih.gov/publications/arh26-4/308-315.htm. Accessed on March 20, 2009.

Bonnie, Richard J., and Mary Ellen O'Connell, eds. *Reducing Underage Drinking: A Collective Responsibility.* Washington, D.C.: National Academy of Sciences, 2004.

Book, Sarah W., M.D., and Carrie L. Randall. "Social Anxiety Disorder and Alcohol Use." *Alcohol Research & Health* 26, no. 2 (2002): 130–135.

Bray, Jeremy W., and Gary A. Zarkin. "Economic Evaluation of Alcoholism Treatment." *Alcohol Research & Health* 29, no. 1 (2006): 27–33.

Breshears, E. M., S. Yeh, and N. K. Young. *Understanding Substance Abuse and Facilitating Recovery: A Guide for Child Welfare Workers.* Rockville, Md.: Substance Abuse and Mental Health Services Administration, 2004.

Brewer, Robert D., M.D., and Monica H. Swahn. "Binge Drinking and Violence." *Journal of the American Medical Association* 294, no. 5 (August 3, 2005): 616–618.

Brewer, Robert D., et al. "The Risk of Dying in Alcohol-Related Automobile Crashes among Habitual Drunk Drivers." *New England Journal of Medicine* 331, no. 8 (August 25, 1994): 513–517.

Brewster, Joan M., et al. "Characteristics and Outcomes of Doctors in a Substance Dependence Monitoring Programme in Canada: Prospective Descriptive Study." *British Medical Journal* 337 (2008). Available online. URL: http://www.bmj.com/cgi/content/full/337/nov03_4/a2098?view=long&pmid=18981018. Accessed May 15, 2009.

Bryson, Chris L., M.D. "Alcohol Screening Scores and Medication Nonadherence." *Annals of Internal Medicine* 149, no. 11 (2008): 795–803.

Bryson, Chris L., M.D., et al. "The Association of Alcohol Consumption and Incident Heart Failure: The Cardiovascular Health Study." *Journal of the American College of Cardiology* 48, no. 2 (2006): 305–311.

Burckell, Lisa A., and Shelley McMain. "Concurrent Personality Disorders and Substance Use Disorders in Women." In *Women & Addiction: A Comprehensive Handbook,* edited by Kathleen T. Brady, Sudie E. Back, and Shelly F. Greenfield, 269–285. New York: Guilford Press, 2009.

Burns, Lucy, and Maree Teesson. "Alcohol Use Disorders Comorbid with Anxiety, Depression and Drug Use Disorders: Findings from the Australian National Survey of Mental Health and Well Being." *Drug and Alcohol Dependence* 68 (2002): 299–307.

Caetano, Raul, M.D. "NESARC Findings on Alcohol Abuse and Dependence." *Alcohol Research & Health* 29, no. 2 (2006): 152–155.

Caetano, Raul, M.D., et al. "Alcohol Consumption among Racial/Ethnic Minorities: Theory and Research." *Alcohol Research & Health* 22, no. 4 (1998): 233–242.

Caetano, Raul, M.D., et al. "Alcohol-Related Intimate Partner Violence among White, Black, and Hispanic Couples in the United States." *Alcohol Research & Health* 25, no. 1 (2001): 58–65.

Caley, Linda, Charles Syms, Luther Robinson, et al. "What Human Service Professionals Know and Want to Know about Fetal Alcohol Syndrome." *Canadian Journal of Clinical Pharmacology* 15, no. 1 (2008): e117–e123.

Calhoun, Patrick S., et al. "Hazardous Alcohol Use and Receipt of Risk-Reduction Counseling among U.S. Veterans of the Wars in Iraq and Afghanistan." *Journal of Clinical Psychiatry* 69, no. 11 (2008): 1,686–1,693.

Carpenter, Christopher. "How Do Zero Tolerance Drunk Driving Laws Work?" *Journal of Health Economics* 23, no. 1 (2004): 61–83.

Carroll, Jane J., and Bryan E. Robinson. "Depression and Parentification among Adults as Related to Parental Workaholism and Alcoholism." *Family Journal: Counseling and Therapy for Couples and Families* 8, no. 4 (2000): 360–367.

Casanueva, Cecilia, Sandra L. Martin, and Desmond K. Runyan. "Repeated Reports for Child Maltreatment among Intimate Partner Violence Victims: Findings from the National Survey of Child and Adolescent Well-Being." *Child Abuse & Neglect* 33, no. 2 (2009): 84–93.

Caspi, Avshalom, et al. "Personality Differences Predict Health-Risk Behaviors in Young Adulthood: Evidence from a Longitudinal Study." *Journal of Personality and Social Psychology* 73 (1997): 1,052–1,063.

Centers for Disease Control and Prevention. "Surveillance for Violent Deaths—National Violent Death Reporting System, 16 States, 2005." *Morbidity and Mortality Weekly Report* 57, no. SS-3 (April 11, 2008).

———. "Youth Risk Behavior Surveillance—United States, 2007." *Morbidity and Mortality Weekly Report* 57, no. SS-4 (June 6, 2008).

Chai, Y. G., et al. "Alcohol and Aldehyde Dehydrogenase Polymorphisms in Men with Type I and Type II Alcoholism." *American Journal of Psychiatry* 162, no. 5 (2005): 1,003–1,005.

Chang, Grace, M.D. "Alcohol Intake and Pregnancy." UpToDate. Available online to subscribers only. URL: http://www.uptodate.com/online/content/topic.do?topicKey=maternal/5807&selectedTitle=2~150&source=search_result. Updated October 8, 2008.

———. "Alcohol-Screening Instruments for Pregnant Women." *Alcohol Research & Health* 25, no. 3 (2001): 204–209.

Chappel, John, M.D., and Garrett O'Connor, M.D. *12-Step Programs.* Addiction Medicine Review Course, Foundations of Addiction Medicine: Evidence & Art. October 6–9, 2004. Slide presentation.

Chen, Chiung M., Mary C. Dugour, M.D., and Hsiao-ye Yo. "Alcohol Consumption among Young Adults Ages 18–24 in the United States: Results from the 2001–2002 NESARC Survey." *Alcohol Research & Health* 28, no. 4 (2004/2005): 269–280.

Chen, Chiung M., and Hsiao-ye Yi. *Surveillance Report #84: Trends in Alcohol-Related Morbidity among Short-Stay Community Hospital Discharges, United States, 1979–2006.* Rockville, Md.: National Institutes of Health, 2008.

Chou, S. Patricia, et al. "Twelve-Month Prevalence and Changes in Driving After Drinking: United States, 1991–1992 and 2001–2002." *Alcohol Research & Health* 29, no. 2 (2006): 145–151.

Clark, Duncan B., M.D. "Childhood Antisocial Behavior and Adolescent Alcohol Use Disorders." *Alcohol Research & Health* 26, no. 2 (2002): 109–115.

Clark, Duncan B., et al. "Physical and Sexual Abuse, Depression and Alcohol Use Disorders in Adolescents: Onsets and Outcomes." *Drug and Alcohol Dependence* 69 (2003): 51–60.

Collins, Kate, and Sanjay Matthew, M.D. "A Review of Generalized Anxiety Disorder." *Perspectives in Clinical Psychiatry: A Clinical Update.* Supplement to *Psychiatric Times,* Issue 2 of 4 (September 2008): 3–8.

Connors, Gerard J., Dennis M. Donovan, and Carlo C. DiClemente. *Substance Abuse Treatment and the Stages of Change.* New York: Guilford Press, 2001.

Corder, R., et al. "Red Wine Procyanidins and Vascular Health." *Nature* 444 (2006): 566.

Crum, Rosa M., M.D., et al. "Depressed Mood in Childhood and Subsequent Alcohol Use Through Adolescence and Young Adulthood." *Archives of General Psychiatry* 65, no. 6 (2008): 702–712.

Cutler, Robert B., and David A. Fishbain. "Are Alcoholism Treatments Effective? The Project MATCH Data." *BMC Public Health* 5, no. 75 (2005). Available online. URL: http://www.biomedcentral.com/1471-2458/5/75. Accessed July 27, 2009.

Darbo, Nancy. "Overview of Issues Related to Coercion in Substance Abuse Treatment: Part I." *Journal of Addictions Nursing* 20, no. 1 (2009): 16–23.

Dawson, Deborah A., Bridget F. Grant, and W. June Ruan. "The Association between Stress and Drinking: Modifying Effects of Gender and Vulnerability." *Alcohol & Alcoholism* 40, no. 5 (2005): 453–460.

Dawson, Deborah, et al. "Recovery from DSM-IV Alcohol Dependence: United States, 2001–2002." *Alcohol Research & Health* 29, no. 2 (2006): 131–142.

Deas, Deborah, M.D., and Suzanne Thomas. "Comorbid Psychiatric Factors Contributing to Adolescent Alcohol and Other Drug Use." *Alcohol Research & Health* 26, no. 2 (2002): 116–121.

De Gottardi, Andrea, M.D., et al. "A Simple Score for Predicting Alcohol Relapse After Live Transplantation: Results from 387 Patients Over 15 Years." *Archives of Internal Medicine* 167 (June 11, 2007): 1,183–1,188.

Desai, Mayur, Robert A. Rosenheck, M.D., and Thomas J. Craig, M.D. "Screening for Alcohol Use Disorders among Medical Outpatients: The Influence of Individual and Facility Characteristics." *American Journal of Psychiatry* 162, no. 8 (August 2005): 1,521–1,526.

Di Castelnuovo, Augusto, et al. "Alcohol Dosing and Total Mortality in Men and Women: An Updated Meta-analysis of 34 Prospective Studies." *Archives of Internal Medicine* 166 (December 11/25, 2006): 2,437–2,445.

Dick, Danielle M., and Arpane Agrawal. "The Genetics of Alcohol and Other Drug Dependence." *Alcohol Research & Health* 31, no. 2 (2008): 111–167.

DiClemente, Carlo C. *Addiction and Change: How Addictions Develop and Addicted People Recover.* New York: Guilford Press, 2003.

DiClemente, Carlo C., Lori E. Bellino, and Tara M. Neavins. "Motivation for Change and Alcoholism Treatment." *Alcohol Research & Health* 23, no. 2 (1999): 86–92.

Dietrich, Richard, Sergey Zimatkin, M.D., and Sergey Pronko, M.D. "Oxidation of Ethanol in the Brain and Its Consequences." *Alcohol Research & Health* 29, no. 4 (2006): 266–273.

Dill, Patricia L., and Elisabeth Wells-Parker. "Court-Mandated Treatment for Convicted Drinking Drivers." *Alcohol Research & Health* 29, no. 1 (2006): 41–48.

Dimich-Ward, Helen, et al. "Occupational Mortality among Bartenders and Waiters." *Canadian Journal of Public Health* 79 (May/June 1988): 194–197.

Doctor, Ronald, Ada Kahn, and Christine Adamec. *The Encyclopedia of Phobias, Fears and Anxiety Disorders.* 3rd ed. New York: Facts On File, 2008.

Doctor, Ronald, and Frank Shirimoto. *Encyclopedia of Traumatic Stress Disorders.* New York: Facts On File, 2009.

Dowd, E. Thomas, and Lorene Rugle, eds. *Substance Abuse: A Practitioner's Guide to Comparative Treatments.* New York: Springer Publishing Co., 1999.

Drake, Robert E., M.D., and Kim T. Mueser. "Co-Occurring Alcohol Use Disorder and Schizophrenia." *Alcohol Research & Health* 26, no. 2 (2002): 99–102.

Drobes, David J. "Concurrent Alcohol and Tobacco Dependence: Mechanisms and Treatment." *Alcohol Research & Health* 26, no. 2 (2002): 136–142.

Dube, Shanta R., et al. "Long-Term Consequences of Childhood Sexual Abuse by Gender of Victim." *American Journal of Preventive Medicine* 28, no. 5 (2005): 430–438.

Du Mont, Janice, et al. "Factors Associated with Suspected Drug-Facilitated Sexual Assault." *Canadian Medical Association Journal* 180, no. 5 (2009): 513–519.

Dunn, W., et al. "Modest Wine Drinking and Decreased Prevalence of Suspected Nonalcoholic Fatty Liver Disease." *Hepatology* 47, no. 6 (2008): 1,947–1,954.

DuPont, Robert L., M.D., and Mark S. Gold, M.D. "Comorbidity and 'Self-Medication.'" In *Dual Disorders: Nosology, Diagnosis, & Treatment Confusion—Chicken or Egg,* edited by Mark S. Gold, M.D., 13–23. Binghamton, N.Y.: Haworth Medical Press, 2007.

DuPont, Robert L., M.D., et al. "Setting the Standard for Recovery: Physicians' Health Programs." *Journal of Substance Abuse Treatment* 36 (2009): 159–171.

Durdle, Heather, and Kevin M. Gorey. "A Meta-Analysis Examining the Relations Among Pathological Gambling, Obsessive-Compulsive Disorder, and Obsessive-Compulsive Traits." *Psychological Reports* 103 (2008): 485–498.

Echebúria, Enrique, Richardo Bravo de Medina, and Javier Aizpiri. "Comorbidity of Alcohol Dependence and Personality Disorders." *Alcohol & Alcoholism* 42, no. 6 (2007): 618–622.

Edenberg, Howard J. "The Genetics of Alcohol Metabolism: Role of Alcohol Dehydrogenase and Aldehyde Dehydrogenase Variants." *Alcohol Research & Health* 30, no. 1 (2007): 5–13.

Edwards, Valerie J., et al. "Relationship between Multiple Forms of Childhood Maltreatment and Adult Mental Health in Community Respondents: Results from the Adverse Childhood Experiences Study." *American Journal of Psychiatry* 160, no. 8 (August 2003): 1,453–1,460.

Ehlers, Cindy L., et al. "The Clinical Course of Alcoholism in 243 Mission Indians." *American Journal of Psychiatry* 161, no. 7 (2004): 1,204–1,210.

Elbogen, Eric B., and Sally C. Johnson, M.D. "The Intricate Link Between Violence and Mental Disorder: Results from the National Epidemiologic Survey on Alcohol and Related Conditions." *Archives of General Psychiatry* 66, no. 2 (2009): 152–161.

Ende, Gabriele, et al. "Monitoring the Effects of Chronic Alcohol Consumption and Abstinence on Brain Metabolism: A Longitudinal Proton Magnetic Resonance Spectroscopy Study." *Biological Psychiatry* 58 (2005): 974–980.

Engels, C. M., E. Rutger, et al. "Alcohol Portrayal on Television Affects Actual Drinking Behavior." *Alcohol & Alcoholism* 44, no. 3 (2009): 244–249.

Eng, Mimy Y., Marc A. Schuckit, and Tom L. Smith. "The Level of Response to Alcohol in Daughters of Alcoholics and Controls." *Drug and Alcohol Dependence* 79 (2005): 83–93.

"Environmental and Contextual Considerations." *Alcohol Research & Health* 28, no. 3 (2004/2005): 155–162.

Epstein, Murray, M.D. "Alcohol's Impact on Kidney Function." *Alcohol Health & Research World* 21, no. 1 (1997): 84–93.

Falk, Daniel E., Hsiao-Ye Yi, and Susanne Hiller-Sturmhofel. "An Epidemiologic Analysis of Co-Occurring Alcohol and Tobacco Use and Disorders: Findings from the National Epidemiologic Survey on Alcohol and Related Conditions." *Alcohol Research & Health* 29, no. 3 (2006): 162–171.

Fals-Stewart, W., K. E. Leonard, and G. R. Birchler. "The Occurrence of Male-to-Female Intimate Partner Violence on Days of Men's Drinking: The Moderating Effects of Antisocial Personality Disorder." *Journal of Consulting and Clinical Psychology* 73 (2005): 239–248.

Fan, Amy Z., et al. "Association of Lifetime Alcohol Drinking Trajectories with Cardiometabolic Risk." *Journal of Clinical Endocrinology & Metabolism* 93 (2008): 154–161.

Fell, James C., and Robert B. Voas. "Mothers Against Drunk Driving (MADD): The First 25 Years." *Traffic Injury Prevention* 7 (2006): 195–212.

Fergusson, David M., Joseph M. Boden, and L. John Horwood. "Tests of Causal Links Between Alcohol Abuse or Dependence and Major Depression." *Archives of General Psychiatry* 66, no. 3 (2009): 260–266.

Flora, David, and Laurie Chassin. "Changes in Drug Use During Young Adulthood: The Effects of Parent Alcoholism and Transition into Marriage." *Psychology of Addictive Behaviors* 19, no. 4 (2005): 352–362.

Flowers, Nicole T., et al. "Patterns of Alcohol Consumption and Alcohol-Impaired Driving in the United States." *Alcoholism: Clinical and Experimental Research* 31, no. 4 (2008): 639–644.

Fluke, J. D., et al. *Rereporting and Recurrence of Child Maltreatment: Findings from NCANDS.* Washington, D.C.: U.S. Department of Health and Human Services, Office of the Assistant Secretary for Planning and Evaluation, 2005.

Frank, Erica, et al. "Alcohol Consumption and Alcohol Counselling Behaviour among U.S. Medical Students: Cohort Study." *British Medical Journal* 337 (2008). Available online. URL: http://www.bmj.com/cgi/content/full/337/nov07_1/a2155?view=long&pmid=18996938. Accessed July 29, 2009.

Franklin, Martin E., et al. "The Child and Adolescent Trichotillomania Impact Project: Descriptive Psychopathology, Comorbidity, Functional Impairment, and Treatment Utilization." *Journal of Developmental & Behavioral Pediatrics* 29 (2008): 493–500.

Freedman, Steven D., M.D., and Michele D. Bishop. "Etiology and Pathogenesis of Chronic Pancreatitis in Adults." Private subscriber service online. URL: http://wwwuptodate.com/online/content/topic.do?topicKey=pancdis/5929&selectedTitle4~79&source=search_result. October 6, 2008. Accessed on March 12, 2009.

Fu, Aiang, M.D., et al. "Shared Genetic Risk of Major Depression, Alcohol Dependence, and Marijuana Dependence." *Archives of General Psychiatry* 59, no. 12 (2002): 1,125–1,132.

Fuchs, C. S., et al. "Alcohol Consumption and Mortality among Women." *New England Journal of Medicine* 332 (1995): 1,245.

Funk, Douglas, Peter W. Marinelli, and Anh D. Le. "Biological Processes Underlying Co-Use of Alcohol and Nicotine: Neuronal Mechanisms, Cross-Tolerance, and Genetic Factors." *Alcohol Research & Health* 29, no. 3 (2006): 186–192.

Galaif, Elisha R., et al. "Gender Differences in the Prediction of Problem Alcohol Use in Adulthood: Exploring the Influence of Family Factors and Childhood Maltreatment." *Journal of Studies on Alcohol* 62, no. 4 (2001): 486–493.

Galanter, Marc, ed. *Alcohol Problems in Adolescents and Young Adults: Epidemiology, Neurobiology, Prevention, and Treatment.* New York: Springer, 2006.

Galen, Luke W., and W. M. Rogers. "Religiosity, Alcohol Expectancies, Drinking Motives and Their Interaction in the Prediction of Drinking among College Students." *Journal of Studies on Alcohol* 65, no. 4 (2004): 469–476.

Garbutt, James C., M.D. "The State of Pharmacotherapy for the Treatment of Alcohol Dependence." *Journal of Substance Abuse Treatment* 36, no. 1 (2009): S15–S23.

Garbutt, James C., M.D., et al. "Efficacy and Tolerability of Long-Acting Injectable Naltrexone: A Randomized Controlled Trial." *Journal of the American Medical Association* 293, no. 13 (April 6, 2005): 1,617–1,625.

Garcia-Andrade, C., T. L. Wall, and C. L. Ehlers. "The Firewater Myth and Response to Alcohol in Mission Indians." *American Journal of Psychiatry* 154 (1997): 983–988.

Garland, Ann, et al. "Diagnostic Profile Associated with Use of Mental Health and Substance Abuse Services Among High-Risk Youths." *Psychiatric Services* 54, no. 4 (April 2003): 562–564.

Garno, Jessica L., et al. "Impact of Childhood Abuse on the Clinical Course of Bipolar Disorder." *British Journal of Psychiatry* 186 (2005): 121–125.

Gentilello, Larry M., M.D. "Alcohol and Injury: American College of Surgeons Committee on Trauma Requirements for Trauma Center Intervention." *Journal of Trauma: Injury, Infection, and Critical Care* 62, Suppl. (2007): S44–S45.

Gentilello, Larry M., et al. "Alcohol Interventions for Trauma Patients Treated in Emergency Departments and Hospitals: A Cost-Benefit Analysis." *Annals of Surgery* 241, no. 4 (2005): 541–550.

George, David T., et al. "Neurokinin 1 Receptor Antagonism as a Possible Therapy for Alcoholism." *Science* 319 (2008): 1,536–1,539.

Gibbs, Deborah A., et al. "Child Maltreatment and Substance Abuse among U.S. Army Soldiers." *Child Maltreatment* 13, no. 3 (2008): 259–268.

Gilbertson, Rebecca, et al. "Effects of Acute Alcohol Consumption in Older and Young Adults: Perceived Impairment Versus Psychomotor Performance." *Journal of Studies on Alcohol and Drugs* 70 (2009): 242–252.

Gilbertson, Rebecca, Robert Prather, and Sara Jo Nixon. "The Role of Selected Factors in the Development and Consequences of Alcohol Dependence." *Alcohol Research & Health* 31, no. 4 (2008): 389–399.

Gilman, Jodi M., et al. "Why We Like to Drink: A Functional Magnetic Resonance Imaging Study of the Rewarding and Anxiolytic Effects of Alcohol." *Journal of Neuroscience* 28, no. 18 (2008): 44,583–44,591.

Gilpin, Nicholas, and George F. Koob. "Neurobiology of Alcohol Dependence: Focus on Motivational Mechanisms." *Alcohol Research & Health* 31, no. 3 (2008): 185–194.

Goh, Siew Simg C., et al. "The Red Wine Antioxidant Resveratrol Prevents Cardiomyocyte Injury Following Ischemia—Reperfusion via Multiple Sites and Mechanisms." *Antioxidants & Redox Signaling* 9, no. 1 (2007): 101–113.

Gold, Mark S., M.D., and Mark D. Aronson, M.D. "Treatment of Alcohol Abuse and Dependence." UptoDate. Available online to subscribers. URL: http://www.uptodate.com/online/content/topic.do?topicKey=subabuse/7484&selected Title=3~150&source=search_result. Accessed on March 13, 2009.

Gold, Mark S., M.D., and Kimberly Frost-Pineda. "Substance Abuse and Psychiatric Dual Disorders: Focus on Tobacco." *Journal of Dual Diagnosis* 1, no. 1 (2004): 15–36.

Gold, Mark S., and L. J. Merlo. *Addiction Research Update 2009.* Paper presented at the 11th Annual Conference of the China Association for Science and Technology International Symposium on Drug Abuse and Addictive Behavior. September 8–10, 2009. Chongqing, P.R. China.

Gold, Mark S., M.D., ed. *Dual Disorders: Nosology, Diagnosis, & Treatment Confusion—Chicken or Egg?* Binghamton, N.Y.: Haworth Medical Press, 2007.

Goldstein, Benjamin, M.D., Nathan Herrmann, M.D., and Kenneth I. Shulman, M.D. "Comorbidity in Bipolar Disorder among the Elderly: Results from an Epidemiological Community Sample." *American Journal of Psychiatry* 163, no. 2 (2006): 319–321.

Gone, Joseph P. "Mental Health Services for Native Americans in the 21st Century United States." *Professional Psychology Research and Practice* 35, no. 1 (2004): 10–18.

Goplerud, Eric, and Laura Jacobus-Kantor. *Improving Criminal Justice Interventions for People with Alcohol Problems.* Washington, D.C.: National Partnership on Alcohol Misuse and Crime, March 2009.

Gorman, Jack M., M.D. *The Essential Guide to Psychiatric Drugs.* 4th ed. New York: St. Martin's Griffin, 2007.

Graham, Noni A., Christopher J. Hammond III, and Mark S. Gold, M.D. "Caffeine in Miscarriages: It's Not Just in the Coffee." *American Journal of Obstetrics & Gynecology* (November 2008). Available online. URL: http://download.journals.elsevierhealth.com/pdfs/journals/0002-9378/PIIS00022937808006066.pdf. Accessed April 10, 2009.

Grant, Bridget F., et al. "The 12-Month Prevalence and Trends in DSM-IV Alcohol Abuse and Dependence: United States, 1991–1992 and 2001–2002." *Alcohol Research & Health* 29, no. 2 (2006): 79–91.

Grant, Bridget F., et al. "Co-Occurrence of 12-Month Alcohol and Drug Use Disorders and Personality Disorders in the United States: Results from the National Epidemiologic Survey on Alcohol and Related Conditions." *Alcohol Research & Health* 29, no. 2 (2006): 121–130.

Grant, Bridget F., et al. "Prevalence and Co-Occurrence of Substance Use Disorders and Independent Mood and Anxiety Disorders: Results from the National Epidemiologic Survey on Alcohol and Related Conditions." *Alcohol Research & Health* 29, no. 2 (2006): 107–120.

Grant, B. F., and D. A. Dawson. "Age at Onset of Alcohol Use and Its Association with DSM-IV Alcohol Abuse and Dependence: Results from the National Longitudinal Alcohol Epidemiologic Survey." *Journal of Substance Abuse* 9 (1997): 103–110.

Grant, Jon E. *Impulse Control Disorders: A Clinician's Guide to Understanding and Treating Behavioral Addictions.* New York: W.W. Norton, 2008.

Grant, Jon E., M.D., and Brian L. Odlaug. "Challenges in Diagnosing and Treating Obsessive-Compulsive Disorder." *Perspectives in Clinical Psychiatry: A Clinical Update.* Supplement to *Psychiatric Times,* Issue 2 of 4 (September 2008): 25–30.

Grant, Jon E., M.D., and Suck Won Kim. "Clinical Characteristics and Psychiatric Comorbidity of Pyromania." *Journal of Clinical Psychiatry* 68, no. 11 (2007): 1,717–1,722.

Green, Carla A. "Gender and Use of Substance Abuse Treatment Services." *Alcohol Research & Health* 29, no. 1 (2006): 55–62.

Greenfield, Lawrence A. *Alcohol and Crime: An Analysis of National Data on the Prevalence of Alcohol Involvement in Crime.* Washington, D.C.: Bureau of Justice Statistics, 1998.

Guindalini, C., et al. "Association of Genetic Variants of Alcohol Dehydrogenase 4 with Alcohol Dependence in Brazilian Patients." *American Journal of Psychiatry* 162, no. 5 (2005): 1,005–1,007.

Grucza, Richard A., and Laura J. Bierut, M.D. "Co-occurring Risk Factors for Alcohol Dependence and Habitual Smoking: Update on Findings from the Collaborative Study on the Genetics of Alcoholism." *Alcohol Research & Health* 29, no. 3 (2006): 172–178.

Grupp, Kitty. "Women with Co-Occurring Substance Abuse Disorders and PTSD: How Women Understand Their Illness." *Journal of Addictions Nursing* 19 (2008): 49–54.

Gunter, Tracy D., et al. "Frequency of Mental and Addictive Disorders among 320 Men and Women Entering the Iowa Prison System: Use of the MINI-Plus." *Journal of the American Academy of Psychiatry Law* 36 (2008): 27–34.

Gunzerath, Lorraine, et al. "National Institute on Alcohol Abuse and Alcoholism Report on Moderate Drinking." *Alcoholism: Clinical and Experimental Research* 28, no. 6 (2004): 829–847.

Haggård-Grann, Ulrika, John Hallqvist, Niklas Långström, and Jette Möller. "The Role of Alcohol and Drugs in Triggering Criminal Violence: A Case–Crossover Study." *Addiction* 101 (2006): 100–108.

Hampton, Tracy. "Interplay of Genes and Environment Found in Adolescents' Alcohol Abuse." *Journal of the American Medical Association* 295, no. 15 (2006): 1,760–1,762.

Harford, Thomas C., and Sharon D. Brooks. "Cirrhosis Mortality and Occupation." *Journal of Studies on Alcohol* 53 (1992): 463–468.

Hasin, Deborah S., et al. "Prevalence, Correlates, Disability, and Comorbidity of DSM-IV Alcohol Abuse and Dependence in the United States: Results from the National Epidemiologic Survey on Alcohol and Related Conditions." *Archives of General Psychiatry* 64, no. 7 (2007): 830–842.

Heilig, Markus, and Mark Egli. "Pharmacological Treatment of Alcohol Dependence: Target Symptoms and Target Mechanisms." *Pharmacology & Therapeutics* 111, no. 3 (2006): 855–876.

Hemmingsson, Tomas, and Gunille Ringback Weitoft. "Alcohol-related Hospital Utilization and Mortality in Different Occupations in Sweden in 1991–1995." *Scandinavian Journal of Work & Environmental Health* 27, no. 6 (2001): 412–419.

Hester, Reid K., and Joseph H. Miller. "Computer-based Tools for Diagnosis and Treatment of Alcohol Problems." *Alcohol Research & Health* 29, no. 1 (2006): 36–40.

Higgins, Stephen T., and Nancy M. Petry. "Contingency Management: Incentives for Sobriety." *Alcohol Research & Health* 23, no. 2 (1999): 122–127.

Hill, Shirley Y., et al. "Disruption of Orbitofrontal Cortex Laterality in Offspring from Multiplex Alcohol Dependence Families." *Biological Psychiatry* 65 (2009): 129–136.

Hingson, R. W., T. Heeren, and M. R. Winter. "Age at Drinking Onset and Alcohol Dependence: Age at Onset, Duration, and Severity." *Archives of Pediatric and Adolescent Medicine* 160, no. 7 (July 2006): 739–746.

Hingson, Ralph, Timothy Heeren, Michael R. Winter, and Henry Wechsler. "Early Age of First Drunkenness as a Factor in College Students' Unplanned and Unprotected Sex Attributable to Drinking." *Pediatrics* 111 (2003): 34–41.

———. "Magnitude of Alcohol-related Mortality and Morbidity among U.S. College Students Ages 18–24: Changes from 1998 to 2001." *Annual Review of Public Health* 26 (2005): 259–279.

Hingson, Ralph, Timothy Heeren, and Ronda Zakocs. "Age of Drinking Onset and Involvement in Physical Fights After Drinking." *Pediatrics* 108 (2001): 872–877.

Hingson, Ralph, and Michael Winter. "Epidemiology and Consequences of Drinking and Driving." *Alcohol Research & Health* 27, no. 1 (2003): 63–78.

Hingson, Ralph W., and Wenxing Zha. "Age of Drinking Onset, Alcohol Use Disorders, Frequent Heavy Drinking, and Unintentionally Injuring Oneself and Others After Drinking." *Pediatrics* 123, no. 6 (2009): 1,477–1,484.

Hirschfeld, Robert, M.D., and Lana A. Vornik. "Bipolar Disorder—Costs and Comorbidity." *American Journal of Managed Care* 11, no. 3 Suppl. (2005): S85–S90.

Hoblyn, Jennifer C., M.D., et al. "Substance Use Disorders as Risk Factors for Psychiatric Hospitalization in Bipolar Disorder." *Psychiatric Services* 60, no. 1 (January 2009): 50–55.

Holder, Harold D. "Community Prevention of Young Adult Drinking and Associated Problems." *Alcohol Research & Health* 28, no. 4 (2004/2005): 245–249.

Hollander, Eric, M.D., Bryann R. Baker, Jessica Kahn, and Dan J. Stein, M.D. "Conceptualizing and Assessing Impulse-Control Disorders." In *Clinical Manual of Impulse-Control Disorders,* edited by Eric Hollander, M.D. and Dan J. Stein, 1–18. Washington, D.C.: American Psychiatric Publishing, 2006.

Howard, A. A., H. H. Arnstein, and M. N. Gourevitch. "Effect of Alcohol Consumption on Diabetes Mellitus: A Systematic Review." *Annals of Internal Medicine* 140 (2004): 211–219.

Howe, David. *Patterns of Adoption: Nature, Nurture and Psychosocial Development.* Oxford, U.K.: Blackwell Science, 1998.

Hulme, T., et al. "Risk Factors for Physical Child Abuse in Infants and Toddlers." *European Journal of Pediatric Surgery* 18, no. 6 (2008): 387–391.

Huppert, Jonathan D., and Moira Ryna. "Generalized Anxiety Disorder." In *Clinical Manual of Anxiety Disorders,* edited by Dan J. Stein, M.D., 147–171. Washington, D.C.: American Psychiatric Press, 2004.

Hutton, Heidi E., et al. "The Relationship between Recent Alcohol Use and Sexual Behaviors: Gender Differences Among Sexually Transmitted Diseases Clinic Patients." *Alcoholism: Clinical and Experimental Research* 32, no. 11 (2008): 2,008–2,015.

Iacono, William G., and Matt McGue. "Minnesota Twin Family Study." *Twin Research* 5, no. 5 (2002): 484–487.

Ibanez, Angela, et al. "Gender Differences in Pathological Gambling." *Journal of Clinical Psychiatry* 64, no. 3 (2003): 295–301.

Ikehara, Satoyo, et al. "Alcohol Consumption, Social Support, and Risk of Stroke and Coronary Heart Disease Among Japanese Men: The JPHC Study." *Alcoholism: Clinical and Experimental Research* 33, no. 4 (2009): 1–8.

Irons, Daniel E., et al. "Mendelian Randomization: A Novel Test for the Gateway Hypothesis and Models of Gene-Environment Interplay." *Development and Psychopathology* 19 (2007): 1,181–1,195.

Israel, Yedy, et al. "Combined Effects of Aldehyde Dehydrogenase Variants and Maternal Mitochondrial Genes on Alcohol Consumption." National Institute of Alcohol Abuse and Alcoholism. Available online. URL: http://pubs.niaaa.nih.gtov/publications/arh294/282-285.htm. Accessed on June 25, 2008.

Jacob, Theodore, and M. Winkle. "Young Adult Children of Alcoholic, Depressed and Nondistressed Parents." *Journal of Studies on Alcohol* 61, no. 6 (2000): 836–844.

Jacobson, Isabel J., et al. "Alcohol Use and Alcohol-Related Problems before and after Military Combat Deployment." *Journal of the American Medical Association* 200, no. 6 (August 13, 2008): 663–673.

Jarman, D. W., T. S. Naimi, S. P. Pickard, W. R. Daley, and A. K. De. "Binge Drinking and Occupation, North Dakota, 2004–2005." *Preventing Chronic Disease* 4, no. 4 (2007).

Johansen, Ditte, et al. "Food Buying Habits of People Who Buy Wine or Beer: Cross-Sectional Study." *British Medical Journal* 332 (2006): 519–522.

Johnson, Bankole A., Norman Rosenthal, Julie A. Capece, et al. "Topiramate for Treating Alcohol Dependence: A Randomized Controlled Trial." *Journal of the American Medical Association* 298, no. 14 (2007): 1,641–1,651.

Johnson, Eric O., and Naomi Breslau. "Sleep Problems and Substance Use in Adolescence." *Drug and Alcohol Dependence* 64 (2001): 1–7.

Johnston, Lloyd D., Patrick M. O'Malley, Jerald G. Bachman, and John E. Schulenberg. *Monitoring the Future: National Results on Adolescent Drug Use. Overview of Key Findings, 2007.* Bethesda, Md.: National Institute on Drug Abuse, 2008.

Johnston, Lloyd D., et al. *Monitoring the Future: National Survey Results on Drug Use, 1975–2007.* Vol. II, *College Students and Adults Age 19–45.* Bethesda, Md.: National Institute on Drug Abuse, 2008.

Jones, K. L., and D. W. Smith. "Recognition of the Fetal Alcohol Syndrome in Early Infancy." *Lancet* 3, no. 2 (1973): 999–1,001.

Joslyn, Geoff. "Chromosome 15q25.1 Genetic Markers Associated with Level of Response to Alcohol in Humans." *Proceedings of the National Academy of Sciences* 105, no. 51 (2008): 20,368–20,373.

Kaltenbach, Tonya, M.D., Seth Crockett, M.D., and Lauren B. Gerson, M.D. "Are Lifestyle Measures Effective in Patients with Gastroesophageal Reflux Disease?" *Archives of Internal Medicine* 166 (May 8, 2006): 965–971.

Karam, E., K. Kypri, and M. Salamoun. "Alcohol Use among College Students: An International Perspective." *Current Opinion in Psychiatry* 20 (2007): 213–221.

Karch, Debra L., et al. "Surveillance for Violent Deaths—National Violent Death Reporting System, 16 States, 2005." *Morbidity and Mortality Weekly Report* 57, SS-3 (April 11, 2008).

Karkoulias, Kiriakos, et al. "The Alcoholic Lung Disease: Historical Background and Clinical Features." *Medicina (Kaunas)* 44, no. 9 (2008): 651–664.

Karpyak, Victor M., et al. "Sequences Variations of the Human MPDZ Gene and Association with Alcoholism in Subjects with European Ancestry." *Alcohol: Clinical and Experimental Research* 33, no. 4 (2009): 712–721.

Kashdan, Todd B., Charlene J. Vetter, and R. Lorraine Collins. "Substance Use in Young Adults: Associations with Personality and Gender." *Addictive Behaviors* 30, no. 2 (2004): 259–269.

Kelley, Michelle L., and William Fals-Stewart. "Psychiatric Disorders of Children Living with Drug-Abusing, Alcohol-Abusing, and Non-Substance-Abusing Fathers." *Journal of the American Academy of Child & Adolescent Psychiatry* 43, no. 5 (May 2004): 621–628.

Kelly, Thomas M. "Psychiatric Disorders among Older Adolescents Treated in Emergency Departments on Weekends: A Comparison with a Matched Community Sample." *Journal of Studies on Alcohol* 64, no. 5 (2003): 616–622.

Kelly, Thomas M., Jack R. Cornelius, and Duncan B. Clark. "Psychiatric Disorders and Attempted Suicide among Adolescents with Substance Use Disorders." *Drug and Alcohol Dependence* 73 (2004): 87–97.

Kerr-Corrêa, Florence, et al. "Patterns of Alcohol Use Between Genders: A Cross-Cultural Evaluation. *Journal of Affective Disorders* 102 (2007): 265–275.

Kershaw, Corey D., M.D., and David M. Guidot, M.D. "Alcoholic Lung Disease." *Alcohol Research & Health* 31, no. 1 (2008): 66–75.

Kessler, Ronald C. "The Epidemiology of Dual Diagnosis." *Biological Psychiatry* 56, no. 10 (2004): 730–737.

———. "The Prevalence and Correlates of Adult ADHD in the United States: Results from the National Comorbidity Survey Replication." *American Journal of Psychiatry* 163, no. 4 (2006): 716–723.

Kessler, Ronald C., et al. "The Prevalence and Correlates of DSM-IV Intermittent Explosive Disorder in the National Comorbidity Survey Replication." *Archives of General Psychiatry* 63 (2006): 669–678.

Kessler, Ronald C., et al. "The Prevalence and Correlates of DSM-IV Pathological Gambling in the National Comorbidity Survey Replication." *Psychological Medicine* 38, no. 9 (2008): 1,351–1,360.

King, Dana E., M.D., Arch G. Mainous III, and Mark E. Geesey. "Adopting Moderate Alcohol Consumption in Middle Age: Subsequent Cardiovascular Events." *American Journal of Medicine* 121 (2008): 201–206.

King, Serena M., et al. "Parental Alcohol Dependence and the Transmission of Adolescent Behavioral Disinhibition: A Study of Adoptive and Non-Adoptive Families." *Addiction* 104 (2009): 578–586.

Kleber, Herbert D., M.D., et al. (Work Group on Substance Use Disorders). *Practice Guidelines for the Treatment of Patients with Substance Use Disorders.* 2nd ed. Washington, D.C.: American Psychiatric Association, 2006.

Kodl, Molly, Steven S. Fu, M.D., and Anne M. Joseph, M.D. "Tobacco Cessation Treatment for Alcohol-Dependent Smokers: When Is the Best Time?" *Alcohol Research & Health* 29, no. 3 (2006): 203–227.

Köhnke, Michael D. "Approach to the Genetics of Alcoholism: A Review Based on Pathophysiology." *Biochemical Pharmacology* 75 (2008): 160–177.

Kool, B., et al. "The Contribution of Alcohol to Falls at Home Among Working-Aged Adults." *Alcohol* 42, no. 5 (2008): 383–388.

Koppes, L., et al. "Moderate Alcohol Consumption Lowers the Risk of Type 2 Diabetes: A Meta-Analysis of Prospective Observational Studies." *Diabetes Care* 28 (2005): 719–725.

Krajicek Bartek, Jean, Marlene Lindeman, and Jane Hokanson Hawks. "Clinical Validation of Characteristics of the Alcoholic Family." *Nursing Diagnosis* 10, no. 4 (1999): 158–168.

Krishnan, K. Ranga Rama. "Psychiatric and Medical Comorbidities of Bipolar Disorder." *Psychosomatic Medicine* 67 (2005): 1–8.

Kroenke, Kurt, M.D., et al. "Anxiety Disorders in Primary Care: Prevalence, Impairment, Comorbidity, and Detection." *Annals of Internal Medicine* 146 (2007): 317–325.

Krueger, Robert F., et al. "Etiologic Connections among Substance Dependence, Antisocial Behavior, and Personality: Modeling the Externalizing Spectrum." *Journal of Abnormal Psychology* 111, no. 3 (2002): 411–424.

Kuehn, Bridget M. "New Therapies for Alcohol Dependence Open Options for Office-Based Treatment." *Journal of the American Medical Association* 298, no. 21 (December 5, 2007): 2,467–2,468.

Kuntsche, Emmanuel, and Marina Delgrande Jordan. "Adolescent Alcohol and Cannabis Use in Relation to Peer and School Factors: Results of Multilevel Analyses." *Drug and Alcohol Dependence* 84 (2006): 167–174.

Kurzthaler, Ilsemarie, et al. "Alcohol and Benzodiazepines in Falls: An Epidemiological View." *Drug and Alcohol Dependence* 79 (2005): 225–230.

LaBrie, Joseph W., et al. "What Men Want: The Role of Reflective Opposite-Sex Normative Preferences in Alcohol Use Among College Women." *Psychology of Addictive Behaviors* 23, no. 1 (2009): 157–162.

Lachenmeier, Dirk W., Fotis Kanteres, and Jürgen Rehm. "Carcinogenicity of Acetaldehyde in Alcoholic Beverages: Risk Assessment Outside Ethanol Metabolism." *Addiction* 104 (2009): 533–550.

Lakins, Nekisha E., Robin A. LaVallee, Gerald D. Williams, and Hsiao-ye Yi. *Surveillance Report #82: Apparent Per Capita Alcohol Consumption: National, State, and Regional Trends, 1977–2005.* Rockville, Md.: National Institutes of Health, August 2007.

Lande, R. Gregory, et al. "Gender Differences and Alcohol Use in the U.S. Army." *Journal of the American Osteopathic Association* 107, no. 9 (2007): 401–407.

Lappalainen, Jaako, et al. "Association between Alcoholism and γ-Amino Butyric Acid α2 Receptor Subtype in a Russian Population." *Alcoholism: Clinical and Experimental Research* 29, no. 4 (April 2005): 493–498.

Larimer, Mary E., et al. "Health Care and Public Service Use and Costs before and after Provision of Housing for Chronically Homeless Persons with Severe Alcohol Problems." *Journal of the American Medical Association* 301, no. 13 (2009): 1,349–1,357.

LaSalle, V. Holland, et al. "Diagnostic Interview Assessed Neuropsychiatric Disorder Comorbidity in 334 Individuals with Obsessive-Compulsive Disorder." *Depression and Anxiety* 19 (2004): 163–173.

Lee, Jung Eun, et al. "Alcohol Intake and Renal Cell Cancer in a Pooled Analysis of 12 Prospective Studies." *Journal of the National Cancer Institute* 99 (2007): 801–810.

Lejoyeux, Michel, et al. "Study of Impulse-Control Disorders among Alcohol-Dependent Patients." *Journal of Clinical Psychiatry* 60, 5 (1999): 302–305.

Leonard, K. E., R. L. Collins, and B. M. Quigley. "Alcohol Consumption and the Occurrence and Severity of Aggression: An Event-based Analysis of Male to Male Barroom Violence." *Aggressive Behavior* 29 (2003): 346–365.

Leonard, Kenneth. "The Role of Drinking Patterns and Acute Intoxication in Violent Interpersonal Behaviors." In *Alcohol and Violence: Exploring Patterns and Responses,* 29–55. Washington, D.C.: International Center for Alcohol Policies, 2008.

Levy Merrick, Elizabeth S., Joanna Volpe-Vartanian, Constance M. Horgan, and Bernard McCann. "Revisiting Employee Assistance Programs and Substance Use Problems in the Workplace: Key Issues and a Research Agenda." *Psychiatric Services* 58, no. 10 (October 2007): 1,262–1,264.

Li, Ting-Kai, M.D. "The Genetics of Alcoholism." *Alcohol Alert* 60 (July 2003): 1–4.

Liang, Lan, and Jidong Huang. "Go Out or Stay In? The Effects of Zero Tolerance Laws on Alcohol Use and Drinking and Driving Patterns Among College Students." *Health Economics* 17 (2008): 1,261–1,275.

Lieber, Charles S., M.D. "Alcohol and Hepatitis C." *Alcohol Research & Health* 25, no. 4 (2001): 245–254.

———. "Relationships between Nutrition, Alcohol Use, and Liver Disease." *Alcohol Research & Health* 27, no. 3 (2003): 220–231.

Lieberman, David A., M.D., et al. "Prevalence of Colon Polyps Detected by Colonoscopy Screening in Asymptomatic Black and White Patients." *Journal of the American Medical Association* 300, no. 12 (2008): 1,417–1,422.

Liu, I-Chao, M.D. "Genetic and Environmental Contributions to the Development of Alcohol Dependence in Male Twins." *Archives of General Psychiatry* 61 (2004): 897–903.

Lloyd, Donald A., and R. Jay Turner. "Cumulative Lifetime Adversities and Alcohol Dependence in Adolescence and Young Adulthood." *Drug and Alcohol Dependence* 93, no. 3 (2008): 217–226.

Lloyd, Gareth. "One Hundred Alcoholic Doctors: A 21-Year Follow-Up." *Alcohol & Alcoholism* 37, no. 4 (2002): 370–374.

Lovinger, David M., and John C. Crabbe. "Laboratory Models of Alcoholism: Treatment Target Identification and Insight into Mechanisms." *Nature Neuroscience* 8, no. 11 (2005): 1,471–1,480.

Maggs, Jennifer L., and John E. Schulenber. "Trajectories of Alcohol Use During the Transition to Adulthood." *Alcohol Research & Health* 28, no. 4 (2004/2005): 195–201.

Maier, Ronald V., M.D. "Controlling Alcohol Problems among Hospitalized Trauma Patients." *Journal of Trauma: Injury, Infection and Critical Care* 59, no. 3 (2005): S1–S2.

Malta, Loretta S., Edward B. Blanchard, and Brian M. Freidenberg. "Psychiatric and Behavioral Problems in

Aggressive Drivers." *Behaviour Research and Therapy* 43 (2005): 1,467–1,484.

Mandell, Wallace, William W. Eaton, James C. Anthony, and Roberta Garrison. "Alcoholism and Occupations: A Review and Analysis of 104 Occupations." *Alcoholism: Clinical and Experimental Research* 16, no. 4 (July/August 1992): 734–746.

Mannuzza, Salvatore, Rachel G. Klein, Nhan L. Truong, et al. "Age of Methylphenidate Treatment Initiation in Children with ADHD and Later Substance Abuse: Prospective Follow-up into Adulthood." *American Journal of Psychiatry* 165, no. 5 (2008): 604–609.

Maraldi, Cinzia, M.D., et al. "Impact of Inflammation on the Relationship among Alcohol Consumption, Mortality, and Cardiac Events: The Health, Aging, and Body Composition Study." *Archives of Internal Medicine* 166 (July 24, 2006): 1,490–1,497.

Mariani, John J., M.D., et al. "A Randomized, Open-Label, Controlled Trial of Gabapentin and Phenobarbital in the Treatment of Alcohol Withdrawal." *American Journal on Addictions* 15 (2006): 76–84.

Marques Fidalgo, Thiago, Evelyn Doering da Silveira, and Dartiu Xavier da Silveira. "Psychiatric Comorbidity Related to Alcohol Use among Adolescents." *American Journal of Drug and Alcohol Abuse* 34 (2008): 83–89.

Martin, Brandon K., et al. "Adherence to Court-Ordered Disulfiram at Fifteen Months: A Naturalistic Study." *Journal of Substance Abuse Treatment* 26 (2004): 233–236.

Martin, Brandon, Laura Mangum, and Thomas P. Beresford, M.D. "Use of Court-Ordered Supervised Disulfiram Therapy at DVA Medical Centers in the United States." *American Journal on Addictions* 14 (2005): 208–212.

Martin, Christopher. "Timing of Alcohol and Other Drug Use." *Alcohol Research & Health* 31, no. 2 (2008): 96–99.

Martin, Christopher, et al. "Polydrug Use in an Inpatient Treatment Sample of Problem Drinkers." *Alcoholism: Clinical and Experimental Research* 20 (1996): 413–417.

Martin, Peter R., Charles K. Singleton, and Susanne Hiller-Sturmhofel. "The Role of Thiamine Deficiency in Alcoholic Brain Disease." *Alcohol Research & Health* 27, no. 2 (2002): 134–142.

Martinez, Diana, et al. "Alcohol Dependence Is Associated with Blunted Dopamine Transmission in the Ventral Striatum." *Biological Psychiatry* 58 (2005): 779–786.

Martino, Steven C., Rebecca L. Collins, and Phyllis L. Ellickson. "Substance Use and Vulnerability to Sexual and Physical Aggression: A Longitudinal Study of Young Adults." *Violence and Victims* 19, no. 5 (2004): 521–540.

Mason, Barbara J. "Rationale for Combining Acamprosate and Naltrexone for Treating Alcohol Dependence." *Journal of Studies of Alcohol* 15 (2005): 148–156.

Mason, Barbara J., Anita M. Goodman, Sylvia Chabac, and Philippe Lehert. "Effect of Oral Acamprosate on Abstinence in Patients with Alcohol Dependence in a Double-Blind, Placebo-Controlled Trial: The Role of Patient Motivation." *Journal of Psychiatric Research* 40 (2006): 382–392.

May, P. A., and J. R. Moran. "Prevention of Alcohol Misuse: A Review of Health Promotion among American Indians." *American Journal of Health Promotion* 9 (1995): 288–299.

McCauley, Jenna, et al. "Rape in Relation to Substance Abuse Problems: Results from a National Sample of College Women." *Addictive Behaviors* 34 (2009): 458–462.

McClure, A. A., et al. "Alcohol-branded Merchandise and Its Association with Drinking Attitudes and Outcomes in U.S. Adolescents." *Archives of Pediatrics & Adolescent Medicine* 163, no. 2 (2009): 211–217.

McClure, Auden C., M.D., Sonya Dal Cin, Jennifer Gibson, and James D. Sargent, M.D. "Ownership of Alcohol-Branded Merchandise and Initiation of Teen Drinking." *American Journal of Preventive Medicine* 30, no. 4 (2006): 277–283.

McCullough, M. J., and C. S. Farah. "The Role of Alcohol in Oral Carcinogenesis with Particular Reference to Alcohol-containing Mouthwashes." *Australian Dental Journal* 53 (2008): 302–305.

McCusker, R. R., B. Fuehrlein, B. A. Goldberger, et al. "Caffeine Content of Decaffeinated Coffee." *Journal of Analytical Toxicology* 30 (2006): 611–613.

McCusker, R. R., B. A. Goldberger, and E. J. Cone. "Caffeine Content of Energy Drinks, Carbonated Sodas, and Other Beverages." *Journal Analy Toxicology* 30 (2006): 112–114.

McDonald, Alden J. III, Nan Wang, and Carlos A. Camargo Jr., M.D. "US Emergency Department Visits for Alcohol-Related Diseases and Injuries Between 1992 and 2000." *Archives of Internal Medicine* 164 (2004): 531–537.

McKay, James R., et al. "The Effectiveness of Telephone-based Continuing Care for Alcohol and Cocaine Dependence: 24-Month Outcomes." *Archives of General Psychiatry* 62 (2005): 199–207.

McKee, Sherry A., et al. "Smoking Status as a Clinical Indicator for Alcohol Misuse in US Adults." *Archives of General Psychiatry* 167 (2007): 716–721.

McKeon, A., M. A. Frye, and Norman Delanty. "The Alcohol Withdrawal Syndrome." *Journal of Neurology, Neurosurgery, & Psychiatry* 79 (2008): 854–862.

McLellan, A. Thomas, et al. "Five Year Outcomes in a Cohort Study of Physicians Treated for Substance Use Disorders in the United States." *British Medical Journal* 337 (2008). Available online. URL: http://www.bmj.com/cgi/content/full/337/nov04_1/a2038?view=long&pmid=18984632. Accessed April 16, 2009.

Merrick, Elizabeth L., et al. "Unhealthy Drinking Patterns in Older Adults: Prevalence and Associated Characteristics." *Journal of the American Geriatric Society* 56, no. 2 (2008): 214–233.

Middleton Fillmore, Kaye, et al. "Moderate Alcohol Use and Reduced Mortality Risk: Systematic Error in Prospective Studies." *Addiction Research and Theory* 14, no. 2 (2006): 1–31.

Miller, J. W., et al. "Binge Drinking and Associated Health Risk Behaviors among High School Students." *Pediatrics* 119, no. 1 (2007): 76–85.

Miller, Laurie, M.D., and Christine Adamec. *The Encyclopedia of Adoption.* 3rd ed. New York: Facts On File, 2006.

Miller, Norman S., M.D., and Mark S. Gold, M.D. "Comorbid Cigarette and Alcohol Addiction: Epidemiology and Treatment." *Journal of Addictive Diseases* 17, no. 1 (1998): 55–66.

Moen, Bente E., M.D., Sverre Sandberg, and Trond Riise. "Drinking Habits and Laboratory Tests in Seamen with and without Chemical Exposure." *Journal of Studies on Alcohol* 53, no. 4 (1992): 364–368.

Mohler-Kuo, M., et al. "Correlates of Rape While Intoxicated in a National Sample of College Women." *Journal of Studies on Alcohol* 65, no. 1 (2004): 37–45.

Mondimore, Francis Mark, M.D. *Bipolar Disorder: A Guide for Patients and Families.* 2nd ed. Baltimore, Md.: Johns Hopkins University Press, 2006.

Monti, Peter M., Tracy O'Leary Tevyaw, and Brian Borsari. "Drinking Among Young Adults: Screening, Brief Intervention, and Outcome." *Alcohol Research & Health* 28, no. 4 (2004/2005): 236–244.

Montooth, Kristi L., Kyle T. Siebenthall, and Andrew G. Clark. "Membrane Lipid Physiology and Toxin Catabolism Underlie Ethanol and Acetic Acid Tolerance in *Drosophila melanogaster.*" *Journal of Experimental Biology* 209 (2006): 3,837–3,850.

Moore, Alison A., M.D. "Alcohol Use, Comorbidity, and Mortality." *Journal of the American Geriatrics Society* 54 (2006): 757–762.

Moore, Alison, et al. "Beyond Alcoholism: Identifying Older, At-risk Drinkers in Primary Care." *Journal of Studies in Alcohol* 63 (2002): 316–324.

Moore, Ernest E., M.D. "Alcohol and Trauma: The Perfect Storm." *Journal of Trauma, Injury, Infection and Critical Care* 59 (2005): S53–S56.

Moos, Rudolf H., and Bernice S. Moos. "Participation in Treatment and Alcoholics Anonymous: A 16-year Follow-up of Initially Untreated Individuals." *Journal of Clinical Psychology* 62, no. 6 (2006): 735–750.

Moos, Rudolf H., Bernice S. Moos, and Christine Timko. "Gender, Treatment and Self-help in Remission from Alcohol Use Disorders." *Clinical Medicine & Research* 4, no. 3 (2006): 163–174.

Moselhy, Hamdy F., George Georgiou, and Ashraf Kahn. "Frontal Lobe Changes in Alcoholism: A Review of the Literature." *Alcohol & Alcoholism* 36, no. 5 (2001): 357–368.

Moussavi, Saba, et al. "Depression, Chronic Diseases, and Decrements in Health: Results from the World Health Surveys." *Lancet* 370 (2007): 851–858.

Mukamal, Kenneth J., M.D. "The Effects of Smoking and Drinking on Cardiovascular Disease and Risk Factors." *Alcohol Research & Health* 29, no. 3 (2006): 199–202.

Mukamal, Kenneth J., M.D., et al. "Alcohol and Risk for Ischemic Stroke in Men: The Role of Drinking Patterns and Usual Beverage." *Annals of Internal Medicine* 142 (2005): 11–19.

Mukamal, Kenneth J., M.D., Stephanie E. Chiuve, and Eric B. Rimm. "Alcohol Consumption and Risk for Coronary Heart Disease in Men with Healthy Lifestyles." *Archives of Internal Medicine* 166 (October 23, 2006): 2,145–2,150.

Mulvey, E. P., et al. "Substance Use and Community Violence: A Test of the Relation at the Daily Level." *Journal of Consulting and Clinical Psychology* 74 (2006): 743–754.

Mundt, Marlon P. *Analyzing the Costs and Benefits of Brief Intervention.* Bethesda, Md.: National Institute of Alcohol Abuse and Alcoholism. Undated. Available online. URL: http://pubs.niaaa.nih.gov/publications/arh291/34-36.htm. Accessed August 4, 2009.

Murphy, Christopher M., et al. "Alcohol Consumption and Intimate Partner Violence by Alcoholic Men: Comparing Violent and Nonviolent Conflicts." *Psychology of Addictive Behaviors* 19, no. 1 (2005): 35–42.

Myers, Mark G., and John F. Kelly. "Cigarette Smoking Among Adolescents with Alcohol and Other Drug Use Problems." *Alcohol Research & Health* 29, no. 3 (2006): 221–227.

Myrick, Hugh, M.D. "Diagnosis of Alcohol Dependence." *Medscape Psychiatry & Mental Health.* Available online to subscribers. URL: http://cme.medscape.com/viewarticle/543758_print. Accessed on May 8, 2009.

Naimi, Timothy S., M.D., et al. "Binge Drinking Among U.S. Adults." *Journal of the American Medical Association* 289 (2003): 70–75.

———. "What Do Binge Drinkers Drink? Implications for Alcohol Control Policy." *American Journal of Preventive Medicine* 33, no. 3 (2007): 188–193.

"Narcissistic Personality Disorder." Mayo Clinic. Available online. URL: http://www.mayoclinic.com/print/narcissistic-personality-disorders.html. Accessed December 16, 2008.

National Center for Health Statistics. *Health, United States, 2008 with Chartbook.* Hyattsville, Md.: National Center for Health Statistics, 2009.

National Center on Addiction and Substance Abuse at Columbia University. *Family Matters: Substance Abuse and the American Family.* New York: National Center on Addiction and Substance Abuse at Columbia University, March 2005.

———. *Women Under the Influence.* Baltimore, Md.: Johns Hopkins University Press, 2006.

National Highway Traffic Safety Administration. *Statistical Analysis of Alcohol-related Driving Trends, 1982–2005.* Springfield, Va.: U.S. Department of Transportation, May 2008.

National Institute on Alcohol Abuse and Alcoholism. *Alcohol: A Women's Issue.* Bethesda, Md.: National Institutes of Health, 2008.

———. "Alcoholic Liver Disease." *Alcohol Alert* 64 (January 2005): 1–5.

———. "Alcohol's Damaging Effects on the Brain." *Alcohol Alert* 63 (October 2004): 1–7.

———. *Alcohol Use and Alcohol Use Disorders in the United States: Main Findings from the 2001–2002 National Epidemiologic Survey on Alcohol and Related Conditions (NESARC).* Bethesda, Md.: National Institutes of Health, January 2006.

———. "Alcohol Research: A Lifespan Perspective." *Alcohol Alert* 74, no. 1 (2008): 1–5.

———. "Alcohol, Violence, and Aggression." *Alcohol Alert* 38 (October 1997).

———. *Harmful Interactions: Mixing Alcohol with Medicines.* Bethesda, Md.: National Institutes of Health, 2007. Available online. URL: http://pubs.niaaa.nih.gov/publications/Medicine/medicine.htm. Downloaded June 27, 2008.

———. "NICHD News Release: New Study Finds Babies Born to Mothers Who Drink Alcohol Heavily May Suffer Permanent Nerve Damage." National Institutes of Health. Available online. URL: http://www.niaaa.hih.gov/NewsEvents/NewsReleases/mothers_alcohol.htm. Accessed March 16, 2009.

———. "Underage Drinking." *Alcohol Alert* 67 (January 2006): 1–7.

National Institute on Alcohol Abuse and Alcoholism National Advisory Council on Alcohol Abuse and Alcoholism Task Force on College Drinking. *High-risk Drinking in College: What We Know and What We Need to Learn.* Bethesda, Md.: National Institutes of Health, April 2002.

Neuner, B., et al. "Trauma Patients' Desire for Autonomy in Medical Decision Making Is Impaired by Smoking and Hazardous Alcohol Consumption—A Bi-national Study." *Journal of International Medical Research* 35 (2007): 609–614.

Neuner, Bruno, et al. "Hazardous Alcohol Consumption and Sense of Coherence in Emergency Department Patients with Minor Trauma." *Drug and Alcohol Dependence* 82 (2006): 143–150.

New, Antonia S., et al. "Low Prolactin Response to Fenfluramine in Impulsive Aggression." *Journal of Psychiatric Research* 38 (2004): 223–230.

Newes-Adeyi, Gabriella, Chiung M. Chen, Gerald D. Williams, and Vivian B. Faden. "Trends in Underage Drinking in the United States, 1991–2003." Bethesda, Md.: National Institute on Alcohol Abuse and Alcoholism, October 2005.

Newlin, David B., et al. "Environmental Transmission of DSM-IV Substance Use Disorders in Adoptive and Step Families." *Alcoholism: Clinical and Environmental Research* 24, no. 12 (December 2000): 1,785–1,794.

Nolen-Hoeksema, Susan. "Gender Differences in Risk Factors and Consequences for Alcohol Use and Problems." *Clinical Psychology Review* 24 (2004): 981–1,010.

Nordback, I., et al. "Is It Long-Term Continuous Drinking or the Post-Drinking Withdrawal Period that Triggers the First Acute Alcoholic Pancreatitis?" *Scandinavian Journal of Gastroenterology* 40, no. 10 (2005): 1,235–1,239.

Nurnberger, John L., M.D., et al. "A Family Study of Alcohol Dependence: Coaggregation of Multiple Disorders in Relatives of Alcohol-dependent Probands." *Archives of General Psychiatry* 61 (December 2004): 1,246–1,256.

Nusbaumer, Michael, and Denise M. Reiling. "Environmental Influences on Alcohol Consumption Practices of Alcoholic Beverage Servers." *American Journal of Drug and Alcohol Abuse* 28, no. 4 (2002): 733–742.

O'Connell, Henry, et al. "Alcohol Use Disorders in Elderly People—Redefining an Age Old Problem in Old Age." *British Medical Journal* 327 (2003): 664–667.

O'Connor, Roisin M., Sherry H. Stewart, and Margo C. Watt. "Distinguishing BAS Risk for University Students' Drinking, Smoking, and Gambling Behaviors." *Personality and Individual Differences* 46 (2009): 514–519.

Office of Applied Studies. "Alcohol Dependence or Abuse among Parents with Children Living in the Home."

NSDUH Report, Substance Abuse and Mental Health Services Administration, February 12, 2004.

———. "Gender Differences in Alcohol Use and Alcohol Dependence or Abuse: 2004 and 2005." *NSDUH Report,* Substance Abuse and Mental Health Services Administration, August 2, 2007.

———. "Participation in Self-help Groups for Alcohol and Illicit Drug Use: 2006 and 2007." *NSDUH Report,* Substance Abuse and Mental Health Services Administration, November 13, 2008.

———. "Quantity and Frequency of Alcohol Use among Underage Drinkers." *NSDUH Report,* Substance Abuse and Mental Health Services Administration, March 31, 2008.

———. "State Estimates of Persons Aged 18 or Older Driving Under the Influence of Alcohol or Illicit Drugs." *NSDUH Report,* Substance Abuse and Mental Health Services Administration, April 17, 2008.

———. "Substance Abuse and Dependence among Women." *NSDUH Report,* Substance Abuse and Mental Health Services Administration, August 5, 2005.

———. "Substance Use and Dependence Following Initiation of Alcohol or Illicit Drug Use." *NSDUH Report,* Substance Abuse and Mental Health Services Administration, March 27, 2008.

Ohannessian, Christine McCauley, and Victor M. Hesselbrock. "Paternal Alcoholism and Youth Substance Abuse: The Indirect Effects of Negative Affect, Conduct Problems, and Risk Taking." *Journal of Adolescent Health* 42, no. 2 (2008): 198–200.

O'Keefe, James H., M.D., Kevin A. Bybee, M.D., and Carl J. Lavie, M.D. "Alcohol and Cardiovascular Health: The Razor-Sharp Double-edged Sword." *Journal of the American College of Cardiology* 50, no. 11 (2007): 1,009–1,014.

O'Malley, Patrick M. *Maturing Out of Problematic Alcohol Use.* Bethesda, Md.: National Institute on Alcohol Abuse and Alcoholism. Undated. Available online. URL: http://pubs.niaaa.nih.gov/publications/arh284/202-204.htm. Accessed August 4, 2009.

O'Malley, Patrick M., and Lloyd D. Johnston. "Epidemiology of Alcohol and Other Drug Use among American College Students." *Journal of Studies of Alcohol* Suppl. 14 (2002): 23–39.

Panuzio, Jillian. "Intimate Partner Aggression Reporting Concordance and Correlates of Agreement among Men with Alcohol Use Disorders and Their Female Partners." *Assessment* 13, no. 3 (2006): 266–279.

Pastor, P. N. and C. A. Reuben. "Diagnosed Attention Deficit Hyperactivity Disorder and Learning Disability: United States, 2004–2006." Hyattsville, Md.: National Center for Health Statistics, Vital and Health Statistics 10 (237), 2008.

Pelucchi, Claudio, et al. "Cancer Risk Associated with Alcohol and Tobacco Use: Focus on Upper Aerodigestive Tract and Liver." *Alcohol Research & Health* 29, no. 3 (2006): 193–198.

Pemberton, Michael R., James D. Colliver, Tania M. Robbins, and Joseph C. Gfroerer. *Underage Alcohol Use: Findings from the 2002–2006 National Surveys on Drug Use and Health.* Rockville, Md.: Substance Abuse and Mental Health Services Administration, Office of Applied Studies, June 2008.

Peres Messas, Guilherme, and Homero Pinto Vallada Filho. "The Role of Genetics in Alcohol Dependence." *Revista Brasileira Psiquiatria* 26, no. 1 (2004): 54–58.

Peterson, Andrew M. "Improving Adherence in Patients with Alcohol Dependence: A New Role for Pharmacists." *American Journal of Health-System Pharmacy* 64, no. 3 (2007): S1–S17.

Petrakis, Ismene L., M.D., et al. "Altered NMDA Glutamate Receptor Antagonist Response in Individuals with a Family Vulnerability to Alcoholism." *American Journal of Psychiatry* 161 (2004): 1,776–1,782.

Petrakis, Ismene L., Charla Nich, and Elizabeth Ralevski. "Psychotic Spectrum Disorders and Alcohol Abuse: A Review of Pharmacotherapeutic Strategies and a Report on the Effectiveness of Naltrexone and Disulfiram." *Schizophrenia Bulletin* 32, no. 4 (2006): 644–654.

Petrakis, Ismene L., M.D., et al. "Comorbidity of Alcoholism and Psychiatric Disorders: An Overview." *Alcohol Research & Health* 26, no. 2 (2002): 81–89.

Pettinati, Helen M., et al. "A Double Blind, Placebo-controlled Trial that Combined Disulfiram and Naltrexone for Treating Co-occurring Cocaine and Alcohol Dependence." *Addictive Behaviors* 33 (2008): 651–667.

Pietrzak, Robert H., et al. "Gambling Level and Psychiatric and Medical Disorders in Older Adults: Results from the National Epidemiologic Survey on Alcohol and Related Conditions." *American Journal of Geriatric Psychiatry* 15, no. 4 (2007): 301–313.

Pinto, Emmanuel, et al. "The *TaqI* A DRD2 Polymorphism in Type II Alcohol Dependence: A Marker of Age at Onset or of a Familial Disease?" *Alcohol* 43 (2009): 1–5.

Podymow, Tiina, et al. "Shelter-based Managed Alcohol Administration to Chronically Homeless People Addicted to Alcohol." *Canadian Medical Association Journal* 174, no. 1 (January 3, 2006): 43–49.

Poelen, Evelien A. P., et al. "Best Friends and Alcohol Consumption in Adolescence: A Within-family Analysis." *Drug and Alcohol Dependence* 88 (2007): 163–173.

Poikolainen, Kari. "Risk Factors for Alcohol Dependence: A Case-Control Study." *Alcohol & Alcoholism* 35, no. 2 (2000): 190–196.

Prescott, Carol A. "Sex Differences in the Genetic Risk for Alcoholism." *Alcohol Research & Health* 273 (2002): 264–273.

Preuss, Ulrich W., M.D., et al. "Predictors and Correlates of Suicide Attempts over 5 Years in 1,237 Alcohol-dependent Men and Women." *American Journal of Psychiatry* 160, no. 1 (January 2003): 56–63.

"Psychosocial Processes and Mechanisms of Risk and Protection." *Alcohol Research & Health* 28, no. 2 (2004/2005): 143–154.

Quertemont, Etienne, and Vincent Didone. "Role of Acetaldehyde in Mediating the Pharmacological and Behavioral Effects of Alcohol." *Alcohol Research & Health* 29, no. 4 (2006): 258–265.

Quigley, Brian M., and Kenneth E. Leonard. "Alcohol Use and Violence among Young Adults." *Alcohol Research & Health* 28, no. 4 (2004/2005): 191–194.

Rasanen, Pirkko, et al. "Schizophrenia, Alcohol Abuse, and Violent Behavior: A 26-year Followup Study of an Unselected Birth Cohort." *Schizophrenia Bulletin* 24, no. 3 (1998): 437–441.

Raskin-White, Helene, and Kristina Jackson. "Social and Psychological Influences on Emerging Adult Drinking Behavior." *Alcohol Research & Health* 28, no. 4 (2004/2005): 182–190.

Ravindran, Lakshmi N., M.D. "Comorbidity and Social Anxiety Disorder: Prognostic Implications." *Perspectives in Clinical Psychiatry: A Clinical Update.* Supplement to *Psychiatric Times.* Issue 2 of 4 (September 2008): 18–21.

Register, Thomas D., et al. "Health Issues in Postmenopausal Women Who Drink." *Alcohol Research & Health* 26, no. 4 (2002): 299–307.

Rehm, Jürgen, et al. "Alcohol-related Morbidity and Mortality." *Alcohol Research & Health* 27, no. 2 (2002): 39–51.

Renna, Francesco. "The Economic Cost of Teen Drinking: Late Graduation and Lowered Earnings." *Health Economics* 16 (2007): 407–419.

Ries, L. A. G., et al., eds. "Surveillance Epidemiology and End Results, Cancer of the Liver and Intrahepatic Duct." *SEER Cancer Statistics Review, 1975–2005.* Bethesda, Md.: National Cancer Institute. Available online. URL: http://seer.cancer.gov/csr/1975_2005/. Downloaded February 1, 2009.

Roche, Ann M., Toby Freeman, and Natalie Skinner. "From Data to Evidence, to Action: Findings from a Systematic Review of Hospital Screening Studies for High Risk Alcohol Consumption." *Drug and Alcohol Dependence* 83 (2006): 1–14.

Roman, Paul M., and Terry C. Blum. "The Workplace and Alcohol Problem Prevention." *Alcohol Research & Health* 26, no. 1 (2002): 49–57.

Romeri, Ester, Allan Baker, and Clare Griffiths. "Alcohol-related Deaths by Occupation, England and Wales, 2001–05." *Health Statistics Quarterly* 25 (Autumn 2007): 6–12.

Rose, Richard J., and Danielle M. Dick. "Gene-Environment Interplay in Adolescent Drinking Behavior." *Alcohol Research & Health* 28, no. 4 (2004/2005): 222–229.

Rotunda, Rob J., Laura West, and Timothy J. O'Farrell. "Enabling Behavior in a Clinical Sample of Alcohol-dependent Clients and Their Partners." *Journal of Substance Abuse Treatment* 26 (2004): 269–276.

Rush, Brian, and Christopher J. Koegl. "Prevalence and Profile of People with Co-occurring Mental and Substance Use Disorders Within a Comprehensive Mental Health System." *Canadian Journal of Psychiatry* 53, no. 12 (2008): 810–821.

Saitz, Richard, M.D. "Unhealthy Alcohol Use." *New England Journal of Medicine* 353, no. 6 (February 10, 2005): 596–607.

Saitz, Richard, M.D., et al. "Brief Intervention for Medical Inpatients with Unhealthy Alcohol Use: A Randomized, Controlled Trial." *Annals of Internal Medicine* 146 (2007): 167–176.

Sampson, H. Wayne. "Alcohol and Other Factors Affecting Osteoporosis Risk in Women." *Alcohol Research & Health* 26, no. 2 (2002): 292–298.

Sartor, Carolyn E., et al. "The Role of Childhood Risk Factors in Initiation of Alcohol Use and Progression to Alcohol Dependence." *Addiction* 102 (2006): 216–225.

Schaeffner, Elke S., M.D., et al. "Alcohol Consumption and the Risk of Renal Dysfunction in Apparently Healthy Men." *Archives of Internal Medicine* 165 (2005): 1,048–1,053.

Scheier, Lawrence M., Sandra C. Lapham, and Janet C'De Baca. "Cognitive Predictors of Alcohol Involvement and Alcohol Consumption–Related Consequences in a Sample of Drunk-Driving Offenders." *Substance Use & Misuse* 43 (2008): 2,089–2,115.

Schiff, Eugene R., M.D., and Nuri Ozden, M.D. "Hepatitis C and Alcohol." *Alcohol Research & Health* 27, no. 3 (2003): 232–239.

Schmidt, Laura, Thomas Greenfield, and Nina Mulia. "Unequal Treatment: Racial and Ethnic Disparities in Alcoholism Treatment Services." *Alcohol Research & Health* 29, no. 1 (2006): 49–54.

Schuckit, M. A. "Biological, Psychological and Environmental Predictors of the Alcoholism Risk: A Longitudinal Study." *Journal of Studies on Alcohol* 59, no. 5 (1998): 485–494.

Schuckit, M. A., and T. L. Smith. "The Relationships of a Family History of Alcohol Dependence, a Low Level of Response to Alcohol and Six Domains of Life Functioning to the Development of Alcohol Use Disorders." *Journal of Studies on Alcohol* 61, no. 6 (2000): 827–835.

Schuckit, Marc A. "Alcohol-use Disorders." *Lancet* 373 (2009): 492–501.

Schuckit, Marc A., M.D. "An Overview of Genetic Influences in Alcoholism." *Journal of Substance Abuse Treatment* 36, no. 1 (2009): S5-S14.

Schuckit, Marc A., M.D., and Victor Hesselbrock. "Alcohol Dependence and Anxiety Disorders: What Is the Relationship?" *Focus: The Journal of Lifelong Learning in Psychiatry* 2, no. 3 (2004): 440–453.

Schumann, Gunter, M.D., et al. "Systematic Analysis of Glutamatergic Neurotransmission Genes in Alcohol Dependence and Adolescent Risky Drinking Behavior." *Archives of General Psychiatry* 65, no. 7 (2008): 826–838.

Schwilke, Eugene W., et al. "Changing Patterns of Drug and Alcohol Use in Fatally Injured Drivers in Washington State." *Journal of Forensic Sciences* 51, no. 5 (2006): 1,191–1,198.

"The Scope of the Problem." *Alcohol Research & Health* 28, no. 2 (2004/2005): 111–120.

Seitz, Helmut K., M.D., and Peter Becker, M.D. "Alcohol Metabolism and Cancer Risk." *Alcohol Research & Health* 30, no. 1 (2007): 38–47.

Shai, I., et al. "Glycemic Effects of Moderate Alcohol Intake among Patients with Type 2 Diabetes: A Multicenter, Randomized Clinical Intervention Trial." *Diabetes Care* 30, no. 12 (2007): 3,011–3,016.

Shankar, Kartik, Martin J. J. Ronis, and Thomas M. Badger. "Effects of Pregnancy and Nutritional Status on Alcohol Metabolism." *Alcohol Research & Health* 30, no. 1 (2007): 55–59.

Shin, S. H., et al. "Relationship between Multiple Forms of Maltreatment by a Parent or Guardian and Adolescent Alcohol Use." *American Journal of Addictions* 18, no. 2 (2009): 226–234.

Shin, Sunny Hyucksun, Erika M. Edwards, and Timothy Heeren. "Child Abuse and Neglect: Relations to Adolescent Binge Drinking in the National Longitudinal Study of Adolescent Health (Add Health) Study." *Addictive Behaviors* 34, no. 3 (2009): 277–280.

Shivani, Ramesh, M.D., R. Jeffrey Goldsmith, M.D., and Robert M. Anthenelli, M.D. "Alcoholism and Psychiatric Disorders: Diagnostic Challenges." *Alcohol Research & Health* 26, no. 2 (2002): 90–98.

Shore, Jay, M.D., Spero M. Manson, and Dedra Buchwald. "Screening for Alcohol Abuse among Urban Native Americans in a Primary Care Setting." *Psychiatric Services* 53, no. 6 (2002): 757–760.

Sigardsson, Sören, Michael Bohman, M.D., and C. Robert Cloninger, M.D. "Replication of the Stockholm Adoption Study of Alcoholism: Confirmatory Cross-fostering Analysis." *Archives of General Psychiatry* 53 (1996): 681–687.

Skipper, Gregory E., et al. "Ethyl Glucuronide: A Biomarker to Identify Alcohol Use by Health Professionals Recovering from Substance Use Disorders." *Alcohol & Alcoholism* 39, no. 5 (July 2004): 445–449.

Skoog, Gunnar, M.D., and Ingmar Skoog, M.D. "A 40-year Follow-up of Patients with Obsessive-compulsive Disorder." *Archives of General Psychiatry* 56 (1999): 121–127.

Sloan, Chantel D., Vicki Sayarath, and Jason H. Moore. "Systems Genetics of Alcoholism." *Alcohol Research & Health* 31, no. 1 (2005): 14–25.

Smith, Gordon S., et al. "Drinking and Recreational Boating Fatalities: A Population-based Case-control Study." *Journal of the American Medical Association* 286, no. 23 (2001): 2,974–2,980.

Smothers, Barbara S., Harold T. Yahr, and Constance E. Ruhl, M.D. "Detection of Alcohol Use Disorders in General Hospital Admissions in the United States." *Archives of Internal Medicine* 164 (2004): 749–756.

Smyer, Michael A., et al. "Childhood Adoption: Long-term Effects in Adulthood." *Psychiatry* 61 (Fall 1998): 191–205.

Snow, Diane, Tonia Smith, and Susan Branham. "Women with Bipolar Disorder Who Use Alcohol and Other Drugs." *Journal of Addictions Nursing* 60 (2008): 19–55.

Snow, Wanda M., et al. "Alcohol Use and Cardiovascular Health Outcomes: A Comparison Across Age and Gender in the Winnepeg Health and Drinking Survey Cohort." *Age and Ageing* 38 (2009): 206–212.

Snyder, Leslie B., et al. "Effects of Alcohol Advertising Exposure on Drinking among Youth." *Archives of Pediatric & Adolescent Medicine* 160 (January 2006): 18–24.

Sonne, Susan C., and Kathleen T. Brady, M.D. "Bipolar Disorder and Alcoholism." *Alcohol Research & Health* 26, no. 2 (2002): 103–189.

Staley, Julie K., et al. "Cortical γ-Aminobuytric Acid Type A-Benzodiazepine Receptors in Recovery from Alcohol Dependence." *Archives of General Psychiatry* 62 (2005): 877–888.

Stewart, Sherry H., Dubravka Gavric, and Pamela Collins. "Women, Girls, and Alcohol." In *Women & Addiction: A Comprehensive Handbook,* edited by Kathleen T. Brady, Sudie E. Back, and Shelly F. Greenfield. New York: Guilford Press, 2009.

Stewart, Scott, and Gerard J. Connors. "Screening for Alcohol Problems: What Makes a Test Effective?" *Alcohol Research & Health* 28, no. 1 (2004/2005): 5–16.

Stinson, Frederick S., et al. "Comorbidity Between DSM-IV Alcohol and Specific Drug Use Disorders in the United States." *Alcohol Research & Health* 29, no. 2 (2006): 94–106.

Streppel, Marinette, et al. "Long-term Wine Consumption Is Related to Cardiovascular Mortality and Life Expectancy Independently." *Journal of Epidemiology and Community Health* (2009). Available online. URL: http://press.psprings.co.uk/jech/april/ch82198pdf. Accessed July 28, 2009.

Subramanian, Rajesh. "Motor Vehicle Traffic Crashes as a Leading Cause of Death in the United States, 2002." *Traffic Safety Facts Research Note* (January 2005).

Substance Abuse and Mental Health Services Administration. *Drug Abuse Warning Network, 2006: National Estimates of Drug-related Emergency Department Visits.* Rockville, Md.: U.S. Department of Health and Human Services, August 2008.

Substance Abuse and Mental Health Services Administration, Office of Applied Studies. *Results from the 2007 National Survey on Drug Use and Health: National Findings.* Rockville, Md.: U.S. Department of Health and Human Services, 2008.

Sullivan, Maria A., and Frances Rudnik-Levin. "Attention Deficit/Hyperactivity Disorder and Substance Abuse: Diagnostic and Therapeutic Considerations." *Annals of New York Academy of Sciences* 931 (2006): 251–270.

Sundell, Laura, et al. "Increased Stroke Risk Is Related to a Binge Drinking Habit." *Stroke* 39 (2008): 3,179–3,184.

Swaroop Vege, Santhi, M.D., and Suresh T. Chari, M.D. "Clinical Manifestations and Diagnosis of Acute Pancreatitis." Official reprint from UpToDate. Private subscriber service online. URL: http://www.uptodate.com/online/content/topic.do?topicKey=pancdis/7667&selectedTitle=3~150&source=search_result. September 22, 2008. Accessed March 12, 2009.

Swift, Robert. "Emerging Approaches to Managing Alcohol Dependence." *American Journal of Health-System Pharmacy* 64, no. 3 (2007): S12-S22.

Szlemko, William J., James W. Wood, and Pamela Jumper Thurman. "Native Americans and Alcohol: Past, Present, and Future." *Journal of General Psychology* 133, no. 4 (2006): 435–451.

Tanasescu, M., et al. "Alcohol Consumption and Risk of Coronary Heart Disease among Men with Type 2 Diabetes." *Journal of the American College of Cardiology* 38, no. 7 (2001): 1,836–1,842.

Tapert, Susan, Lisa Caldwell, and Christina Burke. "Alcohol and the Adolescent Brain: Human Studies." *Alcohol Research & Health* 28, no. 4 (2004/2005): 205–212.

Task Force of the National Advisory Council on Alcohol Abuse and Alcoholism. *High Risk Drinking in College: What We Know and What We Need to Learn: Final Report on Contexts and Consequences.* Washington, D.C.: National Institute on Alcohol Abuse and Alcoholism, April 2002.

Tavares, Hermano, et al. "Factors at Play in Faster Progression for Female Pathological Gamblers: An Exploratory Analysis." *Journal of Clinical Psychiatry* 65, no. 4 (2003): 433–438.

Teplin, Linda A., et al. "Psychiatric Disorders in Youth in Juvenile Detention." *Archives of General Psychiatry* 59 (2002): 1,133–1,143.

Terrell, Francine, et al. "Nationwide Survey of Alcohol Screening and Brief Intervention Practices at US Level I Trauma Centers." *Journal of the American College of Surgeons* 207 (2008): 630–638.

Thatcher, Dawn L., and Duncan B. Clark, M.D. "Adolescents at Risk for Substance Use Disorders: Role of Psychological Dysregulation, Endophenotypes, and Environmental Influences." *Alcohol Research & Health* 31, no. 2 (2008): 168–176.

Theruvathu, Jacob, et al. "Polyamines Stimulate the Formation of Mutagenic 1, N^2-propanodeoxyguluanosine Adducts from Acetaldehyde." *Nucleic Acids Research* 33, no. 11 (2005): 3,513–3,520.

Thomas, Suzanne E., et al. "A Complex Relationship between Co-occurring Social Anxiety and Alcohol Use Disorders: What Effect Does Treating Social Anxiety Have on Drinking?" *Alcohol Clinical and Experimental Research* 32, no. 1 (2008): 77–84.

Thomson, Allan D., and E. Jane Marshall. "The Natural History and Pathophysiology of Wernicke's Encephalopathy and Korsakoff's Psychosis." *Alcohol & Alcoholism* 41, no. 2 (2006): 151–158.

Timberlake, D. S., et al. "College Attendance and Its Effects on Drinking Behaviors in a Longitudinal Study of Adolescents." *Alcoholism: Clinical and Experimental Research* 31, no. 6 (2007): 1,020–1,030.

Tolstrup, Janne, et al. "Prospective Study of Alcohol Drinking Patterns and Coronary Heart Disease in Women and Men." *British Medical Journal* 332 (2006): 1,244–1,248.

Toomey, Traci L. "American Beverage Licensees Attack Mothers Against Drunk Driving." *Addiction* 100 (2005): 1,389–1,391.

Torrey, E. Fuller, M.D. *Surviving Schizophrenia: A Manual for Families, Consumers, and Providers.* New York: Quill, 2001.

Tracy, Sarah W. *Alcoholism in America: From Reconstruction to Prohibition.* Baltimore, Md.: Johns Hopkins University Press, 2005.

Tracy, Sarah W., and Caroline Jean Acker. *Altering American Consciousness: The History of Alcohol and Drug Use in the United States: 1800–2000.* Amherst, Mass.: University of Massachusetts Press, 2004.

Trim, Ryan S., Marc A. Schuckit, and Tom L. Smith. "The Relationships of the Level of Response to Alcohol and Additional Characteristics to Alcohol Use Disorders across Adulthood: A Discrete-time Survival Analysis." *Alcoholism: Clinical and Experimental Research* 33, 9 (2009): 1–9.

Urbano-Marquez, A., et al. "The Greater Risk of Alcoholic Cardiomyopathy and Myopathy in Women Compared with Men." *Journal of the American Medical Association* 274, no. 2 (1995): 149–154.

U.S. Department of Health and Human Services. *The Surgeon General's Call to Action to Prevent and Reduce Underage Drinking.* Washington, D.C.: U.S. Department of Health and Human Services, Office of the Surgeon General, 2007.

U.S. Department of Health and Human Services, Administration on Children, Youth and Families. *Child Maltreatment 2006.* Washington, D.C.: U.S. Government Printing Office, 2008.

Valenstein, Marcia, et al. "Poor Antipsychotic Adherence among Patients with Schizophrenia: Medication and Patient Factors." *Schizophrenia Bulletin* 30, no. 2 (2004): 255–264.

Verduin, Marcia L., M.D., Bryan K. Tolliver, M.D., and Kathleen T. Brady, M.D. "Substance Abuse and Bipolar Disorder." *Medscape Psychiatry and Mental Health* 10, no. 2 (2005).

Virnig, Beth A., et al. "A Matter of Race: Early- versus Late-stage Cancer Diagnosis." *Health Affairs* 28, no. 1 (January/February 2009): 160–168.

Visser, Susanna N., Catherine A. Lesesne, and Ruth Perou. "National Estimates and Factors Associated with Medication Treatment for Childhood Attention-deficit/Hyperactivity Disorder." *Pediatrics* 119 (2007): S99–S106.

Voas, R. B., A. S. Tippetts, and J. C. Fell. "Assessing the Effectiveness of Minimum Legal Drinking Age and Zero Tolerance Laws in the United States." *Accident Analysis and Prevention* 35 (2003): 579–587.

Volk, Heather E., et al. "Evidence for Specificity of Transmission of Alcohol and Nicotine Dependence in an Offspring of Twins Design." *Drug and Alcohol Dependence* 87 (2007): 225–232.

Volpicelli, Joseph R., M.D. "New Options for the Treatment of Alcohol Dependence." *Psychiatric Annals* 35, no. 6 (2005): 484–495.

Vonlaufen, Alain, M.D., et al. "Role of Alcohol Metabolism in Chronic Pancreatitis." *Alcohol Research & Health* 30, no. 1 (2007): 48–54.

Wagenaar, Alexander C., Mildred M. Maldonado-Molina, and Bradley H. Wagenaar. "Effects of Alcohol Tax Increases on Alcohol-related Disease Mortality in Alaska: Time-Series Analyses from 1976 to 2004." *American Journal of Public Health* 99, 1 (2009): 1,464–1,470.

Wagenaar, Alexander C., Traci L. Toomey, and Kathleen M. Lenk. "Environmental Influences on Young Adult Drinking." *Alcohol Research & Health* 28, no. 4 (2004/2005): 230–235.

Wallace, J. M., et al. "Religiosity and Adolescent Substance Abuse: The Role of Individual and Contextual Influences." *Social Problems* 54, no. 2 (2007): 308–327.

Walsh, J. Michael, et al. "Drug and Alcohol Use among Drivers Admitted to a Level-1 Trauma Center." *Accident Analysis & Prevention* 37 (2005): 894–901.

Wang, J., et al. "Moderate Alcohol Drinking Might Be Protective for System Lupus Erythematosus: A Systematic Review and Meta-analysis." *Clinical Rheumatology* 27, no. 12 (2008): 1,557–1,563.

Weintraub, Daniel, M.D. "Dopamine and Impulse Control Disorders in Parkinson's Disease." *Annals of Neurology* 64, Suppl. (2008): S93–S100.

Weiss, Friedbert, and Linda J. Porrino. "Behavioral Neurobiology of Alcohol Addiction: Recent Advances and Challenges." *Journal of Neuroscience* 22, no. 9 (May 1, 2002): 3,332–3,337.

Wells Pence, Brian, et al. "Coping Strategies and Patterns of Alcohol and Drug Use among HIV-infected Patients in the United States Southeast." *AIDS Patient Care and STDs* 22, no. 11 (2008): 869–877.

Whelan, Greg. "A Much Neglected Risk Factor in Elderly Mental Disorders." *Current Opinions in Psychiatry* 16, no. 6 (2003): 609–614.

White, William L. "Pre–A.A. Alcoholic Mutual Aid Societies." *Alcoholism Treatment Quarterly* 19, no. 2 (2001): 1–21.

White, Aaron M. "What Happened? Alcohol, Memory Blackouts, and the Brain." *Alcohol Research & Health* 27, no. 2 (2003): 186–196.

White, A. M., D. W. Jamieson-Drake, and H. S. Swartzwelder. "Prevalence and Correlates of Alcohol-induced Blackouts among College Students: Results of an E-mail Survey." *Journal of American College Health* 51 (2002): 117–131.

Wilens, Timothy E., M.D. "The Nature of the Relationship between Attention-deficit/Hyperactivity Disorder and Substance Use." *Journal of Clinical Psychiatry* 68, no. 11 (2007): S4–S8.

Wilens, Timothy E., et al. "Characteristics of Adults with Attention Deficit Hyperactivity Disorder Plus Substance Use Disorder: The Role of Psychiatric Comorbidity." *American Journal on Addictions* 14 (2005): 319–327.

Wilens, Timothy E., M.D., et al. "Further Evidence of an Association between Adolescent Bipolar Disorder with Smoking and Substance Use Disorders: A Controlled Study." *Drug and Alcohol Dependence* 95, no. 3 (2008): 188–198.

Williams, Jill M., and Douglas Ziedonis. "Addressing Tobacco among Individuals with a Mental Illness or an Addiction." *Addictive Behaviors* 20 (2004): 1,067–1,083.

Wilson, G. Terence. "Eating Disorders and Addictive Disorders." In *Eating Disorders and Obesity: A Comprehensive Handbook,* edited by Christopher G. Fairburn and Kelly D. Brownell, 199–203. New York: Guilford Press, 2002.

Wilson, Jennifer F. "Alcohol Use." *Annals of Internal Medicine* Suppl. (2009): ITC3-1–ITC3-16.

Wollschlaeger, Bernd. "Impulse Control Disorders: A Clinician's Guide to Understanding and Treating Behavioral Addictions." *Journal of the American Medical Association* 300, no. 23 (2008): 2,803–2,804.

World Health Organization. *Alcohol and Interpersonal Violence: Policy Briefing.* Rome, Italy: 2005.

Wright, Clinton B., et al. "Alcohol Intake, Carotid Plaque, and Cognition: The Northern Manhattan Study." *Stroke* 37 (2006): 1,160–1,164.

Xiong, Glen L., M.D., et al. "Wernicke-Korsakoff Syndrome." eMedicine Psychiatry. Available to subscribers online. URL: http://emedicine.medscape.com/article/288379-overview. Accessed March 21, 2009.

Yang, Alice L., M.D., et al. "Epidemiology of Alcohol-related Liver and Pancreatic Disease in the United States." *Archives of Internal Medicine* 168, no. 6 (March 24, 2008): 649–656.

Yoon, Young-Hee, et al. "Accidental Alcohol Poisoning Mortality in the United States, 1996–1998." *Alcohol Research & Health* 27, no. 1 (2003): 110–118.

Yoon, Young-Hee, and Hsiao-ye Yi. *Surveillance Report #83: Liver Cirrhosis Mortality in the United States, 1970–2005.* Baltimore, Md.: National Institutes of Health, August 2008.

Young, Joel L., M.D. *ADHD Grown Up: A Guide to Adolescent and Adult ADHD.* New York: W.W. Norton, 2007.

Zakhari, Samir. "Overview: How Is Alcohol Metabolized by the Body?" *Alcohol Research & Health* 29, no. 4 (2006): 245–254.

Zhang, N., et al. "Moderate Alcohol Consumption May Decrease Risk of Intervertebral Disc Degeneration." *Medical Hypotheses* 71, no. 4 (2008): 501–504.

Zhang, Shumin M., et al. "Alcohol Consumption and Breast Cancer Risk in the Women's Health Study." *American Journal of Epidemiology* 165, no. 6 (2007): 667–676.

Zhang, Yuqing, et al. "Secular Trends in Alcohol Consumption over 50 Years: The Framingham Study." *American Journal of Medicine* 121 (2008): 695–701.

Ziedonis, Douglas, M.D., et al. "Barriers and Solutions to Addressing Tobacco Dependence in Addiction Treatment Programs." *Alcohol Research & Health* 29, no. 3 (2006): 228–235.

Zilberman, Monica L., M.D., et al. "Substance Use Disorders: Sex Differences and Psychiatric Comorbidities." *Canadian Journal of Psychiatry* 48, no. 1 (2003): 5–15.

INDEX

Note: **Boldface** page numbers indicate extensive treatment of a topic. Page numbers followed by *t* indicate tables.

A

abandonment, borderline personality disorder and 205

Abilify. *See* aripiprazole

abstinence **1**. *See also* medication

  as aberrance xviii

  as alcohol dependence treatment xiv, 1, 171, 237

  in alcoholism mutual aid societies 71

  anxiety triggered by 76

  as medical treatment 136

    with alcoholic liver disease 138, 178

    with cirrhosis 104–105

    with liver transplant 143

    with pancreatitis 199

  moderate drinking and 186

  with naltrexone 191–192

  in pregnancy 155

  during Prohibition xxviii

  religiosity and 222–223, 223*t*

  in temperance movement xxiv

  WTCU promotion of xxvii

abuse

  child abuse **101–104**

    adolescent drinking as trigger for 150–151

    in adoption study biases 4

in Adverse Childhood Experiences study 6

alcohol use in 16, 34–35, 150–151

alcohol use disorders in 7, 54, 135, 150, 153

in alcohol use disorders risk 41, 60, 101, 153, 162, 258

in bipolar disorder risk 87

of child with fetal alcohol spectrum disorders 156

codependency and 105–106

consequences of 101

enabling and 135

in narcissistic personality disorder risk 206

repeated 150

state reporting numbers for 299–301

substance abuse and 103*t*

domestic violence

  in Adverse Childhood Experiences study 6

  alcohol use in 16, 34, 65, 145, 147, 150, 263*t*

  children affected by 34–35

  as risk factor for alcohol use disorders 60

elder abuse 15

sexual

  by alcoholic parents 54

  alcohol-related, of women 44

  binge drinking and 101, 154

  borderline personality disorder and 205

  in childhood 7, 60, 101, 153, 154

  impact on adulthood 7, 60, 153

  of older adults 15

  of women, alcohol-related 44

acamprosate 242*t*–243*t*, 244

  abstinence promoted by 1

  in treatment

    for alcohol use disorders 26, 66, 115, 240

    for liver disease treatment 138

    of older adults 131

acetaldehyde **1–2**, 18

  cancer and 93, 96, 139

  in flushing response 50, 162–163

  in pancreatitis 198

  protective effect of 165

acetaminophen 23, 138, 179

acetaminophen and hydrocodone 37

acetaminophen and oxycodone 37